SKELETAL GROWTH FACTORS

SKELETAL GROWTH FACTORS

Editor

Ernesto Canalis, M.D.

Director
Department of Research
St. Francis Hospital and Medical Center
Hartford, Connecticut

Professor
Department of Medicine and Orthopedics
University of Connecticut School of Medicine
Farmington, Connecticut

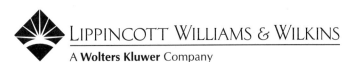

LIPPINCOTT WILLIAMS & WILKINS
A **Wolters Kluwer** Company
Philadelphia · Baltimore · New York · London
Buenos Aires · Hong Kong · Sydney · Tokyo

Acquisitions Editor: Elizabeth Greenspan
Developmental Editor: Julia Seto
Production Editor: W. Christopher Granville
Manufacturing Manager: Kevin Watt
Cover Designer: Christine Jenny
Compositor: Maryland Composition
Printer: Maple Press

© **2000 by LIPPINCOTT WILLIAMS & WILKINS**
530 Walnut Street
Philadelphia, PA 19106 USA
LWW.com

Printed in the USA

Library of Congress Cataloging-in-Publication Data
Skeletal growth factors / edited by Ernesto Canalis.
    p. ; cm
  Includes bibliographical references and index.
  ISBN 0-7817-2474-0
    1. Growth factors. 2. Bones—Growth—Molecular aspects. 3. Bone morphogenetic proteins. 4. Bone cells. I. Canalis, Ernesto.
    [DNLM: 1. Bone Development—physiology. 2. Bone Diseases—physiopathology 3. Growth Substances—physiology. 4. Growth Substances—therapeutic use. WE 200 S62685 2000]
  QP552.G76 S57 2000
  612.7′5—dc21
                          99-052559

10 9 8 7 6 5 4 3 2 1

Contents

Contributing Authors

Matanobu Abe, Ph.D.
Professor
Department of Nutrition
Azabu University School of Veterinary Medicine
Sagamihara 229-8501
Japan

Tamara N. Alliston, Ph.D.
Post Doctoral Scientist
Department of Growth and Development
University of California at San Francisco
521 Parnassus Avenue
San Francisco, California 94143-0640

Melissa Alsina, M.D.
Department of Medicine
Division of Hematology
University of Texas Health Science Center
7703 Floyd Curl Drive
San Antonio, Texas 78284-7880

Andrew Baird, Ph.D.
Ciblex Corporation
11025 Roselle Street
San Diego, California 92121

Roland Baron, D.D.S., Ph.D.
Professor
Departments of Orthopaedics and Cell Biology
Yale University School of Medicine
333 Cedar Street
New Haven, Connecticut 06520-8044

Leslie S. Beasley, M.D.
Resident
Department of Orthopaedics
Hospital for Special Surgery
535 East 70th Street
New York, New York 10021

Vicky A. Blakesley, M.D., Ph.D.
Abbott Laboratories
200 Abbott Park Road
Abbott Park, Illinois 60064–6188

William J. Boyle, M.D.
Amgen, Inc.
Mail Stop 15-2-A-226
1840 DeHavilland Drive
Thousand Oaks, California 91320-1799

Ernesto Canalis, M.D.
Director
Department of Research
St. Francis Hospital and Medical Center
114 Woodland Street
Hartford, Connecticut 06105-1299
Professor of Medicine and Orthopedics
University of Connecticut School of Medicine
Farmington, Connecticut 06030

Yan Chen
Associate Research Scientist
Department of Internal Medicine
Yale University School of Medicine
333 Cedar Street
New Haven, Connecticut 06520–8020

Brian Cho, Ph.D.
Post Doctoral Fellow
Department of Cell Biology
University of Massachusetts Medical School
55 Lake Avenue North
Worcester, Massachusetts 01655

Ung-il Chung, M.D., Ph.D.
Instructor in Medicine
Endocrine Unit
Massachusetts General Hospital and Harvard
*   Medical School*
50 Blossom Street
Boston, Massachusetts 02114

David R. Clemmons, M.D.
Professor
Department of Medicine
University of North Carolina School of Medicine
CB 7170, Room 6111, Thurston-Bowles
Chapel Hill, North Carolina 27599-7170

Tucker Collins, M.D., Ph.D.
Staff Pathology
Department of Pathology
Brigham & Women's Hospital
221 Longwood Avenue
Boston, Massachusetts 02115

Paolo M. Comoglio, M.D.
Division of Molecular Oncology IRCC
Department of Biomedical Sciences
Instituto di Ricerea e Cura del Canero
University of Torino
Str. Provinciale 142, Candialo
10060 Torino
Italy

Cheryl A. Conover, Ph.D.
Professor
Department of Medicine
Mayo Clinic
200 First Street SW
Joseph Building, Room 5-194
Rochester, Minnesota 55905

Françoise Debiais, M.D.
Department of Rheumatology
Jean Bernard Hospital
86021 Poitiers Cedex
France

Rik Derynck, M.D.
Department of Growth and Development
University of California at San Francisco
521 Parnassus Avenue
San Francisco, California 94143–0640

Thomas A. Einhorn, M.D.
Chief
Orthopedic Surgery
Boston Medical Center
Doctors Office Building
Suite 808
720 Harrison Avenue
Boston, Massachusetts 02118-2393

Neal S. Fedarko, M.D.
Division of Geriatric Medicine and Gerontology
Department of Medicine
Johns Hopkins University
5501 Hopkins Bayview Circle
Baltimore, Maryland 21224

Masayuki Funaba, Ph.D.
Assistant Professor
Azabu University School of Veterinary Medicine
Sagamihara 229-8501
Japan

Matthew T. Gillespie, Ph.D.
Senior Research Fellow
Department of Medicine
The University of Melbourne
St. Vincent's Institute of Medical Research
Fitzroy, Victoria, 3065
Australia

Maria Grano, Ph.D.
Associate Professor
Department of Human Anatomy
University of Bari
P. 770 E. Cesare 11
70129 Bari
Italy

Karl L. Insogna, M.D.
Associate Professor
Department of Internal Medicine
Yale University School of Medicine
FITKIN I Room 106
P.O. Box 208020
New Haven, Connecticut 06520-8020

Frederick S. Kaplan, M.D.
Isaac and Rose Nassau Professor of Orthopaedic
    Molecular Medicine
Department of Orthopedics
Hospital of the University of Pennsylvania
3400 Spruce Street
Philadelphia, Pennsylvania 19104

Gerard Karsenty, M.D., Ph.D.
Professor
Department of Molecular and Human Genetics
Baylor College of Medicine
One Baylor Plaza
Houston, Texas 77030

Vicky Kartsogiannis, Ph.D.
Research Officer
Department of Medicine
The University of Melbourne
St. Vincent's Institute of Medical Research
Fitzroy, Victoria, 3065
Australia

Masahiro Kawabata, M.D., Ph.D.
Associate Member
Department of Biochemistry
The Cancer Institute, Japanese Foundation for
    Cancer Research
1-37-1 Kami-ikebukuro
Toshima-ku, Tokyo 170-8455
Japan

L. Lyndon Key, Jr., M.D.
Professor
Department of Pediatrics
Medical University of South Carolina
96 Jonathan Lucas Street
Suite 316
Charleston, South Carolina 29425

Levon M. Khachigian, Ph.D.
Fellow
Centre for Thrombosis and Vascular Research
School of Pathology
The University of New South Wales
Sydney, NSW 2052,
Australia

Anne Klibanski, M.D.
Chief
Neuroendocrine Unit
Massachusetts General Hospital
55 Fruit Street
Boston, Massachusetts 02114

Henry M. Kronenberg, M.D.
Chief
Endocrine Unit
Massachusetts General Hospital
50 Blossom Street
Boston, Massachusetts 02114

David L. Lacey, M.D.
Amgen, Inc.
Mail Stop 15-2-A-226
1840 DeHavilland Drive
Thousand Oaks, California 91320-1799

Mark H.C. Lam, Ph.D.
Research Fellow
Biochemistry and Molecular Biology
The John Curtin School of Medicine
Australian National University
Canberra, 2601
Australia

Derek Le Roith, M.D. Ph.D.
Branch Chief
Clinical Endocrinology Branch
National Institutes of Health, NIDDK
Building 10, Room 8D12
10 Center Drive
Bethesda, Maryland 20892-1758

Jerome Lemonnier, Ph.D.
INSERM U349
Hopital Lariboisiere
2 rue Ambroise Paré
75475 Paris Cedex 10
France

Jane B. Lian, Ph.D.
Professor
Department of Cell Biology
University of Massachusetts Medical School
55 Lake Avenue North
Worcester, Massachusetts 01655-0106

Abderrahim Lomri, Ph.D.
INSERM Unite de Recherche 349
Hopital Lariboisiere
2 rue Ambrose Paré
75475 Paris, Cedex 10
France

Harry C. Lowe, B.H.B., MB.ChB.,
  F.R.A.C.P.
NH & MBC Postgraduate Scholar
Centre for Thrombosis and Vascular Research
School of Pathology
The University of New South Wales
Sydney, NSW 2052,
Australia

Frank P. Luyten, M.D., Ph.D.
Professor and Chairman
Department of Rheumatology
University Hospitals Leuven
Weligerveld I
3231 Pellenberg
Leuven, Belgium

Prema R. Madyastha, Ph.D.
Assistant Professor
Pediatric Endocrinology
Medical University of South Carolina
171 Ashley Avenue
Charleston, South Carolina 29425

Pierre J. Marie, Ph.D.
Director of Research
Cell and Molecular Biology of Bone
INSERM Unite de Recherche 349
Hopital Lariboisiere
2 rue Ambroise Paré
75475 Paris, Cedex 10
France

T. John Martin, M.D., D.Sc.
Director
St. Vincent's Institute of Medical Research
41 Victoria Parade
Fitzroy, 3065, Victoria
Australia

Kohei Miyazono, M.D., Ph.D.
Chief and Member
Department of Biochemistry
The Cancer Institute, Japanese Foundation for
  Cancer Research
1-37-1 Kami-ikebukuro
Toshima-ku Tokyo 170-8455
Japan

Gregory R. Mundy, M.D.
Department of Endocrinology and Metabolism
University of Texas
Health Science Center at San Antonio
7703 Floyd Curl Drive
San Antonio, Texas 778284-7877

Takuya Murata, D.V.M., Ph.D.
Research Associate
Department of Physiology
Fukui Medical University
Matsuoka 910-1193
Japan

Kenji Ogawa, D.V.M., Ph.D.
Research Scientist
Laboratory Animal Research Center
The Institute of Physical and Chemical Research
(RIKEN)
Wako 351-0198
Japan

David M. Ornitz, M.D., Ph.D.
Associate Professor
Department of Molecular Biology and
Pharmacology
Washington University Medical School
660 S. Euclid Avenue
St. Louis, Missouri 63110

Thomas A. Owen
Pfizer Central Research
Box 1170
Groton, Connecticut 06340

Roberto Pacifici, M.D.
Barnes-Jewish Hospital
216 South Kings Highway
St. Louis, Missouri 63110

J. Edward Puzas, Ph.D.
Professor of Orthopaedics
Department of Orthopaedics
University of Rochester School of Medicine
Medical Center, Box 665
601 Elmwood Avenue
Rochester, New York 14642

Louise A. Rafty
Centre for Thrombosis and Vascular Research
School of Pathology
The University of New South Wales
Sydney, NSW 2052,
Australia

William L. Ries, D.D.S., Ph.D.
Professor
Department of Stomatology
Medical University of South Carolina
171 Ashley Avenue
Charleston, South Carolina 29425

Anita B. Roberts, Ph.D.
Chief
Laboratory of Cell Regulation and Carcinogenesis
National Cancer Institute
41 Library Drive; MSC 5055
Building 41; Room C629
Bethesda, Maryland 20892-5055

Pamela Gehron Robey, Ph.D.
Chief
Laboratory of Cell Regulation and Carcinogenesis
NIDCR/National Institutes of Health
Building 30; Room 228
30 Convent Drive MSC 4320
Bethesda, Maryland 20892-0001

Gideon A. Rodan, M.D., Ph.D.
Vice President
Department of Bone Biology and Osteoporosis
Merck Research Laboratories
Sumneytown Pike
West Point, Pennsylvania 19486

G. David Roodman, M.D., Ph.D.
Department of Research/Hematology 151
Audie Murphy VA Hospital
7400 Merton Minter Boulevard
San Antonio, Texas 78284

Clifford J. Rosen, M.D.
St. Joseph Hospital
Maine Center for Osteoporosis Research and
Education
360 Broadway
Bangor, Maine 04401

Vicki Rosen, Ph.D.
Director
Department of Tissue Growth and Repair
Genetics Institute
87 Cambridge Park Drive
Cambridge, Massachusetts 02140

Gemma Sesmilo, M.D.
Research Fellow at MGH and HMS
Neuroendocrine Unit
Massachusetts General Hospital
55 Fruit Street
Boston, Massachusetts 02114

Eileen M. Shore, Ph.D.
Research Assistant Professor
Department of Orthopaedic Surgery
University of Pennsylvania
36th & Hamilton Walk
Philadelphia, Pennsylvania 19104-6081

Natalie Sims, Ph.D.
Departments of Orthopaedics and Cell Biology
Yale University School of Medicine
333 Cedar Street
New Haven, Connecticut 06520-8044

Gary S. Stein, Ph.D.
Professor and Chairman
Department of Cell Biology
University of Massachusetts Medical School
55 Lake Avenue North
Worcester, Massachusetts 01655-0106

Janet L. Stein, Ph.D.
Professor
Department of Cell Biology
University of Massachusetts Medical School
55 Lake Avenue North
Worcester, Massachusetts 01655-0106

Hiromu Sugino, Ph.D.
Professor
The Institute for Enzyme Research
The University of Tokushima
3-18-15 Kuramoto
Tokushima 770-8503
Japan

Kunihiro Tsuchida, M.D., Ph.D.
Associate Professor
The Institute for Enzyme Research
The University of Tokushima
3-18-15 Kuramoto
Tokushima 770-8503
Japan

André J. van Wijnen, Ph.D.
Assistant Professor
Department of Cell Biology
University of Massachusetts Medical School
55 Lake Avenue North
Worcester, Massachusetts 10655-0106

Eleanor C. Weir, B.V.M.S.
Department of Comparative Medicine
Yale University School of Medicine
333 Cedar Street
New Haven, Connecticut 06520-8020

John M. Wozney, Ph.D.
Senior Director
Bone Biology and Applications
Genetics Institute, Inc.
One Burtt Road
Andover, Massachusetts 01810

Gang-Qing Yao, M.D.
Associate Research Scientist
Department of Comparative Medicine
Yale University School of Medicine
333 Cedar Street
New Haven, Connecticut 06520-8020

Alberta Zallone, Ph.D.
University of Bari Policlinico
Piazza Giulio Cesare, II
70124 Bari
Italy

Preface

Recent advances in growth factor biology and their clinical aspects led to the publication of this book on skeletal growth factors.

Skeletal growth factors, polypeptides secreted by bone cells, have a significant function in bone remodeling. The existence of skeletal growth factors was initially reported in 1980 with the discovery that skeletal cells secrete biological activity that stimulates bone cell function and matrix synthesis. Following this discovery, growth factors were isolated and characterized, and it is now known that skeletal cells secrete insulin-like growth factors (IGFs), platelet-derived growth factors (PDGFs), fibroblast growth factors (FGFs), transforming growth factors beta (TGFβs), bone morphogenetic proteins (BMPs), hepatocyte growth factors (HGFs), and cytokines of the interleukin and colony-stimulating factor families.

The reasons why skeletal cells synthesize a variety of growth factors appear to be related to their different biological functions and to their regulation at different levels by distinct agents. Fracture healing, bone mass, and bone development are affected directly by growth factors; for example, IGFs are modest mitogens that increase the differentiated function of the osteoblast, which is important in the maintenance of bone mass.

The book begins with an initial description of basic issues in bone cell biology, then addresses the various growth factors secreted by skeletal cells. A description of the biological role of each factor is followed by a detailed description of the function of the growth factor in the skeleton and a presentation of its clinical relevance. The book is completed with a series of chapters outlining the current knowledge of growth factors on the pathogenesis and therapeutic aspects of metabolic bone disorders, including a chapter discussing the future of growth factors in the treatment of bone disorders.

Leaders in the fields of growth factors and bone cell biology contributed their knowledge and time to the information contained in this book. I am grateful to them. I am also grateful to Joanne Husovski, from Lippincott Williams & Wilkins, for her substantial efforts in the editing and publication of this book.

Ernesto Canalis, M.D.

SKELETAL GROWTH FACTORS

Skeletal Growth Factors,
edited by Ernesto Canalis.
Lippincott Williams & Wilkins, Philadelphia, © 2000.

1

Bone Cells and Their Function

Natalie Sims and Roland Baron

*Departments of Orthopaedics and Cell Biology, Yale University School of Medicine,
New Haven, Connecticut 06520–8044*

Bone is a specialized connective tissue that makes up, together with cartilage, the skeletal system. These tissues serve three functions: (a) mechanical (support and site of muscle attachment for locomotion), (b) protective (for vital organs and bone marrow), and (c) metabolic (as a reserve of ions, especially calcium and phosphate, for the maintenance of serum homeostasis).

The maintenance of both calcium homeostasis and the structural integrity of the skeleton is achieved by the coordinated actions of two major families of bone cells, the osteoblast and the osteoclast lineages. These cells are involved in both bone structural development and the continual turnover of bone matrix during adult life; this participates in the maintenance of calcium homeostasis.

THE OSTEOBLAST AND BONE FORMATION

Osteoblast Structure

The osteoblast is the bone lining cell responsible for the production of the bone matrix constituents collagen and ground substance (Fig. 1.1). Osteoblasts never appear or function individually but are always found in clusters of cuboidal cells along the bone surface (~100 to 400 cells per bone forming site). The osteoblast is characterized morphologically by a round nucleus at the base of the cell (away from the bone surface), an intensely basophilic cytoplasm, and a prominent Golgi complex located between the nucleus

and the apex of the cell. Osteoblasts are always found lining the layer of bone matrix that they are producing but before it is calcified (called, at this point, osteoid tissue). Osteoid tissue exists because of a time lag of approximately 10 days between matrix formation and its subsequent calcification. Behind the osteoblast can usually be found one or two layers of cells: activated mesenchymal cells and preosteoblasts (see below). A mature osteoblast does not divide.

At the ultrastructural level, the osteoblast is characterized by the presence of an extremely well-developed rough endoplasmic reticulum with dilated cisternae, a dense granular content, and the presence of a large, circular Golgi complex comprising multiple Golgi stacks. These organelles are involved in the major activity of the osteoblast: the production and secretion of collagenous and noncollagenous bone matrix proteins. Type I collagen, which makes up 90% of the total matrix protein, is the major protein produced and secreted by osteoblasts (20% of the total protein produced). The major noncollagenous protein produced is osteocalcin, which makes up 1% of the matrix and may play a role in calcium binding and stabilization of hydroxyapatite in the matrix and/or regulation of bone formation, as suggested by increased bone mass in osteocalcin knockout mice (1). Osteoblasts also produce a range of growth factors under a variety of stimuli, including the insulin-like growth factors (IGFs) (2), platelet-derived growth factors (PDGFs) (3), basic fibroblast growth factor (bFGF) (4), transforming growth

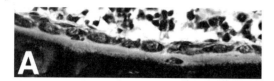

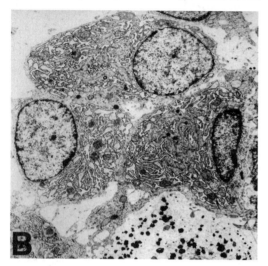

FIG. 1.1. Osteoblasts and osteoid tissue. **A:** Light micrograph of a group of osteoblasts producing osteoid. Note the newly embedded osteocyte. **B:** Electron micrograph of three osteoblasts covering a layer of mineralizing osteoid tissue. Note the prominent Golgi and endoplasmic reticulum characteristic of active osteoblasts.

factor-beta (TGF-β) (5), cytokines (6), and the bone morphogenetic proteins (BMPs) (7), which will be discussed in detail in the chapters to follow.

As mentioned previously, osteoblasts do not operate in isolation and gap junctions are often found between osteoblasts working together on the bone surface. Osteoblasts also appear to communicate with the osteocyte network within the bone matrix (see following) since cytoplasmic processes on the secreting side of the osteoblast extend deep into the osteoid matrix and are in contact with processes of the osteocytes dwelling there.

The plasma membrane of the osteoblast is characteristically rich in alkaline phosphatase (whose concentration in the serum is used as an index of bone formation) and has been shown to have receptors for a wide range of modulators.

Classic endocrine receptors include receptors for parathyroid hormone/parathyroid hormone–related protein (PTH/PTHrP) receptor, thyroid hormone (8), growth hormone (9), insulin (10), progesterone (11), β-adrenergic receptors (12), and receptors for prolactin (13). Osteoblastic nuclear steroid hormone receptors include receptors for estrogens (14,15), androgens (16), vitamin D_3 (17), and retinoids (18). Receptors for paracrine and autocrine effectors include those for epidermal growth factor (EGF) (19), the IGFs (20,21), PDGF (5), TGF-β (22), interleukins (23,24), FGFs (25), and BMPs (26). Osteoblasts also have receptors for several adhesion molecules (integrins) involved in cell attachment to the bone surface (27).

Mechanism of Bone Formation

Bone formation occurs by three coordinated processes: production, maturation, and mineralization of the osteoid matrix. In normal adult bone, these processes occur at the same rate so that the balance between matrix production and mineralization is equal. Initially, osteoblasts deposit collagen rapidly, without mineralization, producing a thickening osteoid seam. This is followed by an increase in the mineralization rate to equal the rate of collagen synthesis. In the final stage, the rate of collagen synthesis decreases and mineralization continues until the osteoid seam is fully mineralized. This time lag (termed the "mineralization lag time" or "osteoid maturation period") appears to be required for osteoid to be modified so that it is able to support mineralization. While this delay is not yet understood, it is likely that either collagen cross-linking occurs or an inhibitor of mineralization, such as matrix gla protein (28), is removed during this time, thus allowing mineralization to proceed.

When bone is formed very rapidly during development and fracture healing or in some metabolic bone diseases, there is no preferential organization of the collagen fibers; this type of bone is called woven bone. Woven bone is characterized by irregular bundles of collagen fibers, large and extremely numerous osteocytes, and delayed and disorderly calcification which occurs in irregularly distributed patches. In lamellar bone, collagen fibers are preferentially arranged to allow the highest density of collagen per unit volume of tissue. The lamellae can be parallel to each other if deposited along a flat surface (trabecular bone and periosteum) or concentric if deposited on a surface surrounding a central blood vessel (cortical bone Haversian system). Woven bone lacks the strength of lamellar bone, and it is for this reason that it is usually replaced by lamellar bone during bone remodeling (see following).

To initiate mineralization in woven bone or in growth plate cartilage, high local concentrations of Ca^{2+} and PO_4^{3-} ions must be reached in order to induce their precipitation into amorphous calcium phosphate, leading to hydroxyapatite crystal formation. This is achieved by membrane-bound matrix vesicles, which originate by budding from the cytoplasmic processes of the chondrocyte or the osteoblast and are deposited within the matrix during its formation (29). In the matrix, these vesicles are the first structure wherein hydroxyapatite crystals are observed. The membranes are very rich in alkaline phosphatase [pyrophosphatase and adenosine triphosphatase (ATPase)] and in acidic phospholipids, which hydrolyze inhibitors of calcification in the matrix including pyrophosphate and ATP, allowing condensation of apatite crystals. Once the crystals are in the matrix environment, they will grow in clusters, which later coalesce to completely calcify the matrix, filling the spaces between and within the collagen fibers. In adult lamellar bone, matrix vesicles are not present and mineralization occurs in an orderly manner through progression of the mineralization front into the osteoid tissue.

Osteoblast function is regulated by a number of endocrine, paracrine, and autocrine factors. Endocrine factors include classical systemic regulators such as vitamin D_3, estrogen, PTH, and others mentioned above. Paracrine and autocrine factors include a wide range of interleukins and growth factors also described above and discussed in detail in the following chapters. Recent research has focused on determining genetic regulators of osteoblast function; one such regulator is Cbfa1 (also known as Osf2). Cbfa1 binds to and activates transcription of most genes expressed in osteoblasts (30). Studies in knockout mice have shown that this factor regulates osteoblast maturation (31,32).

Origin and Fate of the Osteoblast

Osteoblasts originate from local pluripotent mesenchymal stem cells, either bone marrow stromal stem cells (endosteum) or connective tissue mesenchymal stem cells (periosteum). These precursors, with the right stimulation, undergo proliferation and differentiate into preosteoblasts, at which point they are committed to differentiate into mature osteoblasts (Fig. 1.2) although recent evidence suggests that preosteoblast commitment may be more fluid than previously believed (33).

The committed preosteoblast is located in apposition to the bone surface and is usually present in layers below active mature osteoblasts. They are elliptical cells, with an elongated nucleus, and are still capable of proliferation. Preosteoblasts lack the well-developed protein-synthesizing capability of the mature osteoblast and do not have the characteristically localized, mature rough endoplasmic reticulum or Golgi apparatus of the mature cell.

The development of the osteoblast phenotype is a gradual process, with a defined sequence of gene expression and cell activity. In the early stages of osteoblast proliferation, there is expression of the proliferative genes c-myc and c-fos. As osteoblasts begin to lay down osteoid matrix, type I collagen, fibronectin, and some growth factors are expressed. As the cell matures, its function and protein production schedule change. While cells continue to produce type I collagen, they begin producing alkaline phosphatase and then matrix gla protein. Later, collagen production slows, and the wave of alkaline phosphatase production is followed by osteocalcin and osteopontin production (34).

Toward the end of the matrix secreting period, a further step is involved in osteoblast maturation. Approximately 15% of the mature osteoblasts become encapsulated in the new bone matrix and differentiate into osteocytes. In contrast, some cells remain on the bone surface, becom-

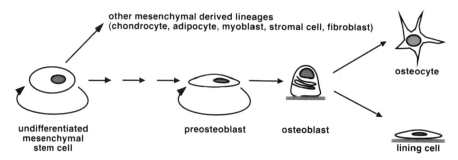

FIG. 1.2. Osteoblast lineage. Osteoblasts originate from undifferentiated mesenchymal cells, which are capable of proliferation and may differentiate into one of a range of cell types. The committed preosteoblast is also capable of proliferation. The mature osteoblast no longer proliferates but can differentiate further into an osteocyte if embedded in the bone matrix or set into a lining cell on the bone surface. See text for details.

ing flat lining cells. The signaling mechanism that determines which cells become osteocytes is not understood.

There is recent evidence that after mechanical stimulation bone lining cells develop ultrastructural features of osteoblastic differentiation and activity, without any cell proliferation (35). By 48 hours after mechanical loading, lining cells became cuboidal, with rounded nuclei and abundant rough endoplasmic reticulum, characteristics of a mature osteoblast. This would provide a mechanism for the rapid osteogenic response seen after mechanical stimuli and is consistent with earlier studies demonstrating increased os-

teoblast activity without cell proliferation following PTH treatment (36).

WITHIN THE MATRIX: THE OSTEOCYTE

The calcified bone matrix is not metabolically inert, and osteocytes are found embedded deep within the bone in small lacunae (Fig. 1.3). All osteocytes are derived from osteoblasts which became trapped in the bone matrix that they produced and that became calcified. Even though the metabolic activity of the osteoblast decreases dramatically once it is fully encased, these cells

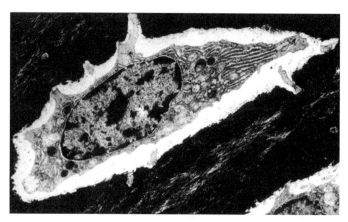

FIG. 1.3. Osteocyte. Electron micrograph of an osteocyte within a lacuna in calcified bone matrix. The cell has a basal nucleus, cytoplasmic extensions, and well-developed Golgi and endoplasmic reticulum.

still produce matrix proteins. Osteocytes have numerous long cell processes rich in microfilaments, which are in contact with cell processes from other osteocytes (there are frequent gap junctions) or with processes from the cells lining the bone surface (osteoblasts or flat lining cells). These processes are organized during the formation of the matrix and before its calcification; they form a network of thin canaliculi permeating the entire bone matrix. Osteocytic canaliculi are not distributed evenly about the cell but are mainly directed toward the bone-forming surface. Between the osteocyte plasma membrane and the bone matrix itself is the periosteocytic space. This space exists both in the lacunae and in the canaliculi, and it is filled with extracellular fluid (ECF), the only source of nutrients for the osteocyte. ECF flow through the canalicular network is altered during bone matrix compression and tension.

Osteocyte morphology varies according to age and functional activity. A young osteocyte has most of the ultrastructural characteristics of the osteoblast from which it was derived, except that there has been a decrease in cell volume and in the importance of the organelles involved in protein synthesis (rough endoplasmic reticulum, Golgi). An older osteocyte, located deeper within the calcified bone, shows a further decrease in cell volume and organelles, and an accumulation of glycogen in the cytoplasm. These cells are able to synthesize small amounts of new bone matrix at the surface of the osteocytic lacunae, which can subsequently calcify. Osteocytes express, in low levels, a number of osteoblast markers, including osteocalcin, osteopontin, osteonectin, and E11 (37,38).

Despite the complex organization of the osteocytic network and its location within the bone matrix, the exact function of these cells remains obscure. Given the structure of the network and the location of osteocytes within lacunae where ECF flow can be detected, it is likely that osteocytes may respond to bone tissue strain and influence bone-remodeling activity by recruiting osteoclasts to sites where bone remodeling is required (39). Osteocyte cellular activity is increased after bone loading; studies in cell culture have demonstrated increased calcium influx and

prostaglandin production by osteocytes after mechanical stimulation (40), but there is no direct evidence for osteocyte signaling to cells on the bone surface in response to bone strain or microdamage.

The fate of the osteocyte is to be phagocytosed and digested together with the other components of bone during osteoclastic bone resorption (41).

THE OSTEOCLAST AND BONE RESORPTION

The osteoclast is the bone lining cell responsible for bone resorption (Fig. 1.4). The osteoclast is a giant multinucleated cell, up to 100 μm in diameter and containing four to 20 nuclei. It is usually found in contact with a calcified bone surface and within a lacuna (Howship's lacunae), which is the result of its own resorptive activity. It is possible to find up to four or five osteoclasts in the same resorptive site, but there are usually only one or two. Under the light microscope, the nuclei appear to vary within the same cell: some are round and euchromatic, and some are irregular in contour and heterochromatic, possibly reflecting the asynchronous fusion of mononuclear precursors. The cytoplasm is ''foamy'' with many vacuoles. The zone of contact with the bone is characterized by the presence of a ruffled border with dense patches on each side (the sealing zone). (42,43).

Characteristic ultrastructural features of this cell are the abundant Golgi complexes around each nucleus, the mitochondria, and transport vesicles loaded with lysosomal enzymes. The most prominent features of the osteoclast are, however, the deep foldings of the plasma membrane in the area facing the bone matrix (ruffled border) and the surrounding zone of attachment (sealing zone). The sealing zone is a ring of contractile proteins that attach the cell to the bone surface, thus sealing off the subosteoclastic bone-resorbing compartment. The attachment of the cell to the matrix is performed via integrin receptors, which bind to specific arginine-glycine-aspartic acid (RGD) sequences in matrix proteins. The plasma membrane in the ruffled border area contains proteins that are also found

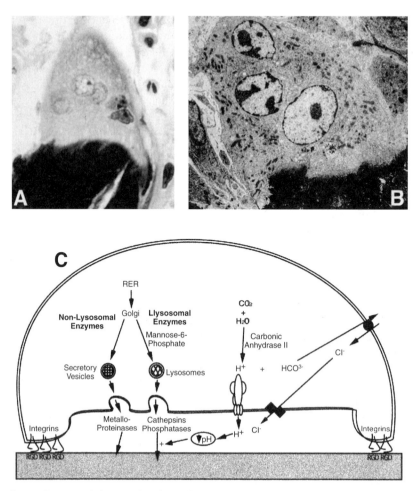

FIG. 1.4. Osteoclasts and the mechanism of bone resorption. Light micrograph **(A)** and electron micrograph **(B)** of an osteoclast, demonstrating the ruffled border and numerous nuclei. **C:** Diagrammatic representation of osteoclastic resorption. The osteoclast forms a sealing zone via integrin-mediated attachment to RGD peptides within the bone matrix, forming a separate compartment between the cell and the bone surface. This compartment is acidified such that an optimal pH is reached for lysosomal enzyme activity and bone resorption. See text for details.

at the limiting membrane of lysosomes and related organelles and a specific type of electrogenic vacuolar proton ATPase involved in acidification. The basolateral plasma membrane of the osteoclast is specifically enriched in Na^+,K^+-ATPase (sodium pumps), HCO_3^-/Cl^- exchangers, and Na^+/H^+ exchangers (44). Also present are numerous ion channels including Na^+, Cl^-, and phosphate channels, calcium-activated K^+ channels, and voltage-activated K^+ and Ca^{2+} channels (45–48).

Lysosomal enzymes such as tartrate-resistant acid phosphatase and cathepsin K are actively synthesized by the osteoclast and found in the endoplasmic reticulum, Golgi, and many transport vesicles. The enzymes are secreted, via the ruffled border, into the extracellular bone-resorbing compartment; they reach a sufficiently high extracellular concentration because this compartment is sealed off. The transport and targeting of these enzymes for secretion at the apical pole of the osteoclast involve mannose-6-phosphate receptors. Furthermore, the cell secretes several matrix metalloproteinases

(MMPs) such as collagenase (MMP-13) and gelatinase B (MMP-9).

Mechanism of Bone Resorption

Osteoclasts resorb bone by acidification and dissolution of hydroxyapatite crystals and proteolysis of the bone matrix within the sealing zone (Fig. 1.4C). Carbonic anhydrase type II produces hydrogen ions within the cell, which are then pumped across the ruffled border membrane via proton pumps, thereby acidifying the extracellular compartment. The ATP and CO_2 are provided by the mitochondria. The basolateral membrane activity exchanges bicarbonate for chloride, thereby avoiding alkalinization of the cytosol. K^+ channels in the basolateral domain and Cl^- channels in the apical ruffled border ensure dissipation of the electrogenic gradients generated by the vacuolar H^+-ATPase. The basolateral sodium pumps might be involved in secondary active transport of calcium and/or protons in association with a Na^+/Ca^{2+} exchanger and/or a Na^+/H^+ antiport. This cell could therefore function in a manner similar to that of kidney tubule intercalated, which also acidify lumens.

Attachment of the osteoclast to the bone surface is essential for bone resorption. This process involves transmembrane adhesion receptors of the integrin family (49). Integrins attach to specific amino acid sequences (mostly RGD sequences) within proteins in or at the surface of the bone matrix. In the osteoclast, $\alpha_v\beta_3$ (vitronectin receptor), $\alpha_2\beta_1$ (collagen receptor), and $\alpha_v\beta_5$ integrins are predominantly expressed (50). Without cell attachment the acidified microenvironment cannot be established and the osteoclast cannot be motile.

After osteoclast adhesion to the bone matrix, $\alpha_v\beta_3$ binding activates cytoskeletal reorganization within the osteoclast, including cell spreading and polarization (51). In most cells, attachment occurs via focal adhesions, where stress fibers (bundles of microfilaments) anchor the cell to the substrate. In osteoclasts, attachment usually occurs via podosomes, clusters of small focal adhesion-like structures. Podosomes are more dynamic structures than focal adhesions

and occur in cells that are highly motile. It is the continual assembly and disassembly of podosomes that allow osteoclast movement across the bone surface during bone resorption. Integrin signaling and subsequent podosome formation are dependent on a number of adhesion kinases including the protooncogene *src*, which, while not required for osteoclast maturation, is required for osteoclast function, as demonstrated by osteopetrosis in the *src* knockout mouse (52). Recently, it has been noted that Pyk2, another member of the focal adhesion kinase family, is also activated by $\alpha_v\beta_3$ during osteoclast attachment and is required for bone resorption (53).

The first process during osteoclastic bone resorption is mobilization of the hydroxyapatite crystals by digestion of their link to collagen via the noncollagenous proteins, and the low pH dissolves the hydroxyapatite crystals, exposing the bone matrix. Then the residual collagen fibers are digested either by cathepsins, now at optimal pH, or activated collagenases. The residues from this extracellular digestion are either internalized or transported across the cell and released at the basolateral domain. Residues may also be released during periods of sealing zone relapse, as probably occurs during osteoclast motility and possibly induced by a calcium sensor responding to the rise of extracellular calcium in the bone-resorbing compartment.

Osteoclast function is regulated both by locally acting cytokines and by systemic hormones. Endocrine regulation of bone resorption may be mediated by osteoblasts; for example, PTH can stimulate osteoblastic production of macrophage colony-stimulating factor (M-CSF) or interleukin (IL)-6, which then act on the osteoclast (54). Other endocrine hormones, such as calcitonin, function directly on osteoclastic receptors (55,56). Other hormones act on osteoclast precursors, such as 1,25-dihydroxyvitamin D_3, to induce proliferation, but are unlikely to act directly on mature osteoclasts since they do not express vitamin D receptors (57,58). While studies of osteoclastic receptors have been limited by the difficulty of obtaining pure osteoclast preparation, osteoclastic receptors for androgens (59), thyroid hormone (60), insulin (61), and glutamate (62) have been demonstrated. The presence of estrogen receptors in osteoclasts remains controversial (63,64). PTH receptors have been demonstrated in osteoclasts (65), but the significance of this finding is unclear since purified osteoclasts do not respond to PTH treatment (66).

A large number of paracrine regulators of osteoclast function act via osteoblast signaling. Some examples include IL-6 and M-CSF (see above), IL-18, which increases osteoclast proliferation via increased osteoblastic production of granulocyte-macrophage colony-stimulating factor (GM-CSF) (67), IL-11 and osteoclast inhibitory factor (OCIF/OPG), described below. IL-6 acts in an autocrine manner on osteoclasts via gp130 (68). Nitric oxide is also an autocrine regulator of osteoclast function (69). Osteoclasts also possess receptors for CSF-1 (70), IGF-1 (71), IL-1 (72), PDGF (73), and activin A (a TGF-β family receptor) (74).

Origin and Fate of the Osteoclast

The osteoclast derives from hematopoietic cells in the mononuclear/phagocytic lineage (Fig. 1.5) (75). Precursor cells fuse at the bone surface to form the multinucleated osteoclast (76). Although this may occur at the early pro-monocyte stage, monocytes and macrophages already committed to their own lineage might still be able to form osteoclasts under the right circumstances.

Recently, a series of papers has described the importance of OCIF (77), also known as osteoprotegerin (OPG) (78), as well as this protein's ligand, osteoclast differentiation factor [ODF; also described independently as osteoprotegerin ligand (OPGL), receptor activator of NF$\kappa\beta$ ligand (RANKL), and tumor necrosis factor–related activation-induced cytokine (TRANCE) (79,80)], in osteoblast-mediated stimulation of osteoclastogenesis. These two proteins act as competitive regulators of bone resorption. ODF, which is expressed in osteoblasts and stromal cells, induces osteoclast formation by direct contact with RANK (also known as TRANCER), a receptor expressed by osteoclast progenitor cells. ODAR is also expressed in mature osteoclasts and has recently been shown to regulate mature osteoclast function as well. In contrast, OPG can act as a decoy RANK-type receptor and competitively inhibits the formation of mature, functional osteoclasts.

Despite its mononuclear/phagocytic origin, the osteoclast membrane expresses distinct markers: it is devoid of several macrophage markers, including Fc and C_3 receptors; like mononuclear phagocytes, however, the osteoclast is rich in nonspecific esterases, synthesizes lysozymes, and expresses mannose-6-phosphate receptors (81). Monoclonal antibodies have been produced that recognize osteoclasts but not macrophages. The osteoclast, unlike macrophages, also expresses millions of copies of the calcitonin and vitronectin receptors, predominantly the integrin $\alpha_v\beta_3$ (49,55,56). Osteoclasts also express high levels of pp60c-src (82), a non-receptor tyrosine kinase involved in osteoclast adhesion (see preceding).

The osteoclast appears to undergo apoptosis

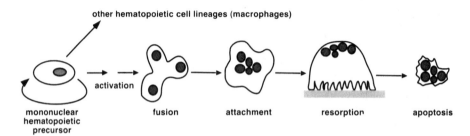

FIG. 1.5. Osteoclast life cycle. The osteoclast is derived from a mononuclear hematopoietic precursor which, upon activation, fuses with other precursors to form a multinucleated cell that attaches to the bone surface and commences resorption. After a cycle of bone resorption, the osteoclast undergoes apoptosis.

after a cycle of resorption (83), characterized by loss of the ruffled border, detachment from the bone surface, and condensation of the nuclear chromatin.

BONE REMODELING

Bone remodeling is the process by which bone is turned over; it is the result of the activity of the cells at the surfaces of bone, mainly the endosteal surface, which includes all trabecular surfaces. Remodeling is traditionally classified in two distinct types: Haversian remodeling within the cortical bone and endosteal remodeling along the trabecular bone surface. This distinction is more morphological than physiological because the Haversian surface is an extension of the endosteal surface, and the cellular events during these two remodeling processes follow exactly the same sequence.

The Remodeling Sequence

Bone formation and bone resorption do not occur along the bone surface at random: they are coordinated as part of the turnover mechanism by which old bone is replaced by new bone. In the normal adult skeleton, bone formation occurs, for the most part, only where bone resorption has already occurred. This basic principle of cellular activity at the remodeling site is the activation–resorption–formation (ARF) sequence (Fig. 1.6) (84,85).

Upon some signal, a locally acting factor released by lining cells, osteocytes, or marrow cells or in response to bone deformation or fatigue-related microfracture activates a group of preosteoclasts. These mononuclear cells attach to the bone via vitronectin receptors and fuse to form a multinucleated osteoclast, which will, in a definite area of the bone surface, resorb the bone matrix. After resorption of the bone, uncharacterized mononuclear cells cover the surface and a cement line is formed. The cement line marks the limit of bone resorption and acts to cement together the old and the new bone. This is termed the ''reversal phase'' and is followed by a period of bone formation. Preosteoblasts are activated, proliferate, and differentiate

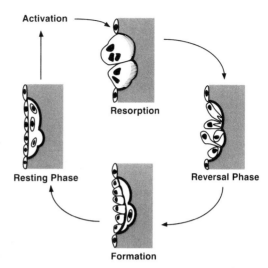

FIG. 1.6. The bone remodeling sequence. The cycle of bone remodeling as it occurs in trabecular bone. See text for details.

into osteoblasts, which move onto the bone surface, forming an initial matrix (osteoid), which becomes mineralized after a time lag (the osteoid maturation period). The basic remodeling sequence is therefore activation-resorption-formation; it is performed by a group of cells called the basic multicellular unit. The complete remodeling cycle takes about 3 months in humans (Fig. 1.7).

For many years it has been accepted that bone resorption and formation are coupled in the same way that matrix formation and calcification are linked. In other words, in the normal adult skeleton, the coupling of bone resorption and formation in remodeling results in equal levels of cellular activity so that bone turnover is balanced: the volume of bone resorbed is equal to the volume formed. This paradigm implies that, for example, a reduction in osteoblast activity would affect a similar reduction in osteoclast activity such that bone volume is maintained. However, a recent paper, in which osteoblast ablation was induced in mature transgenic mice, demonstrated that the dramatic reduction in bone formation is not associated with a reduction in osteoclast activity (86). In these mice, the subsequent osteopenia (bone loss) is striking, and this calls our understanding of bone cell

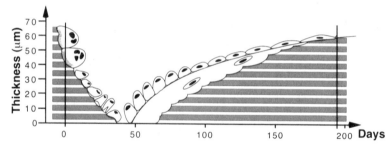

FIG. 1.7. Duration and depth of the phases of the normal cancellous bone remodeling sequence, calculated from histomorphometric analysis of bone biopsy samples from young individuals (From ref. 104, with permission.)

cross-regulation into question. Interestingly, it may also be argued that since osteoblasts are completely absent in this model, they are required to modulate osteoclast activity, or bone resorption could continue in an unregulated manner, thus causing the bone loss observed. In any case, it is clear that studies are needed to define the potential mechanism of the balance of bone cell activity.

Haversian versus Endosteal Bone Remodeling

As previously mentioned, although cortical bone is anatomically different, its remodeling occurs following the same sequence of events. The major difference is that while the average thickness of a trabecula is 150 to 200 μm, the average thickness of the cortex is on the order of 5 to 10 mm. There are no blood vessels in the trabeculae, but the bone envelope system and the osteocyte network are able to carry out enough gaseous exchange, being always relatively close to the surface and the highly vascularized marrow. Consequently, bone remodeling in the trabecular bone will take place along the trabecular surface. On the other hand, the cortical bone itself needs to be vascularized. Blood vessels are first embedded during the histogenesis of cortical bone; the blood vessel and the bone which surrounds it are then called a primary osteon. Later, cortical bone remodeling will be initiated either along the surface of these vascular channels or from the endosteal surface

of the cortex. The remodeling process in cortical bone also follows the ARF sequence. Osteoclasts excavate a tunnel, creating a cutting cone. Again, there is a reversal phase, where mononuclear cells attach and lay down a cement line. Osteoblasts are then responsible for closing the cone, leaving a central canal, centered on blood vessels and surrounded by concentric bone lamellae. For mechanical reasons, all of these Haversian systems are oriented along the longitudinal axis of the bone.

Bone Turnover and Skeletal Homeostasis

In a normal young adult, about 30% of the total skeletal mass is renewed every year (half life = 20 months). In each remodeling unit, osteoclastic bone resorption lasts about 3 days, the reversal 14 days, and bone formation 70 days (total = 87 days). The linear bone formation rate is 0.5 mm/day. During this process, about 0.01 mm^3 of bone is renewed in one given remodeling unit. Theoretically, with balanced matrix deposition and calcification as well as a balance between osteoclast and osteoblast activity, the amount of bone formed in each remodeling unit (and therefore in the total skeleton) equals the amount of bone which was previously resorbed. Thus, the total skeletal mass remains constant. This skeletal homeostasis relies upon a normal remodeling activity. The rate of activation of new remodeling units would then determine only the turnover rate.

SKELETAL DEVELOPMENT—HISTOGENESIS

Anatomically, two types of bone can be distinguished in the skeleton: flat bones (skull bones, scapula, mandible, and ileum) and long bones (tibia, femur, humerus, etc.). These are derived by two distinct types of development, intramembranous and endochondral, respectively, although the development and growth of long bones actually involve both processes. The main difference between intramembranous and endochondral bone formation is the presence of a cartilaginous phase in the latter.

Intramembranous Ossification

During intramembranous ossification, a group of mesenchymal cells within a highly vascularized area of the embryonic connective tissue proliferates, forming early cell condensations within which cells differentiate directly into osteoblasts. These cells will synthesize a woven bone matrix, while at the periphery, mesenchymal cells continue to differentiate into osteoblasts. Blood vessels are incorporated between the woven bone trabeculae and will form the hematopoietic bone marrow. Later, this woven bone will be remodeled by the ARF sequence and progressively replaced by mature lamellar bone.

Endochondral Ossification

Development of long bones begins with condensation of the mesenchyme to form a cartilaginous model of the bone to be formed (Fig. 1.8). Mesenchymal cells undergo division and differentiate into prechondroblasts and then into chondroblasts. These cells secrete the cartilaginous matrix. Like osteoblasts, the chondroblasts be-

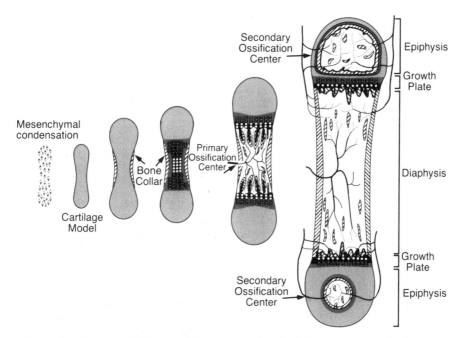

FIG. 1.8. Bone development. Schematic diagram showing the initial stages of endochondral ossification. Bone development begins with mesenchymal condensation to form a cartilage model of the bone to be formed. Following chondrocyte hypertrophy and matrix mineralization, osteoclast activity and vascularization result in formation of the primary and then secondary ossification centers. In mature adult bones, the growth plate is fully resorbed so that one marrow cavity extends the full length of the bone. See text for details.

come progressively embedded within their own matrix, where they lie within lacunae, and they are then called chondrocytes. Unlike osteocytes, however, chondrocytes continue to proliferate for some time, this being allowed in part by the gel-like consistency of cartilage. At the periphery of this cartilage (the perichondrium), the mesenchymal cells continue to proliferate and differentiate. This is called appositional growth. Another type of growth is observed in the cartilage by cell proliferation and synthesis of new matrix between the chondrocytes (interstitial growth).

Beginning in the center of the cartilage model, at what is to become the primary ossification center, chondrocytes differentiate and become hypertrophic. During this process, hypertrophic cells deposit a matrix, where cartilage calcification is initiated by matrix vesicles (87). Once this matrix is calcified, it is partially resorbed by osteoclasts. After resorption and a reversal phase, osteoblasts differentiate in this area and form a layer of woven bone on top of the remaining cartilage. This will later be remodeled into lamellar bone.

The embryonic cartilage is avascular. During its early development, a ring of woven bone is formed at the periphery by intramembranous ossification in the future midshaft area under the perichondrium (which becomes periosteum). Following calcification of this woven bone, blood vessels, preceded by the osteoclasts entering the primary ossification center, will penetrate this bone and the calcified cartilage, forming the blood supply which will allow seeding of the hematopoietic bone marrow and invasion of osteoclasts to resorb the calcified cartilage as described previously.

Secondary ossification centers begin to form at the epiphyseal ends of the cartilaginous model, and by a similar process, trabecular bone and a marrow space are formed at these ends. Between the primary and secondary ossification centers, epiphyseal cartilage (growth plates) remain until adulthood. The continued proliferation and differentiation of chondrocytes, cartilage mineralization, and subsequent remodeling cycles allow longitudinal bone growth to occur such that as new bone is formed, the bone will

reach its final adult shape. There is, however, a progressive decrease in chondrocyte proliferation so that the growth plate becomes thinner, allowing mineralization and resorption to catch up. It is at this point that the growth plates are completely remodeled and longitudinal growth is arrested.

The growth plate demonstrates, from the epiphyseal area to the diaphyseal area, the different stages of chondrocyte differentiation involved in endochondral bone formation (Fig. 1.9). Firstly, there is a proliferative zone, where the chondrocytes divide actively, forming isogenous groups and actively synthesizing the matrix. These cells become progressively larger, enlarging their lacunae in the prehypertrophic and hypertrophic zones. Lower in this area, the matrix of the longitudinal cartilage septa selectively calcifies (zone of provisional calcification). The chondrocytes become highly vacuolated and then die through programmed cell death (apoptosis). Once calcified, the cartilage matrix is resorbed, but only partially, by osteoclasts, leaving the calcified longitudinal septae and blood vessels to appear in the zone of invasion. After resorption, osteoblasts differentiate and form a layer of woven bone on top of the cartilaginous remnants of the longitudinal septa. Thus, the first ARF sequence is complete: the cartilage has been remodeled and replaced by woven bone. The resulting trabeculae are called the primary spongiosum. Still lower in the growth plate, this woven bone is subjected to further remodeling (a second ARF sequence), in which the woven bone and the cartilaginous remnants are replaced with lamellar bone, resulting in the mature trabecular bone called secondary spongiosum.

As chondrocytes mature, the pattern of cellular gene expression changes. For example, proliferating chondrocytes express collagen type II and hypertrophic chondrocytes express collagen type X. Chondrocyte apoptosis appears to be regulated by the ratio of expression of the apoptosis inducer Bax and the antiapoptotic gene Bcl2 (88). Bcl2 inhibits apoptotic pore formation by Bax; a decrease in Bcl2 levels would allow an increase in apoptotic pore formation (89). In the developing growth plate, levels of Bcl2 expression decrease as chondrocytes ma-

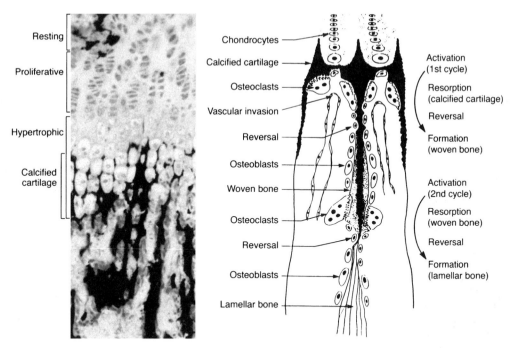

FIG. 1.9. Bone growth and remodeling at the growth plate. The light micrograph demonstrates the zones of chondrocyte differentiation as well as mineralization *(black)*. The schematic representation shows the cellular events occurring at the growth plate in long bones. Note that bone formation in this process occurs by repeated cycles of bone remodeling beginning with resorption of the calcified cartilage matrix.

ture and Bax levels remain unchanged, resulting in a decrease in the ratio Bcl2:Bax and cell death (90,91). Recently, gelatinase B (MMP-9) has also been shown to regulate chondrocyte apoptosis and vascular invasion at the growth plate (92).

Chondrocyte differentiation is regulated by a number of factors, which have recently been described. The first factor shown to control chondrocyte differentiation was PTHrP (93). This factor prolongs chondrocyte proliferation, and in PTHrP knockout mice, the main phenotype is bone shortening caused by premature chondrocyte hypertrophy (94). Targeted overexpression of PTHrP results in the opposite phenotype, with a prolonged delay in chondrocyte maturation (95). PTHrP is part of a genetic signaling cascade, where not only is it regulated by factors expressed earlier in chondrocyte differentiation, such as Indian hedgehog (96) but it also regulates chondrocyte differentiation itself and alters gene expression in more mature chondrocytes (see chapter 25 for a detailed discussion). Other factors which regulate chondrocyte differentiation include the FGFs and BMPs (97–99) (see later chapters for detailed discussions).

Defects in Bone Histogenesis

Congenital defects in bone histogenesis include a variety of chondrodysplasias, which generally are not well characterized due to the range of defects and rarity of the disease. Recently, there has been considerable success at localizing genes that cause skeletal dysplasias, and comparison with transgenic mouse models has revealed a role for these genes in bone histogenesis. One example is Jansen's osteochondrodysplasia, which occurs due to a mutation in the PTH/PTHrP receptor (100). Another is cleidocranial dysplasia, resulting from a mutation in the cbfa1 gene (101), which regulates osteoblast maturation. A range of skeletal abnormalities has been located to various mutations in the three forms of the FGF receptor (102) and to BMP defects (103).

REFERENCES

1. Ducy P, Desbois C, Boyce B, et al. Increased bone formation in osteocalcin-deficient mice. *Nature* 1996; 382:448–452.
2. Canalis E, Pash J, Gabbitas B, et al. Growth factors regulate the synthesis of insulin-like growth factor-I in bone cell cultures. *Endocrinology* 1993;133:33–38.
3. Rydziel S, Shaikh S, Canalis E. Platelet-derived growth factor-AA and -BB (PDGF-AA and -BB) enhance the synthesis of PDGF-AA in bone cell cultures. *Endocrinology* 1994;134:2541–2546.
4. Globus RK, Plouet J, Gospodarowicz D. Cultured bovine bone cells synthesize basic fibroblast growth factor and store it in their extracellular matrix. *Endocrinology* 1989;124:1539–1547.
5. Canalis E, Pash J, Varghese S. Skeletal growth factors. *Crit Rev Eukaryot Gene Expr* 1993;3:155–166.
6. Manolagas S, Jilka R. Bone marrow, cytokines, and bone remodeling. *Mech Dis* 1995;332:305–311.
7. Zhou H, Hammonds RG Jr, Findlay DM, et al. Retinoic acid modulation of mRNA levels in malignant, nontransformed, and immortalized osteoblasts. *J Bone Miner Res* 1991;6:767–777.
8. Rizzoli R, Poser J, Burgi U. Nuclear thyroid hormone receptors in cultured bone cells. *Metabolism* 1986;35: 71–74.
9. Barnard R, Ng KW, Martin TJ, et al. Growth hormone (GH) receptors in clonal osteoblast-like cells. *Endocrinology* 1991;128:1459–1464.
10. Levy JR, Murray E, Manolagas S, et al. Demonstration of insulin receptors and modulation of alkaline phosphatase activity by insulin in rat osteoblastic cells. *Endocrinology* 1986;119:1786–1792.
11. Wei LL, Leach MW, Miner RS, et al. Evidence for progesterone receptors in human osteoblast-like cells. *Biochem Biophys Res Commun* 1993;195:525–532.
12. Moore RE, Smith CK, Bailey CS, et al. Characterization of beta-adrenergic receptors on rat and human osteoblast-like cells and demonstration that beta-receptor agonists can stimulate bone resorption in organ culture. *Bone Miner* 1993;23:301–315.
13. Clement-Lacroix P, Ormandy C, Lepescheux L, et al. Osteoblasts are a new target for prolactin: analysis of bone formation in prolactin receptor knockout mice. *Endocrinology* 1999;140:96–105.
14. Komm BS, Terpening CM, Benz DJ, et al. Estrogen binding, receptor mRNA, and biologic response in osteoblast-like osteosarcoma cells. *Science* 1988;241: 81–84.
15. Eriksen EF, Colvard DS, Nicholas JB, et al. Evidence of estrogen receptors in normal human osteoblast-like cells. *Science* 1988;241:84–86.
16. Colvard D, Spelsberg T, Eriksen E, et al. Evidence of steroid receptors in human osteoblast-like cells. *Connect Tissue Res* 1989;20:33–40.
17. Darwish HM, DeLuca HF. Recent advances in the molecular biology of vitamin D action. *Prog Nucleic Acid Res Mol Biol* 1996;53:321–344.
18. Kindmark A, Torma H, Johansson A, et al. Reverse transcription-polymerase chain reaction assay demonstrates that the 9-cis retinoic acid receptor alpha is expressed in human osteoblasts. *Biochem Biophys Res Commun* 1993;192:1367–1372.
19. Ng KW, Partridge NC, Niall M, et al. Epidermal growth factor receptors in clonal lines of a rat osteogenic sarcoma and in osteoblast-rich rat bone cells. *Calcif Tissue Int* 1983;35:298–303.
20. Bennett A, Chen T, Feldman D, et al. Characterization of insulin-like growth factor I receptors on cultured rat bone cells: regulation of receptor concentration by glucocorticoids. *Endocrinology* 1984;115:1577–1583.
21. Mohan S, Linkhart T, Rosenfeld R, et al. Characterization of the receptor for insulin-like growth factor II in bone cells. *J Cell Physiol* 1989;140:169–176.
22. Kells AF, Schwartz HS, Bascom CC, et al. Identification and analysis of transforming growth factor beta receptors on primary osteoblast-enriched cultures derived from adult human bone. *Connect Tissue Res* 1992;27:197–209.
23. Shelly JA, Laborde AL. Interleukin-1 binding, internalization, and processing in a murine osteoblastic cell line, MC3T3.E1. *Eur Cytokine Netw* 1992;3:469–475.
24. Lacey DL, Erdmann JM, Tan HL, et al. Murine osteoblast interleukin 4 receptor expression: upregulation by 1,25 dihydroxyvitamin D3. *J Cell Biochem* 1993; 53:122–134.
25. Debiais F, Hott M, Graulet AM, et al. The effects of fibroblast growth factor-2 on human neonatal calvaria osteoblastic cells are differentiation stage specific. *J Bone Miner Res* 1998;13:645–654.
26. Koenig BB, Cook JS, Wolsing DH, et al. Characterization and cloning of a receptor for BMP-2 and BMP-4 from NIH-3T3 cells. *Mol Cell Biol* 1994;14:5961–5974.
27. Clover J, Dodds RA, Gowen M. Integrin subunit expression by human osteoblasts and osteoclasts in situ and in culture. *J Cell Sci* 1992;103:267–271.
28. Luo G, Ducy P, McKee MD, et al. Spontaneous calcification of arteries and cartilage in mice lacking matrix GLA protein. *Nature* 1997;386:78–81.
29. Anderson HC. Molecular biology of matrix vesicles. *Clin Orthop* 1995;314:266–280.
30. Ducy P, Zhang R, Geoffroy V, et al. Osf2/Cbfa1: a transcriptional activator of osteoblast differentiation. *Cell* 1997;89:747–754.
31. Otto F, Thornell AP, Crompton T, et al. Cbfa1, a candidate gene for cleidocranial dysplasia syndrome, is essential for osteoblast differentiation and bone development. *Cell* 1997;89:765–771.
32. Komori T, Yagi H, Nomura S, et al. Targeted disruption of Cbfa1 results in a complete lack of bone formation owing to maturational arrest of osteoblasts. *Cell* 1997;89:755–764.
33. Liu F, Malaval L, Aubin JE. The mature osteoblast phenotype is characterized by extensive plasticity. *Exp Cell Res* 1997;232:97–105.
34. Stein GS, Lian JB. Molecular mechanisms mediating proliferation/differentiation interrelationships during progressive development of the osteoblast phenotype. *Endocr Rev* 1993;14:424–442.
35. Chow JW, Wilson AJ, Chambers TJ, et al. Mechanical loading stimulates bone formation by reactivation of bone lining cells in 13-week-old rats. *J Bone Miner Res* 1998;13:1760–1767.

36. Dobnig H, Turner RT. Evidence that intermittent treatment with parathyroid hormone increases bone formation in adult rats by activation of bone lining cells. *Endocrinology* 1995;136:3632–3638.

37. Aarden EM, Wassenaar AM, Alblas MJ, et al. Immunocytochemical demonstration of extracellular matrix proteins in isolated osteocytes. *Histochem Cell Biol* 1996;106:495–501.

38. Wetterwald A, Hoffstetter W, Cecchini MG, et al. Characterization and cloning of the E11 antigen, a marker expressed by rat osteoblasts and osteocytes. *Bone* 1996;18:125–132.

39. Lanyon LE. Osteocytes, strain detection, bone modeling and remodeling. *Calcif Tissue Int* 1993;53(Suppl 1):S102–S106.

40. Ajubi NE, Klein-Nulend J, Alblas MJ, et al. Signal transduction pathways involved in fluid flow-induced PGE2 production by cultured osteocytes. *Am J Physiol* 1999;276:E171–E178.

41. Elmardi AS, Katchburian MV, Katchburian E. Electron microscopy of developing calvaria reveals images that suggest that osteoclasts engulf and destroy osteocytes during bone resorption. *Calcif Tissue Int* 1990; 46:239–245.

42. Baron R, Chakraborty M, Chatterjee D, et al. Biology of the osteoclast. In: Mundy GR, Martin TJ, eds. *Physiology and pharmacology of bone.* New York: Springer, 1993:111–147.

43. Suda T, Takahashi N, Martin TJ. Modulation of osteoclast differentiation. *Endocr Rev* 1992;13:66–80.

44. Baron R, Neff L, Roy C, et al. Evidence for a high and specific concentration of (Na^+, K^+)-ATPase in the plasma membrane of the osteoclast. *Cell* 1986;46: 311–320.

45. Ravesloot JH, Ypey DL, Vrijheid-Lammers T, et al. Voltage-activated K^+ conductances in freshly isolated embryonic chicken osteoclasts. *Proc Natl Acad Sci USA* 1989;86:6821–6825.

46. Ypey DL, Weidema AF, Hold KM, et al. Voltage, calcium, and stretch activated ionic channels and intracellular calcium in bone cells. *J Bone Miner Res* 1992; 7(Suppl 2):S377–S387.

47. Weidema AF, Ravesloot JH, Panyi G, et al. A Ca(2 +)-dependent K(+)-channel in freshly isolated and cultured chick osteoclasts. *Biochim Biophys Acta* 1993; 1149:63–72.

48. Miyauchi A, Hruska KA, Greenfield EM, et al. Osteoclast cytosolic calcium, regulated by voltage-gated calcium channels and extracellular calcium, controls podosome assembly and bone resorption. *J Cell Biol* 1990;111:2543–2552.

49. Davies J, Warwick J, Totty N, et al. The osteoclast functional antigen, implicated in the regulation of bone resorption, is biochemically related to the vitronectin receptor. *J Cell Biol* 1989;109:1817–1826.

50. Zambonin-Zallone A, Teti A, Grano M, et al. Immunocytochemical distribution of extracellular matrix receptors in human osteoclasts: a beta 3 integrin is colocalized with vinculin and talin in the podosomes of osteoclastoma giant cells. *Exp Cell Res* 1989;182: 645–652.

51. Reinholt FP, Hultenby K, Oldberg A, et al. Osteopontin—a possible anchor of osteoclasts to bone. *Proc Natl Acad Sci USA* 1990;87:4473–4475.

52. Soriano P, Montgomery C, Geske R, et al. Targeted disruption of the *c-src* proto-oncogene leads to osteopetrosis in mice. *Cell* 1991;64:693–702.

53. Duong LT, Lakkakorpi PT, Nakamura I, et al. PYK2 in osteoclasts is an adhesion kinase, localized in the sealing zone, activated by ligation of $\alpha_1\beta_3$ integrin, and phosphorylated by Src kinase. *J Clin Invest* 1998; 102:881–892.

54. Martin TJ, Ng KW. Mechanisms by which cells of the osteoblast lineage control osteoclast formation and activity. *J Cell Biochem* 1994;56:357–366.

55. Warshawsky H, Goltzman D, Rouleau MF, et al. Direct in vivo demonstration by radioautography of specific binding sites for calcitonin in skeletal and renal tissues of the rat. *J Cell Biol* 1980;85:682–694.

56. Nicholson GC, Moseley JM, Sexton PM, et al. Abundant calcitonin receptors in isolated rat osteoclasts: biochemical and autoradiographic characterization. *J Clin Invest* 1986;78:355–360.

57. Kurihara N, Gluck S, Roodman GD. Sequential expression of phenotype markers for osteoclasts during differentiation of precursors for multinucleated cells formed in long term human marrow cultures. *Endocrinology* 1990;127:3215–3221.

58. Narbaitz R, Stumpf WE, Sar M, et al. Autoradiographic localization of target cells for 1 alpha,25-dihydroxyvitamin D3 in bones from fetal rats. *Calcif Tissue Int* 1983;35:177–182.

59. Mizuno Y, Hosoi T, Inoue S, et al. Immunocytochemical identification of androgen receptor in mouse osteoclast-like multinucleated cells. *Calcif Tissue Int* 1994; 54:325–326.

60. Abu EO, Bord S, Horner A, et al. The expression of thyroid hormone receptors in human bone. *Bone* 1997; 21:137–142.

61. Lee K. Sonic hedgehog. *Curr Biol* 1998;8:R744.

62. Chenu C, Serre CM, Raynal C, et al. Glutamate receptors are expressed by bone cells and are involved in bone resorption. *Bone* 1998;22:295–299.

63. Collier FM, Huang WH, Holloway WR, et al. Osteoclasts from human giant cell tumors of bone lack estrogen. *Endocrinology* 1998;139:1258–1267.

64. Pederson L, Kremer M, Foged NT, et al. Evidence of a correlation of estrogen receptor level and avian osteoclast estrogen responsiveness. *J Bone Miner Res* 1997;12:742–752.

65. Teti A, Rizzoli R, Zambonin-Zallone A. Parathyroid hormone binding to cultured avian osteoclasts. *Biochem Biophys Res Commun* 1991;174:1217–1222.

66. McSheehy PM, Chambers TJ. Osteoblast-like cells in the presence of parathyroid hormone release soluble factor that stimulates osteoclastic bone resorption. *Endocrinology* 1986;119:1654–1659.

67. Udagawa N, Horwood NJ, Elliott J, et al. Interleukin-18 (interferon-gamma-inducing factor) is produced by osteoblasts and acts via granulocyte/macrophage colony-stimulating factor and not via interferon-gamma to inhibit osteoclast formation. *J Exp Med* 1997;185: 1005–1012.

68. Gao Y, Morita I, Maruo N, et al. Expression of IL-6 receptor and gp130 in mouse bone marrow cells. *Bone* 1998;22:487–493.

69. Sunyer T, Rothe L, Kirsch D, et al. Ca^{2+} or phorbol ester but not inflammatory stimuli elevate inducible nitric oxide synthase messenger ribonucleic acid and nitric oxide (NO) release in avian osteoclasts: autocrine

NO mediates Ca^{2+}-inhibited bone resorption. *Endocrinology* 1997;138:2148–2162.

70. Hofstetter W, Wetterwald A, Cecchini MC, et al. Detection of transcripts for the receptor for macrophage colony-stimulating factor, *c-fms,* in murine osteoclasts. *Proc Natl Acad Sci USA* 1992;89:9637–9641.

71. Hou P, Sato T, Hofstetter W, et al. Identification and characterization of the insulin-like growth receptor in mature rabbit osteoclasts. *J Bone Miner Res* 1997;12: 534–540.

72. Xu LX, Kukita T, Nakano Y, et al. Osteoclasts in normal and adjuvant arthritis bone tissues express the mRNA for both type I and II interleukin-1 receptors. *Lab Invest* 1996;75:677–687.

73. Zhang Z, Chen J, Jin D. Platelet-derived growth factor (PDGF)-BB stimulates osteoclastic bone resorption directly: the role of receptor beta. *Biochem Biophys Res Commun* 1998;251:190–194.

74. Hosoi T, Inoue S, Hoshino S, et al. Immunohistochemical detection of activin a in osteoclasts. *Gerontology* 1996;42(Suppl 1):20–24.

75. Walker DG. Bone resorption restored in osteopetrotic mice by transplants of normal bone marrow and spleen cells. *Science* 1975;190:784–785.

76. Walker DG. Control of bone resorption by hematopoietic tissue. The induction and reversal of congenital osteopetrosis in mice through use of bone marrow and splenic transplants. *J Exp Med* 1975;142:651–663.

77. Tsuda E, Goto M, Mochizuki S, et al. Isolation of a novel cytokine from human fibroblasts that specifically inhibits osteoclastogenesis. *Biochem Biophys Res Commun* 1997;234:137–142.

78. Simonet WS, Lacey DL, Dunstan CR, et al. Osteoprotegerin: a novel secreted protein involved in the regulation of bone density. *Cell* 1997;89:309–319.

79. Lacey DL, Timms E, Tan HL, et al. Osteoprotegerin ligand is a cytokine that regulates osteoclast differentiation and activation. *Cell* 1998;93:165–176.

80. Yasuda H, Shima N, Nakagawa N, et al. Osteoclast differentiation factor is a ligand for osteoprotegerin osteoclastogenesis-inhibitory factor and is identical to TRANCE/RANKL. *Proc Natl Acad Sci USA* 1998;95: 3597–3602.

81. Baron R, Neff L, Brown W, et al. Polarized secretion of lysosomal enzymes: co-distribution of cation-independent mannose-6-phosphate receptors and lysosomal enzymes along the osteoclast exocytic pathway. *J Cell Biol* 1988;106:1863–1872.

82. Horne WC, Neff L, Chatterjee D, et al. Osteoclasts express high levels of pp60$^{c\text{-}src}$ in association with intracellular membranes. *J Cell Biol* 1992;119:1003–1013.

83. Kameda T, Ishikawa H, Tsutsui T. Detection and characterization of apoptosis in osteoclasts in vitro. *Biochem Biophys Res Commun* 1995;207:753–760.

84. Frost HM. *Bone remodeling and its relationship to metabolic bone disease.* Springfield, IL: CC Thomas, 1973.

85. Parfitt AM. The cellular basis of bone remodeling: the quantum concept reexamined in light of recent advances in the cell biology of bone. *Calcif Tissue Int* 1984;36(Suppl 1):S37–S45.

86. Corral DA, Amling M, Priemel M, et al. Dissociation between bone resorption and bone formation in os-

teopenic transgenic mice. *Proc Natl Acad Sci USA* 1998;95:13835–13840.

87. Shukunami C, Ishizeki K, Atsumi T, et al. Cellular hypertrophy and calcification of embryonal carcinoma-derived chondrogenic cell line ATDC5 in vitro. *J Bone Miner Res* 1997;12:1174–1188.

88. Oltvai ZN, Milliman CL, Korsmeyer SJ. Bcl-2 heterodimerizes in vivo with a conserved homolog, Bax, that accelerates programmed cell death. *Cell* 1993;74: 609–619.

89. Antonsson B, Conti F, Ciavatta A, et al. Inhibition of Bax channel-forming activity by Bcl-2. *Science* 1997; 277:370–372.

90. Amling M, Neff L, Tanaka S, et al. Bcl-2 lies downstream of parathyroid hormone–related peptide in a signaling pathway that regulates chondrocyte maturation during skeletal development. *J Cell Biol* 1997;136: 205–213.

91. Wang Y, Toury R, Hauchecorne M, et al. Expression of Bcl-2 protein in the epiphyseal plate cartilage and trabecular bone of growing rats. *Histochem Cell Biol* 1997;108:45–55.

92. Vu TH, Shipley JM, Bergers G, et al. MMP-9/gelatinase B is a key regulator of growth plate angiogenesis. *Cell* 1998;93:411–422.

93. Vortkamp A, Lee K, Lanske B, et al. Regulation of rate of cartilage differentiation by Indian hedgehog and PTH-related protein. *Science* 1996;273:613–622.

94. Amizuka N, Henderson JE, Hoshi K, et al. Programmed cell death of chondrocytes and aberrant chondrogenesis in mice homozygous for parathyroid hormone–related peptide gene deletion. *Endocrinology* 1996;137:5055–5067.

95. Weir EC, Horowitz MC, Baron R, et al. Macrophage colony-stimulating factor release and receptor expression in bone cells. *J Bone Miner Res* 1993;8:1507–1518.

96. Lanske B, Karaplis AC, Lee K, et al. PTH/PTHrP receptor in early development and Indian hedgehog-regulated bone growth. *Science* 1996;273:663–666.

97. Trippel SB, Wroblewski J, Makower AM, et al. Regulation of growth-plate chondrocytes by insulin-like growth-factor I and basic fibroblast growth factor. *J Bone Joint Surg Am* 1993;75:177–189.

98. Kawakami Y, Ishikawa T, Shimabara M, et al. BMP signaling during bone pattern determination in the developing limb. *Development* 1996;122:3557–3566.

99. Shukunami C, Ohta Y, Sakuda M, et al. Sequential progression of the differentiation program by bone morphogenetic protein-2 in chondrogenic cell line ATDC5. *Exp Cell Res* 1998;241:1–11.

100. Schipani E, Kruse K, Juppner H. A constitutively active mutant PTH-PTHrP receptor in Jansen-type metaphyseal chondrodysplasia. *Science* 1995;268:98–100.

101. Mundlos S, Otto F, Mundlos C, et al. Mutations involving the transcription factor Cbfal cause cleidocranial dysplasia. *Cell* 1997;89:773–779.

102. Burke D, Wilkes D, Blundell TL, et al. Fibroblast growth factor receptors: lessons from the genes. *Trends Biochem Sci* 1998;23:59–62.

103. Storm EE, Kingsley DM. Joint patterning defects caused by single and double mutations in members of the bone morphogenetic protein (BMP) family. *Development* 1996;122:3969–3979.

104. Eriksen EF, Axelrod DW, Melsen F. *Bone histomorphometry.* New York: Raven Press, 1994:13–20.

Skeletal Growth Factors,
edited by Ernesto Canalis.
Published by Lippincott Williams & Wilkins, Philadelphia, 2000.

2

Bone Matrix

Neal S. Fedarko and *Pamela Gehron Robey

*Division of Geriatric Medicine and Gerontology, Department of Medicine, Johns Hopkins University, Baltimore, Maryland 21224; and *Craniofacial and Skeletal Diseases Branch, National Institute of Dental and Craniofacial Research, National Institutes of Health, Bethesda, Maryland 20892*

The mineral phase of bone is nucleated, propagated, and remodeled within the scaffolding provided by the extracellular matrix. This organic scaffolding consists primarily of large protein components that have the capacity to form macromolecular aggregates, the organization of which dictates the bone superstructure. Also incorporated into the scaffolding superstructure are relatively small proteins that appear to act in the communication between the matrix and the cells in bone (1). There are no purely "structural" components in the bone matrix. For example, components such as collagen not only provide matrix structure but also generate, through their metabolism, feedback on the state of proliferation and differentiation of the bone cell. Furthermore, many of the so-called structural proteins in the bone matrix possess the sequence motif to interact with integrins and other cell surface receptors; thus, receptor occupancy can provide further feedback between the matrix and the cell.

Bone matrix proteins can be classified as (a) matrix organizers that primarily bind other large extracellular matrix components and cell surfaces, (b) matrix modifiers that bind small molecules/ions that alter the local concentration of these small compounds in the matrix, or (c) matrix messengers, which are specific sequences within the components, or fragments generated from them, that in and of themselves contain signaling information.

For the purpose of understanding the roles of these matrix components, it is appropriate to discuss them in terms of their structure. Broadly speaking, there are three different structural groups. The first group consists of proteins whose structure arises from a repetitive motif (collagen, hyaluronan, decorin, and biglycan) (Fig. 2.1), while the second group consists of proteins whose structure consists of multiple modular domains (versican, thrombospondin, fibronectin, osteonectin, and tenascin) (Fig. 2.2). The third group includes proteins that, at the current level of knowledge, appear to lack either a definable structure (i.e., exist as a random coil) or identifiable modular repeats but do contain amino acid sequences and posttranslational modifications that have been implicated in their respective putative functions (matrix gla protein, osteopontin, bone sialoprotein, and osteocalcin) (Fig. 2.3).

EXTRACELLULAR MATRIX COMPONENTS PRODUCED BY HUMAN OSTEOGENIC CELLS

Bone Matrix Proteins with Repetitive Structure

Collagens

The major organic component of the bone extracellular matrix is type I collagen, accounting for up to 90% of the organic matrix. This interstitial, fibril-forming substance is composed of trimers of two $\alpha 1(I)$ chains and one $\alpha 2(I)$ chain.

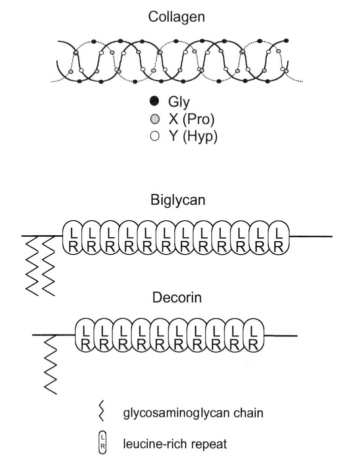

FIG. 2.1. Bone matrix proteins with repetitive structure. The most abundant organic component, collagen, and two other abundant proteins, decorin and biglycan, are constructed of repeated amino acid sequences. Collagen α chains are composed of the triplet repeat sequence Gly-X-Y, where X is often proline and Y is hydroxyproline. The core proteins of decorin and biglycan are tandem repeats of a leucine-rich repeat sequence (L-X-X-L-X-L-X-n-N-k-l-s-x-V-X-X-g-X-f-X-X-l-k-X). Sequences that dictate the addition of glycosaminoglycans are located at the amino terminus of both proteins.

The repetitive motif Gly-X-Y, where X and Y are often proline and its hydroxylated derivative, enables the formation of stable triple helices. The molecular form of collagen secreted into the extracellular matrix is procollagen ($M_r\sim470$ kDa), where the three α chains possess amino- and carboxyl-terminal polypeptide extensions. Collagen fibril formation occurs following cellular secretion and enzymatic removal of the noncollagenous N- and C-terminal extensions. Procollagen processing is influenced by post-translational modifications (hydroxylation of lysyl and prolyl residues and glycosylation) and the binding of other matrix components such as

proteoglycans (2–4). The triple helical molecules of type I collagen form an $\sim$300-nm rigid rod with M_r 300 kDa. The collagen molecules overlap by integral multiples of 67 nm and a gap of 40 nm is left between the quarter-staggered assembly of nonoverlapping collagen molecules. In its role as the major structural component, the collagenous network is stabilized by covalent cross-links within and between the α chains by the formation of somewhat bone-specific deoxypyridinoline cross-links.

The importance of the type I collagen structure in bone matrix metabolism is reflected in observations of the pathophysiological conse-

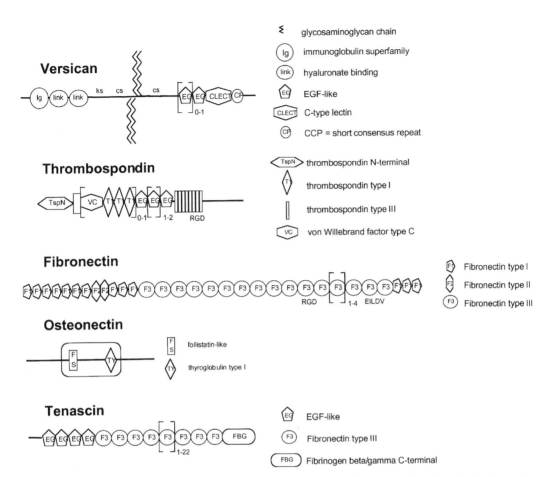

FIG. 2.2. Modular domain proteins. Modular structures are found in many of the abundant extracellular matrix proteins of bone, such as versican, thrombospondin, fibronectin, osteonectin, and tenascin. These modular structures are homologous to other non-connective tissue proteins, such as epidermal growth factor, C-type lectin, von Willebrand factor, fibrinogen, follistatin, and thyroglobulin, as well as modules that are repeated within connective tissue proteins, such as fibronectin types I, II, and III and thrombospondin types I and III repeats.

quences of mutations in the genes that code for it, which cause the brittle bone disorder osteogenesis imperfecta (OI). The mildest form of the disease (type I OI, which presents with minimal to moderate skeletal fragility) arises from mutations that yield either a null allele or mutant collagen chains that are synthesized but not secreted or incorporated into matrix heterotrimers; hence, only half the normal levels of collagen are produced. More severe forms of the disease (types IV, III, and II OI, which present with moderate to severe osseous fragility or perinatal lethality) arise from mutations that not only reduce the level of type I collagen but also yield

structurally aberrant collagen heterotrimers (5,6). Mutations in type I collagen are also associated in vitro with alterations in the levels of other bone matrix components, with some components being reduced (osteonectin, versican, decorin, and biglycan) and others elevated (hyaluronan, fibronectin, and thrombospondin) in the matrix (7–9). Normal collagen metabolism appears to play a role not only in conferring structural integrity but also in cellular feedback and bone cell proliferation/differentiation (10–12).

Type III collagen, which consists of a homotrimer with a triple helical domain of similar size (~1,000 amino acids) to that of type I collagen,

Osteopontin

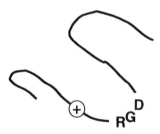

Bone Sialoprotein

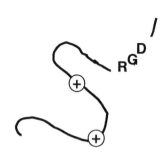

Osteocalcin

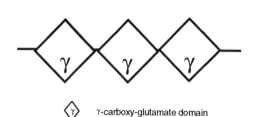

γ-carboxy-glutamate domain

FIG. 2.3. "Structureless" proteins of bone matrix. Although these proteins are not built using a repetitive sequence or modular structures, matrix gla protein, osteopontin, bone sialoprotein, and osteocalcin contain sequences (or modifications thereof) that convey functional activity. Osteopontin and bone sialoprotein contain stretches of acidic residues (aspartic acid and glutamic acid, +) which cause them to bind Ca^{2+} with extremely high affinity. In addition, these proteins contain the RGD (Asp-Gly-Arg) sequence, which allows them to bind to cell surface integrins (Table 2.1). Matrix gla protein (not shown) and osteocalcin are posttranslationally modified by vitamin K–dependent carboxylases to form γ-carboxy glutamic acid, causing these proteins to bind Ca^{2+} with relatively high affinity.

has also been found in bone, though its role in bone matrix metabolism is unclear. It is most likely associated with type I collagen in the matrix produced by preosteogenic cells that have not yet dedicated themselves to the synthesis and deposition of copious amounts of osteoid. In tissues other than bone, data support the hypothesis that the heterotypic interaction of different collagens, specifically types I and III, plays a role in regulating fibril size (13). Studies of transgenic mice provide consistent data in which matrix disorganization and fibril diameter heterogeneity are associated with a point mutation or targeted disruption of the type III collagen gene (14,15). Mutations in the type III collagen gene have been found in patients with Ehlers-Danlos syndrome type IV, where large arteries and bowel suddenly rupture and thin skin and joint hypermobility are also involved (6). The lack of correlation of a bone phenotype to mutations in type III collagen suggests that heterotypic interactions of collagen types in bone are not crucial for regulation of type I collagen fibril diameter.

While the structural and mechanical integrity of bone matrix is highly dependent on the orderly deposition of the collagen fibrils, collagen fibrils, devoid of associated noncollagenous proteins, do not provide an adequate template for physiolocal deposition of mineral. The initiation and propagation of mineralization is dependent on the synthesis of noncollagenous proteins by mature osteoblasts.

Hyaluronan

Hyaluronan (or hyaluronic acid) is comprised of a repeating β-glucuronic acid-β-1,3,-N-acetylglucosamine disaccharide that forms a large glycosaminoglycan chain (>1,000 kDa), which does not appear to have a covalently attached core protein. Hyaluronan is found in bone (16), is synthesized by bone cells in culture, and has been proposed to "capture space" for subsequent matrix deposition (7,8,17,18). Within this context, hyaluronan is a component of "immature" bone matrix, and its increased levels in OI bone matrix are consistent with the early, "immature" bone matrix, being less structurally rigid than the mature, highly collagenous matrices. CD44, which is thought to be a cell surface receptor for hyaluronan (19), has been colocalized with hyaluronan on osteoclasts, osteoblasts, and osteocytes (20). Because of its repetitive disaccharide structure, hylauronan can form extended left-handed helices of 0.8 to 1.0 nm axial rise per disaccharide and three to four disaccharides per turn. A stiff coil behavior is expected for extended hyaluronan sequences, though microdomains containing either left- or right-handed helices are possible (1). The overall stiff coil structure may play an important role in the hydrodynamics of hyaluronan, and the microdomain loops may be involved in its interaction with link proteins and receptors.

Small, Leucine-rich Repeat Proteoglycans

Proteoglycans comprise a family of molecules that possess a core protein to which one or more glycosaminoglycan chains are covalently attached. Decorin and biglycan are interstitial proteoglycans found in many connective tissues, including bone (18,21). Both of them possess leucine-rich repeats, a similar structural motif (circular arch shape) to that of porcine ribonuclease inhibitor (22). Decorin, a 130-kDa proteoglycan with a 45-kDa core protein, has 12 leucine-rich repeats and a single attachment site for a single 40-kDa glycosaminoglycan chain, which can be either chondroitin or dermatan sulfate. Biglycan, a 270-kDa proteoglycan with a 45-kDa core protein, contains ten leucine-rich repeats and two 40-kDa glycosaminoglycan chains, which may be composed of either chondroitin or dermatan sulfate (Fig. 2.1). For both proteoglycans, the glycosaminoglycan attachment site is close to the amino terminus. Decorin binds to (''decorates'') the collagen fibrils (23), while biglycan is found in pericellular areas, including that of osteoblasts and osteocytes (24). The small proteoglycans may act as matrix organizers, orienting and ordering the collagen fibrils, with the protein portion binding to collagen fibrils at specific sites and the glycosaminoglycan chains aggregating to hold the proteins, and hence the collagen fibrils, at defined distances from each other (25). Studies involving in vitro assays have shown that decorin inhibits the growth of collagen fibrils (2,4).

Targeted disruption of the decorin gene in mice yields an abnormal collagen morphology with coarser and more irregular fiber outlines in skin and tendon, suggesting that control of collagen fibril growth and diameter involves decorin (26). Recent evidence indicates that primary calcification in bones follows removal of decorin and fusion of collagen fibrils (27), which may explain the lack of an obvious skeletal phenotype in decorin-deficient mice. Differences in the expression of decorin have been suggested to account for the different phenotypes in two unrelated OI patients with the same mutation in type I collagen (28). In contrast to decorin, targeted disruption of the biglycan gene yields a mouse phenotype with a reduced growth rate and failure to achieve peak bone mass, the low bone mass becoming more pronounced with increasing age (29). This phenotype suggests that biglycan may be a genetic determinant that contributes to peak bone mass.

Both proteoglycans bind transforming growth factor β (TGF-β) (30,31), which is made by bone cells and has been shown to stimulate bone cell proliferation and matrix synthesis (32). However, the effect of binding of this growth factor to these proteoglycans in the extracellular environment on osteoblastic metabolism is not yet clear.

Modular Domain Proteins

Versican

Human bone cells produce a large (~600 kDa) chondroitin sulfate proteoglycan that is versican-like (17). The modular structure of versican consists of an amino-terminal immunoglobulin-like domain, two hyaluronate-link protein-binding domains, multiple domains containing attachment sites for chondroitin sulfate glycosaminoglycan chains, one to two epidermal growth factor (EGF)-like repeats, a C-type lectin domain, and a carboxy-terminal short consensus repeat similar to those found in complement proteins (Fig. 2.1). Although the exact function of bone versican is not known, it has been proposed to act as a space filler in fetal and very young bone, to be replaced by osteoid during later development (18). This versican-like proteoglycan can bind hyaluronan (17). Its biosynthetic level is elevated in fetal and neonatal osteoblast-like cells and decreases with increasing donor age (7,8).

Thrombospondins and Fibronectin

Thrombospondins and fibronectin exemplify proteins found in bone that are composed of various combinations and amounts of modular structures. In addition, they contain the arginine-glycine-aspartate (RGD) cell attachment consensus sequence and are believed to play a role in cell-matrix adhesion via binding to integrin receptors on the cell surface (33).

Thrombospondins comprise a family of M_r 450-kDa, trimeric glycoproteins with five distinct forms and genes isolated thus far. Thrombospondins possess distinct domains that modulate matrix protein interactions, cell attachment, migration, and proliferation (34). Typically, thrombospondin domain structures consist of an amino-terminal thrombospondin domain, followed by a von Willebrand factor type C domain, three thrombospondin type I domains, three to five EGF-like domains, and eight thrombospondin type II repeats (Fig. 2.1). Thrombospondin is synthesized by osteoblastic cells (35), and the various isoforms are expressed at different anatomical sites at different times in bone (36–38). The RGD moiety in thrombospondin is recognized by the $\alpha_v\beta_3$ integrin (39). Thrombospondin can bind to platelet-derived growth factors (PDGFs) (40–42) and can bind and activate latent TGF-β. Recently, it has been found that mice lacking thrombospondin-2 develop long bones with higher density and thicker cortices than normal littermates (43).

Fibronectin is a multifunctional dimeric protein (M_r 450 kDa) that has the capacity to modulate cell migration, cell attachment, and matrix organization. It contains binding domains for fibrin/heparin, gelatin/collagen, and cell surfaces. Of the two cell-binding domains, one involves the RGD motif that binds to the $\alpha_5\beta_1$ integrin, while the other involves a glutamate-

isoleucine-leucine-aspartate-valine (GILRV) moiety, which is bound by $\alpha_4\beta_1$ integrin (44,45). The domain structure of fibronectin consists of modules of fibronectin types I, II, and II repeats, with type I repeats interspersed throughout the molecule (Fig. 2.1). Fibronectin is synthesized by and maintained around osteoblasts during osteogenesis (46). In early bone formation, osteoblasts depend on fibronectin for differentiation signals, while at later stages, the cells depend on fibronectin for survival, becoming apoptotic when antifibronectin antibodies are used to block cellular interactions (47).

Osteonectin

Osteonectin (also termed secreted protein, acidic and rich in cysteine (SPARC), culture shock protein, or BM40), is a 32-kDa Ca^{2+}-binding glycoprotein found in many connective tissues, though relatively high concentrations are present in bone (48). The molecule possesses a cysteine-rich sequence with a follistatin-like domain (thought to be involved in growth factor binding) as well as a carboxy-terminal thyroglobulin type I domain with an EF-hand Ca^{2+}-binding site (Fig. 2.1) (49,50). Osteonectin binds to calcium, hydroxyapatite, and collagen and, therefore, was originally hypothesized to be involved in mineralization of bone (48). Osteonectin inhibits hydroxyapatite crystal growth (51) and binds to collagen types I, II, and IV as well as to thrombospondin (52–54). Calcium and hydroxyapatite binding involve the glutamic acid–rich acidic amino terminus, while binding to collagen involves the carboxy-terminal Ca^{2+}-binding domain and is Ca^{2+}-dependent (55). Osteonectin binds PDGFs, and this binding is not Ca^{2+}-dependent, though it does involve the carboxy-terminal EF hand domain (55,56). Osteonectin expression levels may be related to rapid cell proliferation, matrix remodeling, and epithelial–mesenchymal interactions (54, 57–59). Intact osteonectin and specific structural domains of the protein affect cell morphology by reducing the number of focal contacts and lowering adhesion to extracellular matrix and neighboring cells (60,61); thus, it may be considered an "antiadhesive" matrix component. Targeted disruption of osteonectin in mice yields normal development, a phenotype of severe cataract formation, and low bone mass with increasing age (62).

Tenascin C

Tenascin (also known as hexabrachion and cytotactin) comprises an extracellular matrix family of glycoproteins whose tissue distribution is restricted temporally and spatially. Because of its restricted expression pattern, tenascin is believed to be involved in developmental processes such as morphogenetic cell migration and organogenesis. Tenascin C is a hexameric, multidomain protein with 190- to 240-kDa subunits linked by disulfide bonds (63). The modular structure of tenascin C consists of four amino-terminal EGF-like repeats, eight to 30 fibronectin type III repeats, and a carboxy-terminal fibrinogen β/γ domain (Fig. 2.1). Tenascin is present in developing cartilage and bone, localizing to the condensing mesenchyme of osteogenic cells invading the cartilage (64). It is not detectable in mature bone matrix but is present on periosteal and endosteal surfaces. Tenascin inhibits chondrocyte attachment to fibronectin and by modulating fibronectin–cell interactions may effect cell rounding and condensation (64). Osteoblast proliferation in vitro is similarly modified by treatment with tenascin-C (65). Thus, like osteonectin, tenascin may act as an ''antiadhesive'' component of the bone matrix, playing its role in early bone development. Targeted disruption of tenascin C has no discernible phenotype, with knockout mice exhibiting normal development, life span, and fecundity (66). As with other knockout models where a phenotype is not apparent, molecular redundancy is suggested as an explanation for the lack of effect (67).

"Structureless" Matrix Proteins

Collagen Propeptides

Once procollagen is secreted, the propeptides at the amino and carboxy termini are proteolytically cleaved and deposited in bone matrix.

The amino-terminal propeptides (pN) as well as the carboxy-terminal propeptides (pC) of type I collagen have the capacity to act as feedback regulators of collagen and cellular metabolism. The amino-terminal propeptide decreased collagen synthesis but not degradation or hydroxylation of α chains or synthesis of other noncollagenous proteins (68). Specific binding and uptake of pN, which resulted in the inhibition of polypeptide chain elongation or termination, has been shown (69). pN had a general effect of inhibiting procollagen mRNA translation (70). Further study has shown that reduced collagen levels had no effect on fibronectin but increased immunostaining for thrombospondin and osteonectin (71). In contrast, the carboxy-terminal propeptide of type I collagen (pC) increased collagen synthesis, and the specific sequence responsible was shown to be lysine-threonine-threonine-lysine-serine (KTTKS) (72). Chemical modification of pC led to a decrease in the inhibition of procollagen synthesis in liver stellate cells (73). pC may exert its influence through $\alpha_2\beta_1$ integrin binding to the A domain (74,75). It has been reported that collagen binding to the $\alpha_2\beta_1$ integrin modulated osteoblastic differentiation (76). Recently, it was shown that the procollagen carboxy-terminal proteinase is identical to bone morphogenetic protein-1, a member of a family of proteases implicated in pattern formation during development (77). The role of these bioactive peptides in the formation and maintenance of bone is as yet undefined.

Sialoproteins

The RGD-containing sialoproteins osteopontin and bone sialoprotein (BSP) are produced by osteogenic cells that are reaching maturity, and their deposition leads to the first detectable mineralized matrix, with BSP perhaps being the defining protein of the initiation of bone formation (78).

Osteopontin has an acidic amino terminus with a polyaspartic acid sequence. Similar to BSP, it has sequences for serine phosphorylation, N-linked oligosaccharide attachment, and tyrosine sulfation. The RGD is located in the carboxy-terminal region and is flanked by a thrombin cleavage site. The osteopontin RGD may be bound by $\alpha_v\beta_3$ integrin, the vitronectin receptor, or CD44 (79–82). Immunolocalization of osteopontin revealed the highest density of gold particles associated with electron-dense organic material found at the mineralization front and in "cement lines" (83). Osteopontin is a potent inhibitor of hydroxyapatite formation (84), and reduced mRNA and protein expression levels in Src $-/-$ mice are associated with the inability of osteoclasts to adhere to bone (85).

BSP (along with osteocalcin) is considered a defining noncollagenous protein marker of the mature osteoblast phenotype. Over half of its mass (M_1 70 kDa) is carbohydrate, with the mature protein accounting for only 33 kDa. The amino acid structure of BSP reveals a highly acidic molecule, the first third of which contains a polyglutamic acid sequence and an aspartic acid/glutamic acid–rich region. Consensus sequences for serine phosphorylation and tyrosine sulfation abound, as well as at least four distinct sites for N-linked oligosaccharide modification. The RGD motif in BSP is located near the carboxy terminus. The RGD sequence is recognized by $\alpha_v\beta_3$ (86). BSP is expressed at late stages of osteoblastic differentiation, marks cells in the secretory but not in the proliferative compartment, and has been localized to the sites of earliest mineral deposition (78,87–89).

Because of their inherent polyanionic nature, the sialoproteins can bind calcium and hydroxyapatite, coating the mineral phase of bone and then, via their RGD moieties, enabling cellular adherence to specific sites. Mice lacking a functional osteopontin gene exhibit a phenotype of altered wound healing (90). The disorganized matrix and altered collagen fibrillogenesis (small-diameter collagen fibrils) suggest that osteopontin affects the synthesis and/or turnover of matrix components involved in regulating fibril formation. Targeted disruption of the BSP gene has yet to reveal an apparent phenotype.

The γ-Carboxylated (gla) Proteins Matrix gla Protein and Osteocalcin

There are a number of proteins in bone matrix, including matrix γ-carboxylated (gla) protein (MGP) and osteocalcin, that are posttranslationally modified to contain γ-carboxy glutamic acid, by virtue of the homology of parts of their sequences to certain blood group proteins that are also γ-carboxylated. γ-Carboxylation generates vicinal carboxy groups that convey calcium binding with relatively high affinity to these two proteins. Although they share some sequence homology (thereby allowing γ-carboxylation), their patterns of expression, and most likely their potential functions, diverge considerably.

MGP, with five gla residues, has a molecular weight of ~14 kDa. Its expression begins early in development in many different tissues, including lung, kidney, heart, and bone (91); but the highest levels are found in smooth muscle and in cartilage (92). It is extremely insoluble in normal aqueous solutions, explaining the paucity of studies aimed at unraveling its potential function by conventional analysis. However, generation of a transgenic mouse devoid of MGP expression has been very revealing. MGP-deficient animals exhibited arterial calcification and early calicification of growth, pointing to MGP as a major inhibitor of calcification in soft tissues.

Osteocalcin, a 5-kDa protein with one disulfide bond, comprises 10% to 20% of the noncollagenous proteins in bone, depending on developmental age and the species. Osteocalcin contains three γ-carboxy glutamic acid residues. Levels of osteocalcin are low at early stages of bone formation and increase with increasing age. The function of osteocalcin may be to inhibit mineralization (since osteocalcin inhibits hydroxyapatite crystal growth in solution) until the appropriate temporal and spatial conditions are met (93). It has also been suggested that osteocalcin may function in bone resorption rather than formation (94). Targeted disruption of the osteocalcin gene in mice yielded a phenotype of increased bone mass and strength, suggesting that this small protein normally inhibits bone growth and promotes bone resorption (95). Osteocalcin has recently been found to inhibit osteopontin cross-linking by transglutaminases (96). This suppressive activity of osteocalcin may be involved in suppression of mineralization and excessive calcification via alteration of the cross-linking status of osteopontin and the bone matrix.

Binding Interactions for Matrix Components

Macromolecular Aggregates

The macromolecular interactions that have been reported in the literature for these matrix components, based on in vitro analysis, are summarized in Fig. 2.4. As is evident, the possible permutations for macromolecular binding are numerous. However, the question of which of these interactions is physiologically relevant is for the most part unresolved. Furthermore, there are many conflicting pieces of information, most likely due to differences in the types of assay system used.

As discussed above, numerous matrix components have the capacity to bind to type I collagen, and through these interactions, the bone scaffold is formed after the initiation of hydroxyapatite deposition (78). It has been recently shown that the fibronectin-binding site in type I collagen may regulate the elongation and branching of fibronectin fibrils (97). The roles of the small proteoglycans decorin and biglycan in organizing the collagenous scaffold are of great interest. Using a solid-phase binding assay, decorin was found to interact efficiently only with type IV, and not type I, collagen (98). This is in contrast to a decorin–type I collagen fibrillogenesis assay, which is a solution-phase assay (2).

Decorin has also been shown to bind to fibronectin (99,100) and may have antiadhesive properties by binding to the cell-binding domain of fibronectin (101). Thrombospondin and decorin also interact with an association constant in the nanomolar range (102). In contrast to thrombospondin, which can activate TGF-β, decorin (and mostly likely biglycan) sequesters TGF-β in a latent form (103), which can be released and activated by the action of the appropriate matrix metalloproteinase (104). Other known interactions that are of interest include the binding of versican to hyaluronan (17) and the involvement

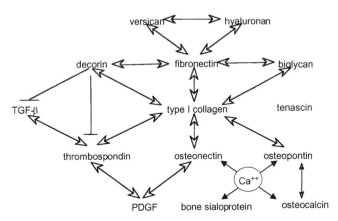

FIG. 2.4. Matrix macromolecular interactions. Following the initiation of hydroxyapatite deposition, the macromolecular scaffolding in bone matrix appears to be dictated in part by the interactions of noncollagenous proteins with type I collagen. Type I collagen (or fibrils) has been reported to interact with fibronectin (97) and decorin and, most likely, with biglycan (2), osteonectin (48), and thrombospondin (35). These interactions are further elaborated on by other interactions between the noncollagenous components, such as between versican and hyaluronan (17), and the interaction of this complex with fibronectin (105). Small leucine repeat sequence proteoglycans (*SLRP*) bind to thrombospondin (102) and fibronectin (100). Furthermore, in addition to collagen cross-linking, matrix can be further stabilized by the development of cross-links between osteopontin and osteocalcin (110). Many of the matrix proteins bind to growth factors, such as transforming growth factor-β (30) and platelet-derived growth factor (111), and others (osteonectin, osteopontin, bone sialoprotein, osteocalcin) have a high affinity for Ca^{2+}.

of versican in hyaluronan binding to fibronectin (105).

Matrix Component and Cell Surface Receptor Interactions

Many of the bone matrix components contain an RGD motif in their coding sequence and thus can interact with integrins on the cell surface. Integrins not only connect to the cytoskeletal elements of the cell but also initiate numerous signal-transduction pathways. Consequently, integrin occupancy enables the matrix composition to influence cellular activity and gene expression (106). Hyaluronan and decorin, components that do not possess an integrin-binding domain, do have other identified cellular receptors. The bone matrix component receptors are summarized in Table 2.1. Recently, the interaction of decorin with the EGF receptor has been described (107–109). Binding of decorin induces dimerization of the EGF receptor, rapid and sustained phosphorylation of the mitogen-activated protein kinase induction of p21, and growth suppression. Thus, decorin may be a novel biological ligand for the EGF receptor. Whether there are specific cell surface receptors for versican, biglycan, osteonectin, MGP, and osteocalcin is as yet unknown. Given the recurrent theme of matrix components possessing both cell-binding domains and domains for binding other matrix components, it is likely that such receptors exist.

SUMMARY

The matrix components of bone consist of three classes of macromolecule. The first group possesses repetitive structural motifs (collagen, hyaluronan, decorin, and biglycan), while the second group possesses a modular domain structure (versican, thrombospondin, fibronectin, osteonectin, and tenascin). In contrast, the structural motifs that convey functionality of the third group (MGP, osteopontin, BSP, and osteocalcin) are not as well defined. Components in the loose interstitial preosteogenic matrix, such as types I and III collagens, versican, and hyaluronan, most likely function early in bone development by providing a space-filling matrix that can be rapidly remodeled. Matrix organizers may function in the nucleation and deposition of hydroxyapatite (BSP) and dictate the structure of the mature collagenous array (type I collagen, decorin, and fibronectin). Other components, such as decorin, biglycan, thrombospondin, fibronectin, osteonectin, and osteocalcin, can also act as matrix modifiers by binding to growth factors and/or calcium ions, thereby regulating local concentrations of these ligands. Some matrix

TABLE 2.1. *Extracellular matrix component receptors*

Matrix	Subunits	RGD[a]	Receptor(s)	Reference
Biglycan	Core protein, CS/DS[b] chains	No	Not known	
Bone sialoprotein	Monomeric	Yes	$\alpha_V\beta_3$	112
Collagen type I	Heterotrimeric	Yes		
Decorin	Core protein, CS/DS chains	No	EGF-R?[c]	107
Fibronectin	Dimeric	Yes	$\alpha_5\beta_1$	33
			$\alpha_V\beta_3$	
Hyaluronan	Repetitive disaccharide chain	No	CD44	19
Osteocalcin	Monomeric	No	Not known	
Matrix gla protein	Monomeric	No	Not known	
Osteonectin	Monomeric	No	Not known	
Osteopontin	Monomeric	Yes	$\alpha_V\beta_3$, CD44	79
Tenascin	Hexameric	Yes	$\alpha_V\beta_3$?	63
Thrombospondin	Trimeric	Yes	$\alpha_V\beta_3$, CD34	39
Versican	Core protein, CS chains	No	Not known	

[a] RGD, arginine-glycine-aspartate.
[b] CS/DS, chrondroitin sulfate/dermatan sulfate.
[c] EGF-R, epidermal growth factor receptor.

proteins are considered adhesive macromolecules (collagen, fibronectin, osteopontin, BSP), while others are sometimes termed "antiadhesive" (versican, thrombospondin, osteonectin, and tenascin). Thus, there is considerable overlap between the various groups of matrix components in their biological "activities." The complexity in the number and type of binding interactions between the various matrix components and the secreting cells conveys to bone its unique function of providing a stable yet dynamic structure.

REFERENCES

1. Gehron Robey P, Boskey AL. The biochemistry of bone. In: Marcus R, Feldman D, eds. *Osteoporosis.* New York: Raven Press, 1996;95–184.
2. Brown DC, Vogel KC. Characteristics of the in vitro interaction of a small proteoglycan of bovine tendon with type I collagen. *Matrix* 1989;9:468–478.
3. Fessler JH, Fessler LI. Biosynthesis of procollagen. *Annu Rev Biochem* 1978;47:129.
4. Vogel C, Paulsson M, Heinegard D. Specific inhibition of type I and type II collagen fibrillogenesis by the small proteoglycan of tendon. *Biochem J* 1984;223:587–597.
5. McKusick V. Osteogenesis imperfecta. In: McKusick VA, ed. *Heritable disorders of the connective tissue.* St. Louis: CV Mosby, 1992:90–144.
6. Prockop D, Kivirikko K. Collagens: molecular biology, diseases, and potentials for therapy. *Annu Rev Biochem* 1995;64:403–434.
7. Fedarko NS, Moerike M, Brenner R, et al. Extracellular matrix formation by osteoblasts from patients with osteogenesis imperfecta. *J Bone Miner Res* 1992;7:921–930.
8. Fedarko NS, Vetter U, Weinstein S, et al. Age-related changes in hyaluronan, proteoglycan, collagen and osteonectin synthesis by human bone cells. *J Cell Physiol* 1992;151:215–227.
9. Fedarko NS, Gehron Robey P, Vetter U. Extracellular matrix stoichiometry in osteoblasts from patients with osteogenesis imperfecta. *J Bone Miner Res* 1995;10:1122–1129.
10. Celic S, Katayama Y, Chilco P, et al. Type I collagen influence on gene expression in UMR106-06 osteoblast-like cells is inhibited by genistein. *J Endocrinol* 1998;158:377–388.
11. Fedarko NS, D'Avis P, Frazier C, et al. Cell proliferation of human fibroblasts and osteoblasts in osteogenesis imperfecta: influence of age. *J Bone Miner Res* 1996;11:1705–1712.
12. Shi S, Kirk M, Kahn A. The role of type I collagen in the regulation of the osteoblast phenotype. *J Bone Miner Res* 1996;11:1139–1145.
13. Birk D, Mayne R. Localization of collagen types I, III and V during tendon development. Changes in collagen types I and III are correlated with changes in fibril diameter. *Eur J Cell Biol* 1997;72:352–361.
14. Liu X, Wu H, Byrne M, et al. Type III collagen is crucial for collagen I fibrillogenesis and normal cardiovascular development. *Proc Natl Acad Sci USA* 1997;94:1852–1856.
15. Quaglino D, Toman D, Crumbrugghe BD, et al. Transgenic mice expressing a col3a1 mutation at a crosslinking position exhibit structural alterations at sites of wound healing. *Matrix Biol* 1994;14:512–513.
16. Oohira A, Nogami H. Elevated accumulation of hyaluronate in the tubular bones of osteogenesis imperfecta. *Bone* 1989;10:409–413.
17. Fedarko NS, Gehron Robey P, Termine J. High performance liquid chromatographic separation of hyaluronan and four proteoglycans produced by human bone cell culture. *Anal Biochem* 1990;188:398–407.
18. Fisher L. The nature of proteoglycans of bone. In: Butler TW, ed. *The chemistry and biology of mineralized tissues.* Birmingham: EBSCO Media, 1985:188–196.
19. Culty M, Shizari M, Thompson EW, et al. Binding and degradation of hyaluronan by human breast cancer cell lines expressing different forms of CD44: correlation with invasive potential. *J Cell Physiol* 1994;160:275–286.
20. Noonan K, Stevens J, Tammi R, et al. Spatial distribution of CD44 and hyaluronan in the proximal tibia of the growing rat. *J Orthop Res* 1996;14:573–581.
21. Almond A, Brass A, Sheehan J. Deducing polymeric structure from aqueous molecular dynamics simulations of oligosaccharides: predictions from simulations of hyaluronan tetrasaccharides compared with hydrodynamic and X-ray fibre diffraction data. *J Mol Biol* 1998;284:1425–1437.
22. Fisher L, Termine J, Young M. Deduced protein sequence of bone small proteoglycan I, biglycan, shows homology with proteoglycan II, decorin and several nonconnective tissue proteins in a variety of species. *J Biol Chem* 1989;264:4571–4576.
23. Weber I, Harrison R, Iozzo R. Model structure of decorin and implications for collagen fibrillogenesis. *J Biol Chem* 1996;271:31767–31770.
24. Fleischmajer R, Fisher L, MacDonald E, et al. Decorin interacts with fibrillar collagen of embryonic and adult human skin. *J Struct Biol* 1991;106:82–90.
25. Bianco P, Fisher L, Young M, et al. Expression and localization of the two small proteoglycans biglycan and decorin in developing skeletal and nonskeletal tissues. *J Histochem Cytochem* 1990;38:1549–1559.
26. Scott J. Extracellular matrix, supramolecular organisation and shape. *J Anat* 1995;187:259–269.
27. Danielson K, Baribault H, Holmes D, et al. Targeted disruption of decorin leads to abnormal collagen fibril morphology and skin fragility. *J Cell Biol* 1997;136:729–743.
28. Hoshi K, Kemmotsu S, Takeuchi Y, et al. The primary calcification in bones follows removal of decorin and fusion of collagen fibrils. *J Bone Miner Res* 1999;14:273–280.
29. Dyne K, Valli M, Forlino A, et al. Deficient expression of the small proteoglycan decorin in a case of severe/lethal osteogenesis imperfecta. *Am J Med Genet* 1996;63:161–166.
30. Xu T, Bianco P, Fisher L, et al. Targeted disruption of the biglycan gene leads to an osteoporosis-like phenotype in mice. *Nat Genet* 1998;24:78–82.

31. Ruoslahti E, Yamaguchi Y. Proteoglycans as modulators of growth factor activities. *Cell* 1991;64:867–869.

32. Yamaguchi T, Mann D, Ruoslahti E. Negative regulation of transforming growth factor-beta by the proteoglycan decorin. *Nature* 1990;346:281–284.

33. Gehron Robey P, Young MF, Flanders KC, et al. Osteoblasts synthesize and respond to transforming growth factor-type beta (TGF-beta) in vitro. *J Cell Biol* 1987;105:457–463.

34. D'Souza S, Ginsberg M, Plow E. Arginyl-glycyl-aspartic acid (RGD), a cell adhesion motif. *Trends Biochem* 1991;16:246–250.

35. Asch A, Nachman R. Thrombospondin: phenomenology to function. *Prog Hemostasis Thromb* 1989;9:157–176.

36. Gehron Robey P, Young MF, Fisher LW, et al. Thrombospondin is an osteoblast-derived component of mineralized extracellular matrix. *J Cell Biol* 1989;108:719–727.

37. Grzesik WJ, Gehron Robey P. Bone matrix RGD glycoproteins: immunolocalization and interaction with human primary osteoblastic bone cells in vitro. *J Bone Miner Res* 1994;9:487–496.

38. Tooney P, Sakai T, Sakai K, et al. Restricted localization of thrombospondin-2 protein during mouse embryogenesis: a comparison to thrombospondin-1. *Matrix Biol* 1998;17:131–143.

39. Tucker R, Adams J, Lawler J. Thrombospondin-4 is expressed by early osteogenic tissues in the chick embryo. *Dev Dyn* 1995;203:477–490.

40. Lawler J, Duquette M, Whittaker C, et al. Identification and characterization of thrombospondin-4, a new member of the thrombospondin gene family. *J Cell Biol* 1993;120:1059–1067.

41. Hogg P, Hotchkiss K, Jimenez B, et al. Interaction of platelet-derived growth factor with thrombospondin 1. *Biochem J* 1997;326:709–716.

42. Schultz-Cherry S, Chen H, Mosher D, et al. Regulation of transforming growth factor-beta activation by discrete sequences of thrombospondin 1. *J Biol Chem* 1995;270:7304–7310.

43. Schultz-Cherry S, Ribeiro S, Gentry L, et al. Thrombospondin binds and activates the small and large forms of latent transforming growth factor-beta in a chemically defined system. *J Biol Chem* 1994;269:26775–26782.

44. Kyriakides TR, Zhu YH, Smith LT, et al. Mice that lack thrombospondin 2 display connective tissue abnormalities that are associated with disordered collagen fibrillogenesis, an increased vascular density, and a bleeding diathesis. *J Cell Biol* 1998;140:419–430.

45. Guan J, Hynes R. Lymphoid cells recognize an alternatively spliced segment of fibronectin via the integrin receptor alpha 4 beta 1. *Cell* 1990;60:53–61.

46. Mould A, Wheldon L, Komoriya A, et al. Affinity chromatographic isolation of the melanoma adhesion receptor for the IIICS region of fibronectin and its identification as the integrin alpha 4 beta 1. *J Biol Chem* 1990;265:4020–4024.

47. Weiss R, Reddi A. Appearance of fibronectin during the differentiation of cartilage, bone and bone marrow. *J Cell Biol* 1981;88:630–638.

48. Globus R, Doty S, Lull J, et al. Fibronectin is a survival factor for differentiated osteoblasts. *J Cell Sci* 1998;111:1385–1393.

49. Termine J, Belcourt H, Coma F, et al. Mineral and collagen-binding proteins of fetal calf bone. *J Biol Chem* 1981;256:10403–10408.

50. Bolander ME, Young MF, Fisher LW, et al. Osteonectin cDNA sequence reveals potential binding regions for calcium and hydroxyapatite and shows homologies with both a basement membrane protein (SPARC) and a serine proteinase inhibitor (ovomucoid). *Proc Natl Acad Sci USA* 1988;85:2919–2923.

51. Hohenester E, Maurer P, Timpl R. Crystal structure of a pair of follistatin-like and EF-hand calcium-binding domains in BM-40. *EMBO J* 1996;16:3778–3786.

52. Romberg R, Werness P, Riggs B, et al. Inhibition of hydroxyapatite crystal growth by bone-specific and other calcium-binding proteins. *Biochemistry* 1986;25:1176–1180.

53. Clezardin P, Malaval L, Ehrensperger A, et al. Complex formation of human thrombospondin with osteonectin. *Eur J Biochem* 1988;175:275–284.

54. Kelm RJ, Mann K. The collagen binding specificity of bone and platelet osteonectin is related to differences in glycosylation. *J Biol Chem* 1991;266:9632–9639.

55. Sage E, Vernon R, Decker J, et al. Distribution of the calcium binding protein SPARC in tissues of embryonic and adult mice. *Histochem Cytochem* 1989;37:819–829.

56. Gohring W, Sasaki T, Heldin C, et al. Mapping of the binding of platelet-derived growth factor to distinct domains of the basement membrane proteins BM-40 and perlecan and distinction from the BM-40 collagen-binding epitope. *Eur J Biochem* 1998;255:60–66.

57. Raines E, Lane T, Iruela-Arispe M, et al. The extracellular glycoprotein SPARC interacts with platelet-derived growth factor (PDGF)-AB and -BB and inhibits the binding of PDGF to its receptors. *Proc Natl Acad Sci USA* 1992;89:1281–1285.

58. Holland P, Harper S, McVey J, et al. In vivo expression of mRNA for the calcium binding protein SPARC (osteonectin) revealed by in situ hybridization. *J Cell Biol* 1987;105:473–482.

59. Tremble P, Lane T, Sage E, et al. SPARC, a secreted protein associated with morphogenesis and tissue remodeling induces expression of metalloproteinases in fibroblasts through a novel extracellular matrix-dependent pathway. *J Cell Biol* 1993;121:1433–1441.

60. Wewer U, Albrechtsen R, Fisher L, et al. Osteonectin/SPARC/BM40 in human decidua and carcinoma tissue characterized by de novo formation of basement membrane. *Am J Pathol* 1988;132:345–355.

61. Lane T, Sage E. The biology of SPARC, a protein that modulates cell–matrix interactions. *FASEB J* 1994;8:163–173.

62. Sage H, Johnson C, Bornstein P. Characterization of a novel serum albumin-binding glycoprotein secreted by endothelial cells in culture. *J Biol Chem* 1984;259:3993–4007.

63. Gilmour D, Lyon G, Carlton M, et al. Mice deficient for the secreted glycoprotein SPARC/osteonectin/BM40 develop normally but show severe age-onset cataract formation and disruption of the lens. *EMBO J* 1998;17:1860–1870.

64. Seiffert M, Beck S, Schermutzki F, et al. Mitogenic and adhesive effects of tenascin-C on human hematopoietic cells are mediated by various functional domains. *Matrix Biol* 1998;17:47–63.

65. Mackie E, Thesleff I, Chiquet-Ehrismann R. Tenascin is associated with chondrogenic and osteogenic differentiation in vivo and promotes chondrogenesis in vitro. *J Cell Biol* 1987;105:2569–2579.

66. Mackie E, Ramsey S. Modulation of osteoblast behaviour by tenascin. *J Cell Sci* 1996;109:1597–1604.

67. Forsberg E, Hirsch E, Frohlich L, et al. Skin wounds and severed nerves heal normally in mice lacking tenascin-C. *Proc Natl Acad Sci USA* 1996;93:6594–6599.

68. Chiquet-Ehrismann R, Hagios C, Matsumoto K. The tenascin gene family. *Perspect Dev Neurobiol* 1994; 2:3–7.

69. Weistner AM, Krieg T, Horlein D, et al. Inhibiting effect of procollagen peptides on collagen biosynthesis in fibroblasts cultures. *J Biol Chem* 1979;254:7016–7023.

70. Horlein D, McPherson JM, Goh SH, et al. Regulation of protein synthesis: translational control by procollagen-derived fragments. *Proc Natl Acad Sci USA* 1981; 8:6163–6167.

71. McPherson JM, Horlein D, Abbott-Brown D, et al. Inhibition of protein synthesis in vitro by procollagen-derived fragments is associated with changes in protein phosporylation. *J Biol Chem* 1982;257:8557–8560.

72. Fouser L, Sage EH, Clark J, et al. Feedback regulation of collagen gene expression: a Trojan horse approach. *Proc Natl Acad Sci USA* 1991;88:10158–10162.

73. Katayama K, Armendariz-Borunda J, Raghow R, et al. A pentapeptide from type I procollagen promotes extracellular matrix production. *J Biol Chem* 1993;268: 9941–9944.

74. Ma X, Svegliati-Baroni G, Poniachik J, et al. Collagen synthesis by liver stellate cells is released from its normal feedback regulation by acetaldehyde-induced modification of the carboxy-terminal propeptide of procollagen. *Alcohol Clin Exp Res* 1997;21:1204–1211.

75. Davies D, Tuckwell DS, Weston SA, et al. Molecular characterization of integrin–procollagen C–propeptide interactions. *Eur J Biochem* 1997;246:274–282.

76. Weston SA, Hulmes DJ, Mould AP, et al. Identification of integrin alpha 2 beta 1 as cell surface receptor for the carboxyl-terminal propeptide of type I procollagen. *J Biol Chem* 1994;269:20982–20986.

77. Takeuchi A, Katayama K, Matsumoto T. Differentiation and cell surface expression of transforming growth factor-beta receptors are regulated by interaction with collagen in murine osteoblastic cells. *J Biol Chem* 1996;271:3938–3944.

78. Kessler E, Takahara K, Biniaminov L, et al. Bone morphogenetic protein-1: the type I procollagen C-proteinase. *Science* 1996;271:360–362.

79. Riminucci M, Bradbeer JN, Corsi A, et al. Vis-a-vis cells and the priming of bone formation. *J Bone Miner Res* 1998;13:1852–1861.

80. Reinholt FP, Hultenby K, Oldberg A, et al. Osteopontin—a possible anchor of osteoclasts to bone. *Proc Natl Acad Sci USA* 1990;87:4473–4475.

81. Rudzki Z, Jothy S. CD44 and the adhesion of neoplastic cells. *Mol Pathol* 1997;50:57–71.

82. Ue T, Yokozaki H, Kitadai Y, et al. Co-expression of osteopontin and CD44v9 in gastric cancer. *Int J Cancer* 1998;79:127–132.

83. Weber GF, Ashkar S, Cantor H. Interaction between CD44 and osteopontin as a potential basis for metastasis formation. *Proc Assoc Am Physicians* 1997;109: 1–9.

84. Chen J, McKee M, Nanci A, et al. Bone sialoprotein mRNA expression and ultrastructural localization in fetal porcine calvarial bone: comparisons with osteopontin. *Histochem J* 1994;26:67–78.

85. Hunter G, Kyle C, Goldberg H. Modulation of crystal formation by bone phosphoproteins: structural specificity of the osteopontin-mediated inhibition of hydroxyapatite formation. *Biochem J* 1994;300:723–728.

86. Chackalaparampil I, Peri A, Nemir M, et al. Cells in vivo and in vitro from osteopetrotic mice homozygous for c-src disruption show suppression of synthesis of osteopontin, a multifunctional extracellular matrix protein. *Oncogene* 1996;12:1457–1467.

87. Flores ME, Norgard M, Heinegard D, et al. RGD-directed attachment of isolated rat osteoclasts to osteopontin, bone sialoprotein, and fibronectin. *Exp Cell Res* 1992;201:526–530.

88. Bianco P, Fisher L, Young M, et al. Expression of bone sialoprotein (BSP) in developing human tissues. *Calcif Tissue Int* 1991;49:421–426.

89. Bianco P, Riminucci M, Bonucci E, et al. Bone sialoprotein (BSP) secretion and osteoblast differentiation: relationship to bromodeoxyuridine incorporation. *J Histochem Cytochem* 1993;41:183–191.

90. Riminucci M, Silvestrini G, Bonucci E, et al. The anatomy of bone sialoprotein immunoreactive sites in bone as revealed by combined ultrastructural histochemistry and immunohistochemistry. *Calcif Tissue Int* 1995;57: 277–284.

91. Liaw L, Birk DE, Ballas CB, et al. Altered wound healing in mice lacking a functional osteopontin gene (spp1). *J Clin Invest* 1998;101:1468–1478.

92. Hale JE, Fraser JD, Price PA. The identification of matrix Gla protein in cartilage. *J Biol Chem* 1988;263: 5820–5824.

93. Luo G, D'Souza R, Hogue D, et al. The matrix Gla protein gene is a marker of the chondrogenesis cell lineage during mouse development. *J Bone Miner Res* 1995;10:325–334.

94. Price P, Williamson M. Excessive mineralization with growth plate closure in rats on chronic warfarin treatment. *Proc Natl Acad Sci USA* 1982;79:7734–7738.

95. Lian J, Dunn K, Key L. In vitro degradation of bone particles by human monocytes is decreased with the depletion of the vitamin K-dependent bone protein from the matrix. *Endocrinology* 1986;118:1636–1641.

96. Ducy P, Desbois C, Boyce B, et al. Increased bone formation in osteocalcin-deficient mice. *Nature* 1996; 382:448–452.

97. Kaartinen M, Pirjenon A, Linnala-Kankkunen A, et al. Transglutaminase-catalyzed cross-linking of osteopontin is inhibited by osteocalcin. *J Biol Chem* 1997;272: 22736–22741.

98. Dzamba D, Wu H, Jaenisch R, et al. Fibronectin binding sites in type I collagen regulate fibronectin fibril formation. *Matrix* 1993;13:6.

99. Bidanset DJ, Guidry C, Rosenberg LC, et al. Binding of the proteoglycan decorin to collagen type VI. *J Biol Chem* 1992;267:5250–5256.

100. Schmidt G, Hausser H, Kresse H. Interaction of the small proteoglycan decorin with fibronectin. *Biochem J* 1991;280:411–414.

101. Schmidt G, Robenek R, Harrach R, et al. Interaction

of small dermatan sulfate proteoglycan from fibroblasts with fibronectin. *J Cell Biol* 1987;266:1683–1691.

102. Winnemöller M, Schmidt G, Kresse H. Influence of decorin on fibroblast adhesion to fibronectin. *Eur J Cell Biol* 1991;54:10–17.

103. Winnemöller M, Schön P, Vischer P, et al. Interactions between thrombospondin and the small proteoglycan decorin: interference with cell attachment. *Eur J Cell Biol* 1992;59:47–55.

104. Teicher B, Ikebe M, Ara G, et al. Transforming growth factor-beta 1 overexpression produces drug resistance in vivo: reversal by decorin. *In Vivo* 1997;11:463–472.

105. Imai K, Hiramatsu A, Fukushima D, et al. Degradation of decorin by matrix metalloproteinases: identification of the cleavage sites, kinetic analyses and transforming growth factor-beta 1 release. *Biochem J* 1997;22:809–814.

106. Yamagata M, Yamada KM, Masahiko Y, et al. Chondroitin sulfate proteoglycan (PG-M-like proteoglycan) is involved in the binding of hyaluronic acid to cellular fibronectin. *J Biol Chem* 1986;261:13526–13535.

107. Dedhar S. Integrins and signal transduction. *Curr Opin Hematol* 1999;6:37–43.

108. Iozzo R, Moscatello D, McQuillan D, et al. Decorin is a biological ligand for the epidermal growth factor receptor. *J Biol Chem* 1999;274:4489–4492.

109. Moscatello D, Santra M, Mann D, et al. Decorin suppresses tumor cell growth by activating the epidermal growth factor receptor. *J Clin Invest* 1998;101:406–412.

110. Santra M, Mann D, Mercer E, et al. Ectopic expression of decorin protein core causes a generalized growth suppression in neoplastic cells of various histogenetic origin and requires endogenous p21, an inhibitor of cyclin-dependent kinases. *J Clin Invest* 1997;100:149–157.

111. Ritter N, Farach-Carson M, Butler W. Evidence for the formation of a complex between osteopontin and osteocalcin. *J Bone Miner Res* 1992;7:877–885.

112. Sage E, Bassuk J, Yost J, et al. Inhibition of endothelial cell proliferation by SPARC is mediated through a Ca^{2+}-binding EF-hand sequence. *J Cell Biochem* 1995;57:127–140.

113. Fisher LW, McBride OW, Termine JD, et al. Human bone sialoprotein. Deduced protein sequence and chromosomal localization. *J Biol Chem* 1990;265:2347–2351.

Skeletal Growth Factors,
edited by Ernesto Canalis.
Published by Lippincott Williams & Wilkins, Philadelphia, 2000.

3

Biology of Growth Factors

Derek Le Roith and *Vicky A. Blakesley

*Clinical Endocrinology Branch, NIDDK, National Institutes of Health,
Bethesda, Maryland 20892-1758
Abbott Laboratories, Abbott Park, Illinois 60064-6188

The transduction of extracellular signals to the nucleus, such that the cell responds in a physiological manner, is accomplished by activation of a number of membrane-spanning cell surface receptors. These receptors transmit specific signals via intracellular signal-transduction pathways to affect other cytoplasmic signal cascades and nuclear transcription factors that lead to changes in cell behavior. In this overview, we discuss the following cell surface receptors and their signaling pathways: tyrosine kinase receptors, G protein–coupled or serpentine receptors, cytokine receptors, and cell adhesion receptors such as integrins. For each group of receptors, we present examples to illustrate structural and functional concepts and the major signaling pathways employed. Traditionally, each type of receptor has been associated with specific signaling pathways. However, it has become apparent that many of the signaling pathways of one type, such as tyrosine kinase–activated pathways, are often controlled by signaling pathways emanating from another receptor family, such as G protein–coupled receptors. The complex aspect of crosstalk between receptor signaling cascades will be addressed, again using a few examples to illustrate general concepts. Our goal is to give in "broad strokes" an overview and introduction to the chapters that follow on various aspects of bone biology. We do not attempt to be comprehensive; rather, we include references to excellent recent reviews on the various topics to which the reader may refer if more in-depth knowledge on a particular aspect is required.

TYROSINE KINASE RECEPTORS

Classes and Structures of Tyrosine Kinase Receptors

The transmembrane tyrosine kinase receptor family is comprised of a large number of receptors that are activated by various growth factors and hormones. The family can be divided into various subclasses based on whether the active receptor is a dimer and on the structures of the extracellular domain and the catalytic domain (Fig. 3.1). The extracellular ligand-binding region contains cysteine-rich domains in classes I and II, whereas in classes III and IV immunoglobulin domains are the hallmarks of the extracellular domain. All members of the family have highly conserved tyrosine kinase domains in the cytoplasmic region (1). Ligand binding and dimerization of two receptor molecules activate those receptors composed of a single polypeptide chain (class I), such as epidermal growth factor (EGF) receptor. Activation leads to intermolecular autophosphorylation and enhanced tyrosine kinase activity (2). Class II receptors, for example, the insulin and insulin-like growth factor-I (IGF-I) receptors, exist as oligomers (two $\alpha_2\beta_2$ proteins) in the unstimulated state. Ligand binding leads to conformational changes in the receptors that activate intermolecular autophosphorylation and increase the receptor tyrosine kinase activities (3).

Each subclass of tyrosine kinase receptors consists of several members; for example, class I contains the ErbB (also known as HER) growth

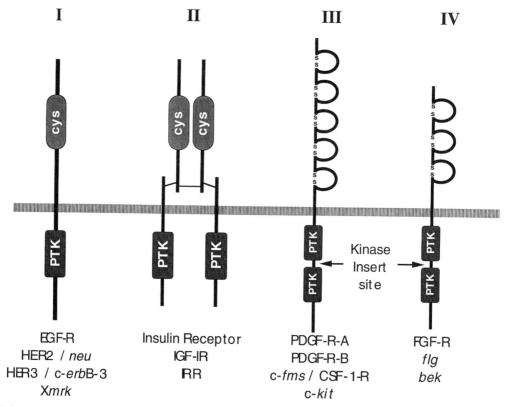

FIG. 3.1. Classes of receptor tyrosine kinases (RTK). The receptors in classes I and II have cysteine-rich domains (cys) in their extracellular regions. The receptors in classes III and IV have several immunoglobulin-like motifs in the extracellular regions, and the intracellular kinase domains have a short insert. Newly described members have been added to the classification of Yarden and Ullrich (2).

factor receptors. ErbB-1 binds EGF, transforming growth factor-α (TGF-α), vaccinia virus growth factor, and amphiregulin (4). ErbB-3 and ErbB-4 bind the multiple isoforms of the Neu differentiation factor, whereas ErbB-2 has no known ligand. Each ErbB receptor isoform can form homodimers to activate downstream signaling pathways. Furthermore, homodimer and heterodimer combinations of the ErbB proteins may exist, giving rise to different proliferative potentials (5). Further enhancement of intracellular signaling can occur by transactivation between receptors of the various subclasses of the tyrosine kinase receptor family (5).

The insulin receptor, the IGF-I receptor, and the insulin receptor–related receptor (IRR) belong to the insulin receptor family or class II of

tyrosine kinase receptors. The insulin and IGF-I receptors are similar in overall structure, and the position of many of the cysteine residues thought to be involved in disulfide bond formation are conserved. In fact, hybrids may occur between the insulin and IGF-I receptors, resulting in a receptor composed of one insulin hemireceptor and an IGF-I hemireceptor (6). Both naturally occurring and in vitro–produced hybrids demonstrate a higher affinity for IGF-I than for insulin. IGF-I can bind these hybrid receptors and activate the metabolic responses of the insulin receptor hemireceptor by intramolecular transphosphorylation. The relative contribution of this signaling is likely small because the levels of naturally occurring hybrids are relatively small compared with the levels of insulin or IGF-I receptors; however, activation of hybrid receptors may allow for modulation of the metabolic actions of IGF-I (7).

Signaling via Tyrosine Kinase Receptors

Receptor protein tyrosine kinases (PTKs) are activated by an intermolecular mechanism (8). The monomeric receptors, such as the EGF receptor, dimerize following ligand interaction. Following dimerization, intrinsic catalytic activity is stimulated, leading to autophosphorylation of the cytoplasmic domains of the PTKs. The exact mechanism by which this occurs has been under recent investigation. Results of crystallographic studies support the "stabilization of the open loop" theory. Based on similarities with the unphosphorylated insulin and fibroblast growth factor (FGF) receptors, which have highly mobile activation loops (A loops) in their catalytic domains, the A loop of the EGF receptor is also likely to be highly mobile (9). When the A loop is stabilized in the open position, adenosine triphosphate (ATP) is bound and transphosphorylation can proceed. Further stabilization of the A loop in the open state occurs with the insulin receptor when the three tyrosine residues in the catalytic domain are phosphorylated. Thereafter, the insulin receptor is fully activated and capable of phosphorylating endogenous substrates on tyrosine residues (10).

Transmembrane tyrosine kinase receptors share several features with regard to activation of the receptors and intracellular signaling pathways. Ligand binding to the extracellular domain of the receptor triggers a specific conformational change that results in autophosphorylation of the receptor and enhanced tyrosine kinase activity toward endogenous substrates. Docking sites for endogenous substrates are created by the phosphorylation of tyrosine residues on the cytoplasmic regions of the receptor. Growth factor receptor-bound protein-2 (Grb2), an Src homology-2 (SH2) and SH3 domain–containing adapter protein, associates directly with some growth factor receptors, such as the EGF receptor (11), and indirectly via protein intermediates with other growth factor receptors, such as the insulin and IGF-I receptors. Mamma-

lian son-of-sevenless (mSOS) is bound to the SH3 domain of Grb2, thus recruiting it to the inner surface of the plasma membrane. mSOS in turn activates Ras by exchanging guanosine triphosphate (GTP) for guanosine diphosphate (GDP), thereby activating the Ras/Raf/mitogen-activated protein (MAP) kinase pathway (Fig. 3.2) (12). Other substrates known to interact with various growth factor receptors include members of the insulin/IGF-I receptor family of substrates (IRS-1, IRS-2, IRS-3, and IRS-4), SHC, protein tyrosine phosphatase-1D (PTP-1D or Syp), and phospholipase C (PLC). Several of these substrates are docking proteins for lipid or protein kinases or phosphatases. The docking proteins of the IRS family are essential for IGF-I and insulin receptor action. The IRS proteins interact with several proteins, including phosphoinositide 3′-kinase (PI3′-K) and PTP-1D/Syp, thereby activating other downstream signaling pathways (13,14). The downstream cascades emanating from Ras and PI3′-K are numerous and varied, and while each growth factor tyrosine kinase receptor has been shown to activate each of these pathways, the use appears to be selective in specific cell types. This selectivity may reflect the multiple signals being generated by different receptors. For example, while both platelet-derived growth factor (PDGF) and insulin activate their respective receptors and thus PI3′-K equally in adipocytes, only insulin results in translocation of the glucose transporters to the cell surface, a biological function dependent on PI3′-K (15).

Three parallel pathways involving Ras and Ras-related proteins are known to transduce intracellular signaling of the tyrosine kinase receptors. GTP loading of the Ras protein triggers a cascade of serine/threonine protein kinases and dual threonine/tyrosine protein kinases that ultimately results in activation of the MAP kinases (16). The known mammalian MAP kinases, c-Jun N-terminal kinase (JNK) or stress-activated protein kinase (SAPK), p38 kinase, and the extracellular signal–regulated kinases (Erks), possess overlapping substrate specificities with a minimal consensus sequence of $\zeta \times [S/T] P$, where ζ is proline or an aliphatic amino acid. The Erks bind the 90-kDa ribosomal S6 protein

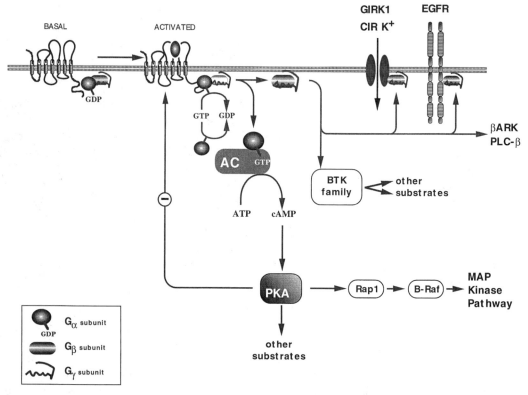

FIG. 3.2. G protein–coupled receptor signaling. Agonist binding to the serpentine receptor leads to the exchange of GDP for GTP in Gα. Activated Gα dissociates from Gβγ and from the receptor, with the two subunits then acting on downstream effectors. Activated Gα activates adenylyl cyclase *(AC)*, which converts adenosine triphosphate *(ATP)* to cyclic adenosine monophosphate *(cAMP)*. Elevated cAMP regulates multiple downstream pathways, some of which are mediated by protein kinase A *(PKA)*. PKA and β-adrenergic kinase *(bARK)* also phosphorylate serpentine receptors, leading to their inactivation and, in effect, acting as a negative feedback loop. Gβγ interacts with and regulates the activity of several proteins, including potassium channels (GIRK1, CIR K[+]), βARK, phospholipase Cβ, the epidermal growth factor receptor *(EGFR)*, and members of the BTK family.

kinase (Rsk); several transcription factors, including Elk-1, c-Myc, and Ets-2 (17); and the recently identified MAP kinase signal-integrating kinases MNK-1 and MNK-2, the latter being activated by the Erks and p38 but not by JNK (18). MNK-1 in turn phosphorylates the ribosomal protein eIF-4E, which is involved in mRNA translation and activated by insulin stimulation (19).

The pathways emanating from the tyrosine kinase receptors are multiple and varied. This chapter has described only a few of the known substrates and pathways. Heretofore unknown proteins which are components of these pathways will undoubtedly be identified. With each

new discovery of substrate and the delineation of the contribution on intracellular signaling involving those substrates, the possibility exists of finding the key to understanding specific diseases resulting from perturbations of important signaling cascades.

SERINE/THREONINE KINASE RECEPTORS

Structures of Serine/Threonine Kinase Receptors

Serine/threonine (ser/thr) kinase receptors are transmembrane proteins with a short, cysteine-rich extracellular domain and an intracellular kinase domain with specificity toward serine and threonine residues. The best-characterized members of the ser/thr kinase receptor superfamily are those that serve as receptors for members of the TGF-β family of growth and differentiation factors. These receptors have many features in common (20). Based on primary amino acid sequence and differing functional properties, the family has been grouped into two classes: type I and type II.

Signaling via Serine/Threonine Kinase Receptors

The exact class of receptor that binds each ligand and the complete assembly of the receptor complex varies, but a description of the activation by TGF-β serves to demonstrate general mechanisms for this receptor family. A heterodimeric receptor is formed by recruitment of a type I receptor (TβRI) upon TGF-β binding to a type II receptor (TβRII) (21). TβRII is itself a constitutively active kinase, and once TβRI is recruited to the complex, the TβRII phosphorylates serine and threonine residues in the highly conserved glycine rich segment (GS) domain of the TβRI (22). Once phosphorylated, the heterodimeric receptor is competent to signal to downstream target proteins. Mutational analyses of key amino acids in the GS domains confirm that the type I receptor is the downstream signaling protein of the receptor complex (23). Both the type I and type II receptors are required for appropriate functioning of the ser/thr kinase receptors, based on results of studies using mutant type I and type II receptors. Some studies indicate that a higher-order receptor structure, such as that of heterotetramers, is essential for signal transduction by these ser/thr kinase receptors (24).

Downstream signaling targets of the ser/thr kinase receptors are being identified by yeast two-hybrid and genetic screens. To date, several proteins have been identified that may be substrates for these receptors, such as TGF-β receptor–interacting protein-1 (TRIP-1), farnesyltransferase-α, FK506/rapamycin-binding protein (FKBP-12), apolipoprotein J/clusterin, TGF-β-activated kinase (TAK-1), and

MADR (mothers against dpp-related proteins) (22). Of these proteins, only a handful have been confirmed to associate with the type I and type II TGF-β receptors in mammalian cells. Three of these proteins are known to be involved in other signaling mechanisms but have yet to be firmly established in signaling from the ser/thr kinase receptors.

Farnesyltransferase-α is the regulatory subunit of the enzyme that catalyzes farnesylation of the C terminus of Ras, a modification that is essential for Ras association with the inner aspect of plasma membrane and for Ras function (25). There is no firm evidence that TGF-β receptor signaling involves farnesylation of Ras. However, since the α subunit is also a regulatory subunit for other isoprenyltransferases, this signaling molecule may indeed play a role in ser/thr kinase receptor signaling. TAK-1, the second putative signaling molecule, has been identified and shown to be regulated by TGF-β in a time- and dose-dependent manner (26). Active TAK-1 mediates a transcriptional response that is typical of TGF-β, and kinase-deficient TAK-1 disrupts this TGF-β induction of transcription.

The most convincing data for potential downstream targets of these ser/thr kinase receptors are for members of the MADR family. Mutations of the human MADR2 and MADR4 have been identified in colorectal and pancreatic tumors, respectively (27). In functional studies, it appears that the MADR proteins impart some of the specificity of signaling from specific ligands via TGF-β receptors. The specificities observed correlate well with the phosphorylation of specific MADR proteins in response to stimulation by specific ligands. Furthermore, ligand stimulation results in MADR protein translocation to the nucleus, where presumably MADR proteins serve to modify transcription of target genes. It is unknown if phosphorylation of the MADR proteins is essential for movement of the molecule into the nucleus and its subsequent interactions. It has also not been determined which kinase(s) actually phosphorylates the MADR proteins or, in fact, if the ser/thr kinase receptor catalyzes this reaction.

Another interesting group of proteins within this family is the bone morphogenetic proteins (BMPs), which were originally identified as inducers of bone and cartilage formation but recently have been found to regulate growth, differentiation, chemotaxis, and apoptosis in monocytes, epithelial cells, mesenchymal cells, and neuronal cells (28). BMPs belong to the TGF-β superfamily and signal the cells via activation of specific ser/thr kinase receptors (29–32). The cytoplasmic substrates for these receptors are called Smads, and several of the seven identified Smads form homo- and hetero-oligomers (33). They interact transiently with the receptors and, following heterodimerization, migrate to the nucleus, where they apparently affect gene transcription.

G PROTEIN–COUPLED RECEPTORS

The function of the family of G protein–coupled receptors (GPCRs) is to transduce extracellular signals as diverse as photons, amine neurotransmitters, odorants, proteases, ions, and hormones to specific intracellular effectors. The family of GPCRs, with over 2,000 members described thus far, can be classified into three subfamilies based on structural homologies: the first group consists of rhodopsin and rhodopsin-like receptors; the second subfamily includes receptors for parathyroid hormone (PTH), calcitonin, corticotrophin-releasing hormone, secretin, glucagon, and other related peptides; and the third family consists of the calcium-sensing receptor and metabotropic glutamate receptors. The GPCRs themselves do not possess any intrinsic enzymatic activity but are coupled to effector proteins in a large complex comprised of $\alpha\beta\gamma$ subunits that transmit the signal to appropriate downstream kinases and phosphatases.

Structure of G Protein–coupled Receptors

The most characteristic structural feature common to all members of the family of GPCRs is the presence of seven highly conserved sequences of between 20 and 27 hydrophobic amino acid residues, which are predicted to form seven transmembrane α helices connected by loops of various lengths (34). All GPCRs have an extracellular N-terminal tail, the seven transmembrane domains (TM1 to TM7), three extra-

cellular loops, three intracellular loops, and the C-terminal tail that lies within the cytoplasmic space. The N- and C-terminal segments vary widely in length. The N-terminal segment contains consensus sites for N-linked glycosylation, whereas the C-terminal tail has a conserved cysteine (Cys) residue in the C-terminal tail that is a site for fatty acylation. Palmitoylation at this Cys may serve to anchor the tail to the inner aspect of the plasma membrane, thereby forming a fourth intracellular loop. There are ser/thr residues in the third intracellular loop (I-3) and the C-terminal tail (I-4) that are sites for phosphorylation by kinases, as well as extracellular disulfide bonds. The α helices span the membrane and form a relatively compact bundle with a central cavity, this structure likely aided by disulfide bonds that form between extracellular loop 2 (E2) and the junction between E1 and the third transmembrane helix (TM3). The structures have led to this family of receptors being referred to as heptahelical "serpentine" receptors.

Ligand-binding sites on the receptor are variable and dependent on the class of ligands and receptors. Glycoprotein hormones, including luteinizing hormone (LH), follicle-stimulating hormone (FSH), thyroid-stimulating hormone (TSH), and human chorionic gonadotropin (hCG), are large and initially bind with high affinity to the large (350 to 400 amino acid residues) N-terminal segment (35). Secondarily, they interact with extracellular loops 1 to 3 (E1–3) and activate the receptor. Not surprisingly, therefore, mutations in E1–3 may result in constitutive activation. PTH has a similar two-step binding–activation process. Initially, PTH binds to the N-terminal domain and then activates its receptor via specific interactions with TM3 and E2. These interactions differ from those seen with biogenic amines, for example, those that enter and bind the transmembrane core directly.

Ligand binding and activation of the GPCRs is associated with a conformational change that is transmitted to the cytoplasmic side of the receptor (36). This results in a physical interaction between the receptor and the heterotrimeric ($\alpha\beta\gamma$) guanine nucleotide–binding regulatory proteins (G proteins). The GDP-bound G protein heterotrimer dissociates the GDP and binds GTP to the G protein α subunit, thereby releasing the G protein $\beta\gamma$ heterodimer (G$\beta\gamma$). GTP-bound G protein α subunits and $\beta\gamma$ complexes independently initiate intracellular signaling cascades. G protein α subunits can be subdivided in part based on their effector interactions, that is, stimulatory (G$_s$), inhibitory (G$_{i/o}$), or coupling (G$_q$) actions. G$_s$ proteins stimulate adenylyl cyclase, G$_{i/o}$ proteins frequently inhibit adenylyl cyclase, and G$_{q/11}$ proteins frequently couple receptors to PLC isoenzymes. The G$\beta\gamma$ heterodimer also interacts with effectors, although less is known about the specific mechanisms of the interactions. They have been shown to effect adenylyl cyclase, PLC-β, some ser/thr kinases, and several protein tyrosine kinases (37). The G$\beta\gamma$ heterodimer thus released from the $\alpha\beta\gamma$ heterotrimers, following activation of muscarinic receptors, for example, stimulates the activity of Akt/protein kinase B (PKB), a powerful antiapoptotic ser/thr kinase, via the PI3'-K pathway. The PI3'-K activation by G$\beta\gamma$ is also required for activation of the MAP kinase pathway.

Desensitization of G Protein–coupled Receptors

Unique to this family of receptors are the mechanisms involved in desensitization that have been well characterized by Lefkowitz (38). One mechanism is the phosphorylation of serine residues in the third cytoplasmic loop (I-3) and the C-terminal tail of the receptor. This causes a conformational change in the receptor such that its interaction with the G-protein complex is impaired. Serine phosphorylation occurs following elevation of cyclic adenosine monophosphate (cAMP) and activation of protein kinase A (PKA) or diacylglycerol, in the case of protein kinase C (PKC). Heterologous desensitization is the description given to this type of event since it may also occur following activation of other receptor-mediated signaling. Homologous desensitization, a second mechanism of desensitization, follows activation of the specific receptor by an agonist and consists of a rapid, two-step process whereby the activated receptor is phosphorylated by a specific G protein receptor kinase (GRK), such as β-adrenergic receptor kinase (βARK) in the case of the β-adrenergic receptor. This phosphorylation is followed by binding of a member of the arrestin family, which prevents G-protein binding. Six arrestins have thus far been characterized. Targeting of a GRK to the receptor involves the binding of a G$\beta\gamma$, which is prenylated and membrane-bound, and a membrane phosphatidylinositol bisphosphate.

GPCRs may internalize both via classical clathrin-coated and nonclathrin-coated vesicle pathways (39). It is becoming evident that the arrestin proteins are important for internalization in that arrestins can bind clathrin. Phosphorylation of the receptor facilitates the binding of arrestins (40). Whether arrestin binding to clathrin affects receptor downregulation is still undefined.

Receptor endocytosis appears to be important for the process of "resensitization" following removal of the agonist (41). The endocytotic vesicle, in which the receptor is sequestrated, contains phosphatase activity, primarily a membrane-associated phosphatase of the protein phosphatase-2A (PP-2A) family (42). Dephosphorylation of the receptor results in rapid resensitization. Endocytosis is also important for certain signaling responses to activated GPCRs, especially those mediated by G$\beta\gamma$, but not for activation of the cAMP and PLC pathways. Interestingly, whereas GPCRs may activate the Ras/Raf/MAP kinase pathways at all levels, internalization of the receptor is apparently important for the activation of MAP kinase kinase (MEK) and Erk1 only, not for the activation of upstream components such as Raf. Finally, other novel substrates for the GPCRs include tubulin, which is phosphorylated by the GRKs, and microtubules, which associate with GRKs. The functional significance of these findings is yet to be determined (43).

Signaling Mechanisms of G Protein–Coupled Receptors

The multiple transmembrane-spanning domains of the GPCRs cluster into a bundle to form a hydrophobic pocket for specific ligand binding. Certain amino acids in these hydrophobic domains are critical for specific ligand interactions (44,45). Regions of the GPCRs critical for transducing the signal generated by ligand binding are found in the second and third cytoplasmic loops (I-2 and I-3) and the proximal C-terminal tail (I-4). These loops form a binding site for the G proteins (46,47). It has been proposed that following ligand binding the receptor undergoes a conformational change that unmasks key intracellular amino acid residues of the GPCR, thereby allowing interaction of the G proteins and certain enzymes with the receptor (Fig. 3.2). For example, ligand binding to β_2-adrenergic receptors that are associated with the G_s proteins causes activation of the heterotrimeric G protein by replacement of GDP by GTP via a change in relative affinities of the guanine nucleotides for the $G\alpha$ subunit (48). The GTP-loaded $G\alpha$ dissociates from the $G\beta\gamma$, liberating the active $G\alpha$-GTP and the stable $G\beta\gamma$ heterodimer. The $G\alpha$-GTP subunit activates adenylyl cyclase, leading to elevation of intracellular cAMP (49,50). cAMP then leads to multiple intracellular responses, some of which are mediated by PKA. Control of this process occurs at multiple levels, leading to receptor desensitization and downregulation. Firstly, $G\alpha$ has inherent GTPase activity and can hydrolyze the GTP to GDP, thereby returning the G_s protein to the inactive heterotrimeric state. Secondly, the receptor becomes phosphorylated by PKA and βARK, which reduces its ability to activate G proteins (51). Thirdly, the phosphorylated receptor becomes a binding site for the proteins of the arrestin family that cause desensitization of the receptor, as described previously.

As a second example, it has been shown recently that lysophosphatidic acid (LPA), a bioactive intercellular lipid with mitogenic, cytoskeletal remodeling, and chemotactic properties, binds to at least two different receptors. These GPCRs can bind to at least three distinct G proteins, including G_q, G_i, and $G_{12/13}$. By coupling with different effectors, LPA-induced activation of its receptors can induce intracellular signals via PLC (G_q proteins), Ras·GTP accumulation and inhibition of adenylyl cyclase (pertussis

toxin–sensitive G_i proteins), and Rho activation (pertussis toxin–insensitive $G_{12/13}$ proteins). The exact mechanisms by which LPA receptors induce these signals and integrate with receptor systems using the same intracellular effector molecules remain to be fully elucidated.

GPCRs are involved in normal growth and tumorigenesis, and recently the pathways connecting these receptors to the nucleus have been elucidated in some detail (52). The family of MAP kinases has been shown to be major players in tumorigenic signaling, and GPCRs activate MAP kinases. These effects were not seen with G_{aq}, G_s, G_{ui2} (53) or G_{12} and suggested that $G\beta\gamma$ heterodimers may be responsible (54). Indeed, $G\beta\gamma$ heterodimers activate MAP kinase via a Ras-dependent pathway by inducing accumulation of GTP-bound Ras (55).

CYTOKINE RECEPTORS

Structure and Classes of Cytokine Receptors

The cytokine receptor superfamily comprises many members with common structural features in the extracellular domain (Fig. 3.3) (56). These receptors lack intrinsic enzyme activity; instead, they are bound to one of several cytoplasmic Janus kinases (JAKs). Some family members are comprised of a single protein chain, whereas others have multiple protein subunits (57). Class I receptors are comprised of a single transmembrane protein and include receptors for growth hormone (GH), prolactin (Prl), erythropoietin (EPO), thrombopoietin, and granulocyte-specific colony-stimulating factor (G-CSF). Class II receptors are multimeric proteins and the class is subdivided into subclasses. Class IIa receptors share the common γ_c subunit and include receptors for interleukins (ILs) -2, -4, -7, -9, and -15. Class IIb receptors have a β_c subunit and include receptors for IL-3, IL-5, and granulocyte-macrophage colony-stimulating factor (GM-CSF). Class IIc are receptors that share the gp130 subunit and include receptors for IL-6, IL-11, oncostatin M (OSM), leukemia inhibitory factor (LIF), ciliary neurotrophic factor (CNTF), and cardiotrophin. Class III receptors are those for

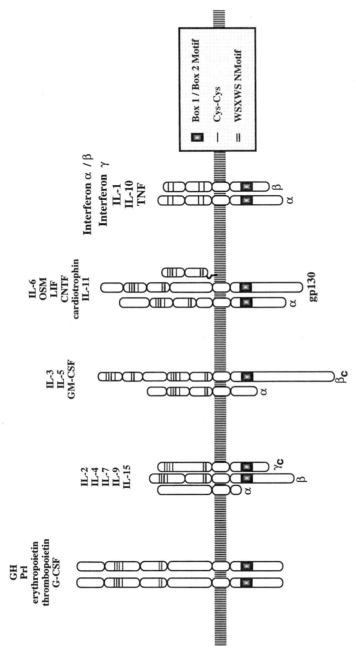

FIG. 3.3. Structure of cytokine receptors showing the formation of homodimers, heterodimers, and heterotrimers. Shown are the receptors for growth hormone (*GH*), prolactin (*Prl*), granulocyte colony-stimulating factor (*G-CSF*), granulocyte-macrophage colony-stimulating factor (*GM-CSF*), interleukins (*IL*), oncostatin M (*OSM*), ciliary neurotrophic factor (*CNTF*), leukemia inhibitory factor, and tumor necrosis factor (*TNF*).

tumor necrosis factor (TNF), interferon (IFN), and IL-1 and IL-10. Lastly, a few hematopoietic growth factors, that is, colony-stimulating factor-I (CSF-I), stem cell factor (SCF), and hepatocyte growth factor (HGF), are ligands for tyrosine kinase receptors that do not bind any of the cytokine receptors (58,59).

Ligand binding and receptor activation have been well characterized for some of the cytokine receptors. The human GH (hGH) receptor (class I) shares some structural features with the hematopoietic cytokine receptors (class II) in that it is comprised of multiple subunits and lacks intrinsic kinase activity. The hGH receptor does not have a WSXWS motif but rather a YGEFS motif, which may be important for the specificity of ligand binding (60). hGH binds to its receptor with a stoichiometry of one molecule of the ligand to two receptor molecules. hGH binds each receptor molecule sequentially via two independent sites. This results in dimerization of the receptors, which is followed by activation of the endogenous protein tyrosine kinase substrate JAK2. Elucidation of this process helped to explain the "bell-shaped" biological curve observed in cells treated with hGH, whereby very high concentrations of ligand inhibit function by preventing the dimerization process (61).

Signaling via Cytokine Receptors

Cytokine receptors are phosphorylated on tyrosine residues following ligand-induced activation but do not possess intrinsic kinase activity. The tyrosine phosphorylation is due to activation of the associated JAKs that are necessary for cytokine signaling. JAK homology domains that appear to be unique to this family of proteins are located in the N-terminal region. It has been postulated that the JAK homology domains determine the protein–protein interactions that govern the function of the individual cytokine receptor pathways. The exact mechanisms by which cytokine binding activates JAKs is not known; however, it has been hypothesized that induction of homo- or heterodimerization of receptor components causes the juxtaposition of their cytoplasmic domains, thereby activating JAK (62). JAKs interact directly with the membrane proximal domain of the receptor that contains the essential box1/box2 motifs (63).

The JAK family of kinases, including JAKs 1–3 and TYK2, are expressed at varying levels in different cells and tissues, and their activation pattern seems to vary appropriately with the levels of kinases expressed. Each cytokine receptor activates a different set of JAKs. For example, JAK2 is activated following stimulation with GH. However, if the stimulus is IL-2, IL-4, IL-7, or IL-9, then JAK1 and JAK3 are phosphorylated (64). The various permutations that are possible given the formation of these heterostructural complexes makes it possible for individual cells to respond to the wide array of circulating cytokines with high specificity. Evidence for the obligatory role of JAK1 and JAK2 was obtained by the generation of mice lacking the genes that encode these two proteins. JAK1-deficient mice are runted at birth, fail to nurse, and die perinatally. Furthermore, cytokine receptors of the class II type and those that use the γ_c subunit or the gp130 subunit for signaling are inactivated by the absence of JAK1. JAK2-deficient mice show embryonic lethality due to absent erythropoiesis. The responses to erythropoietin (EPO), thrombopoietin, IL-3, and GM-CSF are absent; however, responses to IFN-α/β and IL-6 are unaffected. These results suggest that JAK1 and JAK2 are essential for signaling through a wide variety of cytokine receptors.

The interaction of JAKs with members of the STAT (signal transducers and activators of transcription) family is critical for cytokine receptor signal transduction. The seven known STATs (STATs 1–4, STATs 5a and 5b, and STAT6) are activated by more than 30 different polypeptides (65). Recently, it has been shown that the STATs are substrates for the JAKs (Fig. 3.4) (66). It has been hypothesized that the specificity of phosphorylation of each particular STAT protein by a JAK is determined by the composition of the receptor complex. For example, GH receptor complexes phosphorylate STAT5 and IL-4 receptor complexes phosphorylate STAT6, while IL-6 receptor complexes phosphorylate both STAT1 and STAT3. The multiple STAT proteins that are substrates for particular cytokine receptors may well explain the pleiotropic responses seen with some cytokines. Following tyrosine phosphorylation, the STATs dimerize into homo- and heterodimers via reciprocal SH2–phosphotyrosine interactions and translocate to the nucleus, where the dimers bind the DNA through IFN-γ-activated sequence (GAS)-like sequences and stimulate transcription of downstream genes (67). In addition, some of the STATs, such as STAT1 and STAT3, must be serine-phosphorylated, with this phosphorylation apparently requiring activation of the MAP kinases in order to be fully activated (68). The specific serine kinase responsible for phosphorylating these STATs has not been identified. However, serine phosphorylation appears important in forming and maintaining homo- and heterodimers of STAT1 and STAT3. Other STATs, such as STAT2, are fully active with only tyrosine phosphorylation. STATs may have essential and nonessential roles in the cellular response to cytokine responses. In mice deficient for STAT5a and STAT5b, either individually or combined, responses to EPO were normal. Combined STAT5a/b mutant mice responded less well to IL-3 and GM-CSF, whereas this combination led to ovarian dysfunction due to interference with Prl receptor signaling and a phenotype comparable to the GH receptor–deficient mouse. Thus, while STAT5a and STAT5b are redundant, the STAT5 proteins are essential for Prl and GH receptor responses (69).

Other signaling pathways activated by cytokine receptors include PI3'-K, vav, and Ras (70,71) (Fig. 3.4). These pathways represent possible interception points whereby cytokines can elicit trans-signaling with cascades used by other types of receptor. Some specific examples are given below (see Crosstalk Between Receptor Signaling Pathways).

CELL ADHESION RECEPTORS

Cell–substrate Adhesion Complexes

Integrins, cadherins, selectin, and immunoglobulin superfamily members are crucial in the maintenance of cellular structure. Generally, cell–extracellular matrix (ECM) adhesions contain integrin-type receptors, whereas cell–cell adhesions involve cadherins. Studies of the supramolecular complexes that link the intracellular cytoskeletal proteins through integrins to the ECM have provided evidence of substrates that may be modified and activated by ligand-bound integrins. These supramolecular complexes include focal contact proteins (e.g., α-actinin, talin, and filamin) that have been shown to interact directly with the cytoplasmic domains of the various integrin subtypes (72,73). These interactions direct the assembly of actin filaments via the formation of complex structures comprised of vinculin, paxillin, p130^{Cas}, Src, Crk, and focal adhesion kinase (FAK), to list a few of the proteins identified in focal adhesion complexes. The exact mechanisms by which integrins direct the assembly of the cytoskeleton have not been fully elucidated; however, it is apparent that the composition of focal adhesion complexes varies depending on the state of integrin aggregation, ligand occupancy, and/or the phosphorylation of proteins within the complex.

Classes and Structures of Cell Adhesion Receptors

The integrin family of receptors is comprised of transmembrane proteins composed of noncovalently bound α- and β-subunit heterodimers (74). The α subunits ($\sim$1,000 amino acids) are larger than the β subunits ($\sim$750 amino acids). The majority of the receptor complex is extracellular, with both the α and β subunits possessing only small cytoplasmic domains. Integrins interact with ligands in the ECM, such as the vitronectins, collagens, and fibronectins (75). The interaction of integrins with extracellular proteins led not only to reorganization of the cytoskeleton, as noted above, but also to activation of kinase signaling cascades, gene expression, and growth, establishing this family of transmembrane proteins as bona fide signaling receptors (76). In addition, the extracellular domains of the integrins bind to other cell surface receptors, including intercellular adhesion molecule-1 (ICAM-1) and vascular cell adhesion molecule-1 (VCAM-1). These interactions result in activation of intracellular signaling cascades (76–79).

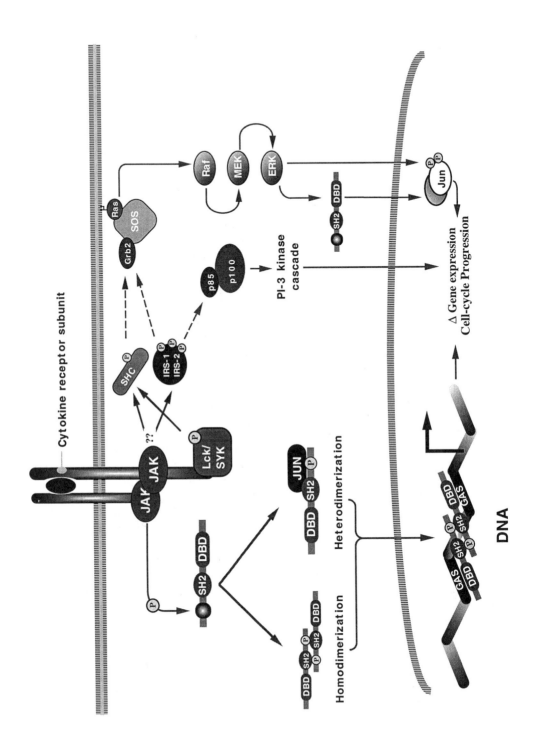

Signaling Molecules of the Integrin-mediated Adhesion Complex

Ligand binding to integrins results in increased tyrosine phosphorylation of several proteins located in focal adhesion complexes, such as paxillin, FAK, p130^{Cas}, and tensin. The tyrosine phosphorylation of the integrin subunits themselves is also affected. It is clear that ligand-induced tyrosine phosphorylation of proteins in the focal adhesion complex activates signal-transduction cascades. FAK has an important role in signal transduction of the focal adhesion complex. FAK is a 125-kDa protein that is non-myristylated and does not bind directly to phospholipid membranes. It binds to the short cytoplasmic domains of the β subunits of integrin via its amino-terminal "integrin-binding" region and a carboxy-terminal region named FAT (80,81). The intrinsic kinase of FAK is activated by adhesion of the cell to the extracellular matrix (ECM) (82). FAK associates with various proteins in focal adhesion complexes. Some of these interactions, such as FAK–p130^{Cas}, are constitutive, whereas other interactions, such as FAK–Src, are induced by tyrosine phosphorylation or integrin aggregation. The interactions occur via motifs that are conserved in many signal-transduction proteins. Phosphotyrosine residues and proline-rich regions of one protein interact with the SH2 and SH3 domains of other proteins, respectively. The SH3 domains of p130^{Cas} and a newly discovered member of the Rho GTPase-activating protein family referred to as GRAF (GTPase regulator associated with FAK) bind with high affinity to the proline-rich region of FAK that lies proximal to the FAK catalytic domain (83,84). When cells interact with the ECM and form focal adhesions, p130^{Cas} and paxillin are phosphorylated on tyrosine residues, allowing for the interaction of p130^{Cas} and Src via SH2 domains with Crk and paxillin. An inducible interaction of Src and FAK occurs following integrin interaction with the ECM (85,86). FAK undergoes autophosphorylation on tyrosine residue 397 (Tyr^{397}), thereby creating a high-affinity phosphotyrosine-binding site for the SH2 domains of proteins of the Src family kinases, such as Src, Fyn, and PI3′-K (87). The phosphorylation of tyrosine residues in the catalytic and C-terminal domains, such as Tyr^{925}, is important for interactions with Grb2 (88), which may activate the Ras/Raf/MAP kinase pathway.

Other protein kinases that are activated by integrin-mediated cell adhesion include the MAP kinases p42 and p44 (Erk1 and Erk2 in mammalian cells) (Fig. 3.5) (87). The pathway(s) of activation could involve Grb2 or PI3′-K, both of which associate with FAK, or IRS-1, which interacts with integrin $\alpha\nu\beta$1 (89). Another potential pathway is via PKC, which is activated upon cell adherence to fibronectin (90). SHC, another adapter protein, couples $\alpha\nu\beta$3 and subsets of β_1 integrins to the Ras signaling pathway and gene expression of immediate-early genes such as c-*fos*. Adapter proteins, such as Nck and Crk, that

---

FIG. 3.4. Signal-transduction cascades activated by cytokine receptors. Cytokine receptors lack intrinsic kinase activity, with the associated Janus kinase *(JAK)* being activated upon ligand binding. JAK then phosphorylates members of the signal transduction and activators of transcription (STAT) protein family. Tyrosine phosphorylation of STAT proteins induces dimerization through the binding of Src homology *(SH)* 2 domains, present in the N-terminal half of the protein, to SH2-binding domains. STATs form homodimers and heterodimers within the STAT family (STAT1, STAT2, STAT3, STAT4, STAT5a, STAT5b, and STAT6). Alternatively, STATs may dimerize with proteins other than STATs, such as Jun. STAT dimers translocate to the nucleus, where STATs control transcription through the binding of the STAT DNA-binding domain *(DBD)* to γ-interferon-activated sequences *(GAS)* present in gene promoters. Other pathways may also be activated by cytokine receptors; for example, the MAP kinase cascade may be activated by insulin receptor substrate *(IRS)*-1 or Shc-Grb2. IRS-1 may also couple the cytokine receptors to the phosphatidylinositol-3′-kinase pathway, via the association of the p85 regulatory subunit to tyrosine-phosphorylated IRS-1. The Src-like kinases Lck and SYK bind to the C-terminal regions of some cytokine receptors and participate in cytokine receptor signal transduction possibly by phosphorylating Shc.

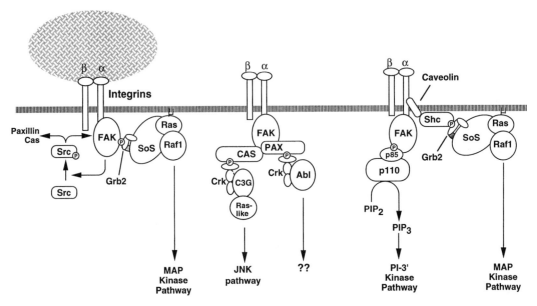

FIG. 3.5. An example of signal-transduction pathways emanating from adhesion complexes. Integrin activation after binding to the extracellular matrix is associated with activation of multiple signal-transduction pathways. The Ras–MAP kinase pathway can be activated via several mechanisms: binding of Grb2 to focal adhesion kinase *(FAK)*, binding of Grb2 to tyrosine-phosphorylated Shc, or indirectly via the phosphatidylinositol-3'-kinase pathway. The increased tyrosine phosphorylation of Cas and paxillin associated with FAK activation creates binding sites for the SH2 domains of the Crk adapter proteins, thus activating the c-Jun N-terminal kinase *(JNK)* pathway, while the nonreceptor tyrosine kinase Abl has been implicated in oncogenic transformation.

bind p130^{Cas} may also lead to activation of Ras and Ras-like proteins via their associations with the nucleotide exchange proteins mSOS and C3G (91,92).

In addition to integrin activation of FAK, growth factors such as PDGF and IGF-I, for example, activate FAK, suggesting that there is an integration of signals between the integrins and growth factor receptors. Since wortmannin, a fungal product that inhibits PI3'-K, blocks PDGF-stimulated FAK activity, it has been suggested that at least some of the signaling pathways involved in growth factor activation of FAK are mediated by PI3'-K (93). This provides functional evidence supporting the finding that a number of proteins involved in growth factor signal-transduction pathways accumulate in focal adhesion complexes (94).

CROSSTALK BETWEEN RECEPTOR SIGNALING PATHWAYS

The most exciting aspect of recent studies of growth factor receptor signaling has been the elucidation that no one system signals in isolation. Trans-signaling or receptor crosstalk signaling is an area of intense study. Trans-signaling may occur directly at the level of cell surface receptors or through their downstream signaling intermediates. To illustrate this growing area of investigation, we highlight a number of different examples that have recently been described. Further examples of receptor crosstalk have been reviewed (95).

Tumor cell motility involves cell attachment to the ECM, allowing cellular migration and invasion (96). While integrins are essential for this process, they are not sufficient. Tumor cells expressing the integrin $\alpha\nu\beta5$, which facilitates adhesion to vitronectin, also require tyrosine kinase receptor-mediated signaling for motility on vitronectin. IGF-I stimulates the colocalization of $\alpha\nu\beta5$ integrin and α-actinin, implicating both the IGF-I receptor and the actin cytoskeleton as necessary for cell migration (97). Similarly, PKC activators also facilitate $\alpha\nu\beta5$ integrin-dependent cell spreading and migration on vitronectin (98).

GPCRs produce cellular responses similar to those of growth factor receptors via activation of the MAP kinase cascade (99). While GPCR activation may induce this pathway via G$\beta\gamma$-heterodimer signaling mechanisms, the GPCR may also activate the growth factor receptor tyrosine kinase activity independent of ligand binding. Examples of this mechanism include the thrombin receptor inducing autophosphorylation of the EGF receptor in Rat-1 fibroblasts and autophosphorylation of the PDGF receptor by angiotensin II treatment of smooth muscle (100,101). The convergence of these different classes of receptors on mitogenesis was previously attributed to common intermediate substrates such as G protein–mediated Src activation affecting the Grb2/SHC/p21^{ras} pathway (102), but it appears that direct receptor transsignaling may also occur (103). Interestingly, one mechanism that may be common to these processes is Src activation, which has been shown to directly autophosphorylate the IGF-I receptor (104). Not all crosstalk between membrane receptors involves stimulation of the said pathways; in fact, TNF-α inhibits insulin signaling by decreasing the tyrosine phosphorylation of the insulin receptor and IRS-I (105). The mechanism whereby TNF-α inhibits the insulin receptor–IRS-1 signaling pathway may involve activation of the ceramide pathway following sphingomyelinase activation (106).

An interesting example of common signaling pathways between different classes of receptors is the role of the IRS-1 and IRS-2 molecules. Originally discovered as major substrates in insulin and IGF-I receptor signaling, these molecules apparently also play roles in cytokine receptor signaling (Fig. 3.6). Activated insulin and IGF-I receptors phosphorylate IRS-1 and IRS-2 on tyrosine residues and then use them as interfaces with SH2 domain–containing proteins. These interactions bring the SH2 domain–containing proteins into close proximity with the receptors, promoting phosphorylation and subsequent signaling via the appropriate downstream cascades (107). In addition, the IRS proteins are phosphorylated by the JAKs,

themselves activated by various cytokines, including IL-2, IL-4, IL-9, IL-13, LIF, IFN-α, IFN-β, IFN-γ, and GH (108). GH has been shown to activate the Ras/MEK/Erk pathway, an effect that is blocked by both PD098059 and wortmannin, which block MEK and PI3'-K, respectively. These effects may originate at the level of IRS phosphorylation (109). Traditionally it was thought that activated STATs were involved exclusively in cytokine receptor signaling pathways; however, STATs are also physiologically relevant to tyrosine kinase receptors. STAT5 has been found to be a direct substrate of the insulin receptor, whereas STAT1 and STAT3 may be activated directly by the EGF receptor without the need of JAK activation (110,111).

A third example of crosstalk between receptor signaling cascades is that of cAMP, first identified as a secondary messenger of GPCRs. cAMP commonly inhibits growth factor–stimulated cell growth in fibroblasts and smooth muscle cells. The mechanism that has been proposed to explain these findings includes cAMP inhibition of growth factor–induced activation of the Erks (112). However, in some cells, cAMP may enhance the activation of Erks. In PC12 cells, cAMP induces differentiation by activation of MAP kinase and the transcription factor Elk-1. The pathways leading to this event include PKA activation of Rap1 (a small G protein), which in turns activates B-Raf (113). Thus, in specific cell types, GPCRs via cAMP may utilize the MAP kinase pathway to induce differentiation and inhibit proliferation.

An important aspect of cell biology is cancer growth, and breast cancer represents an interesting example of where growth factor signaling and steroid hormone effects interact. During late stages of breast cancer progression, progesterone may upregulate the responsiveness of the cells to EGF. Progesterone upregulates the EGF receptor, c-ErbB2, and c-ErbB3 receptors and enhances STAT5 protein levels and the subsequent phosphorylation of JAK2 and SHC. These effects result in activation of the MAP kinase pathway and increased cyclin D1 and cyclin E levels. Breast cancer cell growth provides a clear demonstration of synergy between a steroid hor-

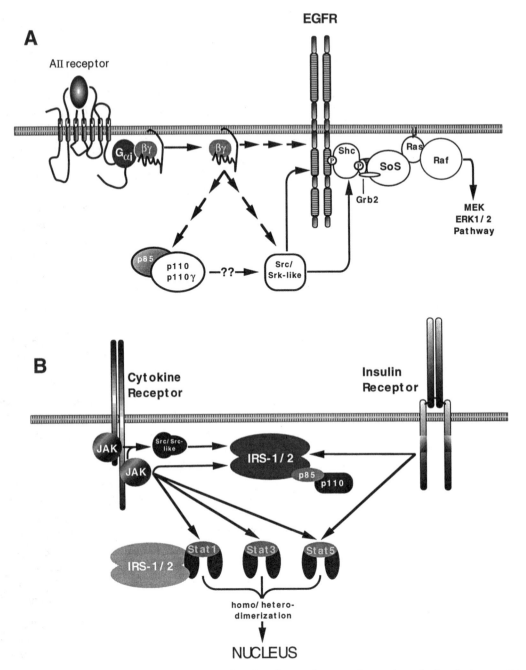

FIG. 3.6. Examples of crosstalk between the signaling pathways of receptors. In the first example **(A)**, the utilization of the mitogenic epidermal growth factor receptor *(EGFR)* by the β2-adrenergic receptor to activate the Ras–MAP kinase cascade is outlined. Gβγ influences EGFR activity by activating Src kinase, which phosphorylates and activates the EGFR kinase. Gβγ activates Src kinase by two possible mechanisms, either binding directly to Src or indirectly by activation of the phosphatidylinositol-3′-kinase pathway (shown are the p85 regulatory and p110 catalytic subunits). Crosstalk also occurs between cytokine receptors (growth hormone receptor, interleukin-4 receptor) and class II receptor tyrosine kinases (insulin and insulin-like growth factor-I receptors). Insulin, growth hormone, and interleukin-4 induce the tyrosine phosphorylation of insulin receptor substrate-1 *(IRS-1)*, either by direct interaction and phosphorylation (insulin receptor) or indirectly through Src/Src-like kinase (cytokines). STAT5 is a substrate of the insulin receptor, while STAT1 may interact directly with IRS-1.

mone response and a growth factor receptor response (114).

CONCLUSIONS

This brief review illustrates the diversity and complexity of signaling mechanisms by which extracellular signals are transduced intracellularly. It is our hope that we were able to impress on the reader the presence of both the common signaling pathways used by the various families of receptors and the intricacies of trans-signaling or crosstalk between the signaling pathways. While these pathways are still being uncovered, it is clear that they are critical for the normal function of all cells and tissues, including the skeletal system. Furthermore, understanding the normal physiology of signal transduction will enable us to understand the derangements involved in pathological states and lead to more appropriate therapeutic modalities for such common diseases as osteoporosis.

REFERENCES

1. Ullrich A, Schlessinger J. Signal transduction by receptors with tyrosine kinase activity. *Cell* 1990;61: 203–212.
2. Yarden Y, Ullrich A. Molecular analysis of signal transduction by growth factors. *Biochemistry* 1988;27: 3113–3119.
3. Le Rotih D, Werner H, Beitner-Johnson D, et al. Molecular and cellular aspects of the insulin-like growth factor I receptor. *Endocr Rev* 1995;16:143–163.
4. Rusch V, Mendelsohn J, Dmitrovsky E. The epidermal growth factor receptor and its ligands as therapeutic targets in human tumors. *Cytokine Growth Factor Rev* 1996;7:133–141.
5. Tzahar E, Waterman H, Chen X, et al. A hierarchical network of interreceptor interactions determines signal transduction by New differentiation factor/neuregulin and epidermal growth factor. *Mol Cell Biol* 1996;16: 5276–5287.
6. Soos MA, Field CE, Siddle K. Purified hybrid insulin–insulin-like growth factor-I receptors bind insulin-like growth factor-I, but not insulin, with high affinity. *Biochem J* 1993;290:419–426.
7. Frattali AL, Pessin JE. Relationship between alpha subunit ligand occupancy and beta subunit autophosphorylation in insulin–insulin-like growth factor-1 hybrid receptors. *J Biol Chem* 1993;268:7393–7400.
8. Lemmon MA, Schlessinger J. Regulation of signal transduction and signal diversity by receptor oligomerization. *Trends Biochem Sci* 1994;19:459–463.
9. Hubbard SR, Mohammadi M, Schlessinger J. Autoregulatory mechanisms in protein-tyrosine kinases. *J Biol Chem* 1998;273:11987–11990.
10. Weiss A, Schlessinger J. Switching signals on or off by receptor dimerization. *Cell* 1998;94:277–280.
11. Rozakis-Adcock M, Fernley R, Wade J, et al. The SH2 and SH3 domains of mammalian Grb2 couple the EGF receptor to the Ras activator mSos1 (see comments). *Nature* 1993;363:83–85.
12. Crews CM, Erikson RL. Extracellular signals and reversible protein phosphorylation: what to Mek of it all. *Cell* 1993;74:215–217.
13. Myers MG Jr, Backer JM, Sun XJ, et al. IRS-1 activates phosphatidylinositol 3′-kinase by associating with src homology 2 domains of p85. *Proc Natl Acad Sci USA* 1992;89:10350–10354.
14. Myers MG Jr, Sun XJ, Cheatham B, et al. IRS-1 is a common element in insulin and insulin-like growth factor-I signaling to the phosphatidylinositol 3′-kinase. *Endocrinology* 1993;132:1421–1430.
15. Kotani K, Carozzi AJ, Sakaue H, et al. Requirement for phosphoinositide 3-kinase in insulin-stimulated GLUT4 translocation in 3T3-L1 adipocytes. *Biochem Biophys Res Commun* 1995;209:343–348.
16. Seger R, Krebs EG. The MAPK signaling cascade. *Faseb J* 1995;9:726–735.
17. Yang BS, Hauser CA, Henkel G, et al. Ras-mediated phosphorylation of a conserved threonine residue enhances the transactivation activities of c-Ets1 and c-Ets2. *Mol Cell Biol* 1996;16:538–547.
18. Waskiewicz AJ, Flynn A, Proud CG, et al. Mitogen-activated protein kinases activate the serine-threonine kinases Mnk1 and Mnk2. *EMBO J* 1997;16:1909–1920.
19. Lin TA, Kong X, Haystead TA, et al. PHAS-I as a link between mitogen-activated protein kinase and translation initiation (see comments). *Science* 1994;266: 653–655.
20. Attisano L, Wrana JL, Lopez-Casillas F, et al. TGF-beta receptors and actions. *Biochem Biophys Acta* 1994;1222:71–80.
21. Wrana JL, Attisano L, Wieser R, et al. Mechanism of activation of the TGF-beta receptor. *Nature* 1994;370: 341–347.
22. Attisano L, Wrana JL. Signal transduction by members of the transforming growth factor-beta superfamily. *Cytokine Growth Factor Rev* 1996;7:327–339.
23. Wieser R, Wrana JL, Massague J. GS domain mutations that constitutively activate T beta R-I, the downstream signaling component in the TGF-beta receptor complex. *EMBO J* 1995;14:2199–2208.
24. Weis-Barcia F, Massague J. Complementation between kinase-defective and activation-defective TGF-beta receptors reveals a novel form of receptor cooperativity essential for signaling. *EMBO J* 1996;15: 276–289.
25. Andres DA, Goldstein JL, Ho YK, et al. Mutational analysis of alpha-subunit of protein farnesyltransferase. Evidence for a catalytic role. *J Biol Chem* 1993; 268:1383–1390.
26. Yamaguchi K, Shirakabe K, Shibuya H, et al. Identification of a member of the MAPKKK family as a potential mediator of TGF-beta signal transduction. *Science* 1995;270:2008–2011.
27. Eppert K, Schere SW, Ozcelik H, et al. MADR2 maps to 18q21 and encodes a TGFbeta-regulated MAD-related protein that is functionally mutated in colorectal carcinoma. *Cell* 1996;86:543–552.

28. Hogan BL. Bone morphogenetic proteins: multifunctional regulators of vertebrate development. *Genes Dev* 1996;10:1580–1594.

29. Ten Dijke P, Yamashita H, Sampath TK, et al. Identification of type I receptors for osteogenic protein-1 and bone morphogenetic protein-4. *J Biol Chem* 1994;269:16985–16988.

30. Rosenzweig BL, Imamura T, Okadome T, et al. Cloning and characterization of a human type II receptor for bone morphogenetic proteins. *Proc Natl Acad Sci USA* 1995;92:7632–7636.

31. Nohno T, Ishikawa T, Saito T, et al. Identification of a human type II receptor for bone morphogenetic protein-4 that forms differential heteromeric complexes with bone morphogenetic protein type I receptors. *J Biol Chem* 1995;270:22522–22526.

32. Koenig BB, Cook JS, Wolsing DH, et al. Characterization and cloning of a receptor for BMP-2 and BMP-4 from NIH 3T3 cells. *Mol Cell Biol* 1994;14:5961–5974.

33. Wu RY, Zhang Y, Feng XH, et al. Heteromeric and homomeric interactions correlate with signaling activity and functional cooperativity of Smad3 and Smad4/DPC4. *Mol Cell Biol* 1997;17:2521–2528.

34. Ji TH, Gorssmann M, Ji I. G protein–coupled receptors. I. Diversity of receptor–ligand interactions. *J Biol Chem* 1998;273:17299–17302.

35. Grossmann M, Weintraub BD, Szkudlinski MW. Novel insights into the molecular mechanisms of human thyrotropin action: structural, physiological, and therapeutic implications for the glycoprotein hormone family. *Endocr Rev* 1997;18:476–501.

36. Gether U, Kobilka BK. G protein–coupled receptors. II. Mechanism of agonist activation. *J Biol Chem* 1998;273:17979–17982.

37. Skiba NP, Bae H, Hamm HE. Mapping of effector binding sites of transducin alpha-subunit using G alpha t/G alpha i 1 chimeras. *J Biol Chem* 1996;271:413–424.

38. Lefkowitz RJ. G protein–coupled receptors. III. New roles for receptor kinases and beta-arrestins in receptor signaling and desensitization. *J Biol Chem* 1998;273:18677–18680.

39. Luttrell LM, Daaka Y, Della Rocca GJ, et al. G protein–coupled receptors mediate two functionally distinct pathways of tyrosine phosphorylation in rat 1 a fibroblasts. Shc phosphorylation and receptor endocytosis correlate with activation of Erk kinases. *J Biol Chem* 1997;272:31648–31656.

40. Sibley DR, Strasser RH, Benovic JL, et al. Phosphorylation/dephosphorylation of the beta-adrenergic receptor regulates its functional coupling to adenylate cyclase and subcellular distribution. *Proc Natl Acad Sci USA* 1986;83:9408–9412.

41. Zhang J, Barak LS, Winkler KE, et al. A central role for beta arrestins and clathrin-coated vesicle-mediated endocytosis resensitization in two distinct cell types. *J Biol Chem* 1997;272:27005–27014.

42. Pitcher JA, Payne ES, Csortos C, et al. The G-protein-coupled receptor phosphatase: a protein phosphatase type 2A with a distinct subcellular distribution and substrate specificity. *Proc Natl Acad Sci USA* 1995;92:8343–8347.

43. Pitcher JA, Hall RA, Daaka Y, et al. The G protein–coupled receptor kinase 2 is a microtubule-associated protein kinase that phosphorylates tubulin. *J Biol Chem* 1998;273:12316–12324.

44. Schertler GF, Villa C, Henderson R. Projection structure of rhodopsin. *Nature* 1993;362:770–772.

45. Dohlman HG, Caron MG, Strader CD, et al. Identification and sequence of a binding site peptide of the beta 2-adrenergic receptor. *Biochemistry* 1988;27:1813–1817.

46. O'Dowd BF, Hantowich M, Regan JW, et al. Site-directed mutagenesis of the cytoplasmic domains of the human beta 2-adrenergic receptor. Localization of regions involved in G protein-receptor coupling. *J Biol Chem* 1988;263:15985–15992.

47. Suryanarayana S, von Zastrow M, Kobilka BK. Identification of intramolecular interactions in adrenergic receptors. *J Biol Chem* 1992;267:21991–21994.

48. Lambright DG, Noel JP, Hamm HE, et al. Structural determinants for activation of the alpha-subunit of a heterotrimeric G protein (see comments). *Nature* 1994;369:621–628.

49. Taussig R, Quarmby LM, Gilman AG. Regulation of purified type I and type II adenylylcyclases by G protein beta gamma subunits. *J Biol Chem* 1993;268:9–12.

50. Chen J, DeVivo M, Dingus J, et al. A region of adenylyl cylcase 2 critical for regulation by G protein beta gamma subunits. *Science* 1995;268:1166–1169.

51. Hausdorff WP, Bouvier M, O'Dowd BF, et al. Phosphorylation sites on two domains of the beta 2-adrenergic receptor are involved in distinct pathways of receptor desensitization. *J Biol Chem* 1989;264:12657–12665.

52. Gutkind JS. The pathways connecting G protein–coupled receptors to the nucleus through divergent mitogen-activated protein kinase cascades. *J Biol Chem* 1998;273:1839–1842.

53. Crespo P, Xu N, Simonds WF, et al. Ras-dependent activation of MAP kinase pathway mediated by G-protein beta gamma subunits (see comments). *Nature* 1994;369:418–420.

54. Clapham DE, Neer EJ. G protein beta gamma subunits. *Annu Rev Pharmacol Toxicol* 1997;37:167–203.

55. Koch WJ, Hawes BE, Allen LF, et al. Direct evidence that Gi-coupled receptor stimulation of mitogen-activated protein kinase is mediated by G beta gamma activation of p21ras. *Proc Natl Acad Sci USA* 1994;91:12706–12710.

56. Ihle JN, Witthuhn BA, Quelle FW, et al. Signaling through the hematopoietic cytokine receptors. *Annu Rev Immunol* 1995;13:369–398.

57. Stahl N, Yancopoulos GD. The alphas, betas, and kinases of cytokine receptor complexes. *Cell* 1993;74:587–590.

58. Sato N, Miyajima A. Multimeric cytokine receptors: common versus specific function. *Curr Opin Cell Biol* 1994;6:174–179.

59. Taga T, Kishimoto T. Signaling mechanisms through cytokine receptors that share signal transducing receptor components. *Curr Opin Immunol* 1995;7:17–23.

60. Baumgartner JW, Wells CA, Chen CM, et al. The role of the WSXWS equivalent motif in growth hormone receptor function. *J Biol Chem* 1994;269:29094–29101.

61. Staten NR, Byatt JC, Krivi GG. Ligand-specific dimerization of the extracellular domain of the bovine

growth hormone receptor. *J Biol Chem* 1993;268: 18467–18473.

62. Davis S, Aldrich TH, Stahl N, et al. LIFR beta and gp130 as heterodimerizing signal transducers of the tripartite CNTF receptor. *Science* 1993;260:1805–1808.

63. Quelle FW, Sato N, Witthuhn BA, et al. JAK2 associates with the beta c chain of the receptor for granulocyte-macrophage colony-stimulating factor, and its activation requires the membrane-proximal region. *Mol Cell Biol* 1994;14:4335–4341.

64. Ihle JN. The Janus protein tyrosine kinase family and its role in cytokine signaling. *Adv Immunol* 1995;60: 1–35.

65. Horvath CM, Darnell JE. The state of the STATs: recent developments in the study of signal transduction to the nucleus. *Curr Opin Cell Biol* 1997;9:233–239.

66. Quelle FW, Thierfelder W, Witthuhn BA, et al. Phosphorylation and activation of the DNA binding activity of purified Stat 1 by the Janus protein-tyrosine kinases and the epidermal growth factor receptor. *J Biol Chem* 1995;270:20775–20780.

67. Gupta S, Yan H, Wong LH, et al. The SH2 domains of Stat1 and Stat2 mediate multiple interactions in the transduction of IFN-alpha signals. *EMBO J* 1996;15: 1075–1084.

68. Wen Z, Zhong Z, Darnell JE Jr. Maximal activation of transcription by Stat1 and Stat3 requires both tyrosine and serine phosphorylation. *Cell* 1995;82:241–250.

69. Teglund S, McKay C, Schuetz E, et al. Stat5a and Stat5b proteins have essential and nonessential, or redundant, roles in cytokine responses. *Cell* 1998;93: 841–850.

70. Satoh T, Nakafuku M, Miyajima A, et al. Involvement of ras p21 protein in signal-transduction pathways from interleukin 2, interleukin 3, and granulocyte-macrophage colony-stimulating factor, but not from interleukin 4. *Proc Natl Acad Sci USA* 1991;88:3314–3318.

71. Miura O, Miura Y, Nakamura N, et al. Induction of tyrosine phosphorylation of Vav and expression of Pim-1 correlates with Jak2-mediated growth signaling from the erythropoietin receptor. *Blood* 1994;84: 4135–4141.

72. Parsons JT. Integrin-mediated signalling: regulation by protein tyrosine kinases and small GTP-binding proteins. *Curr Opin Cell Biol* 1996;8:146–152.

73. Schwartz MA, Schaller MD, Ginsberg MH. Integrins: emerging paradigms of signal transduction. *Annu Rev Cell Dev Biol* 1995;11:549–599.

74. Hynes RO. Integrins: versatility, modulation, and signaling in cell adhesion. *Cell* 1992;69:11–25.

75. Burridge K, Turner CE, Romer LH. Tyrosine phosphorylation of paxillin and pp125FAK accompanies cell adhesion to extracellular matrix: a role in cytoskeletal assembly. *J Cell Biol* 1992;119:893–903.

76. Meredith JE Jr., Winitz S, Lewis JM, et al. The regulation of growth and intracellular signaling by integrins. *Endocr Rev* 1996;17:207–220.

77. Yamada KM, Geiger B. Molecular interactions in cell adhesion complexes. *Curr Opin Cell Biol* 1997;9: 76–85.

78. Clark EA, Brugge JS. Integrins and signal transduction pathways: the road taken. *Science* 1995;268:233–239.

79. Geiger B, Yehuda-Levenberg S, Bershadsky AD. Molecular interactions in the submembrane plaque of cell–cell and cell–matrix adhesions. *Acta Anat* 1995; 1654:46–62.

80. Miyamoto S, Teramoto H, Coso OA, et al. Integrin function: molecular hierarchies of cytoskeletal and signaling molecules. *J Cell Biol* 1995;131:791–805.

81. Schaller MD, Parsons JT. Pp125FAK-dependent tyrosine phosphorylation of paxillin creates a high-affinity binding site for Crk. *Mol Cell Biol* 1995;15:2635–2645.

82. Guan JL, Shalloway D. Regulation of focal adhesion-associated protein tyrosine kinase by both cellular adhesion and oncogenic transformation. *Nature* 1992; 358:690–692.

83. Polte TR, Hanks SK. Interaction between focal adhesion kinase and Crk-associated tyrosine kinase substrate p130Cas. *Proc Natl Acad Sci USA* 1995;92: 10678–10682.

84. Burbelo PD, Miyamoto S, Utani A, et al. P190-B, a new member of the Rho GAP family, and Rho are induced to cluster after integrin cross-linking. *J Biol Chem* 1995;270:30919–30926.

85. Nojima Y, Morino N, Mimura T, et al. Integrin-mediated cell adhesion promotes tyrosine phosphorylation of p130Cas, a Src homology 3-containing molecule having multiple Src homology 2-binding motifs. *J Biol Chem* 1995;270:15398–15402.

86. Schaller MD, Otey CA, Hildebrand JD, et al. Focal adhesion kinase and paxillin bind to peptides mimicking beta integrin cytoplasmic domains. *J Cell Biol* 1995;130:1181–1187.

87. Chen Q, Kinch MS, Lin TH, et al. Integrin-mediated cell adhesion activates mitogen-activated protein kinases. *J Biol Chem* 1994;269:26602–26605.

88. Schlaepfer DD, Hanks SK, Hunter T, et al. Integrin-mediated signal transduction linked to Ras pathway by GRB2 binding to focal adhesion kinase. *Nature* 1994; 372:786–791.

89. Vuori K, Ruoslahti E. Association of insulin receptor substrate-1 with integrins. *Science* 1994;266:1576–1578.

90. Vuori K, Ruoslahti E. Activation of protein kinase C precedes alpha 5 beta 1 integrin-mediated cell spreading on fibronectin. *J Biol Chem* 1993;268:21459–21462.

91. Wary KK, Mainiero F, Isakoff SJ, et al. The adaptor protein Shc couples a class of integrins to the control of cell cycle progression. *Cell* 1996;87:733–743.

92. Schlaepfer DD, Broome MA, Hunter T. Fibronectin-stimulated signaling from a focal adhesion kinase–c-Src complex: involvement of the Grb2, p130cas, and Nck adaptor proteins. *Mol Cell Biol* 1997;17: 1702–1713.

93. Rankin S, Hooshmand-Rad R, Claesson-Welsh L, et al. Requirement for phosphatidylinositol 3′-kinase activity in platelet-derived growth factor-stimulated tyrosine phosphorylation of p125 focal adhesion kinase and paxillin. *J Biol Chem* 1996;271:7829–7834.

94. Plopper GE, McNamee HP, Dike LE, et al. Convergence of integrin and growth factor receptor signaling pathways within the focal adhesion complex. *Mol Cell Biol* 1995;6:1349–1365.

95. Castellino AM, Chao MV. Trans-signaling by cytokine and growth factor receptors. *Cytokine Growth Factor Rev* 1996;7:297–302.

96. Akiyama SK, Olden K, Yamada KM. Fibronectin and integrins in invasion and metastasis. *Cancer Metastasis Rev* 1995;14:173–189.

97. Brooks PC, Klemke RL, Schon S, et al. Insulin-like growth factor receptor cooperates with integrin alpha v beta 5 to promote tumor cell dissemination in vivo. *J Clin Invest* 1997;99:1390–1398.

98. Lewis JM, Cheresh DA, Schwartz MA. Protein kinase C regulates alpha v beta 5-dependent cytoskeletal associations and focal adhesion kinase phosphorylation. *J Cell Biol* 1996;134:1323–1332.

99. Van Biesen T, Luttrell LM, Hawes BE, et al. Mitogenic signaling via G protein–coupled receptors. *Endocr Rev* 1996;17:698–714.

100. Daub H, Weiss FU, Wallasch C, et al. Role of transactivation of the EGF receptor in signalling by G-protein-coupled receptors. *Nature* 1996;379:557–560.

101. Linseman DA, Benjamin CW, Jones DA. Convergence of angiotensin II and platelet-derived growth factor receptor signaling cascades in vascular smooth muscle cells. *J Biol Chem* 1995;270:12563–12568.

102. Luttrell LM, van Biesen T, Hawes BE, et al. G beta gamma subunits mediate mitogen-activated protein kinase activation by the tyrosine kinase insulin-like growth factor 1 receptor. *J Biol Chem* 1995;270:16495–16498.

103. Dikic I, Tikiwa G, Lev S, et al. A role for Pyk2 and Src in linking G-protein-coupled receptors with MAP kinase activation. *Nature* 1996;383:547–550.

104. Peterson JE, Kulik G, Jelinek T, et al. Src phosphorylates the insulin-like growth factor type I receptor on the autophosphorylation sites. Requirement for transformation by src. *J Biol Chem* 1996;271:31562–31571.

105. Hotamisligil GS, Murray DL, Choy LN, et al. Tumor necrosis factor alpha inhibits signaling from the insulin receptor. *Proc Natl Acad Sci USA* 1994;91:4854–4858.

106. Peraldi P, Hotamisligil GS, Buurman WA, et al. Tumor necrosis factor (TNF)-alpha inhibits insulin signaling through stimulation of the p55 TNF receptor and activation of sphingomyelinase. *J Biol Chem* 1996;271:13018–13022.

107. White MF. The IRS-1 signaling system. *Curr Opin Genet Dev* 1994;4:47–54.

108. Chen XH, Patel BK, Wang LM, et al. Jak 1 expression is required for mediating interleukin-4-induced tyrosine phosphorylation of insulin receptor substrate and Stat6 signaling molecules. *J Biol Chem* 1997;272:6556–6560.

109. Hodge C, Liao J, Stofega M, et al. Growth hormone stimulates phosphorylation and activation of elk-1 and expression of c-fos, egr-1, and junB through activation of extracellular signal-regulated kinases 1 and 2. *J Biol Chem* 1998;273:31327–31336.

110. Ridderstrale M, Degerman E, Tornqvist H. Growth hormone stimulates the tyrosine phosphorylation of the insulin receptor substrate-1 and its association with phosphatidylinositol 3-kinase in primary adipocytes. *J Biol Chem* 1995;270:3471–3474.

111. Uddin S, Yenush L, Sun XJ, et al. Interferon-alpha engages the insulin receptor substrate-1 to associate with the phosphatidylinositol 3′-kinase. *J Biol Chem* 1995;270:15938–15941.

112. Cook SJ, McCormick F. Inhibition by cAMP of Ras-dependent activation of Raf (see comments). *Science* 1993;262:1069–1072.

113. Vossler MR, Yao H, York RD, et al. cAMP activates MAP kinase and Elk-1 through a B-Raf- and Rap1-dependent pathway. *Cell* 1997;89:73–82.

114. Lange CA, Richer JK, Shen T, et al. Convergence of progesterone and epidermal growth factor signaling in breast cancer. Potentiation of mitogen-activated protein kinase pathways. *J Biol Chem* 1998;273:31308–31316.

Skeletal Growth Factors,
edited by Ernesto Canalis.
Lippincott Williams & Wilkins, Philadelphia, © 2000.

4

Mechanisms of Action of Skeletal Growth Factors in Osteoblasts

Gary S. Stein,* Thomas A. Owen, André J. van Wijnen, Brian Cho, Janet L. Stein, and Jane B. Lian

*Department of Cell Biology, University of Massachusetts Medical School, Worcester, Massachusetts 01655; and *Pfizer Central Research, Groton, Connecticut 06340*

The mechanisms that govern bone formation during both development and remodeling must be understood within the context of responsiveness to growth factors and steroid hormones that control proliferation and differentiation of osteoprogenitor cells. Proliferation of osteoblast lineage cells is mediated by a sequential expression of genes that respond to an integrated cascade of regulatory signals that license osteoblastic cells to proliferate or render bone cells quiescent. In this chapter, we focus on functional interrelationships of growth factors and steroid hormones with cell cycle checkpoints that interface growth regulatory mechanisms with commitment to expression of the skeletal phenotype.

REQUIREMENTS FOR CELL CYCLE AND GROWTH CONTROL OF OSTEOBLAST PROLIFERATION AND DIFFERENTIATION

Growth control in osteoblasts must support competency for proliferation and cell cycle progression within several biologically defined parameters. *In vivo,* proliferation of osteoprogenitor cells occurs for formation of the embryonic skeleton and expansion of the bone stem cell population. While bone stem cells and differentiated osteoblasts and osteocytes are then rendered quiescent, the osteoprogenitor cells reinitiate a limited extent of proliferation on demand during skeletal remodeling or fracture repair.

(Fig. 4.1) schematically illustrates the *in vivo* location of bone-forming cells and their proliferative status.

It is necessary to account for the induction, synthesis, activation, and suppression of the complex and interrelated regulatory factors associated with control of osteoprogenitor cell proliferation *in vivo* that are necessary for bone tissue development, turnover, and repair. Equally important is an explanation for repression of postproliferative bone phenotypic genes in early-stage proliferating osteoblasts, with the apparent exception of genes required for extracellular matrix biosynthesis. The induction of differentiated phenotypes occurs concomitantly with downregulation of proliferation in numerous cell types. Control of these reciprocal regulatory events may, in part, reside in the representation and activity of cell cycle and growth-regulatory proteins, which are involved in both positive and negative control (1–4).

MECHANISMS MEDIATING COMPETENCY FOR PROLIFERATION AND CELL CYCLE PROGRESSION

Checkpoints Govern Cell Cycle Progression

From a historical perspective, early indications that modifications in gene expression are required to support initiation of proliferation, entry into S phase, and mitosis were obtained

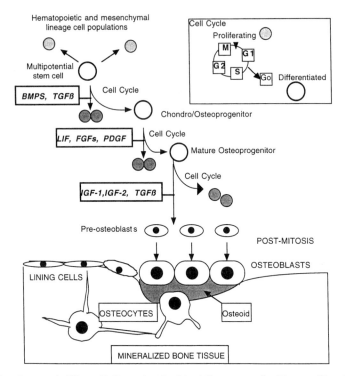

FIG. 4.1. *Proliferation and differentiation of osteoblast lineage cells.* The proliferative capacity and responsiveness of potential bone-forming cells to growth factors and cytokines are indicated beginning with the undifferentiated stem cells. Osteoblasts originate from the mesenchyme, which gives rise to cells for numerous tissue phenotypes (e.g., fibroblasts, adipocytes, myoblasts, skeletal cells). As mesenchymal stem cells commit to the chondrogenic or the osteogenic lineage, cells share similar growth responsiveness but then diverge under transcriptional control. Maturation of osteoprogenitor cells, either from marrow stroma or residing in the periosteum, is indicated in relation to morphological organization of the developing bone tissue. The developmental sequence of cellular differentiation, from preosteoblast to postmitotic surface osteoblast and then to either the mature osteocyte in its lacunae in mineralized bone matrix or a quiescent lining cell on the surface, is characterized by a temporal expression of phenotypic genes. Shaded cells reflect proliferating cells in the cell cycle and open circles illustrate the cell that exits from the cell cycle to the next stage of differentiation, which can be stimulated to proliferate or further differentiate.

from inhibition studies. First observed was the necessity of transcription and protein synthesis for DNA replication and mitotic division (5,6). Restriction points late in G_1 and G_2 for competency to initiate S phase and mitosis were mapped (7–9). Subsequently, by the combined application of gene expression inhibitors and modulation of growth factor levels in cultured cells, a mitogen-dependent (growth factor/cytokine-responsive) period was defined early in G_1, in which competency for proliferation is established, and a late G_1 restriction point

was identified, in which competency for cell cycle progression is attained (9).

Checkpoints have been identified which govern passage through G_1 and G_2 (Fig. 4.2), where competency for cell cycle traverse is monitored (7,8,10). The first evidence for these checkpoints was provided by the observation of delayed entry into S phase or mitosis following exposure to radiation or carcinogens. Editing functions are operative and decisions for continued proliferation, growth arrest, or apoptotic cell death are executed at these regulatory junctures

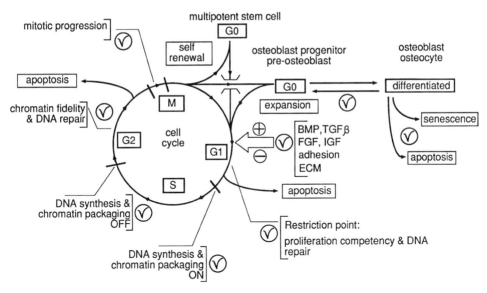

FIG. 4.2. *Multiple checkpoints control cell cycle progression in bone cells.* The cell cycle is regulated by several critical cell cycle checkpoints (indicated by checkmarks), at which competency for cell cycle progression is monitored. Entry into and exit from the cell cycle is controlled by growth-regulatory factors (e.g., cytokines, growth factors, cell adhesion, and/or cell–cell contact) that determine self-renewal of stem cells and expansion of precommitted progenitor cells. The biochemical parameters associated with each cell cycle checkpoint are indicated. Options for defaulting to apoptosis during G_1 and G_2 are evaluated by surveillance mechanisms that assess fidelity of structural and regulatory parameters of cell cycle control. Apoptosis also occurs in mature differentiated bone cells.

(11). Here, long-standing fundamental questions deal with the requirement of proliferation for the onset of differentiation as well as the extent to which proliferation and postproliferative expression of cell and tissue phenotypic genes are overlapping or mutually exclusive. Knowledge of control that is operative at cell cycle checkpoints is rapidly increasing. The complexity of the surveillance mechanisms which govern decisions for cell cycle progression is becoming increasingly apparent. We are now aware of multiple checkpoints during S phase which monitor regulatory events associated with DNA replication, histone biosynthesis, and fidelity of chromatin assembly. Mitosis is similarly controlled by an intricate series of checkpoints that are responsive to biochemical and structural parameters of chromosome condensation, mitotic apparatus assembly, chromosome alignment, chromosome movement, and cytokinesis (12–14). Similarly, checkpoints prior to S phase monitor genome integrity, nucleotide precursor pools, and mitogen availability prior to the decision to commit to DNA synthesis (15,16).

Multiple, Interdependent Cycles Control Proliferation

Several interdependent cycles are functionally linked to control of proliferation (Figs. 4.2, 4.3). The first is a stringent growth-regulated series of sequential biochemical and molecular events that support genomic replication and mitotic division. The second is a cascade of cyclin-containing growth-regulatory factors that transduce growth factor–mediated signals into discrete phosphorylation events, controlling expression of genes responsible for both initiation of proliferation and competency for cell cycle progression. Other cell cycle–related regulatory loops involve chromosome condensation, spindle assembly, metabolism and assembly of

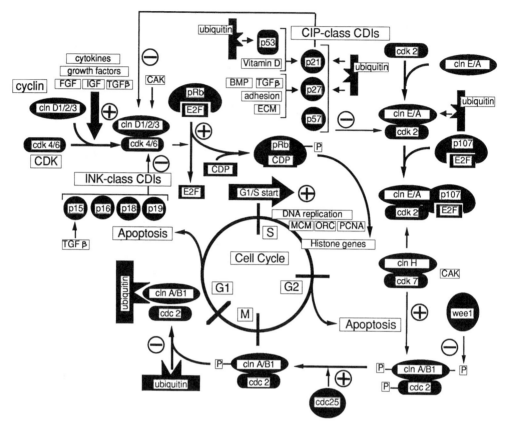

FIG. 4.3. *Regulation of the cell cycle in bone cells by cyclin-dependent kinases (CDKs) and tumor-suppressor proteins.* Competency for cell cycle progression is determined by CDKs, which monitor intracellular levels of cyclins, and CDK inhibitory proteins (*CKI/CDIs*). CDKs mediate phosphorylation of the retinoblastoma (*pRB*) class of tumor-suppressor proteins (i.e., pRB/p105, p107, and p130), which results in activation of E2F and CAAT-displacement protein (*CDP*)/cut-homeodomain transcription factors. These E2F-dependent and independent mechanisms induce expression of genes required for the G$_1$/S phase transition. Commitment to initiate DNA replication at the start of S phase is regulated in part by licensing factors, minute chromosome maintenance proteins (*MCMs*), origin recognition complex (*ORC*), and proliferating cell nuclear antigen (*PCNA*). Newly replicated DNA is packaged by histones into nucleosomes. Regulation of histone gene expression which is functionally coupled to DNA replication involves complexes of CDP and pRB. The activities of CDKs are influenced by phosphorylation [e.g., wee1 or CDK-activating kinase (*CAK*)], dephosphorylation (cdc25), ubiquitin-dependent proteolysis, and induction of p21 by the tumor-suppressor protein p53. Options for apoptosis are indicated within the context of cell cycle regulatory factors. Bone-related growth factors [e.g., fibroblast growth factor (*FGF*), insulin-like growth factor (*IGF*), transforming growth factor β (*TFG-β*), and platelet-derived growth factor (*PDGF*)] and cytokines induce the activities of CDKs, which mediate the G$_0$/G$_1$ transition. Vitamin D and transforming TGF-β-dependent cell signaling pathways upregulate CDIs (e.g., p21 and p27), which blocks cell cycle progression and supports differentiation in the presence of tissue-specific regulatory factors.

cdc2, and assembly/disasembly of DNA replication factor complexes [replicators and potential initiator proteins (17–26)]. It is becoming increasingly evident that each step in the regulatory cycles governing proliferation is responsive to multiple signaling pathways and has multiple regulatory options. The diversity in cyclin–cyclin-dependent kinase (cdk) complexes accommodates control of proliferation under multiple biological circumstances and provides functional redundancy as a compensatory mechanism. Similarly, several inhibitors of cyclin–cdk complexes bind to and regulate multiple cyclin–cdk-containing complexes at several checkpoint (27,28). The regulatory events associated with these proliferation-related cycles support control within the contexts of (a) responsiveness to a broad spectrum of positive and negative mitogenic factors, (b) cell–cell and cell–extracellular matrix interactions, (c) monitoring genomic integrity and invoking DNA repair and/or apoptotic mechanisms if required, and (d) competency for differentiation. Perturbation of any of these cell cycle regulatory elements can result in unregulated or neoplastic growth.

Phosphorylation-dependent Signaling Pathways Mediate Cell Cycle and Growth Control

Cell cycle competency and progression are controlled by an integrated cascade of phosphorylation-dependent regulatory signals (29,30) (Fig. 4.3). Growth factor–receptor interactions facilitate phosphorylation-dependent signaling pathways that, in turn, phosphorylate growth-regulatory transcription factors. Concomitant with the signal-transduction cascades is the accumulation and activation of cyclin–cdk complexes, also by phosphorylation-dependent pathways. Cyclins are synthesized, activated, and degraded in a cell cycle–dependent manner and function as regulatory subunits of cdks. The cdks phosphorylate a broad spectrum of structural proteins and transcription factors (TFs), including TFIIH, to mediate sequential parameters of cell cycle control. Certain cyclin–cdk complexes, including components of TFIIH, phosphorylate RNA polymerase II (31–34), while others colocalize with DNA replication foci (35,36). These findings support a direct role for cell cycle regulatory kinase activity in basal transcription and DNA synthesis, respectively. The emerging concept is that the cyclins and cdks are responsive to regulation by the phosphorylation-dependent signaling pathways associated with activities of the early-response genes, which are upregulated following mitogen stimulation of

proliferation [reviewed in (30,37,38), summarized in Fig. 4.3)]. Cyclin-dependent phosphorylation activity is functionally linked to activation and suppression of both p53 and retinoblastoma (RB)–related tumor-suppressor genes, which mediate transcriptional events involved with passage into S and M phases. p53 accumulates in response to stress, inducing arrest at G_1 or G_2. Growth arrest is, in part, due to induction of the cyclin-dependent kinase inhibitor of proteins (CKI) p21, which can interact with multiple cyclin–cdk complexes. The activities of the cdks are downregulated by a series of inhibitors (designated CDIs) and mediators of ubiquitination, which signal destabilization and/or destruction of these regulatory complexes in a cell cycle–dependent manner (39).

Particularly significant is the accumulating evidence for functional interrelationships between activities of cyclin–cdk complexes and growth arrest at G_1 and G_2 checkpoints, when editing and repair are monitored following DNA damage (Fig. 4.3). It is at these times and in relation to these processes that apoptotic cell death is invoked as a compensatory mechanism. Cells arrested at G_1 or G_2 attempt to repair DNA damage prior to progression through restriction points. It is believed that when damage is extensive or repair is not completed by mechanisms that are operative at the restriction point, apoptosis may be induced. Failure to arrest cell cycle progression in response to DNA damage prior to S phase can result in the propagation of a mutation by failure to correctly repair the altered and/or damaged base or nucleic acid prior to DNA replication. Incorporation of mutations in the form of point lesions, insertions, and deletions can also occur as DNA replication errors during S phase unless repair machinery can correct the lesions. Typical genetic lesions that occur due to defective G_2 and M checkpoints can include nondisjunction, aneuploidy, and endoreduplication.

During G_1, expression of genes associated with deoxynucleotide biosynthesis is upregulated (e.g., thymidine kinase, thymidylate synthase, dihydrofolate reductase) in preparation for DNA synthesis (40–42). As cells progress through G_1, regulatory factors required for initiation of DNA replication are sequentially expressed and/or activated. Following stimulation of quiescent cells to proliferate, expression of the fos/jun-related early-response genes is induced early in G_1, playing a pivotal role in activation of subsequent cell cycle regulatory events. In S phase, DNA replication is paralleled by, and functionally coupled with histone gene expression, providing the necessary basic chromosomal proteins (H1, H4, H3, H2A, and H2B) for packaging newly replicated DNA into chromatin (43,44). During G_2, regulatory factors for mitosis are synthesized, and modifications of chromatin structure to support mitotic chromosome condensation occur [reviewed in (38)]. Mitosis involves sequential remodeling of genomic architecture from uncondensed chromatin to highly condensed chromosomes and back to chromatin. These processes include: assembly and subsequent disassembly of the mitotic apparatus, alignment and separation of condensed chromosomes, breakdown and reformation of the nuclear membrane, return of chromatin to uncondensed status, and modifications in activities of factors required for reinitiation of cell cycle progression, quiescence, or differentiation.

As the sophistication of experimental approaches for dissection of promoter elements and characterization of cognate regulatory factors increases, there is an emerging recognition of cyclic modifications in occupancy of the promoter domains and protein–protein interactions that control cell cycle progression. The coupling of histone gene transcription with DNA synthesis involves transcription factor complexes that include cyclins, tumor-suppressor proteins, and transcriptional activators as well as inhibitory factors. The changes observed in the site II cell cycle regulatory promoter element of the histone gene illustrate such changes in factor occupancy and activities that are functionally linked to activation, suppression, and subtle modifications in levels of expression which are proliferation-dependent (45–50).

Although considerable attention has been directed to experimentally addressing transcriptional regulatory mechanisms that are associated with cell cycle and growth control, the importance of regulation at posttranscriptional and posttranslational levels should not be underestimated. For example, cell cycle–dependent modifications in histone mRNA processing and histone phosphorylation and acetylation contribute to linkage of histone regulation with DNA replication and the S phase of the cell cycle (9,51–54). Compartmentalization and sequestration of cell cycle regulatory factors and/or cognate gene transcripts, as well as phosphorylation or ubiquitination, are necessary for proper cell cycle regulation (55–57).

Specialized Cells Have Unique Cell Cycle Regulatory Requirements

Consistent with the stringent requirement for fidelity of DNA replication and repair to execute proliferation, cell cycle stage-specific modifications of regulatory factors have been observed to parallel physiological changes and perturbations in growth control. Some striking examples of physiological changes are regulatory mechanisms that support developmental transitions during early embryogenesis, when DNA replication and mitotic division occur in rapid succession in the absence of significant G_1 or G_2 periods. In contrast, proliferation in somatic cells of the adult requires passage through a cell cycle with G_1, S, G_2, and mitotic periods that are operative and necessary. Often, a prolonged G_1 period provides support for long-term quiescence of cells and tissues while retaining the competency to reinitiate proliferation for tissue remodeling and renewal. In contrast, terminally differentiated or senescent cells are typically unable to reenter the cell cycle. Stem cells require complex control of proliferation competency to modulate commitments for cell cycle progression, quiescence, or differentiation. Thus, responsiveness of stem cells to cell growth and tissue-specific regulatory factors must be stringently monitored to maintain a balance between proliferation and differentiation. Adult tissues and organs (e.g., epithelial cells) have distinct layers of self-renewing cells that are typically associated with a basement membrane. As cells divide, progeny cells progress toward the surface and develop differentiated phenotypes. Interactions with basement membrane and/or distal cell–cell interactions influence the competency of cells to proliferate or differentiate.

The abrogated components of growth control in transformed and tumor cells are associated with defective regulation of cyclin–cdk complexes. Characteristic inactivation of cdk inhibitors and p53 has been associated with progressive stages of neoplasia and specific tumors [reviewed in (30,37)]. Frequently, the hallmark of tumor tissue is coexpression of cell growth and tissue-specific genes rather than mutually exclusive expression or cell division out of the normal context of cell–extracellular matrix interactions. Consequently, tumor cells provide us with valuable insight into rate-limiting regulatory steps in cell cycle and cell growth control. In addition, we are increasing our opportunity to therapeutically rectify proliferative disorders in a targeted manner. Particularly challenging is the possibility of restoring fidelity of regulatory mechanisms operative at cell cycle checkpoints, when responses to apoptotic signals prevent accumulation and phenotypic expression of mutations associated with growth control perturbations.

Cell Cycle Regulatory Factors Contribute to Control of Differentiation

Because acquisition of tissue-specific phenotypes is frequently associated with growth arrest, it is necessary to understand the involvement of cell cycle regulatory factors in mechanisms that ensure exit from the cell cycle as a prerequisite for differentiation (Figs. 4.1, 4.2). These mechanisms include dephosphorylation of RB family members, stabilization of p53, decreased representation or activity of cyclin–cdk complexes, and activities of CDIs during differentiation and senescence. While interrelationships between cell cycle regulatory factors and carcinogenesis are well established (38,58–60), there is growing awareness of functional linkages between factors that control cell cycle progression with postproliferative events that mediate the onset and maintenance of differentiation.

In addition to the well-documented role of RB proteins in transcriptional control of E2F-regulated genes, it is becoming evident that there are high levels of RB in postmitotic cells (58,61–65). Further support for significant contributions of RB-related p105, p107, and p130 factors to postproliferative phenotype development is provided by abrogated neural development (66–70), adipogenesis (70–72), myogenesis (62,73–75), chondrogenesis, and limb development (76), as well as aberrant embryogenesis in RB gene overexpression and/or ablation studies. Inhibition of wild-type p53 function or expression of E2F in senescent cells can induce DNA synthesis, supporting a role for p53 in maintaining senescence and inhibition of E2F function during quiescence and senescence (77–80).

Examples of contributions by cdks to postproliferative (kinase activity) regulation include cdk5 in differentiating neurons (81–83) as well as cdk7, cdc2, cdk2, and cdk4 in several cell types (59,84–87) including osteoblasts (88). There is increasing evidence for phenotype-restricted postproliferative upregulation of cyclins with developmental consequences. Examples are enhanced expression of cyclin E in differentiating osteoblasts (88,89), cyclin DI inhibition of B and T cells (90), and cyclin D–mediated constraints on differentiation of breast and neural cells (91–94). Taken together, there is emerging evidence for functional involvement of factors that control the cell cycle in fidelity of growth suppression and the orchestration of gene regulatory mechanisms that are required for initiating and sustaining expression of phenotypic genes.

Our understanding of factors that are components of regulatory patterns supporting proliferation and postproliferative gene expression is rapidly expanding, and recent findings have been comprehensively reviewed (95).

FUNCTIONAL INTERRELATIONSHIPS OF GROWTH FACTORS WITH REGULATORY PARAMETERS OF CELL CYCLE AND GROWTH CONTROL

Throughout the lifespan of a vertebrate organism, there is a need for a tightly coupled interplay between cell growth and differentiation for the development and maintenance of the skeleton. During embryogenesis, there is a demand for rapid growth in size as well as for formation of specific spatial patterns. Following birth and continuing until adult size is reached, there is again the need for skeletal growth along a predetermined pattern as well as the need for constant skeletal remodeling to maintain mineral homeostasis and the occasional repair of a fracture. Throughout the adult lifespan, bone remodeling and fracture repair continue, but the mechanisms controlling these activities must be adapted to a changing hormonal environment. In all cases, these physiological changes are controlled by extracellular signals that result in modulation of gene expression and, ultimately, determination of the phenotype of the cell.

A large part of this physiological control of cell phenotype must occur at a point where entry into and departure from the cell cycle is mediated. Control of entry into the cell cycle allows for proliferation of the cells needed for growth in size, those required at a particular time and skeletal site to carry out remodeling, and those responsible for the rapid repair of skeletal fractures. In complementary processes, the spatial and temporal control of exit from the cell cycle dictates the pattern of expression of genes controlling the phenotype of the mature cell required at a particular time and skeletal site. This stringent control of the cell cycle also minimizes the possibility of an uncontrolled cell proliferative response to the multitude of growth factors available to the skeleton, with the resulting formation of osteosarcomas.

Initiation of, controlled passage through, and exit from the cell cycle are tightly controlled by a series of phosphorylation-dependent biochemical pathways (described previously) that ultimately integrate the many signals from the extracellular environment into a decision about gene expression, which subsequently determines the cell phenotype. It is becoming increasingly evident that the interactions of cyclins, cdks, kinase inhibitors, and phosphatases are responsive to pathways invoked by early-response genes, activate and/or suppress transcription factors including nuclear hormone receptors, and are ulti-

mately responsible for progression through the G_1 and G_2 cell cycle checkpoints as well as the decision to enter the cell cycle or to exit it to a state of differentiation or apoptosis in response to damage or as an integral part of pattern formation.

The growth and differentiation factors which govern the remodeling and maintenance of the skeleton continue to be investigated in order to further elucidate their interrelationships with the biochemical pathways controlling the cell cycle. Members of the transforming growth factor (TGF)-β superfamily, including the bone morphogenetic proteins (BMPs), are among the primary effectors of skeletal patterning and homeostasis (96–98). Members of this protein family bind to cell surface receptors that possess intrinsic serine/threonine kinase activity. Upon ligand-induced activation, the kinase activity associated with these receptors phosphorylates various SMAD proteins (SMADs 1–8), which can associate with and regulate each other's activities, ultimately directing association with various transcription factors and thereby directly regulating gene expression (99,100) (Fig. 4.4A). One of these TGF-β signaling pathways has recently been shown to directly interact with the vitamin D receptor, a nuclear hormone receptor that mediates the expression of many bone-associated genes and functions in control of calcium metabolism. In this case, SMAD3 was found to function as a coactivator for gene transactivation by the vitamin D receptor (101). This ability of receptors for TGF-β family members to regulate the SMAD proteins by phosphorylation, along with the widely varying tissue distribution of the SMADs, results in a tremendous number of combinations of signal integration possibilities which can affect both the regulatory pathways involved in cell cycle progression [e.g., interactions with AP-1 and SP-1 responsive genes (102) and induction of the cdk inhibitors p15 and p21 (103,104)] as well as those involved in bone cell phenotype expression [e.g., interactions with the vitamin D receptor (101)]. Further complexity in this regulation has recently been shown with the report of a vitamin D–responsive element in the promoter of the human TGF-β2 gene (105). This potential feedback loop between a tran-

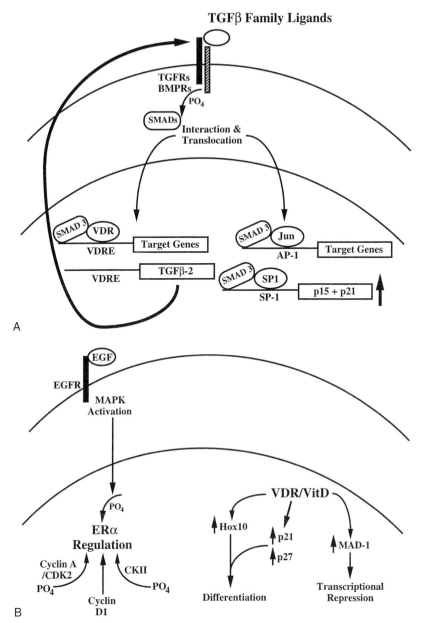

FIG. 4.4. Impact of skeletal growth and differentiation factors on cell cycle control. **A:** Ligands of the transforming growth factor (*TGF-β*) superfamily bind and signal through a heterodimer of type I and type II receptors. One consequence of receptor activation is the phosphorylation of members of the SMAD family. These proteins then interact and translocate to the nucleus, where they function as regulators of transcription for genes involved in cell cycle progression, such as p15 and p21, as well as co-activators of the vitamin D receptor, which regulates transcription of a number of skeletal phenotype genes. Also impacting this pathway is the vitamin D regulation of the expression of one of the ligand family members, TGF-*β*2. **B:** DNA binding and transcriptional regulation by estrogen receptor *α* (*ERα*) has been shown to be affected by a number of different pathways involved in cell cycle regulation. ERα is phosphorylated following activation of the mitogen-activated protein kinase (*MAPK*) pathway by the epidermal growth factor receptor (*EGFR*) and by the cyclin A–cdk2 complex as well as casein kinase II (*CKII*). Conversely, the vitamin D receptor, another nuclear hormone receptor, has been shown to increase the abundance of the cyclin-dependent kinase inhibitors (CKIs) p21 and p27. It also causes increased expression of the homeobox protein *Hox10*, overexpression of which can lead to differentiation, and of the Mad-1 protein, a member of the Mad-Max transcriptional repressor complex. *Continued*

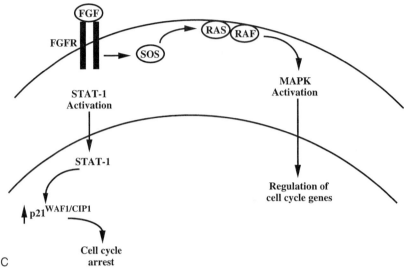

C

FIG. 4.4. *Continued.* **C:** Binding of fibroblast growth factors (*FGFs*) to their cell surface receptors can activate the Ras-Raf pathway and its resulting signaling via activated MAPK, finally regulating the expression of a variety of cell cycle–related genes. Activation of an FGF receptor can also result in the activation and nuclear translocation of the transcription factor STAT-1. Activation of STAT-1, in turn, increases the expression of p21[WAF1/CIP1], which ultimately results in cell cycle withdrawal and growth arrest.

scriptional effector and the gene encoding the ligand for a receptor which upregulates the effector's transcriptional activity would provide a cell with exquisitely fine control of its cell cycle with respect to proliferation versus differentiation state.

Interactions of the vitamin D receptor with target genes can also impinge on the direct control of the cell cycle. The best evidence for direct effects comes from studies aimed at identifying target genes for vitamin D action during the differentiation of U937 myelomonoblastic cells. One of the genes induced by vitamin D encodes p21[WAF1/CIP1], a member of a group of small proteins termed cyclin-dependent kinase inhibitors (CKIs) (106). These proteins inhibit the activity of the cyclin–CDK complexes, causing cells to undergo G_1 arrest and to withdraw from the cell cycle. A similar study in pancreatic cancer–derived cells showed p21 as well as another CKI, p27, to increase in abundance during vitamin D blockade of cell proliferation (107). The screen for vitamin D target genes in U937 cells also found the homeobox HoxA10 gene and the gene

encoding the basic helix-loop-helix-zip protein Mad1 (108). HoxA10 was subsequently shown to induce differentiation following overexpression in these cells (109). Mad1 is a member of the Mad-Max transcriptional repressor complex and has recently been shown to be associated with the histone deacetylase activity required to repress transcription (110). The induction of these CKIs and transcription factors by vitamin D clearly demonstrates how signaling via ligand activation of the vitamin D receptor directly impacts multiple pathways which dictate progression through and exit from the cell cycle to a differentiated state (Fig. 4.4B).

Nuclear hormone receptors are also themselves targets for regulatory signals from the mitogen-activated protein (MAP) kinase and cdk pathways, thereby affecting, in association with specific ligand binding and cofactor recruitment, the activation and/or repression of genes responsible for decisions about cell cycle progression and differentiation. For example, estrogen receptor α (ERα) is directly phosphorylated by creatine kinase II, resulting in its increased ability to bind DNA (111). Similarly, an effect of cyclin A, which is dependent on cdk activity (112), as well as a cdk-independent effect of cyclin D1 (94) have been reported to activate and enhance transcriptional competency of ERα. Additional evidence is being uncovered that ERα can also be phosphorylated and thereby activated by MAP kinase which has itself been activated following signaling from the epidermal growth factor receptor (113,114). This ligand-independent activation of ERα adds additional complexity to the ability of the estrogen receptor transcriptional modulation pathways to influence the proliferation/differentiation state of cells in many target tissues (Fig. 4.4B).

Activation of receptors which signal through tyrosine kinase domains also results in a variety of effects on skeletal growth and differentiation through modulation of the cell cycle in cells responsible for control of longitudinal bone growth as well as for maturation of newly differentiated bone. Members of the fibroblast growth factor (FGF) family signal to cells involved in skeletal formation and differentiation through four different cell surface receptors, which have intrinsic tyrosine kinase activities (115). Various studies have recently demonstrated that activation of this tyrosine kinase results in the phosphorylation of a number of cellular substrates, which, as a complex, target the nucleotide exchange factor Sos to the cell membrane. This results in activation of the Ras/Raf signaling pathway, which transduces signals to the nucleus via the MAP kinase pathway, thereby affecting a variety of cell cycle decision points (116–119). FGF receptors which are mutated in human chondrodysplasias also specifically activate the transcription factor STAT1 (120). This activation results in an increased expression of the CKI p21$^{WAF1/CIP1}$, with a resulting withdrawal from the cell cycle and subsequent growth arrest. This mechanism through which the FGFs directly influence cell cycle progression has very clear implications for regulating the extent of longitudinal bone growth as well as for modulating the effects of the FGFs on the differentiation, remodeling, and ossification at the growth plate (Fig. 4.4C).

CONCLUSIONS AND PERSPECTIVES

There is emerging recognition for interrelationships between control of genes that regulate the cell cycle and the initiation as well as sustained physiological responsiveness of genes that are functionally linked to the skeletal phenotype. Examples include, but are not restricted to, involvement of cyclins and cdks in postproliferative bone tissue-specific gene expression, coupling of TGF-β signaling pathways with vitamin D–mediated transcriptional regulation, and crosstalk between cyclin inhibitors and vitamin D responsiveness. The challenge we now face is to further refine our understanding of mechanisms that interface the activities of skeletal growth factors with components of gene expression during bone cell growth and differentiation. The outcome will be additional insight into the regulatory cues that are essential for skeletal development and aberrant in bone metabolic disorders and tumors.

ACKNOWLEDGMENTS

Components of the work reported in this chapter were supported by National Institutes of Health grants AR45688, AR45689, and DE12528. Its contents are solely the responsibility of the authors and do not necessarily represent the official views of the National Institutes of Health. The authors thank Steve Smock (Pfizer Central Research) for illustrations and are appreciative of the editorial assistance from Elizabeth Bronstein with organization of the manuscript.

REFERENCES

1. Stein GS, Lian JB, Stein JL, et al. Transcriptional control of osteoblast growth and differentiation. *Physiol Rev* 1996;76:593–629.
2. Owen TA, Aronow M, Shalhoub V, et al. Progressive development of the rat osteoblast phenotype in vitro: reciprocal relationships in expression of genes associated with osteoblast proliferation and differentiation during formation of the bone extracellular matrix. *J Cell Physiol* 1990;143:420–430.
3. Stein GS, van Wijnen AJ, Hushka DR, et al. Molecular mechanisms controlling the cell cycle and proliferation–differentiation interrelationships. In: Quesenberry PJ, Stein GS, Forget BG, Weissman SM, eds.

Stem cell biology and gene therapy. New York: Wiley-Liss, 1998:41–80.

4. Stein GS, van Wijnen AJ, Frenkel B, et al. Gene expression: the regulatory and regulated mechanisms. In: Stein GS, Baserga R, Giordano A, Denhardt DT, eds. *Cell cycle and growth control: the molecular basis of cell cycle and growth control.* New York: Wiley-Liss, 1998:183–224.

5. Terasima T, Yasukawa M. Synthesis of G1 protein preceding DNA synthesis in cultured mammalian cells. *Exp Cell Res* 1966;44:669–672.

6. Baserga R, Estensen RD, Petersen RO. Inhibition of DNA synthesis in Ehrlich ascites cells by actinomycin D. II. The presynthetic block in the cell cycle. *Proc Natl Acad Sci USA* 1965;54:1141–1148.

7. Sherr CJ. Mammalian G1 cyclins. *Cell* 1993;73: 1059–1065.

8. Dowdy SF, Hinds PW, Louie K, et al. Physical interaction of the retinoblastoma protein with human D cyclins. *Cell* 1993;73:499–511.

9. Pardee AB. G1 events and regulation of cell proliferation. *Science* 1989;246:603–608.

10. Nurse P. Ordering S phase and M phase in the cell cycle. *Cell* 1994;79:547–550.

11. White E. Tumour biology. p53, guardian of Rb [news; comment]. *Nature* 1994;371:21–22.

12. Hinchcliffe EH, Li C, Thompson EA, et al. Requirement of Cdk2-cyclin E activity for repeated centrosome reproduction in *Xenopus* egg extracts [see comments]. *Science* 1999;283:851–854.

13. Zimmerman W, Sparks CA, Doxsey SJ. Amorphous no longer: the centrosome comes into focus. *Curr Opin Cell Biol* 1999;11:122–128.

14. Doxsey S. The centrosome—a tiny organelle with big potential [news; comment]. *Nat Genet* 1998;20:104–106.

15. Planas-Silva MD, Weinberg RA. The restriction point and control of cell proliferation. *Curr Opin Cell Biol* 1997;9:768–772.

16. Zavitz KH, Zipursky SL. Controlling cell proliferation in differentiating tissues: genetic analysis of negative regulators of G1→S-phase progression. *Curr Opin Cell Biol* 1997;9:773–781.

17. Stillman B. Cell cycle control of DNA replication. *Science* 1996;274:1659–1664.

18. Hamlin JL, Mosca PJ, Levenson VV. Defining origins of replication in mammalian cells. *Biochim Biophys Acta* 1994;1198:85–111.

19. Muzi-Falconi M, Kelly TJ. Orp1, a member of the Cdc18/Cdc6 family of S-phase regulators, is homologous to a component of the origin recognition complex. *Proc Natl Acad Sci USA* 1995;92:12475–12479.

20. Clyne RK, Kelly TJ. Genetic analysis of an ARS element from the fission yeast *Schizosaccharomyces pombe. EMBO J* 1995;14:6348–6357.

21. Dubey DD, Kim SM, Todorov IT, et al. Large, complex modular structure of a fission yeast DNA replication origin. *Curr Biol* 1996;6:467–473.

22. Gavin KA, Hidaka M, Stillman B. Conserved initiator proteins in eukaryotes [see comments]. *Science* 1995; 270:1667–1671.

23. Gossen M, Pak DT, Hansen SK, et al. A *Drosophila* homolog of the yeast origin recognition complex [see comments]. *Science* 1995;270:1674–1677.

24. Leatherwood J, Lopez-Girona A, Russell P. Interaction of Cdc2 and Cdc18 with a fission yeast ORC2-like protein. *Nature* 1996;379:360–363.

25. Carpenter PB, Mueller PR, Dunphy WG. Role for a *Xenopus* Orc2-related protein in controlling DNA replication. *Nature* 1996;379:357–360.

26. Wohlgemuth JG, Bulboaca GH, Moghadam M, et al. Physical mapping of origins of replication in the fission yeast *Schizosaccharomyces pombe. Mol Cell Biol* 1994;5:839–849.

27. Harper JW, Adami GR, Wei N, et al. The p21 Cdk-interacting protein Cip1 is a potent inhibitor of G1 cyclin-dependent kinases. *Cell* 1993;75:805–816.

28. Xiong Y, Hannon GJ, Zhang H, et al. p21 is a universal inhibitor of cyclin kinases. *Nature* 1993;366:701–704.

29. Hartwell LH, Culotti J, Pringle JR, et al. Genetic control of the cell division cycle in yeast. *Science* 1974; 183:46–51.

30. Hartwell LH, Weinert TA. Checkpoints: controls that ensure the order of cell cycle events. *Science* 1989; 246:629–634.

31. Shiekhattar R, Mermelstein F, Fisher RP, et al. Cdk-activating kinase complex is a component of human transcription factor TFIIH. *Nature* 1995;374:283–287.

32. Serizawa H, Makela TP, Conaway JW, et al. Association of Cdk-activating kinase subunits with transcription factor TFIIH. *Nature* 1995;374:280–282.

33. Edwards MC, Wong C, Elledge SJ. Human cyclin K, a novel RNA polymerase II-associated cyclin possessing both carboxy-terminal domain kinase and Cdk-activating kinase activity. *Mol Cell Biol* 1998;18:4291–4300.

34. Rickert P, Corden JL, Lees E. Cyclin C/CDK8 and cyclin H/CDK7/p36 are biochemically distinct CTD kinases. *Oncogene* 1999;18:1093–1102.

35. Xiong Y, Zhang H, Beach D. D type cyclins associate with multiple protein kinases and the DNA replication and repair factor PCNA. *Cell* 1992;71:505–514.

36. Pagano M, Theodoras AM, Tam SW, et al. Cyclin D1-mediated inhibition of repair and replicative DNA synthesis in human fibroblasts. *Genes Dev* 1994;8:1627–1639.

37. Hunter T, Pines J. Cyclins and cancer II: cyclin D and cdk inhibitors come of age. *Cell* 1994;79:573–582.

38. MacLachlan TK, Sang N, Giordano A. Cyclins, cyclin-dependent kinases and cdk inhibitors: implications in cell cycle control and cancer. *Crit Rev Eukaryot Gene Expr* 1995;5:127–156.

39. Koepp DM, Harper JW, Elledge SJ. How the cyclin became a cyclin: regulated proteolysis in the cell cycle *Cell* 1999;97:431–434.

40. King RW, Jackson PK, Kirschner MW. Mitosis in transition [see comments]. *Cell* 1994;79:563–571.

41. Pardee AB, Keyomarsi K. Modification of cell proliferation with inhibitors. *Curr Opin Cell Biol* 1992;4: 186–191.

42. Johnson LF. G1 events and the regulation of genes for S-phase enzymes. *Curr Opin Cell Biol* 1992;4: 149–154.

43. Azizkhan JC, Jensen DE, Pierce AJ, et al. Transcription from TATA-less promoters: dihydrofolate reductase as

a model. *Crit Rev Eukaryot Gene Expr* 1993;3:229–254.

44. Plumb M, Stein J, Stein G. Coordinate regulation of multiple histone mRNAs during the cell cycle in HeLa cells. *Nucleic Acids Res* 1983;11:2391–2410.

45. van Wijnen AJ, van Gurp MF, de Ridder MC, et al. CDP/*cut* is the DNA-binding subunit of histone gene transcription factor HiNF-D: a mechanism for gene regulation at the G_1/S phase cell cycle transition point independent of transcription factor E2F. *Proc Natl Acad Sci USA* 1996;93:11516–11521.

46. Vaughan PS, Aziz F, van Wijnen AJ, et al. Activation of a cell-cycle-regulated histone gene by the oncogenic transcription factor IRF-2. *Nature* 1995;377:362–365.

47. van Wijnen AJ, Aziz F, Grana X, et al. Transcription of histone H4, H3, and H1 cell cycle genes: promoter factor HiNF-D contains CDC2, cyclin A, and an RB-related protein. *Proc Natl Acad Sci USA* 1994;91:12882–12886.

48. Stein G, Lian J, Stein J, et al. Altered binding of human histone gene transcription factors during the shutdown of proliferation and onset of differentiation in HL-60 cells. *Proc Natl Acad Sci USA* 1989;86:1865–1869.

49. Holthuis J, Owen TA, van Wijnen AJ, et al. Tumor cells exhibit deregulation of the cell cycle histone gene promoter factor HiNF-D. *Science* 1990;247:1454–1457.

50. Pauli U, Chrysogelos S, Stein G, et al. Protein-DNA interactions in vivo upstream of a cell cycle–regulated human H4 histone gene. *Science* 1987;236:1308–1311.

51. Harris ME, Bohni R, Schneiderman MH, et al. Regulation of histone mRNA in the unperturbed cell cycle: evidence suggesting control at two posttranscriptional steps. *Mol Cell Biol* 1991;11:2416–2424.

52. Marzluff WF, Pandey NB. Multiple regulatory steps control histone mRNA concentrations. *Trends Biochem Sci* 1988;13:49–52.

53. Morris TD, Weber LA, Hickey E, et al. Changes in the stability of a human H3 histone mRNA during the HeLa cell cycle. *Mol Cell Biol* 1991;11:544–553.

54. Peltz SW, Brewer G, Bernstein P, et al. Regulation of mRNA turnover in eukaryotic cells. *Crit Rev Eukaryot Gene Expr* 1991;1:99–126.

55. Zambetti G, Stein J, Stein G. Targeting of a chimeric human histone fusion mRNA to membrane-bound polysomes in HeLa cells. *Proc Natl Acad Sci USA* 1987;84:2683–2687.

56. Birnbaum MJ, van Zundert B, Vaughan PS, et al. Phosphorylation of the oncogenic transcription factor interferon regulatory factor 2 (IRF2) in vitro and in vivo. *J Cell Biochem* 1997;66:175–183.

57. Pagano M. Cell cycle regulation by the ubiquitin pathway. *FASEB J* 1997;11:1067–1075.

58. Weinberg RA. The retinoblastoma protein and cell cycle control. *Cell* 1995;81:323–330.

59. Kranenburg O, de Groot RP, Van der Eb AJ, et al. Differentiation of P19 EC cells leads to differential modulation of cyclin-dependent kinase activities and to changes in the cell cycle profile. *Oncogene* 1995;10:87–95.

60. Marks PA, Richon VM, Rifkind RA. Cell cycle regulatory proteins are targets for induced differentiation of transformed cells: molecular and clinical studies employing hybrid polar compounds. *Int J Hematol* 1996;63:1–17.

61. Yen A, Varvayanis S, Platko JD. 12-*O*-Tetradecanoylphorbol-13-acetate and staurosporine induce increased retinoblastoma tumor suppressor gene expression with megakaryocytic differentiation of leukemic cells. *Cancer Res* 1993;53:3085–3091.

62. Gu W, Schneider JW, Condorelli G, et al. Interaction of myogenic factors and the retinoblastoma protein mediates muscle cell commitment and differentiation. *Cell* 1993;72:309–324.

63. Kiyokawa H, Richon VM, Rifkind RA, et al. Suppression of cyclin-dependent kinase 4 during induced differentiation of erythroleukemia cells. *Mol Cell Biol* 1994;14:7195–7203.

64. Szekely L, Jin P, Jiang WQ, et al. Position-dependent nuclear accumulation of the retinoblastoma (RB) protein during in vitro myogenesis. *J Cell Physiol* 1993;155:313–322.

65. Cordon-Cardo C, Richon VM. Expression of the retinoblastoma protein is regulated in normal human tissues. *Am J Pathol* 1994;144:500–510.

66. Jacks T, Fazeli A, Schmitt EM, et al. Effects of an *Rb* mutation in the mouse. *Nature* 1992;359:295–300.

67. Clarke AR, Maandag ER, van Roon M, et al. Requirement for a functional Rb-1 gene in murine development. *Nature* 1992;359:328–330.

68. Lee EY, Chang CY, Hu N, et al. Mice deficient for Rb are nonviable and show defects in neurogenesis and haematopoiesis. *Nature* 1992;359:288–294.

69. Slack RS, Miller FD. Retinoblastoma gene in mouse neural development. *Dev Genet* 1996;18:81–91.

70. Lee EY, Hu N, Yuan SS, et al. Dual roles of the retinoblastoma protein in cell cycle regulation and neuron differentiation. *Genes Dev* 1994;8:2008–2021.

71. Morgenbesser SD, Williams BO, Jacks T, et al. p53-dependent apoptosis produced by Rb-deficiency in the developing mouse lens [see comments]. *Nature* 1994;371:72–74.

72. Chen PL, Riley DJ, Chen Y, et al. Retinoblastoma protein positively regulates terminal adipocyte differentiation through direct interaction with C/EBPs. *Genes Dev* 1996;10:2794–2804.

73. Schneider JW, Gu W, Zhu L, et al. Reversal of terminal differentiation mediated by p107 in Rb−/− muscle cells. *Science* 1994;264:1467–1471.

74. Novitch BG, Mulligan GJ, Jacks T, et al. Skeletal muscle cells lacking the retinoblastoma protein display defects in muscle gene expression and accumulate in S and G2 phases of the cell cycle. *J Cell Biol* 1996;135:441–456.

75. Wiman KG. The retinoblastoma gene: role in cell cycle control and cell differentiation. *FASEB J* 1993;7:841–845.

76. Cobrinik D, Lee MH, Hannon G, et al. Shared role of the pRB-related p130 and p107 proteins in limb development. *Genes Dev* 1996;10:1633–1644.

77. Johnson DG, Schwarz JK, Cress WD, et al. Expression of transcription factor E2F1 induces quiescent cells to enter S phase. *Nature* 1993;365:349–352.

78. Kowalik TF, DeGregori J, Schwarz JK, et al. E2F1 overexpression in quiescent fibroblasts leads to induc-

tion of cellular DNA synthesis and apoptosis. *J Virol* 1995;69:2491–2500.

79. Bond JA, Blaydes JP, Rowson J, et al. Mutant p53 rescues human diploid cells from senescence without inhibiting the induction of SDI1/WAF1. *Cancer Res* 1995;55:2404–2409.

80. Gire V, Wynford-Thomas D. Reinitiation of DNA synthesis and cell division in senescent human fibroblasts by microinjection of anti-p53 antibodies. *Mol Cell Biol* 1998;18:1611–1621.

81. Nikolic M, Dudek H, Kwon YT, et al. The cdk5/p35 kinase is essential for neurite outgrowth during neuronal differentiation. *Genes Dev* 1996;10:816–825.

82. Tsai LH, Takahashi T, Caviness VS Jr, et al. Activity and expression pattern of cyclin-dependent kinase 5 in the embryonic mouse nervous system. *Development* 1993;119:1029–1040.

83. Ohshima T, Ward JM, Huh CG, et al. Targeted disruption of the cyclin-dependent kinase 5 gene results in abnormal corticogenesis, neuronal pathology and perinatal death. *Proc Natl Acad Sci USA* 1996;93:11173–11178.

84. Bartkova J, Zemanova M, Bartek J. Expression of CDK7/CAK in normal and tumor cells of diverse histogenesis, cell-cycle position and differentiation. *Int J Cancer* 1996;66:732–737.

85. Dobashi Y, Kudoh T, Toyoshima K, et al. Persistent activation of CDK4 during neuronal differentiation of rat pheochromocytoma PC12 cells. *Biochem Biophys Res Commun* 1996;221:351–355.

86. Gao CY, Bassnett S, Zelenka PS. Cyclin B, p34cdc2, and H1-kinase activity in terminally differentiating lens fiber cells. *Dev Biol* 1995;169:185–194.

87. Jahn L, Sadoshima J, Izumo S. Cyclins and cyclin-dependent kinases are differentially regulated during terminal differentiation of C2C12 muscle cells. *Exp Cell Res* 1994;212:297–307.

88. Smith E, Frenkel B, MacLachlan TK, et al. Post-proliferative cyclin E-associated kinase activity in differentiated osteoblasts: inhibition by proliferating osteoblasts and osteosarcoma cells. *J Cell Biochem* 1997;66:141–152.

89. Smith E, Frenkel B, Schlegel R, et al. Expression of cell cycle regulatory factors in differentiating osteoblasts: postproliferative up-regulation of cyclins B and E. *Cancer Res* 1995;55:5019–5024.

90. Bodrug SE, Warner BJ, Bath ML, et al. Cyclin D1 transgene impedes lymphocyte maturation and collaborates in lymphomagenesis with the myc gene. *EMBO J* 1994;13:2124–2130.

91. Fantl V, Stamp G, Andrews A, et al. Mice lacking cyclin D1 are small and show defects in eye and mammary gland development. *Genes Dev* 1995;9:2364–2372.

92. Sicinski P, Donaher JL, Parker SB, et al. Cyclin D1 provides a link between development and oncogenesis in the retina and breast. *Cell* 1995;82:621–630.

93. Han EK, Begemann M, Sgambato A, et al. Increased expression of cyclin D1 in a murine mammary epithelial cell line induces p27kip1, inhibits growth, and enhances apoptosis. *Cell Growth Differ* 1996;7:699–710.

94. Zwijsen RM, Wientjens E, Klompmaker R, et al. CDK-

independent activation of estrogen receptor by cyclin D1. *Cell* 1997;88:405–415.

95. Stein GS, Baserga R, Giordano A, et al., eds. *Cell cycle and growth control.* New York: Wiley-Liss, 1998.

96. Sakou T. Bone morphogenetic proteins: from basic studies to clinical approaches. *Bone* 1998;22:591–603.

97. Karsenty G. Genetics of skeletogenesis. *Dev Genet* 1998;22:301–313.

98. Wozney JM, Rosen V. Bone morphogenetic protein and bone morphogenetic protein gene family in bone formation and repair. *Clin Orthop* 1998;346:26–37.

99. Derynck R, Zhang Y, Feng XH. Smads: transcriptional activators of TGF-beta responses. *Cell* 1998;95:737–740.

100. Heldin CH, Miyazono K, ten Dijke P. TGF-beta signalling from cell membrane to nucleus through SMAD proteins. *Nature* 1997;390:465–471.

101. Yanagisawa J, Yanagi Y, Masuhiro Y, et al. Convergence of transforming growth factor-beta and vitamin D signaling pathways on SMAD transcriptional coactivators. *Science* 1999;283:1317–1321.

102. Zhang Y, Feng XH, Derynck R. Smad3 and Smad4 cooperate with c-Jun/c-Fos to mediate TGF-beta-induced transcription [published erratum appears in *Nature* 1998;396:491]. *Nature* 1998;394:909–913.

103. Datto MB, Yu Y, Wang XF. Functional analysis of the transforming growth factor beta responsive elements in the WAF1/Cip1/p21 promoter. *J Biol Chem* 1995;270:28623–28628.

104. Li JM, Nichols MA, Chandrasekharan S, et al. Transforming growth factor beta activates the promoter of cyclin-dependent kinase inhibitor p15INK4B through an Sp1 consensus site. *J Biol Chem* 1995;270:26750–26753.

105. Wu Y, Craig TA, Lutz WH, et al. Identification of 1 alpha,25-dihydroxyvitamin D3 response elements in the human transforming growth factor beta 2 gene. *Biochemistry* 1999;38:2654–2660.

106. Liu M, Lee MH, Cohen M, et al. Transcriptional activation of the Cdk inhibitor p21 by vitamin D3 leads to the induced differentiation of the myelomonocytic cell line U937. *Genes Dev* 1996;10:142–153.

107. Kawa S, Nikaido T, Aoki Y, et al. Vitamin D analogues up-regulate p21 and p27 during growth inhibition of pancreatic cancer cell lines. *Br J Cancer* 1997;76:884–889.

108. Freedman LP. Transcriptional targets of the vitamin D3 receptor-mediating cell cycle arrest and differentiation. *J Nutr* 1999;129:581S–586S.

109. Rots NY, Liu M, Anderson EC, et al. A differential screen for ligand-regulated genes: identification of HoxA10 as a target of vitamin D3 induction in myeloid leukemic cells. *Mol Cell Biol* 1998;18:1911–1918.

110. Laherty CD, Yang WM, Sun JM, et al. Histone deacetylases associated with the mSin3 corepressor mediate mad transcriptional repression. *Cell* 1997;89:349–356.

111. Tzeng DZ, Klinge CM. Phosphorylation of purified estradiol-ligandeed estrogen receptor by casein kinase II increases estrogen response element binding but does not alter ligand stability. *Biochem Biophys Res Commun* 1996;223:554–560.

112. Trowbridge JM, Rogatsky I, Garabedian MJ. Regulation of estrogen receptor transcriptional enhancement

by the cyclin A/Cdk2 complex. *Proc Natl Acad Sci USA* 1997;94:10132–10137.

113. Bunone G, Briand PA, Miksicek RJ, et al. Activation of the unliganded estrogen receptor by EGF involves the MAP kinase pathway and direct phosphorylation. *EMBO J* 1996;15:2174–2183.

114. Kato S, Endoh H, Masuhiro Y, et al. Activation of the estrogen receptor through phosphorylation by mitogen-activated protein kinase. *Science* 1995;270:1491–1494.

115. De Luca F, Baron J. Control of bone growth by fibroblast growth factors. *Trends Endocrinol Metab* 1999; 10:61–65.

116. Klint P, Claesson-Welsh L. Signal transduction by fibroblast growth factor receptors. *Front Biosci* 1999;4: D165–177.

117. Kanai M, Goke M, Tsunekawa S, et al. Signal transduc- tion pathway of human fibroblast growth factor recep- tor 3. Identification of a novel 66-kDa phosphoprotein. *J Biol Chem* 1997;272:6621–6628.

118. Klint P, Kanda S, Claesson-Welsh L. Shc and a novel 89-kDa component couple to the Grb2-Sos complex in fibroblast growth factor-2-stimulated cells. *J Biol Chem* 1995;270:23337–23344.

119. LaVallee TM, Prudovsky IA, McMahon GA, et al. Ac- tivation of the MAP kinase pathway by FGF-1 corre- lates with cell proliferation induction while activation of the Src pathway correlates with migration. *J Cell Biol* 1998;141:1647–1658.

120. Su WC, Kitagawa M, Xue N, et al. Activation of Stat1 by mutant fibroblast growth-factor receptor in thanato- phoric dysplasia type II dwarfism. *Nature* 1997;386: 288–292.

Skeletal Growth Factors,
edited by Ernesto Canalis.
Lippincott Williams & Wilkins, Philadelphia, © 2000.

5

In Vitro and *In Vivo* Models to Study Growth Factor Actions in Bone

J. Edward Puzas

Department of Orthopaedics, University of Rochester School of Medicine and Dentistry, Rochester, New York 14642

Factor modulation of cell phenotype is one of the key points of regulation of any cellular process. It is the means by which cells communicate with each other over short distances and occasionally long distances. Moreover, it is also the way cells respond to their immediate environment. There is no better illustration of the action of growth factors on cell behavior than what occurs in the skeleton.

As we know, bone is a rich source of a number of regulatory growth factors. These factors are present to coordinate timing events between bone-resorbing and bone-forming cells during a remodeling episode. They also mediate skeletal development and are involved in healing (i.e., fracture healing).

Cell and animal models have played a key role in uncovering the actions of bone active factors. It has been through assays developed with cells and animals that we have been able to understand the overall workings of the skeleton. It has also been possible to utilize these findings in devising therapeutic protocols to control, in part, bone metabolism in humans.

IN VITRO MODELS

Isolated cells and cell lines that are freshly prepared, immortalized, and/or cloned have played a critical role in uncovering the mechanistic pathways that control bone metabolism. Specifically, osteoblast and osteoclast cell models are the mainstay of the biochemical and molecular investigations of the skeleton.

Osteoblast Models

The osteoblast lineage is now a well-defined cell pathway composed of three identifiable phenotypes. They are the preosteoblast (or osteoprogenitor cell), the mature functioning osteoblast, and the osteocyte. Nontransformed, highly enriched cell models exist for each phenotype.

Preosteoblast and Osteoblast Phenotype

The preosteoblast is characterized by a number of unique features. First, these cells are located near bone-forming surfaces. That is, they are usually present at sites where active, mature osteoblasts synthesize bone. Their appearance is that of an elongated cell with an elongated nucleus. Most often they are found in a stratum a few cell layers distant from active osteoblasts. Second, they have the capacity to divide. Frequently, mitotic figures can be found in these cells. Third, these cells usually stain less intensely for alkaline phosphatase and there is no evidence of a developed rough endoplasmic reticulum. In other words, they have not yet acquired all of the characteristics of mature osteoblasts.

Preosteoblasts give rise to osteoblasts at two distinct sites, the endosteum and the periosteum.

Endosteal preosteoblasts are active on trabecular and endocortical bone surfaces. They are derived from the stromal group of cells that, along with the hematopoietic group, populate marrow spaces. These stromal cells are self-renewing and with each cell division have the capacity to create a determined osteoprogenitor cell (DOPC), which will ultimately become a mature osteoblast and an inducible osteoprogenitor cell (IOPC) that will retain stem cell potentiality. The nomenclature of DOPC and IOPC was coined by Friedenstein et al. (1).

The ultrastructural and histological features of osteoblasts underscore the fact that these cells are very active metabolically. They contain an extensive rough endoplasmic reticulum comprised of polysomal structures that stain intensely basophilic. The predominant genes that are transcribed and translated in these cells deal with the synthesis of an extracellular matrix, that is, collagenous and noncollagenous matrix proteins. Nearly 20% of the total protein produced by osteoblasts is type I collagen. This is extraordinary when one considers the number of genes that need to be expressed for an osteoblast to remain viable. The predominant noncollagen protein secreted by osteoblasts is osteocalcin or bone gla protein (BGP), which makes up approximately 1% of extracellular matrix protein. Moreover, a host of regulatory factors is produced and deposited in bone by osteoblasts. These include the family of bone morphogenetic proteins (BMPs), beta transforming growth factors (TGF-βs), insulin-like growth factors (IGFs), platelet-derived growth factors (PDGFs), and basic fibroblast growth factor (bFGF) among others. Though these proteins represent a minor component of the extracellular matrix, they play a critical role in bone remodeling.

All osteoblasts are mononuclear, with the nucleus positioned eccentrically opposite the rough endoplasmic reticulum. The nuclear material is similar to that in other eukaryotic cells and remains in a diffuse, uncondensed state during interphase. There are usually one to three nucleoli. A mature, functioning osteoblast does not divide.

A characteristic of osteoblasts which can be

demonstrated histochemically is the presence of a substantial amount of the enzyme alkaline phosphatase. Bone-specific alkaline phosphatase has been localized to the plasma membrane of osteoblasts, and although it is known to be present in large amounts, its true function has not yet been determined.

Preosteoblast and Osteoblast Cell Models

Models for preosteoblastic cells exist mainly as freshly isolated cells from many skeletal sites. Virtually any bone cell isolate that is propagated in culture loses some of its differentiated characteristics and becomes progenitor in nature. However, specific techniques have been developed to enrich isolated cells for preosteoblasts. These usually include sequential enzymatic digestion from a periosteal or endosteal tissue that contains all forms of the osteoblast lineage. Early work by Peck et al. (2,3), Wong and Cohn (4), and Hefley et al. (5) pioneered these isolation techniques. In fact, with the innovations employed by Hefley et al. (5), it was possible to prepare highly enriched subpopulations from sequentially digested, microdissected segments of parietal bone. In order to eliminate contaminating cells derived from sources such as calvarial suture lines and underlying chondrocranium and fibrous elements, these investigators used only the uniform flat regions of the calvarial parietal bones (Fig. 5.1). Five cell fractions from timed sequential digestions of the parietal segments

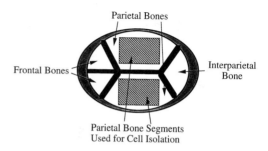

FIG. 5.1. Diagrammatic representation of a neonatal rat calvarium. Isolated bone cells enriched for preosteoblasts and osteoblasts can be prepared from parietal bone segments. Use of these well-defined plates of bone avoids contamination by suture line cells and chondrocytes.

were routinely obtained. Fraction 1 was composed primarily of fibrous elements of the periosteum on both the endocranial and ectocranial surfaces of the calvarium. Fraction 2 was a mixture of fibroblasts and preosteoblasts. Fraction 3 was predominantly preosteoblasts. Fraction 4 was a mixture of preosteoblasts and osteoblasts. Fraction 5 was a mature subpopulation of osteoblasts immediately adjacent to the bone on the parietal segments. The only cells remaining in the segments after digestion were the occasional osteocyte embedded in the bone.

Figures 5.2–5.4 demonstrate some of the biochemical characteristics of the isolated fractions. Figure 5.2 shows an example of the alkaline phosphatase content of cells isolated from calvarial segments. Note that the fibrous cells in fraction 1 have very low levels, the preosteoblasts in fraction 3 have low but detectable levels, and the osteoblasts in fraction 5 have quite high levels. These biochemical findings parallel the histochemical localization of alkaline phosphatase in calvarial tissue sections.

Figure 5.3 shows the amount of collagen synthesized by each cell phenotype as a percentage

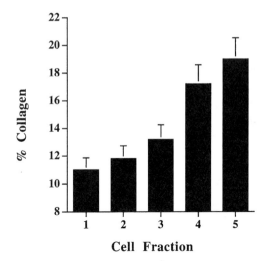

FIG. 5.3. Collagen synthesis in isolated bone cells. Cell fractions are as described in Fig. 5.2. Fraction 5 cells (osteoblasts) synthesize predominantly type I collagen. Nearly 20% of the total protein synthesized is collagen.

of the total protein produced. Again, it is evident that osteoblasts in fraction 5 produce the most collagen, approaching 20% of their total protein production. All of the collagen is type I.

Panels A and B of Fig. 5.4 demonstrate the sensitivity of the different fractions to 1,25-dihydroxyvitamin D_3 and parathyroid hormone (PTH). It is of interest to note that the mature, fully functioning osteoblast may not be the cell most sensitive to bone target hormones such as vitamin D and PTH. Apparently, the progenitor cell population, i.e., fraction 3 cells, is the most sensitive cell type in the calvarium. Although not immediately obvious, it does make sense that preosteoblasts would possess the greatest potential for modifying their phenotype and, thus, might be the most sensitive to endocrine regulation. A mature, fully functioning osteoblast that produces large amounts of collagen and growth factors and is responsible for mineralization is not as pliable a phenotype as a less differentiated cell type.

Osteocyte Phenotype

An osteocyte is an osteoblast which has become encased in calcified bone. During the pro-

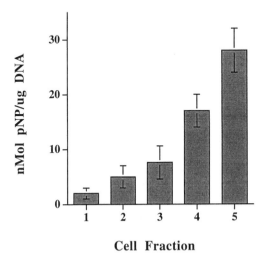

FIG. 5.2. Alkaline phosphatase activity of bone cells isolated from neonatal rat calvaria. Cell fraction 1 represents predominantly fibroblasts, cell fraction 3 predominantly preosteoblasts, and cell fraction 5 predominantly mature osteoblasts. Alkaline phosphatase–specific activity is highest in mature osteoblasts.

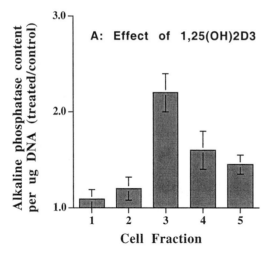

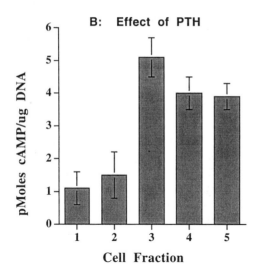

FIG. 5.4. Hormonal sensitivity (**A**, 1,25(OH)$_2$D$_3$; **B**, parathyroid hormone) for cells isolated from neonatal rat calvaria. Panels **A** and **B** demonstrate that fraction 3 cells (preosteoblasts) are the most sensitive bone cell type in the calvarium to vitamin D and parathyroid hormone.

cess of bone formation, the osteoblast determines its own fate by calcifying itself inside a lacuna. Approximately 15% of osteoblasts eventually become osteocytes. Although not all osteoblasts survive as osteocytes, all osteocytes originated from osteoblasts. As the cell becomes encased in bone, its metabolic activity decreases substantially due to a lack of nutrient diffusion. The only source of nutrients and gas exchange to which the osteocyte has access is through small bone canals known as canaliculi. These channels are the remnants of cellular processes from an osteoblast. The canaliculi form an extensive array of connecting tubules, and may serve as a communication and a nutrient network.

Osteocyte Cell Models

By the very nature of the osteocyte and its location, very few isolated cell models for this phenotype have been developed. However, the most recent attempt to create an osteocyte cell line has utilized a clever animal model along with molecular methods to clone a phenotype with many characteristics of an osteocyte. This work was performed by Kato et al. (6) and has been recently reviewed by Bonewald (7).

The strategy for preparing this cell line involved the creation of a transgenic mouse that contained the simian virus 40 (SV40) large T-antigen oncogene downstream of the osteocalcin promoter, the logic being that cells that express the largest amounts of osteocalcin (i.e., osteocytes) would have the strongest stimulus to be immortalized. Isolated bone cells were prepared from long bones by sequential enzyme digestion, and clones with high osteocalcin levels and low alkaline phosphatase levels were selected. The clone that was most fully characterized, MLO-Y4 (mouse long bone osteocyte Y4), produced extensive dendritic processes, was positive for osteopontin and connexin 43, and was negative for the osteoblast factor OSF-2 (Cbfa1). It remains to be seen how useful MLO-Y4 cells will be for the study of osteocyte physiology.

Another method that has been used for osteocyte isolation utilizes specific antibodies for selecting subpopulations of bone cell types from a complex mixture of isolated cells (8). In these types of study, antibodies to discrete stages of bone cell differentiation were used for cell sorting, identification of maturational stages, and even the discovery of previously unknown cell surface markers.

Osteocyte cultures have been used for a variety of studies; however, the most interesting feature of these cells appears to be their response to mechanical stimuli (9). Most investigators now recognize that osteocytes, by virtue of their location and intercommunication pathways, are in an ideal environment to detect and respond to mechanical stimuli. Numerous studies in "stretched" osteocytes have been performed, looking at prostaglandin production, ion fluxes, gene expression, etc. (10,11). As this is still a relatively new area in the use of a specific bone cell model, much new information is likely to be forthcoming.

Endosteal Versus Periosteal Bone Cell Models

Osteoblastic bone formation occurs on two different types of bone surface: the endosteal surface and the periosteal surfaces. Although both of these surfaces are lined with active bone cells, they effectively serve two different functions in the skeleton. Endosteal surfaces, and by extension the endosteal bone volume, are the reservoir for the maintenance of serum calcium and phosphate levels. It is at these surfaces that osteoclastic and osteoblastic regulatory pathways intersect to control bone resorption and formation. Conversely, periosteal surfaces on the cortex of bone are predominantly responsible for mechanical support. Rarely, if ever, is there osteoclastic activity on periosteal surfaces in a normal adult skeleton. This osseous surface is strictly populated by bone-forming cells. Given the different nature of these bone surfaces, one might expect that the osteoblasts that populate them would be different, and indeed they are. Early work by Baylink et al. (12) showed that the bone formation response to a restoration of calcium in the diet was qualitatively different on the endosteum than on the periosteum. Moreover, hormonal regulation of osteoblasts on these two surfaces also appears to be different (13).

The qualitative difference in osteoblast phenotype between endosteal and periosteal sites raises an important issue with regard to cell models. As most all freshly isolated osteoblast preparations utilize periosteal bone, care must be taken in drawing conclusions about what might occur on an endosteal surface.

Transformed Osteoblast Cell Models

Transformed osteoblast models are numerous. In the American Type Culture Collection alone, there are 88 cell lines derived from osteosarcomas. The species represented are human, rat, mouse, canine, and feline. Moreover, there are also many hundreds of genetically engineered bone-derived cell clones that express a multitude of regulatory factors. The BMPs, colony-stimulating factors (CSFs), TGF-βs, etc. are all available in clonal cell lines.

Perhaps the most widely used transformed osteoblast models are ROS 17/2.8, UMR 106, MC3T3E1, SAOS, and U2OS, with over 1,500 reports published using these cells models. Although these cells are derived from bone and retain many of the characteristics of osteoblasts, a number of published reports have identified aberrations in their behavior. Thus, although these models can be convenient and easy to use, care in the interpretation of data as they relate to normal skeletal biology must be taken when working with such cells.

Osteoclast Models

Osteoclasts and Their Genesis

The osteoclast is a giant, multinucleated cell that, when resorbing bone, demonstrates a polarity defined by a ruffled border that is composed of extensive interdigitated villi in direct contact with bone. Osteoclasts vary between 30 to 100 μ in diameter and may contain as many as ten to 20 nuclei per cell. Active osteoclasts have an extensive mitochondria, lysosomes, and a well-developed Golgi apparatus. These are also mobile cells that frequently migrate across a bony surface during the process of bone resorption. *In vitro* characteristics associated with the formation of authentic osteoclasts include multinuclearity, tartrate-resistant acid phosphatase positivity, bony attachment, the ability to form resorption lacunae in bone wafers, and hormone sensitivity (both stimulatory with PTH and inhibitory with calcitonin).

The osteoclast is derived from the macrophage lineage and, thus, is a member of the hematopoietic stem cell family. The regulatory pathway for osteoclastogenesis utilizes many of the early steps found in all macrophagic cell differentiation.

Isolated Osteoclast Models

Osteoclast isolation procedures were pioneered during the 1970s. The predominant feature of these cells, that is, their large size, was used as a basis for their separation. Recovery of the cells by curetting long bone dissections or with enzymatic digestions produced a complex mixture of cellular elements from the marrow spaces of bone. However, sedimentation techniques through isopycnic and gradient solutions were used to obtain small but relatively pure populations of isolated osteoclasts from these mixtures of cells. The earliest successful isolations were performed from rabbits (14–16), rats (17), and chickens (18).

Avian osteoclast isolations were further enhanced by two innovative techniques involving placing the animals on low-calcium diets to generate larger numbers of osteoclasts (19) and brief exposures to calcitonin to aid in the release of the cells from the bone surface (20). Nevertheless, viability of cells isolated in this manner was always an issue, with a number of investigators documenting only an approximate 10% viability in such preparations.

Perhaps the technique that generated the highest viability with the highest purity was described by Collin-Osdoby et al. (21). In this method, highly purified (though not necessarily viable) osteoclasts were used to create osteoclast-specific monoclonal antibodies, which were then coupled to small magnetic beads. Dispersed cells from chick marrow would adhere and engulf the coated beads and collection of the cells in a magnetic field could be effected. Purity on the order of 95% could be achieved, with a viability as high as 99%. However, the yields were modest, with only a few hundred thousand cells available per animal. Still, for the preparation of cDNA libraries and for more so-phisticated molecular methods, this procedure was more than satisfactory.

For those investigators who wish to study the actions of factors and hormones on osteoclast activity, purified cells are not necessary. In fact, highly purified cells might not be responsive since we now know that stromal cell or osteoblast interaction with osteoclasts is required for activity. This is the case for almost all factors except the newly discovered OPGL/RANKL/ODF/TRANCE family (see following).

Isolation and quantification methods such as those described by Murrills et al. (22,23) prove satisfactory for exploring osteoclast regulation. However, one caveat in the use of osteoclasts for studying hormone regulation is the apparent insensitivity of avian osteoclasts to calcitonin. Although mammalian osteoclasts are known to be extremely sensitive to calcitonin, with an almost complete cessation of activity when exposed to concentrations in the picogram per milliliter range, avian osteoclasts have been shown to be refractory to the hormone (24). Thus, if avian cells are selected as a model, they should not be used for calcitonin studies.

Emerging Models of Osteoclast Activity

The discovery of, perhaps, the final mediator of osteoclastogenesis has opened a wide door into devising cell models for studying bone resorption *in vitro*. Identification of the molecules known as ODF (osteoclast differentiation factor), OPGL (osteoprotegerin ligand), RANKL (receptor activator of NFκB ligand), and/or TRANCE (tumor necrosis factor–related activation-induced cytokine) has opened the possibility that monocyte or macrophage cell lines can be induced to form osteoclasts by the simple addition of a factor(s). The ability to produce a virtually pure population of cells undergoing differentiation into functional osteoclasts would greatly enhance our ability to uncover other regulatory pathways in osteoclastogenesis.

IN VIVO MODELS

Bone-Formation Models

The investigation of bone formation in an animal model can encompass a broad range of experimentation. Normal bone development in mice and chick embryos has given rise to a complex picture of the role of morphogenetic proteins. Studies of genetically altered mice have revealed the existence of unique transcription factors specific for bone. Implant models in rabbits, dogs, rats, mice, and sheep have been extensively used to bridge the gap from basic investigation to clinical utility.

Staged examination of skeletal development in embryos has uncovered a complex interaction between the BMPs, a family of paracrine regulators known as hedgehog molecules [Indian hedgehog (IHH); and sonic hedgehog (SHH)], and PTH-related peptide (PTHrP). From studies in mice and chicks, we are beginning to understand the interaction between differentiation-inducing agents such as BMP-6, BMP-7, and IHH and differentiation-inhibiting agents such as PTHrP (25–27).

In a study documenting the similarities and differences between fetal and postnatal skeletal development of the expression of BMP-6 and IHH, Helms et al. (28) showed that a critical interaction occurred between these molecules for normal bone formation. Moreover, another expressed protein, gli, also appeared to be centrally involved in sending and receiving the IHH signal (28–30). In almost all of the skeletal tissues examined, the expression domains of IHH and BMP-6 were coincident or adjacent to each other and the entire region was interspersed with gli-expressing cells. This observation supported the role of gli as a negative regulator of IHH and BMP-6, as suggested by Roberts et al. (31).

Upon sexual maturity, transcripts for IHH, BMP-6, and gli are no longer detectable, yet in this mouse model there remains an active growth plate and endochondral bone formation process. This suggests that these primordial regulatory factors are critical for early skeletal patterning but not necessary to sustain the endochondral process once it is under way. Such a finding has a large implication in therapeutic approaches to dealing with skeletal defects. That is, many of the late-stage regulatory factors, such as growth hormone, the IGFs, TGF-β, etc., may not be the appropriate molecules to regenerate the early forms of bone. A reversion to embryonic factors

may be the only way to re-create many of the osseous elements necessary for clinical problems.

The use of bead implantation into developing chick embryos has also opened up new avenues of investigation regarding skeletal development. These types of studies have shown that BMPs play direct roles in regulating the spatial distribution of chondrogenic mesenchyme and in controlling the location of joints and diaphyseal regions of long bones once the chondrogenesis begins to occur (32).

Genetically altered mice have been a major asset in discovering the many pathways involved in skeletal development. Perhaps this is best demonstrated in the sequence of reports related to Cbfa1, an osteoblast transcription factor. Cbfa1 (also known as OSF-2) is a transcriptional activator of osteoblasts that is under the control of BMPs and vitamin D (33,34). Animals that are devoid of Cbfa1 (i.e., Cbfa1 $-/-$) do not survive after birth, and thus, the role of this transcription factor in skeletal development has been difficult to study. However, with the advent of modern molecular techniques, it has been possible to devise an animal model that effectively shuts down the production of Cbfa1 upon maturation of the osteoblast phenotype. This was done by creating a Cbfa1 DNA-binding domain that had a higher affinity for the DNA-binding element than the authentic Cfba1 factor did. This protein was termed DeltaCbfa1. Upon the terminal differentiation of osteoblasts, DeltaCbfa1 expression would occur and the further development of the cells would be blocked. This animal model side-stepped the issue of perinatal lethality of the Cbfa1 knockout. The results of the study indicate that DeltaCbfa1-expressing mice have a normal skeleton at birth but develop an osteopenic phenotype thereafter. Dynamic histomorphometric studies show that this phenotype is caused by a major decrease in the bone formation rate in the face of a normal number of osteoblasts, thus indicating that once osteoblasts are differentiated, Cbfa1 regulates their function (35).

The use of animal models to study bone and cartilage formation in "implant" types of study dates back to the 1960s. The importance of these types in experiments is that they provide results that bear directly on the design of human clinical trials. One of the best examples of the use of animals for these types of study is the assessment of the role of factors and other proteins on bone formation during skeletal fusions. In these cases, an animal model has been able to predict what will occur in the human situation by uncovering pathogenic mechanisms, predisposing factors, and degree of difficulty in performing surgery.

Using these models, Boden et al. (36) were able to identify yet another factor that mediates the effects of the BMPs in inducing bone formation. Using rat calvarial bone cell cultures as a screening tool, they examined genes induced by the BMPs during osteoblast differentiation. A novel intracellular protein, LIM-mineralization protein (LMP-1), was discovered that was upstream of the induction of other soluble factors that induced new bone formation. Inhibition of LMP-1 synthesis blocked osteoblast differentiation, while overexpression of LMP-1 was sufficient to induce *de novo* bone nodule formation *in vitro* and in subcutaneous implants. Further investigations using rabbits, dogs, rats, and guinea pigs have been quite successful at elucidating other complex pathways of bone formation (37–40).

The appropriateness of an animal model can many times determine if experiments will be successful. For example, size, skeletal anatomy, similarity to human biology, healing potential, availability, ease of housing, uniformity, previous data, maintenance costs, etc. are all factors that need to be weighed in selecting which model to use. A careful consideration of these criteria will prevent the wasteful and unethical use of animals in a bone-formation model.

Bone-Resorption Models

Recent reports have shown that the myeloid and B lymphocyte transcription factor PU.1 plays a critical role in osteoclast formation (41). In mutant mice that are devoid of this transcription factor, no macrophages of any kind develop nor do osteoclasts form. The animals develop osteopetrosis and a skeletal sclerosis character-

ized by dense bone, small marrow spaces, and a lack of remodeling. Thus, disruptions at the earliest stages of macrophage development are an indication that osteoclast formation is dependent on points of regulation that exist in the formative pathways of myeloid cell differentiation. So far, the earliest identified step in myeloid development and subsequent osteoclastogenesis is the step that is inhibited as a result of PU.1 deletion.

A second transcription factor, c-fos, has also been implicated in osteoclast formation. A deletion in c-fos causes a form of osteopetrosis that can be reversed by myeloid cell transplantation. However, c-fos deletion does not interfere with the formation of active macrophages, whereas PU.1 deletion prevents macrophage formation everywhere. Interestingly, c-fos deletion is associated with a substantial increase in the number of macrophages (42). This suggests that c-fos regulates a branch point in the osteoclast differentiation pathway and is downstream from the PU.1-regulated step.

Other mutations in humans and other species have further delineated the osteoclast pathway. The *op/op* mouse, known to have a deficiency in the hematopoietic regulatory protein CSF-1 (43), has no osteoclasts and almost no macrophages. This deficiency is curable by injections of CSF-1. Because in this mutant model most phagocytic cells are nonfunctional, the CSF-1 control point is probably downstream of PU.1 and upstream of c-fos.

Mice which lack c-SRC also have osteopetrosis (44) but not because of a lack of osteoclastogenesis. Instead, these animals have an abundant number of cells with an osteoclast phenotype yet are not competent to resorb bone. Similar observations have been made in animals with mutations in carbonic anhydrase (45) and the proton pump H^+-ATPase (46). These enzymes seem to function in the late stages of osteoclastogenesis, as they essentially affect the mature cell. Thus, a number of the control points for osteoclastogenesis, from the earliest developmental stages to the final functions of the cell, are being uncovered.

Most recently, a new family of transcription factors involved in controlling the genes used by osteoclasts in the process of bone resorption has been discovered. They are the NFκB/Rel/IκB molecules (reviewed in 47). NFκB was originally characterized as a lymphoid-specific transcription factor involved in B-lymphocyte maturation. However, subsequent work has shown that a number of immunological and matrix degradation pathways are under its control. The two key members of the NFκB family are NFκB1 (the gene is termed p50) and NFκB2 (the gene is termed p52). NFκB1 and NFκB2 can dimerize with another pair of factors known as RelA and RelB. The subsequent heterodimer makes up the active transcription factor that can translocate into the nucleus and activate specific gene transcription. However, this does not occur until an inhibitory protein (IκB) is dissociated from the heterodimer and degraded. That is, in an inactive cell, all three components (NFκB, Rel, and IκB) are complexed in the cytosol. Upon activation of specific receptors involved in bone resorption, the IκB subunit is phosphorylated and targeted for proteosome degradation by subsequent ubiquitination. (Ubiquitination is the process by which ubiquitin side chains are added to terminal lysine residues in proteins destined for removal.) This liberates the NFκB/Rel dimer and allows it to enter the nucleus and evoke a response.

In animals that have been genetically manipulated to knock out both NFκB1 and NFκB2, severe osteopetrosis develops because osteoclast-mediated bone resorption does not occur (48). Deleting either NFκB1 or NFκB2 alone does not lead to the defect. This suggests that there is a redundancy in the action of these factors. A summary of these pathways is presented in Fig. 5.5.

The most interesting facet of this regulatory pathway is the potentially large number of steps at which it would be possible to intervene and control bone resorption. A number of pharmaceuticals, protease inhibitors, and gene therapy protocols could be used to block osteoclastogenesis or osteoclastic activity. For example, sulfasalazine and glucocorticoid hormones interfere with IκB degradation (49,50), thereby preventing translocation of the NFκB/Rel complex into the nucleus. Although direct experiments using this strategy for the prevention of bone resorption have not yet been attempted, it is conceivable that targeting the proteosome in osteoclasts

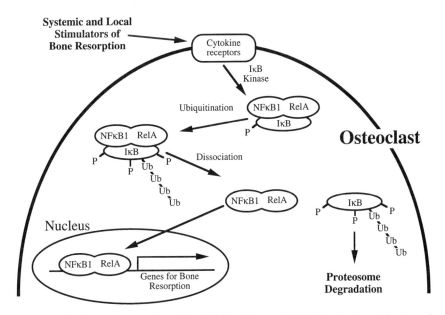

FIG. 5.5. Diagrammatic representation of the NFκB pathway. Cell activation leads to phosphorylation of IκB and its ultimate degradation. This allows the NFκB transcription factor to translocate into the nucleus and stimulate genes needed in the process of bone resorption.

may be a mechanism to prevent bone loss. The same holds true for genetic alteration of NFκB, Rel, or IκB. Any one of a number of strategies may be used to interfere with this pathway. Altering the NFκB or Rel molecules, inactivating the IκB protein kinase, altering the phosphorylation sites on IκB, removing the ubiquitination sites on IκB, and altering the nuclear translocation signals on NFκB are all potential targets for controlling osteoclast differentiation.

SUMMARY

In vitro and *in vivo* models have been indispensable in uncovering the complex workings of the skeleton. Through the basic research performed with these model systems it has been possible to devise human therapeutic protocols for arthritis, osteoporosis, and metastasis of cancers to bone. All of these protocols have produced Food and Drug Administration–approved medications or are in clinical trials. Thus, our dependence on cellular and animal models up to the present time has proven well worth the effort. This will not change in the future.

REFERENCES

1. Friedenstein AY, Chailakhyan RK, Latsinik NY, et al. Stromal cells responsible for transferring the microenvironment of the hemopoietic tissues. *Transplantation* 1974;17:331–340.
2. Peck WA, Carpenter J, Messinger K, et al. Cyclic 3'5'-adenosine monophosphate in isolated bone cells. Response to low concentrations of parathyroid hormone. *Endocrinology* 1973;92:692–698.
3. Peck WA, Carpenter J, Messinger K. Cyclic 3'5'-adenosine monophosphate in isolated bone cells. II. Response to adenosine and parathyroid hormone. *Enodocrinology* 1974;94:148–158.
4. Wong GL, Cohn DV. Target cells in bone for parathormone and calcitonin are different: enrichment for each cell type by sequential digestion of mouse calcaria and selective adhesion to polymeric surfaces. *Proc Natl Acad Sci USA* 1975;72:3167–3171.
5. Hefley T, Cushing J, Brand JS. Enzymatic isolation of cells from bone: cytotoxic enzymes of bacterial collagenase. *Am J Physiol* 1981;240:C234–C241.
6. Kato Y, Windle JJ, Koop BA, et al. Establishment of an osteocyte-like cell line, MLO-Y4. *J Bone Miner Res* 1997;12:2014–2023.
7. Bonewald LF. Establishment and characterization of an osteocyte-like cell line, MLO-Y4 *J Bone Miner Metab* 1999;17:61–65.
8. Aubin JE, Turksen K. Monoclonal antibodies as tools for studying the osteoblast lineage. *Microsc Res Tech* 1996;33:128–140.
9. Mikuni-Takagaki Y. Mechanical responses and signal transduction pathways in stretched osteocytes. *J Bone Miner Metab* 1999;17:57–60.
10. Ajubi NE, Klein-Nulend J, Alblas MJ, et al. Signal transduction pathways involved in fluid flow-induced PGE2 production by cultured osteocytes. *Am J Physiol* 1999; 276:E171–E178.
11. Kawata A, Mikuni-Takagaki Y. Mechanical transduction in stretched osteocytes—temporal expression of immediate early and other genes. *Biochem Biophys Res Commun* 1998;246:404–408.
12. Drivdahl RH, Liu CC, Baylink DJ. Regulation of bone repletion in rats subjected to varying low-calcium stress. *Am J Physiol* 1984;246:R190–R196.
13. Turner RT, Colvard DS, Spelsberg TC. Estrogen inhibition of periosteal bone formation in rat long bones: down-regulation of gene expression for bone matrix proteins. *Endocrinology* 1990;127:1346–1351.
14. Nelson R, Bauer G. Isolation of osteoclasts by velocity sedimentation at unit gravity. *Calcif Tissue Res* 1977; 22:303–309.
15. Chambers T. Phagocytosis and trypsin-resistant glass adhesion by osteoclasts in culture. *J Pathol* 1979;127: 55–64.
16. Chambers T, Magnus C. Calcitonin alters behaviour of isolated osteoclasts. *J Pathol* 1982;136:27–34.
17. Hefley T, Stern P. Isolation of osteoclasts from fetal rat long bones. *Calcif Tissue Int* 1982;34:480–490.
18. Osdoby P, Martini M, Caplan A. Isolated osteoclasts and their presumed progenitor cells, the monocyte, in culture. *J Exp Zool* 1982;244:331–340.
19. Zambonin-Zallone A, Teti A, Primavera M. Isolated osteoclasts in primary culture: first observation on structure and survival in culture media. *Anat Embryol* 1982; 165:405–415.
20. Gay C, Ito M, Schraer H. Carbonic anhydrase activity in isolated osteoclasts. *Metab Bone Dis Relat Res* 1983; 5:33–39.
21. Collin-Osdoby P, Oursler M, Webber D, et al. Osteoclast-specific monoclonal antibodies coupled to magnetic beads provide a rapid and efficient method of purifying avian osteoclasts. *J Bone Miner Res* 1991;6: 1353–1362.
22. Murrills RJ, Dempster DW. The effects of stimulators of intracellular cyclic AMP on rat and chick osteoclasts in vitro: validation of a simplified light microscope assay of bone resorption. *Bone* 1990;11:333–344.
23. Murrills RJ, Shane E, Lindsay R, et al. Bone resorption by isolated human osteoclasts in vitro: effects of calcitonin. *J Bone Miner Res* 1989;4:259–268.
24. Arnett TR, Dempster DW. A comparative study of disaggregated chick and rat osteoclasts in vitro: effects of calcitonin and prostaglandins. *Endocrinology* 1987;120: 602–608.
25. Bitgood MJ, McMahon AP. Hedgehog and Bmp genes are coexpressed at many diverse sites of cell–cell interaction in the mouse embryo. *Dev Biol* 1995;172: 126–138.
26. Lanske B, Karaplis AC, Lee K, et al. PTH/PTHrP receptor in early development and Indian hedgehog–regulated bone growth. *Science* 1996;273:663–666.
27. Vortkamp A, Lee K, Lanske B, et al. Regulation of

rate of cartilage differentiation by Indian hedgehog and PTH-related protein. *Science* 1996;273:613–622.

28. Iwasaki M, Le AX, Helms JA. Expression of Indian hedgehog, bone morphogenetic protein 6 and gli during skeletal morphogenesis. *Mech Dev* 1997;69:197–202.

29. Dominguez M, Brunner M, Hafen E, et al. Sending and receiving the hedgehog signal: control by the *Drosophila* Gli protein Cubitus interruptus. *Science* 1996;272: 1621–1625.

30. Marigo V, Johnson RL, Vortkamp A, et al. Sonic hedgehog differentially regulates expression of GLI and GLI3 during limb development. *Dev Biol* 1996;180:273–283.

31. Roberts DJ, Johnson RL, Burke AC, et al. Sonic hedgehog is an endodermal signal inducing Bmp-4 and Hox genes during induction and regionalization of the chick hindgut. *Development* 1995;121:3163–3174.

32. Macias D, Ganan Y, Sampath TK, et al. Role of BMP-2 and OP-1 (BMP-7) in programmed cell death and skeletogenesis during chick limb development. *Development* 1997;124:1109–1117.

33. Ducy P, Zhang R, Geoffroy V, et al. Osf2/Cbfa1: a transcriptional activator of osteoblast differentiation. *Cell* 1997;89:747–754.

34. Owen MJ, Karsenty G. New developments in bone formation. *Curr Opin Nephrol Hypertens* 1998;7:363–366.

35. Ducy P, Starbuck M, Priemel M, et al. A Cbfa1-dependent genetic pathway controls bone formation beyond embryonic development. *Genes Dev* 1999;13:1025–1036.

36. Boden SD, Liu Y, Hair GA, et al. LIMP-1, a LIM-domain protein, mediates BMP-6 effects on bone formation. *Endocrinology* 1998;139:5125–5134.

37. Guizzardi S, Di Silverstre M, Scandroglio R, et al. Implants of heterologous demineralized bone matrix for induction of posterior spinal fusion in rats. *Spine* 1992; 17:701–707.

38. Lovel TP, Dawson EG, Nilsson OS, et al. Augmentation of spinal fusion with bone morphogenetic protein in dogs. *Clin Orthop Rel Res* 1989;243:266–274.

39. Ragini P, Lindholm S. Interaction of allogeneic demineralized bone matrix and porous hydroxyapatite bioceramics in lumbar interbody fusion in rabbits. *Clin Orthop Rel Res* 1991;272:292–299.

40. Singh SH, Kirkaldy-Willis WH. Experimental anterior spinal fusion in guinea pigs: a histologic study of the changes in the anterior and posterior elements. *Can J Surg* 1972;15:239–248.

41. Tondravi MM, McKercher S, Anderson K, et al. Osteopetrosis in mice lacking haematopoietic transcription factor PU.1. *Nature* 1997;386:81–84.

42. Grigoriadis AE, Wang Z, Cecchini MG, et al. c-Fos: a key regulator of osteoclast-macrophage lineage determination and bone remodeling. *Science* 1994;266:443–448.

43. Kodama H, Yamasaki A, Nose M, et al. Congenital osteoclast deficiency in osteopetrotic (op/op) mice is cured by injections of macrophage colony stimulating factor. *J Exp Med* 1991;173:269–272.

44. Soriano P, Montgomery C, Geske R, et al. Targeted disruption of the c-src proto-oncogene leads to osteopetrosis in mice. *Cell* 1991;64:693–702.

45. Sly WS, Hewett-Emmett D, Whyte MP, et al. Carbonic anhydrase II deficiency identified as the primary defect in the autosomal recessive syndrome of osteopetrosis with renal tubular acidosis and cerebral calcification. *Proc Natl Acad Sci USA* 1983;80:2752–2756.

46. Yamamoto T, Kurihara N, Yamaoka K, et al. Bone marrow–derived osteoclast-like cells from a patient with craniometaphyseal dysplasia lack expression of osteoclast-reactive vacuolar proton pump. *J Clin Invest* 1993; 91:362–367.

47. Verma IM, Stevenson JK, Schwarz EM, et al. Rel/NF-κB/IκB family: intimate tales of association and dissociation. *Genes Dev* 1995;9:2723–2735.

48. Iotsova V, Caamano J, Loy J, et al. Osteopetrosis in mice lacking NF-kappaB1 and NF-kappaB2. *Nat Med* 1997;3:1285–1289.

49. Scheinman RI, Cogswell PC, Lofquist AK, et al. Role of transcriptional activation of IκBα in mediation of immunosuppression by glucocorticoids. *Science* 1995; 270:283–286.

50. Wahl C, Liptay S, Adler G, et al. Sulfasalazine: a potent and specific inhibitor of nuclear factor kappa B. *J Clin Invest* 1998;101:1163–1174.

Skeletal Growth Factors,
edited by Ernesto Canalis.
Lippincott Williams & Wilkins, Philadelphia, © 2000.

6

Insulin-like Growth Factors

Their Binding Proteins and Growth Regulation

David R. Clemmons

*Department of Medicine, University of North Carolina School of Medicine,
Chapel Hill, North Carolina 27599-7170*

The family of insulin-like growth factors (IGFs) consists of the polypeptide ligands of IGF-I, IGF-II, and insulin. These peptides bind to three separate receptors. The insulin receptor has high affinity for insulin and much lower affinity (greater than 100-fold reduction) for IGF-I and IGF-II. The IGF-I receptor, in contrast, has 500-fold greater affinity for IGF-I than insulin and a 20-fold reduction in affinity for IGF-II (1). The mannose-6-phosphate/IGF-II receptor has the highest affinity for IGF-II, an 80-fold lower affinity for IGF-I, and no affinity for insulin. These receptors, particularly the IGF-I receptor, are ubiquitously present in almost all tissues; therefore, almost all cell types in the human body are responsive to IGF-I.

IGF-I is produced in peripheral tissues as well as in the liver (2). The liver is the source of 80% of the IGF-I peptide in blood, but production by peripheral tissues is an important stimulus of systemic growth. Following tissue injury, specific cell types in the damaged area synthesize IGF-I, and this increase in locally synthesized IGF-I is an important part of the repair response (3). This response does not require plasma IGF-I, and animals that have been hypophysectomized respond appropriately, even though their serum IGF-I concentrations are low.

The ability to genetically manipulate animals has resulted in greater understanding of the role of locally produced IGF-I in regulating growth *in vivo* (4). Results from these studies have highlighted the need for understanding both the systemic endocrine effects of IGF-I, which can be demonstrated by *in vivo* infusion experiments or selective gene targeting of IGF-I expression in the liver, and the local effects, which can be analyzed by deletion of IGF-I expression in peripheral tissues. A more complete picture of how these two systems are coordinated is currently being developed.

Recent research has focused on the structural relationship between IGF-I and insulin, their respective receptors, and the signaling systems that they utilize. These hormones diverged from a common ancestral precursor, and separate mechanisms were developed for controlling their concentrations in extracellular fluids. Insulin does not bind to binding proteins, and its levels fluctuate rapidly with changes in carbohydrate intake. In contrast, IGF-I that is bound to IGF binding protein-3 (IGFBP-3) (the principal binding protein for IGF-I in serum) has a half-life of approximately 16 hours (5). Although the amount of free IGF-I that is available to bind to receptors may be under more short-term regulation, this stable resevoir of IGF-I provides a mechanism for providing sufficient peptide to receptors to result in long-term growth stimulation. Further distinctions between insulin and

IGF-I have been determined at the receptor level. The hormones have two distinct receptors. While both receptors activate common signaling elements, specific differences have also been identified (6).

IGF-I was originally discovered based on its ability to stimulate sulfation of proteoglycans present in cartilage and cartilage DNA synthesis. Using bioassays based on this model, it was possible to purify the factor and to determine its amino acid sequence. Similarly, those investigating the insulin-like activity of serum utilized bioassays to purify this material and determine its sequence. Comparison of the sequences showed that both peptides were structurally homologous. Thus, they were named "insulin-like growth factors" because of their homologies and the evolutionary linkage to proinsulin (7). Current studies are focusing on the receptor signal-transduction mechanisms of each hormone, the capacity of IGFBPs to modify IGF-I action *in vitro* and *in vivo,* and the relative roles and *in vivo* actions of autocrine/paracrine regulation of IGF-I action as compared to its endocrine effects.

INSULIN-LIKE GROWTH FACTOR-I GENE AND PROTEIN STRUCTURES

IGF-I is a complex gene with six exons (8). The gene is complex because it has multiple promoters. In addition, alternative splicing of mRNA occurs, and the two major forms have been detected in cells and tissues, termed IGF-I-A and IGF-I-B. When the number of transcripts in tissues is analyzed, at least four specific transcripts are often detected, the most abundant being 6 kb. The abundance of this transcript and of a small, 0.9-kb transcript appears to be regulated in the liver by growth hormone (GH) (9). Fetal and tissue-specific promoters for IGF-I transcripts have also been identified, and the fetal promoters are active at specific times during development. The other major variables that account for transcripts of different sizes are the polyadenylation sites and regulation of processing of 3′–untranslated mRNA extensions (10).

The mature IGF-I polypeptide contains 70 amino acids compared to 67 in IGF-II. The A and B portions of the peptide chains are similar in length (Fig. 6.1), and the sequences of the regions of IGF-I are 41% and 43% homologous with proinsulin. IGF-I contains a D amino acid extension beyond the termination of the A peptide. IGF-I and IGF-II are secreted as single chains, and there is no cleavage as occurs in the processing of proinsulin to insulin. Analysis of forms of IGF-I has shown that peptides with the E-terminal peptide extensions can be detected in certain cell culture supernatants, and variable processing of the E-peptide region of both IGF-I and IGF-II resulting in peptides of different lengths has been reported to occur in serum (11).

The exact amino acids that account for IGF-I binding to IGFBPs and receptors have been identified (12). Tyrosines 24, 60, and, to some extent, 31 are critical for receptor recognition. The primary receptor-binding site occurs between positions 24 and 37. The corresponding amino acids in IGF-II are tyrosines 27 and 59, with no residue comparable to Tyr[31]. In contrast, amino acids 3, 4, 15, and 16 of the B-chain region of IGF-I are extremely important for IGFBP affinity (13). The comparable residues are present in IGF-II at positions 6, 7, 18, and 19. In addition, residues 49, 50, and 51 of the A chain of IGF-I are critical for recognition by four of the six high-affinity binding proteins. The comparable residues in IGF-II are positions 48, 49, and 50. The C-peptide region is greatly divergent between IGF-I and IGF-II. There are three disulfide linkages that are conserved in IGF-I, IGF-II, and proinsulin. Computer modeling studies have indicated that the tertiary structure of IGF-I is similar to that of insulin (14). An alternatively processed form of IGF-I, termed des-1–3-IGF-I, is detectible in serum (15). A protease that cleaves native IGF-I to the des-1–3-IGF-I form has also been detected in serum (16). The importance of this cleavage is that des-IGF-I binds poorly to several of the IGFBPs, and this may be a mechanism for further activating IGF-I in serum.

INSULIN-LIKE GROWTH FACTOR-I RECEPTOR

IGF-I receptors are detectable in cell types derived from all three embryonic lineages. The

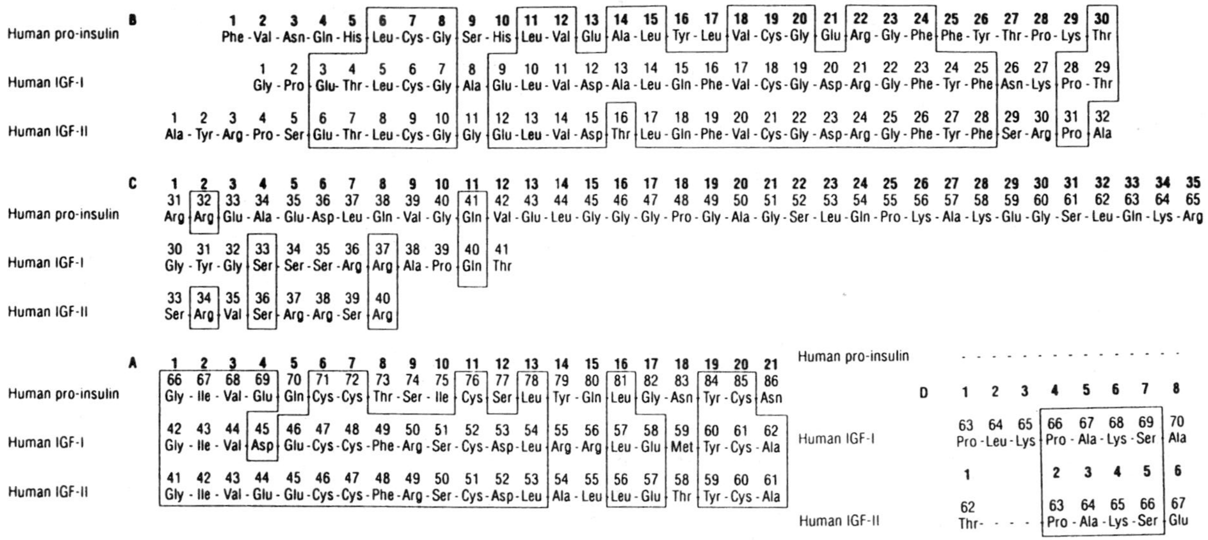

FIG. 6.1. Amino acid sequence alignment of proinsulin, insulin-like growth factor I (IGF-I) and IGF-II. The structural domains of each of the three proteins are shown using the nomenclature *B*, *C*, *A*, and *D*. There is a great deal of homology in the *B* and *A* regions among the three family members. Notably, however, there are amino acid differences between proinsulin and IGF-I in positions 3, 4, 15, and 16 of the IGF-I B region. Similarly, residues 49, 50, and 51 of the A region are distinct. These are significant because these residues are important for IGF binding protein association. Similarly, tyrosine-31, which is important for IGF-I receptor association, is not present in proinsulin. The D-peptide extensions of IGF-I and IGF-II are not present in proinsulin, which has a much longer C domain.

B region

Human pro-insulin (1–30): Phe(1)-Val(2)-Asn(3)-Gln(4)-His(5)-Leu(6)-Cys(7)-Gly(8)-Ser(9)-His(10)-Leu(11)-Val(12)-Glu(13)-Ala(14)-Leu(15)-Tyr(16)-Leu(17)-Val(18)-Cys(19)-Gly(20)-Glu(21)-Arg(22)-Gly(23)-Phe(24)-Phe(25)-Tyr(26)-Thr(27)-Pro(28)-Lys(29)-Thr(30)

Human IGF-I (1–29): Gly(1)-Pro(2)-Glu(3)-Thr(4)-Leu(5)-Cys(6)-Gly(7)-Ala(8)-Glu(9)-Leu(10)-Val(11)-Asp(12)-Ala(13)-Leu(14)-Gln(15)-Phe(16)-Val(17)-Cys(18)-Gly(19)-Asp(20)-Arg(21)-Gly(22)-Phe(23)-Tyr(24)-Phe(25)-Asn(26)-Lys(27)-Pro(28)-Thr(29)

Human IGF-II (1–32): Ala(1)-Tyr(2)-Arg(3)-Pro(4)-Ser(5)-Glu(6)-Thr(7)-Leu(8)-Cys(9)-Gly(10)-Gly(11)-Glu(12)-Leu(13)-Val(14)-Asp(15)-Thr(16)-Leu(17)-Gln(18)-Phe(19)-Val(20)-Cys(21)-Gly(22)-Asp(23)-Arg(24)-Gly(25)-Phe(26)-Tyr(27)-Phe(28)-Ser(29)-Arg(30)-Pro(31)-Ala(32)

C region

Human pro-insulin (31–65): Arg(31)-Arg(32)-Glu(33)-Ala(34)-Glu(35)-Asp(36)-Leu(37)-Gln(38)-Val(39)-Gly(40)-Gln(41)-Val(42)-Glu(43)-Leu(44)-Gly(45)-Gly(46)-Gly(47)-Pro(48)-Gly(49)-Ala(50)-Gly(51)-Ser(52)-Leu(53)-Gln(54)-Pro(55)-Leu(56)-Ala(57)-Leu(58)-Glu(59)-Gly(60)-Ser(61)-Leu(62)-Gln(63)-Lys(64)-Arg(65)

Human IGF-I (30–41): Gly(30)-Tyr(31)-Gly(32)-Ser(33)-Ser(34)-Ser(35)-Arg(36)-Arg(37)-Ala(38)-Pro(39)-Gln(40)-Thr(41)

Human IGF-II (33–40): Ser(33)-Arg(34)-Val(35)-Ser(36)-Arg(37)-Arg(38)-Ser(39)-Arg(40)

A region

Human pro-insulin (66–86): Gly(66)-Ile(67)-Val(68)-Glu(69)-Gln(70)-Cys(71)-Cys(72)-Thr(73)-Ser(74)-Ile(75)-Cys(76)-Ser(77)-Leu(78)-Tyr(79)-Gln(80)-Leu(81)-Glu(82)-Asn(83)-Tyr(84)-Cys(85)-Asn(86)

Human IGF-I (42–62): Gly(42)-Ile(43)-Val(44)-Asp(45)-Glu(46)-Cys(47)-Cys(48)-Phe(49)-Arg(50)-Ser(51)-Cys(52)-Asp(53)-Leu(54)-Arg(55)-Arg(56)-Leu(57)-Glu(58)-Met(59)-Tyr(60)-Cys(61)-Ala(62)

Human IGF-II (41–61): Gly(41)-Ile(42)-Val(43)-Glu(44)-Glu(45)-Cys(46)-Cys(47)-Phe(48)-Arg(49)-Ser(50)-Cys(51)-Asp(52)-Leu(53)-Ala(54)-Leu(55)-Leu(56)-Glu(57)-Thr(58)-Tyr(59)-Cys(60)-Ala(61)

D region

Human pro-insulin: (absent) - - - - - - - -

Human IGF-I (positions 1–8): Pro(63)-Leu(64)-Lys(65)-Pro(66)-Ala(67)-Lys(68)-Ser(69)-Ala(70)

Human IGF-II: Thr(62)- - - Pro(63)-Ala(64)-Lys(65)-Ser(66)-Glu(67) receptor number is tightly controlled within a range of 20,000 to 35,000 per cell. Hormonal regulation of receptor number occurs, and hormones such as GH, follicle-stimulating hormone (FSH), luteinizing hormone (LH), progesterone, estradiol, and thyroxine have been shown to alter receptor expression (17). Similarly, growth factors such as platelet-derived growth factor (PDGF), epidermal growth factor (EGF), fibroblast growth factor (FGF), and angiotensin II can upregulate receptor expression in specific cell types (18,19). Following hormone binding, there is some downregulation of receptor number, but the rate of internalization is substantially less than that which occurs with the EGF or insulin receptors. Whether this is due to IGFBPs in the pericellular environment has not been determined. The structure of the receptor is shown in Fig. 6.2. It is a heterotetrameric glycoprotein composed of two ligand-binding subunits, termed α subunits, which contain 706 amino acids, and two β subunits, which contain 627 amino acids. The membrane-spanning domain is located in the β subunits. The C-terminal end of the β subunit contains intrinsic tyrosine kinase activity. This tyrosine kinase domain is 84% homologous with the insulin receptor tyrosine kinase domain and is located between positions 906 and 929. The receptor is synthesized as a single polypeptide and then cleaved to generate the α and β subunits. The affinity of the receptor is approximately 10^{-9} M, and IGF-II binds it with sixfold lower affinity (6). The tyrosine kinase domain contains an adenosine triphosphate (ATP)–binding motif and a catalytic lysine at position 1003. Following ligand binding, the receptor is activated and undergoes a conformational change, following which the tyrosine kinase is activated. It then transphosphorylates the opposite β subunit. The most critical residues that need to be autophosphorylated during activation are tyrosines 1149, 1150, and 1151 (20). Substitution for these tyrosines results in abolition of IGF-I signaling. Other tyrosines that appear to be important include 1131, 1135, 1136, 1316, 1250, and 1251. Following phosphorylation of critical tyrosines, the activated receptor can bind to and phosphorylate specific intracellular signaling molecules. Chimeric receptors that contain $\alpha\beta$ dimers of the IGF-I receptor and insulin receptor have been identified (21). These receptor subtypes are present in increased amounts in specific tissues, such as placenta. This receptor subtype has a much higher affinity for IGF-I than does insulin and its subtype is upregulated in states of insulin resistance, such as type II diabetes.

Overexpression of the IGF-I receptor can result in cellular transformation. Specifically, expression of 10^6 receptors per cell results in a marked diminution in the requirement for exogenous growth factors, such as EGF and PDGF, and transformation by certain tumor viruses, such as large T antigen induction by the cellular transforming simia virus 40 (SV40), results in alteration in transforming activity that is IGF-I receptor–dependent (22). Cells bearing enhanced receptor numbers can grow in soft agar and form tumors in nude mice, whereas cells that bear a normal receptor number cannot.

The receptor is also extremely important for normal growth and development. Mice that have had the receptor deleted by homologous recombination are born at approximately 40% normal size and are not viable after birth (23). Receptor expression is important for IGF-I to be able to inhibit apoptosis. Cells that are forced to undergo apoptosis, such as hematopoietic cells, which are interleukin-3-dependent, are protected from apoptosis by exposure to IGF-I following interleukin-3 removal from culture medium. If the IGF-I receptor is deleted, they undergo massive apoptosis. Mutation of specific tyrosines within the β subunit can result in loss of IGF-I-mediated signaling, a reduction in IGF-I-stimulated cell growth, refractoriness to SV40 or receptor overexpression–induced cellular transformation, and the ability of IGF-I to inhibit apoptosis (24).

RECEPTOR-MEDIATED SIGNAL TRANSDUCTION

Following activation of the intrinsic tyrosine activity, phosphorylation of the triple tyrosine domain of the receptor results in the binding of an important docking protein, insulin receptor substrate-1 (IRS-1), to the receptor (25). Other

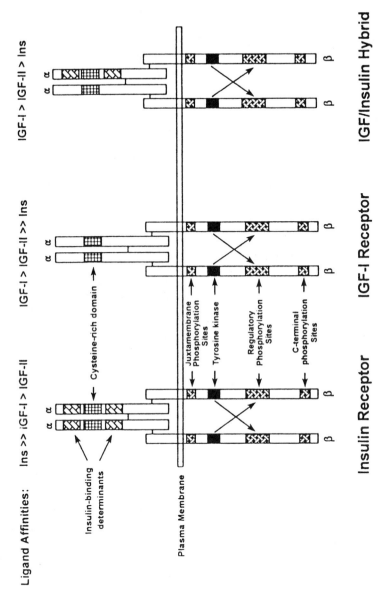

FIG. 6.2. Insulin-like growth factor I (*IGF-I*) receptor, insulin, and hybrid receptors. The domain structure of each receptor is shown. The extracellular binding domain in the IGF-I receptor is substantially smaller than the determinants of insulin binding. The location of tyrosine kinase activity is similar within both β subunits, and regulatory phosphorylation sites, as well as C-terminal phosphorylation sites, are in similar proximity, although the exact residues that are phosphorylated by each kinase may differ. An IGF/insulin hybrid receptor is also shown.

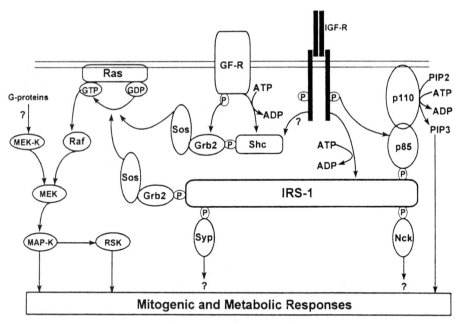

FIG. 6.3. Insulin-like growth factor I *(IGF-I)* receptor–linked signal-transduction pathways. The signaling pathways for typical growth factor receptors as well as for the IGF-I receptor are shown. As shown in the diagram, the IGF-I receptor often signals by activating the docking protein IRS-1. This protein can activate either the mitogen-activated protein *(MAP)* kinase pathway or the phosphatidylinositol *(PI)* 3-kinase pathway. However, direct activation of the MAP kinase pathway can also occur through Shc, as shown.

homologous proteins, IRS-2, IRS-3, and IRS-4, have also been identified (26). Following IRS-1 binding to the receptor, several sites are phosphorylated, which create docking motifs for intracellular proteins that contain Src homology-2 (SH2) domains (Fig. 6.3). These domains contain approximately 100 amino acids and share similarity to the cellular oncogene C-Src. Other proteins that have been shown to bind directly to the phosphorylated tyrosines on IRS-1 include Nck, Grb-2, and Shc (27). Grb-2 activation results in activation of a ras-activating protein termed son of sevenless (SOS), and this complex leads to P-21 ras activation. This, in turn, activates raf and the downstream components of the mitogen-activated protein (MAP) kinase signaling pathway, which is extremely important for the mitogenic activity of IGF-I. IRS-1 also activates binding of the two major subunits of phosphatidylinositol (PI) 3-kinase. This binding results in catalytic activation of PI 3-kinase, generation of inositol triphosphate, and the sub-

sequent activation of protein tyrosine kinase B. This kinase activates p-70 S-6 kinase and glycogen synthetase kinase, a regulator of glucose transport. This pathway is extremely important for IGF-I stimulation of cell motility and inhibition of apoptosis. The activated IGF-I receptor can also directly phosphorylate Shc, and this can lead to Grb-2 activation. An additional receptor-activated signaling molecule that is activated is Crk, a Grb-2-like protein, and Crk can activate the ras–MAP kinase pathway. Other signaling pathways that are activated include protein kinase C, phospholipase C, and the calcium-permeable ion channels (28,29).

THE QUESTION OF INSULIN VERSUS INSULIN-LIKE GROWTH FACTOR-I RECEPTOR SPECIFICITY

A great deal of attention has been focused on comparing the components of the signaling pathways that are activated by insulin and IGF-I.

Some intermediary substances, such as IRS-1 and IRS-2, are activated by both receptors; however, certain specific properties have been identified for each pathway. The first and most important specific property is the known differential affinity of the two receptors (for example, of the insulin receptor having 200 greater affinity for insulin than does IGF-I and the IGF-I receptor having 500-fold greater affinity for IGF-I similar to insulin). Although the kinase domains are approximately 84% identical, not all of the residues that are autophosphorylated are similar. Activation of Crk-2 by activated IGF-I receptor is specific and does not occur with the insulin receptor (30). Likewise, insulin receptor activation results in dephosphorylation of tyrosine residues on focal adhesion kinase, whereas the IGF-I receptor does not have this effect (31). Activated IRS-1 also binds to different phosphorylated tyrosine domains within each receptor. Activation of Src kinase results in phosphorylation of the IGF-I receptor but not the insulin receptor. Finally, gene targeting experiments have shown that the phenotypes resulting from the deletion of each receptor are quite different from each other, but how these differences are mediated, beyond the known receptor ligand-binding selectivity, remains to be determined.

INSULIN-LIKE GROWTH FACTOR-II/MANNOSE-6-PHOSPHATE RECEPTOR

This receptor is a single-chain glycoprotein containing 2,451 amino acids. It binds to mannose-6-phosphate residues on lysosomal enzymes and to IGF-II, at a separate binding site. The extracellular domain is composed of three sets of 15 repeating motifs, with motifs seven to nine containing the mannose-6-phosphate-binding site and motif 11 containing the IGF-II binding region (32). This receptor functions to translocate newly synthesized lysosomal enzymes to endosomes. Once it recycles to the cell surface, it binds to mannose-6-phosphate-containing extracellular glycoproteins, which are then entocytosed into endosomes. An important protein that binds to this receptor is latent transforming growth factor β (TGF-β). This binding

is required for TGF-β activation (33). The receptor binds IGF-II with an affinity of 1.3 nM. The affinity for IGF-I is 80-fold lower. The receptor is rapidly recycled from endosomes to the cell surface, and recycling can be stimulated by insulin.

The extracellular portion of the receptor is proteolytically cleaved and can be detected in extracellular fluids. Mutation of this receptor results in mice that die at 17 days *in utero* (34). They develop severe edema and are larger than fetuses of a comparable age. If the IGF-II gene is also deleted, the animals survive. This suggests that the IGF-II receptor has an important scavenging function that prevents accumulation of toxic levels of IGF-II and, possibly, IGF-I. Whether this receptor has an important growth-regulatory function is unclear. It does not contain intrinsic kinase activity. Certain cell types that express this receptor have been shown to grow in response to IGF-II. The cytoplasmic portion of the receptor does contain specific residues that are important for binding of GTP-binding proteins (35). In addition, it contains residues that are phosphorylated by intracellular kinases; however, a specific signaling pathway that is linked to specific functions of IGF-II has not been identified.

INSULIN-LIKE GROWTH FACTOR BINDING PROTEINS

The IGFBPs comprise a family of six proteins that have high affinity for IGF-I and IGF-II. In each case, this affinity is greater than that of the IGF-I receptor for IGF-I (1). Since one or more members of this family is present in all extracellular fluids, they have the capacity to control the amount of IGF-I and IGF-II available to bind to receptors. Other major functions of the IGFBPs include transporting the IGFs in the vasculature, controlling their access to extravascular tissue, controlling tissue localization and distribution, and direct IGF-independent effects.

Compared to the IGFs, the IGFBPs have a simpler gene structure. They are composed of four exons (36). Their protein structures also show a great deal of similarity. Eighteen cysteines are present in five of the six forms of

TABLE 6.1. *Affinities of the insulin-like growth factor binding proteins (IGFBPs) for insulin-like growth factor I (IGF-I) and IGF-II*

IGFBP	Affinity ($K_a \times 10^9$) L/M	
	IGF-I	IGF-II
IGFBP-1	1.1	1.2
IGFBP-2	3.4	10.9
IGFBP-3	8.9	22.1
IGFBP-4	2.6	6.0
IGFBP-5	38	41
IGFBP-6	0.1	4.4

IGFBPs, and only IGFBP-6 has 16 cysteines. IGFBP-4 has two additional cysteines. If the cysteine structure is disrupted, IGF-I or IGF-II binding is markedly attenuated. The affinities of each of the proteins for IGF-I and IGF-II are shown in Table 6.1. The only major discrepancy between IGF-I and IGF-II binding is IGFBP-6, which has a 40-fold higher affinity for IGF-II than does IGF-I. There is a great deal of conservation across species in the N-terminal and C-terminal thirds of each of the IGFBPs, and, likewise, there is a great deal of homology among the six members of the family in each of these regions. In contrast, the mid-third of each protein is not conserved among the six forms. Two of the proteins are *N*-glycosylated, IGFBP-3 and IGFBP-4, and the glycosylation sites occur in this middle third of the sequence. IGFBP-5 and IGFBP-6 undergo *O*-glycosylation. There is an Arg-Gly-Asp sequence near the carboxyl terminus of IGFBP-1 and IGFBP-2. There is a region of sequence in IGFBP-3 and IGFBP-5 in which ten of 18 amino acids are basic. This sequence accounts for heparin, glycosaminoglycan, and extracellular matrix (ECM) binding of each protein.

CONTROL OF INSULIN-LIKE GROWTH FACTOR-I SYNTHESIS IN TISSUES

Connective tissue cells are a major source of IGF-I that is synthesized in peripheral tissues. *In situ* hybridization studies have indicated that fibroblasts or fibroblast-like cells are often the source of IGF-I mRNA within tissues such as dermis, lung, and skeletal muscle (2). In the liver, the nonparenchymal cells as well as parenchymal cells are a major source, but in the gut the myofibroblasts, in blood vessels the smooth muscle cells, and in cartilage the prechondrocytes as well as fibroblasts are major sources of this peptide. Regulation of IGF-I synthesis by fibroblasts has been shown to occur in peripheral tissues in animals in response to GH. Likewise, regulation in cartilage shows that both FGF and GH are potent stimulants of IGF-I synthesis by prechondrocytes (37).

IGF-I is an important factor for erythropoiesis, and erythroid precursor cells have been shown to synthesize IGF-I. Its synthesis in these cells can be stimulated by both GH and erythropoietin. Granulocyte precursor cells also synthesize IGF-I mRNA, and this synthesis is stimulated by granulocyte macrophage and colony-stimulating factor (38).

IGF-I is expressed in ovaries, and expression is stimulated by GH and FSH. Thecal cells of the early follicle contain abundant IGF-I mRNA. Other cells in the reproductive tract that express IGF-I include oviductal cells and endometrium. Progesterone is a potent stimulant of IGF-I synthesis by stromal cells in the endometrium. In the testes, IGF-I mRNA is expressed in Leydig cells, and Leydig cell expression is upregulated by LH.

Most of the brain IGF-I arises from synthesis within the central nervous system (CNS). The major sites of synthesis of IGF-I mRNA are Purkinje cells of the cerebellum, the olfactory bulb, the hippocampus, and the retina (39). Astroglial cells in the cerebellum are also an important site of synthesis. Following synthesis, IGF-I can be transported along the axons and dendrites.

In skeletal muscle, IGF-I is synthesized in satellite cells and myoblasts. Following ischemic or toxic injury, there is a marked increase in IGF-I mRNA expression (40). Similarly, in the nervous system, following denervation, there is significant IGF-I synthesis by neurons (3). The wave of skeletal muscle IGF-I synthesis that occurs following injury coincides with increased cell division. Work-induced hypertrophy in hypophysectomized rats leads to an increase in IGF-I synthesis by skeletal muscle and cardiac muscle, and IGF-I production is stimulated in states of cardiac hypertrophy that are induced in experimental animals (41). Blood vessel, endothelial, and smooth muscle cells synthesize IGF-I, and synthesis is markedly increased with either pressure overload or denudation injury (42).

Changes in IGF-I expression in the liver correlate extremely well with changes in plasma concentrations. There is low hepatic expression in hypophysectomized animals, and it increases after GH administration (43). Nutritional deprivation results in a major decrease in IGF-I mRNA in the liver, which can be restored with refeeding.

IGF-I is expressed at low levels in fetal kidney. Immunohistochemical staining shows moderate amounts of IGF-I in the proximal and distal tubules, and in adult animals it is localized in the collecting ducts. Overexpression of IGF-I in the kidneys results in enhanced renal growth, and after unilateral nephrectomy, there is an increase in IGF-I in the contralateral kidney as it undergoes compensatory growth (44). The interstitial cells are the primary site of synthesis of IGF-I during this response.

CONTROL OF SERUM INSULIN-LIKE GROWTH FACTOR-I CONCENTRATIONS

Initial conclusions regarding the physiological role of IGF-I in controlling growth had to rely on inferences made from changes in plasma levels that occurred after administration of GH to GH-deficient humans or other animals. From these studies, several important variables that determine IGF-I concentrations were identified. IGF-I concentrations are low at birth (between 20 and 60 ng/ml) and rise to peak values (between 600 and 1,100 ng/ml) at puberty (45). They fall 2.5-fold during the second decade, reaching a mean value of 350 ng/ml by age 20 years. The rate of decline then slows, and a 50% reduction occurs between 20 and 60 years. This series of changes correlates closely with changes in endogenous GH secretion that occur during the same periods. There is an important genetic determinant of plasma IGF-I. Studies in twins show that approximately 40% of each individual's IGF-I variability can be accounted for on the basis of an undefined genetic factor that is linked to height (46).

A more direct relationship between plasma IGF-I and GH secretion has been identified by measuring IGF-I values in childhood GH deficiency (GHD). Most children with proven GHD have values that are below the 95% confidence interval for age, and a normal age-adjusted IGF-I value in childhood is strong evidence against the presence of GHD (47). However, because other variables control IGF-I secretion, such as nutritional intake, a low value does not definitively prove that GHD is present. Administration of GH to patients with GHD results in a substantial rise in IGF-I within the first 4 to 6 hours and a peak at 24 hours. Part of the change in IGF-I in response to GH is due to increased synthesis in tissues, but part is also due to an increase in the principal IGFBP in serum, IGFBP-3, and a third protein that binds IGF-I and IGFBP-3, termed acid-labile subunit (ALS). Since the synthesis of ALS and IGFBP-3 is also GH-dependent and since they function to prolong the half-life of IGF-I from less than 6 minutes to 16 hours, clearly the ability of GH to induce their synthesis also results in a substantial change in plasma IGF-I. In states of GH excess, such as acromegaly, IGF-I values are uniformly increased (48). IGF-I measurements have been used extensively in monitoring treatment and correlate well with residual GH secretion in most patients.

Thyroxine is also an important controller of IGF-I concentrations. Patients with hypothyroidism have low values that increase with thyroxine replacement (49). Prolactin has a weak stimulatory effect on plasma IGF-I if severe GHD is also present. In addition to GH, the most important variable controlling plasma IGF-I concentrations is nutrient intake. Restriction of either intake or calories results in substantial reduction in IGF-I, which will remain suppressed until optimal nutritional repletion is given (50). Total fasting results in refractoriness to GH after 3 days, showing that the nutritional stimulus is primary (51). Severe catabolic conditions that are partly dependent on nutrient intake or inadequate processing of nutrients, such as hepatic failure, inflammatory bowel disease, or renal failure, result in low serum IGF-I concentrations. Patients with poorly controlled diabetes mellitus have low or normal IGF-I that rises to the normal range with adequate insulin treatment, and in type I diabetes, there is a correlation between hemoglobin A1C and IGF-I (52).

CONTROL OF INSULIN-LIKE GROWTH FACTOR BINDING PROTEIN CONCENTRATIONS IN SERUM

Four forms of intact IGFBP are relatively abundant in serum. IGFBP-3 is the most abundant and has the highest affinity for IGF-I and IGF-II. It accounts for 75% of the IGF carrying capacity in serum. Plasma concentrations of IGFBP-3 are regulated by GH. They are low in patients with GHD and increase following GH treatment (53). This increase is partly due to a direct effect of GH on IGFBP-3 synthesis, but it is also due to the fact that GH increases ALS and IGF-I concentrations and that both proteins function to prolong the half-life of IGFBP-3. ALS is an 88-kDa glycoprotein that contains leucine-rich domains that are responsible for binding to IGFBP-3. Although ALS is increased by GH, it is not increased by IGF-I. The molar concentration of IGFBP-3 in serum is generally equal to the sum of IGF-I and IGF-II concentrations; therefore, it is usually saturated. Plasma IGFBP-3 and ALS levels are elevated in acromegaly and low in GHD (54,55). Age is also an important determinant of IGFBP-3, and values vary in a manner similar to IGF-I.

The abundance of intact IGFBP-3 is also regulated by protease activity. Several proteases that degrade IGFBP-3 and are present in serum have been described, including prostate-specific antigen (PSA) and plasmin (56). Protease activity is abundant in human pregnancy serum, but it is also present in GH-deficient states (57). Proteolytic cleavage results in the appearance of a 32-kDa fragment that has substantially reduced affinity for IGF-I. An important function of this protease may be to cleave IGFBP-3 and liberate IGF-I from the IGFBP-3/ALS complex, thus allowing greater extravascular equilibration through binding to lower-molecular-weight forms of IGFBPs that are more freely diffusible out of the vascular space.

The next most abundant IGFBP in plasma is IGFBP-2. Since it does not bind to ALS, it has a half-life of 90 min and is present in substantially lower concentrations than is IGFBP-3. IGFBP-2 concentrations are inversely related to GH, being low in acromegaly and high in GHD (58). IGFBP-2 can freely cross capillary barriers. It is also degraded by a protease, and its fragments have markedly reduced affinity for IGF-I. Hepatocytes are the major source of IGFBP-2 in blood (59). One of the major stimuli of IGFBP-2 in serum is IGF-I, and concentrations rise three- to fourfold after IGF-I administration. Plasma IGFBP-2 concentrations are also elevated in patients with tumors that produce IGF-II. Nutrient restriction results in increases in plasma IGFBP-2, as does poorly controlled diabetes, and prolonged nutrient deprivation will result in a two- to threefold increase. This is primarily dependent on restricted protein content, rather than restricted calories. This increase in IGFBP-2 with nutrient restriction and a decrease in IGFBP-3 results in a shift in the proportion of IGF-I bound to IGFBP-2 as opposed to that bound to IGFBP-3.

The third most abundant protein serum is IGFBP-1. IGFBP-1 circulates in substantially lower concentrations than does IGFBP-2, and its levels fluctuate widely throughout the day. Its synthesis is markedly suppressed by insulin; therefore, following a meal, there is a 3.5- to 4.0-fold reduction, and concentrations increase four- to sixfold during an overnight fast (60). The major site of synthesis of blood IGFBP-1 is the liver, although kidney and maternal placenta and uterus are sources of this peptide (61). Hepatic synthesis is under the control of insulin, but hormones such as GH and cortisol also have effects (62). IGFBP-1 in plasma is also unsaturated. IGFBP-1 concentrations decrease in experimental animals following insulin administration, and this is due to a direct effect on gene transcription (63). IGFBP-1 crosses intact capillary beds, and the amount that crosses is proportionate to insulin concentrations (64). Because of its wide fluctuation after meals and following administration of insulin, IGFBP-1 has been proposed to have a glucoregulatory function. In states of severe diabetes, there is enhanced phosphorylation of IGFBP-1, which leads to an increased affinity for IGF-I, which further attenuates the ability of IGF-I to enhance insulin sensitivity (65). Administration of large concentrations of IGFBP-1 to hypophysectomized rats results in a slight increase in glucose concentration, suggesting that it may have a glucoregulatory function, and IGFBP-1 may contribute to the insulin resistance that occurs in diabetes (66). IGFBP-1 concentrations are also increased in catabolic states and, along with IGFBP-2, IGFBP-I becomes the major binding component in serum.

IGFBP-4 concentrations correlate with changes in bone physiology, are low in states of high bone turnover, and are increased by vitamin D and sunlight exposure (67). IGFBP-5 exists in serum mostly as proteolytic fragments. The major proteolytic fragment of IGFBP-5, the 22-kDa form, is GH-dependent.

BIOLOGICAL ACTIONS OF INSULIN-LIKE GROWTH FACTOR-I

IGF-I has been shown to control DNA synthesis in multiple cell types in culture. There is an extensive list of cell types that have been shown to respond to IGF-I addition. The biological actions that have been analyzed include DNA synthesis, protein synthesis, increases in cell size, effects on carbohydrate metabolism (e.g., glucose transport, glucose oxidation, lipid synthesis), mitogenesis, and inhibition of cell death. Other processes that have been analyzed include cell cycle progression, differentiation, and migration.

One of the most commonly studied effects is the ability of IGF-I to stimulate DNA synthesis. IGF-I acts principally by stimulating entry into the cell cycle from the latter part of the G_1 phase (68). In some systems, its presence is required for all 12 hours of G_1. IGF-I is not as potent in stimulating quiescent cells to enter G_1 as other growth factors, such as PDGF or FGF, but once they have entered the cell cycle, it is often sufficient to stimulate progression through S phase. In some cell types, it is possible to activate autocrine-secreted IGF-I by exposing cells to growth factors that increase IGF-I synthesis, such as EGF or PDGF, or by viral transformation with C-myb or SV40 (69). If an antibody is added that prevents autocrine-stimulated IGF-I from binding to the receptor, then the cellular DNA synthesis response does not occur.

The complete list of cell types that are IGF-I-responsive is beyond the scope of this chapter (70). Some examples of interesting model systems are discussed herein. Cartilage has been extensively studied because IGF-I is produced by prechondrocytes, and prechondrocytes respond to GH with a large increase in IGF-I synthesis (71). However, as prechondrocytes differentiate into chondrocytes and hypertrophic chondrocytes, their rates of IGF-I synthesis are diminished, as is their degree of GH responsiveness. Triiodothyronine is also a potent stimulant of IGF-I synthesis by cartilage, and this results in progression of maturation of chondrocytes. Skin is a system wherein the effect of paracrine-produced IGF-I has been studied. IGF-I is produced abundantly by dermal fibroblasts but not by skin epithelial cells, which possess abundant IGF-I receptors. Paracrine fibroblast-synthesized IGF-I presumably acts on the skin epithelial cells, in the basal germinal layer to stimulate rapid proliferation. In skeletal muscle, IGF-I is not only a potent mitogen but also a potent differentiation factor. Thus, early in myogenic differentiation, premyoblast precursors and satellite cells synthesize abundant IGF-I. This leads to myoblast proliferation and to rapid differentiation of myoblasts into myocytes (72). Although myocytes maintain high rates of IGF-I synthesis, they fuse and become nondividing cells. Thus, IGF-I, by stimulating proliferation, actually enhances the rate of differentiation and ultimately slows cell division. In muscle, in addition to stimulating the differentiation program, IGF-II may function to inhibit apoptosis that occurs during transition from proliferation to differentiation in myoblast lines, thus increasing the final number of differentiated myocytes (73). In the nervous system, IGF-I stimulates not only DNA synthesis in oligodendrocytes and glial cells but also neurite outgrowth and myelin synthesis in terminally differentiated neurons (74). IGF-I is also a potent inhibitor of apoptosis in the CNS during development. In other systems, IGF-I has been shown to be a potent inhibitor of cell death. These include hematopoietic cells, myeloid precursors, ovarian follicular cells, myoblasts, and neurons (32).

EFFECTS ON SPECIALIZED FUNCTIONS

IGF-I and IGF-II stimulate specialized functions in many types of cell, such as steroid production by ovarian granulosa cells, in which case its effects are synergistic with those of FSH (75). It also stimulates steroid production by adrenal cortical cells in synergy with corticotropin (76). It stimulates testosterone secretion from Leydig cells, acting synergistically with LH. Thyroglobulin production by thyroid follicular cells is increased by IGF-I and enhances the effect of thyroid-stimulating hormone (TSH) (77). GH secretion by pituitary cells is inhibited by IGF-I. Histamine release from β cells is stimulated in response to immunoglobulin E (IgE), and this is potentiated by IGF-I. IGF-I specifically stimulates IGFBP-5 synthesis by muscle cells. Other specific proteins whose synthesis is stimulated by IGF-I include elastin by smooth muscle cells (78), crystallin by lens epithelial cells (79), and cholesterol side chain cleavage enzyme by adrenal corticol cells (80).

ROLE IN METABOLISM *IN VITRO*

IGF-I has been shown to stimulate glucose uptake, glycolysis, glucose oxidation by fat cells and skeletal muscle cells, and glycogen synthesis by skeletal muscle and liver cells. These effects can be mediated by the insulin receptor if high concentrations are used; however, if low concentrations are used, often the IGF-I receptor or hybrid receptors are capable of mediating these responses. In connective tissue cells, IGF-I is a potent stimulant of protein synthesis, ECM component synthesis, cell migration, and proteoglycan and collagen synthesis. IGF-I is a potent stimulant of cell migration, by both chemotaxis and chemokinesis. It is not angiogenic but stimulates the synthesis of angiogenic peptides, such as vascular endothelial growth factor.

ROLE IN TRANSFORMED CELL GROWTH

Since IGF-I is a potent inhibitor of apoptosis, it has been proposed that it will facilitate the growth of tumor cells *in vitro* and in experimental animal models. Several experiments have indicated that an intact IGF-I receptor is necessary for cellular transformation (81). Absence of the IGF-I receptor has been shown to limit the growth of C-6 glioma cells and MCF-7 breast carcinoma cells (82). Often in these models, however, IGF-I receptors have to be overexpressed in order to facilitate tumor cell formation. IGF-I receptor number is increased in some tumor model systems, such as Wilms' tumor, small cell carcinoma of the lung, and uterine cancer (83). Transgenic mice that overexpress IGF-II have a higher rate of tumor formation, and some viral transformation models, such as SV40 T-antigen induction of pancreatic tumor cell growth, require IGF-II for continued growth.

CONTROL OF INSULIN-LIKE GROWTH FACTOR-I ACTION AND CELLS IN TISSUES BY IGFBPs

IGFBPs are ubiquitously present in all cells and tissues and have a high affinity for IGF-I and IGF-II; therefore, they regulate their functions by controlling access to receptors. The most important determinant of their capacity to regulate the degree of receptor occupancy is their affinity, although other variables, such as binding to their own receptors, which lead to IGF-independent actions, can play roles.

REGULATION OF INSULIN-LIKE GROWTH FACTOR BINDING PROTEIN AFFINITY

The affinity of each binding protein is between two and 50-fold greater than that of the type I receptor for IGF-I (Table 6.1). The biological implication of this high affinity is that in their soluble forms the binding proteins will prevent receptor association. Variables that lower affinity to levels that are much less than the receptor, such as proteolysis, function to allow a sudden increase in the amount of receptor-associated IGF-I. In contrast, variables that lower their affinities into a range that approximates the receptor may result in prolonged, enhanced diffusion of IGF-I and IGF-II onto receptors, and either process may result in enhancement of IGF-I action. Variables that inhibit proteolytic cleavage may result in inhibition of IGF-I actions.

PROTEOLYSIS

Proteolytic cleavage of IGFBP-3 results in the appearance of a 32-kDa fragment that has a 20-fold reduction in affinity for IGF-I (84). Proteolysis is easily detectable in pregnancy serum and following nutritional deprivation. The nature of this protease is unknown, although a significant amount of data supports the hypothesis that it is a cation-dependent serine protease. Matrix metalloproteinases, such as MMP-1, MMP-2, and MMP-9, degrade several forms of IGFBPs, including IGFBP-3, and account for some portion of the serum protease activity that is noted during pregnancy (85). Several well-defined proteases, including plasmin, cathepsin D, and PSA, have been shown to degrade IGFBP-3 (59). Proteolytic activity is also present in other extracellular fluids, including lymph, follicular fluid, peritineal fluid, and amniotic fluid. Proteases have also been identified that cleave IGFBP-2 and IGFBP-4 (86,87). These proteases have the unique property of cleaving these forms of IGFBP poorly, unless IGF-I or IGF-II is bound to the binding proteins, and then cleavage proceeds rapidly. IGFBP-5 is cleaved by a cation-dependent, 95-kDa serine protease that is present in cell culture supernatants from connective tissue cell types. IGFBP-3 and IGFBP-5 have also been shown to be cleaved by MMP-2 and MMP-9. In general, fragments that are generated from these forms of binding protein have very low affinity, and blocking proteolytic cleavage by creating protease-resistance mutant forms of IGFBP-4 and IGFBP-5 has been shown to inhibit the actions of IGF-I *in vitro* (88).

PHOSPHORYLATION

IGFBP-1, -3, and -5 have been shown to be phosphorylated on serine residues. IGFBP-1 is phosphorylated at positions 101, 119, and 169 (89). Casiene kinase-2 is one of the two kinases that can phosphorylate IGFBP-1. Phosphorylation of this protein results in a sixfold enhancement of affinity (90). Different distributions of the phosphorylated forms of IGFBP-1 have been detected in physiological fluids (90,91). During poorly controlled diabetes, there is a very highly phosphorylated IGFBP-1 that predominates, and this is believed to result in lower free IGF-I concentrations. IGFBP-3 is phosphorylated at positions 111 and 113, and its phosphorylation can be enhanced by IGF-I (92).

ADHERENCE TO CELL SURFACE, EXTRACELLULAR MATRIX, AND GLYCOSAMINOGLYCANS

Both IGFBP-3 and IGFBP-5 have been shown to adhere to cell surfaces. Proteoglycan-containing cell surface proteins may be an important cell surface binding component for each protein. IGF-I that is bound to cell-associated IGFBP-3 is in more favorable equilibrium with receptors since IGFBP-3 binding to cells lowers its affinity by approximately tenfold. Specific receptors have been postulated to exist for IGFBP-3. The type V TGF-β receptor has been shown to bind to IGFBP-3. IGFBP-5 binding to ECM or to proteoglycans results in an eightfold reduction in affinity (93). Non-proteoglycan-containing components of the ECM have been shown to bind to IGFBP-5, such as plasminogen activator inhibitor-1. Localization of IGFBP-5 in the ECM or pericellular environment may be an important means for focally concentrating IGF-I and IGF-II and making them more accessible to receptors.

EFFECTS OF SPECIFIC FORMS OF INSULIN-LIKE GROWTH FACTOR BINDING PROTEINS ON IGF ACTION

Most published studies have shown that addition of IGFBP-1 to cells in culture with IGF-I, using at least a 4:1 molar excess of IGFBP-1, results in inhibition of IGF-I actions. This is particularly true if highly phosphorylated, high-affinity forms of IGFBP-1 are utilized. IGFBP-1 in such systems has been shown to inhibit DNA synthesis, glucose incorporation and transport, and the steroidogenic response of human granulosa cells to IGF-I (1). Using different conditions, some investigators have shown that IGFBP-1 can enhance the effects of IGF-I. In general, this requires dephosphorylated forms of IGFBP-1 that are added in equimolar ratios with IGF-I or less. The DNA synthesis response of smooth muscle cells, keratinocytes, and fibroblasts to IGF-I has been shown to be potentiated by IGFBP-1 (94,95). IGFBP-1 has direct effects in stimulating the migration of Chinese hamster ovary cells by binding to the $\alpha5\beta1$ integrin receptor through its RGD sequence (96).

IGFBP-2 has been shown to be inhibitory in most *in vitro* test systems, including inhibition of DNA synthesis in chick embryo fibroblasts and rat astroglial cells as well as human lung carcinoma cells (1). IGFBP-2 inhibits protein synthesis in Madin Darby bovine kidney cells.

IGFBP-3 has been shown to inhibit IGF-I-stimulated glucose incorporation of fat cells and DNA synthesis in fibroblasts. This requires a 5:1 molar ratio of IGFBP-3 to IGF-I (97). It also inhibits aminoisobutyric acid (AIB) transport into muscle cells. If IGFBP-3 is preincubated with muscle cells or fibroblasts, however, it can potentiate both AIB uptake and IGF-I-stimulated DNA synthesis (98). IGFBP-3 binds directly to the type V TGF-β receptor, and direct addition can attenuate the mitogenic effects of FGF (99). TGF-β is believed to cause part of its growth-inhibitory effect in breast carcinoma cells by inducing the synthesis and secretion of IGFBP-3 (100). IGFBP-3 can also be localized in the nucleus, and this nuclear localization is thought to mediate some of its direct growth-inhibitory actions.

IGFBP-4 has been consistently shown *in vitro* to be inhibitory of IGF-I action. Several differentiated functions that are stimulated by IGF-I have been shown to be inhibited by IGFBP-4, including the generation of cyclic adenosine monophosphate, protein synthesis, glycogen synthesis, and the steroidogenic response of granulosa cells (1).

IGFBP-5 has been shown to inhibit IGF-I action if added at high concentration to extracellular fluids. If it is allowed to equilibrate with ECM and IGF-I is added, it can potentiate the effects of IGF-I on fibroblasts, osteoblasts, chondrocytes, and muscle cells (1). IGFBP-5 binds to ECM with the highest affinity of all of the IGFBPs.

IGFBP-6 preferentially inhibits the response to IGF-II in bone and neuroblastoma cells. In summary, the IGFBPs are important modulators of IGF action *in vitro* and have been shown to control or modulate many different types of physiological responses.

ACTIONS OF INSULIN-LIKE GROWTH FACTOR-I *IN VIVO*

The initial hypotheses regarding IGF actions were deduced from experiments using hypophysectomized animals. Hypophysectomy was shown to result in a low serum IGF-I, and administration of GH reversed this low serum concentration and resulted in balanced growth of all tissues. Similarly, GH excess that was induced by implanting GH-producing tumors resulted in generalized tissue overgrowth and high circulating IGF-I. Subsequently, adequate IGF-I was purified to administer to animals. This was shown to result in balanced growth in hypophysectomized rats (101). A rate-limiting factor was the amount of IGF-I that could be infused since at very high concentrations it induced hypoglycemia. If animals were made catabolic by nutritional deprivation, administration of IGF-I resulted in a partial reversal of the catabolism (102). Systemic infusions of IGF-I into animals also showed that it would improve would healing and recovery of renal function after kidney injury, as well as stimulate whole-body protein synthesis. Stimulation of renal and splenic growth appeared to be preferential to changes in skeletal growth. However, the growth of all tissues was enhanced. IGF-I was shown to stimulate glomerular filtration rate, to be trophic for gut epithelial proliferation, and to increase gut length (103). IGF-I administration to diabetic animals showed that it stimulated glucose utilization, peripheral glucose uptake, and glycerol synthesis and suppressed hepatic glucose output, possibly due to suppression of glucagon and GH (104).

Two of the IGFBPs have been shown in direct *in vivo* infusion experiments to modify the effects of IGF-I. When IGFBP-1 was administered with IGF-I at high concentrations, it attenuated the growth response to IGF-I in hypophysectomized rats (105). Similarly, administration of a large excess of IGFBP-1 to normal rats resulted in a transient, 6% increase in plasma glucose concentrations (66). In contrast, administration of IGFBP-1 with IGF-I, using a 4:1 molar ratio of IGF-I to IGFBP-1, to wounds resulted in accelerated reepithelialization and formation of granulosa tissue, suggesting that, when administered locally, it could potentiate its effects (106). IGFBP-3 has also been administered with IGF-I to animal models. Administration of the combination results in enhancement of protein synthesis in hypophysectomized rats and increased bone formation in estrogen-deficient rats (107). A polyclonal antibody that functions much like an IGFBP has also been shown to enhance the effects of IGF-I on growth in experimental animals when administered concomitantly (108).

TRANSGENIC ANIMAL STUDIES

Creation of transgenic animals that overexpressed IGF-I showed that it would stimulate somatic growth. The effect of IGF-I was greater in animals that had had GH secretion deleted (109). If IGF-I was expressed adequately, these animals would grow at a rate that was comparable to normal, control animals. There was some disproportionate increase in kidney, liver, pancreas, and spleen size, however. Brain size appears to be particularly sensitive to IGF-I transgene expression, and, if it is deliberately overexpressed in the brain, disproportionate increase in brain and cranial size can be induced (110). One major difference between IGF-I and GH transgenic animals is the change in liver size. Animals that are deficient in GH, even with normal growth of other tissues, consistently have smaller, hypoplastic livers (109). A major conclusion of these studies is that a majority of

growth-promoting effects of GH are mediated by IGF-I and that autocrine/paracrine expression may be as important as increases in plasma concentrations for normal growth.

IGFBP transgenic animals have been prepared that overexpress IGFBPs 1 and 3. Enhanced expression of IGFBP-1 results in slight growth retardation if a high level of expression can be achieved in liver (111). Similarly, if high levels of expression are achieved in brain, there is organ-specific growth retardation (112). Very high hepatic expression can also result in modest glucose intolerance. In IGFBP-3 transgenic animals, in contrast, there is an increase in liver, spleen, and kidney size, although total body weight is not significantly greater than in control animals (113).

Homologous recombination experiments have also been very revealing in terms of trying to determine the effects of IGF-I and IGF-II on growth and the effects of the binding proteins in whole-animal model systems. Deletion of the IGF-I gene results in animals that are 60% of normal birth weight and length (4). These animals have a high juvenile mortality rate, and only 10% survive to adulthood. The animals that do survive have significant growth retardation and reach only 30% of normal adult size. Deletion of IGF-II results in small animals at birth, but these animals grow normally postnatally and do not have a low survival rate (114). Deletion of the IGF-I receptor results in an animal that is 45% of normal size at birth (23). None survive birth, and all have hypoplastic diaphragms with poor skeletal muscle cell formation. They are unable to take a normal inspiration. They have multiple skeletal and skin defects, indicating that the IGF-I receptor is necessary for normal muscle, skin, and bone development *in utero*. Deletion of IGFBP-2 results in animals that are born with large spleens, but no other changes in organ growth have been noted (115). Body size is unchanged at birth and remains normal throughout juvenile development. Deletion of IGFBP-4, however, results in a 15% reduction in size at birth, and this difference persists postnatally, although there is no further deceleration in growth rate (116).

AUTOCRINE/PARACRINE REGULATION OF INSULIN-LIKE GROWTH FACTOR-I–MEDIATED GROWTH

Initial studies of IGF-I expression showed that it occurred in connective tissue cells in multiple organs, raising the question of whether this locally produced IGF-I was important for normal growth (2). Likewise, following injury, fibroblasts and fibroblast-like cells, as well as macrophages, were shown to express IGF-I preferentially in the area of injury (117). Regulation of this response to injury was completely independent of pituitary GH since it occurred normally in hypophysectomized animals (3). The wave of IGF-I expression following injury occurs during times of peak cell replication and migration responses, raising the question of whether it is a normal component of this response (118). Overexpression of IGFBP-1 in the brain has clearly shown that local production of IGF-I by the brain is important for maintenance of normal brain size. GH administration to hypophysectomized animals resulted in IGF-I transcript increases not only in liver but also in multiple peripheral tissues, suggesting that autocrine/paracrine stimulation of growth locally may be an important component of the balanced growth response to GH administration (70). Taken together, all of these facts suggest that local expression of IGF-I may be an important regulator of growth.

A recent experimental animal model has further elucidated the relative importance of autocrine/paracrine-produced IGF-I compared to blood-transported IGF-I that originates from the liver. Using a Cre lox expression system, Yakar et al. (119) targeted IGF-I gene expression in the liver. These animals had plasma IGF-I concentrations that were only 20% of normal. In spite of this lowering of serum IGF-I concentrations, the animals grew normally postnatally, suggesting that autocrine/paracrine-produced IGF-I was sufficient for normal statural growth. Since the expression of IGF-I in peripheral tissues is under GH control, this experiment did not distinguish between the portion of autocrine/paracrine growth regulated by GH and

that regulated by other factors. However, it does suggest that a major source of blood IGF-I is the liver and that this endocrine-transported IGF-I does not have to be completely normal in order to achieve normal adult size.

EFFECTS OF INSULIN-LIKE GROWTH FACTOR-I IN HUMANS

Many of the effects of IGF-I that have been shown to occur in experimental animals have been replicated in humans. Administration of a large dose of IGF-I results in hypoglycemia, and IGF-I is approximately one-twelfth as potent as insulin on a molar basis in reducing glucose and free fatty acid levels (120). Administration of lower doses suppresses insulin, but euglycemia is maintained, suggesting that there is either enhancement of insulin action or a direct effect of IGF-I on glucose transport (121). At high infusion rates, protein breakdown can be decreased, but at lower infusion rates, the primary effect is on protein synthesis. These infusion rates also suppress GH and glucagon, which may contribute to enhanced glucose sensitivity. Administration of IGF-I to catabolic subjects results in decreased catabolism, and if IGF-I is given concomitantly with GH, the effect of IGF-I is accentuated (122). IGF-I can partially reverse the effect of glucocorticoids on protein catabolism. Cholesterol is lowered in response to acute IGF-I infusion, as is potassium, and the glomerular filtration rate increases 15% (123). The combination of GH and IGF-I has a greater effect on decreasing protein oxidation in GH-deficient subjects than does either substance given alone. The effects of IGF-I administration on bone metabolism are reviewed in chapter 7.

In diabetes, administration of IGF-I improves insulin sensitivity 2.8-fold as assessed by the minimum model (124). Longer-term studies showed that administration of IGF-I to subjects with type I or type II diabetes for 12 weeks results in a substantial reduction in hemoglobin A1C and improvement in insulin sensitivity. IGF-I also suppresses apolipoprotein B-100 levels and triglycerides, as well as plasminogen activator inhibitor-1.

Administration of IGF-I to patients who have mutations in the GH receptor results in improved nitrogen and phosphate retention and decreases in glucose and insulin (125). Long-term administration subcutaneously to these subjects results in improved growth velocity, and an accelerated growth is maintained through 5 years of treatment (126).

In summary, IGF-I is a potent stimulant of anabolic effects *in vivo*. Synthesis of IGF-I in peripheral tissues as well as liver appears to be required for a normal, balanced growth response to GH administration. Transgenic animal models have been extremely important in validating the original somatomedin hypothesis. In addition to its important growth-promoting actions, IGF-I is an important regulator of normal intermediary metabolism, and current studies are attempting to dissect the proportion of insulin action that is accentuated by IGF-I and whether insulin-independent effects of IGF-I on metabolism occur. The results of these studies should lead to a new and better understanding of the role of this important growth factor in maintaining somatic growth and in altering intermediary metabolism in ways that promote growth.

REFERENCES

1. Jones JI, Clemmons DR. Insulin like growth factor and their binding proteins: biologic actions. *Endocr Rev* 1995;16:3–34.
2. Han VKM, D'Ercole AJ, Lund PK. Cellular location of somatomedin (insulin-like growth factor) messenger RNA in the human fetus. *Science* 1987;236:193–197.
3. Hansson HA, Dahlin LB, Danielsen N, et al. Evidence indicating trophic importance of IGF-I in regenerating peripheral nerves. *Acta Physiol Scand* 1986;126:609–613.
4. Baker J, Liu JP, Robertson EJ, et al. Role of insulin like growth factors in embryonic and postnatal growth. *Cell* 1993;75:83–94.
5. Guler H-P, Zapf J, Schmid C, et al. Insulin-like growth factors I and II in healthy man. Estimations of half-lives and production rates. *Acta Endocrinol (Copenh)* 1989;121:753–758.
6. LeRoith D, Werner H, Beitner-Johnson D, et al. Molecular and cellular aspects of the insulin-like growth factor-I receptor. *Endocr Rev* 1995;16:143–163.
7. Rinderknecht E, Humbel RE. The amino acid sequence of human insulin-like growth factor I and its structural homology with proinsulin. *J Biol Chem* 1978;253:2769–2776.
8. Ullrich A, Gray A, Tam AW, et al. Insulin-like growth

factor-I receptor primary structure: comparison with insulin receptor suggests structural determinants that define functional specificity. *EMBO J* 1986;5:2503–2512.
9. Murphy LJ, Bell GI, Duckworth ML, et al. Identification, characterization, and regulation of complementary dexoxyribonucleic acid which evokes insulin-like growth factor I. *Endocrinology* 1987;121:684.
10. Hepler JE, Van Wyk JJ, Lund PK. Different half lives of insulin-like growth factor-I mRNA that differ in length of 3' untranslated sequence. *Endocrinology* 1990;127:155.
11. Conover CA, Baker BK, Hintz RL. Cultured human fibroblasts secrete insulin-like growth factor-I A. *J Clin Endocrinol Metab* 1989;69:25–30.
12. Cascieri MA, Chicchi GC, Applebaum J, et al. Mutants of human insulin like growth factor I with reduced affinity for the type I insulin like growth factor receptor. *Biochemistry* 1988;27:3229–3233.
13. Clemmons DR, Dehoff MH, Busby WH, et al. Competition for binding to insulin-like growth factor (IGF) binding protein-2, 3, 4, and 5 by the IGFs and IGF analogs. *Endocrinology* 1992;131:890–895.
14. Blundell TL, Bedarkar S, Rinderknecht E, et al. Insulin-like growth factor: a model for tertiary structure accounting for immunoreactivity and receptor binding. *Proc Natl Acad Sci USA* 1978;75:180–184.
15. Sara V, Carlsson-Skwirut C, Anderson C, et al. Characterization of somatomedin from fetal brain: identification of a variant form of insulin-like growth factor-I. *Proc Natl Acad Sci USA* 1986;83:4904–4907.
16. Yamamoto H, Murphy LJ. Generation of des 1-3 insulin-like growth factor-I in serum by acid protease. *Endocrinology* 1994;135:2432.
17. Hernandez ER. Regulation of the genes for insulin-like growth factor (IGF) I and II and their receptors by steroids and gonadotrophins in the ovary. *J Steroid Biochem Mol Biol* 1995;53:219–221.
18. Hernandez-Sanchez C, Werner H, Roberts CT, et al. Differential regulation of insulin-like growth factor-I receptor gene expression by IGF-I and basic fibroblast growth factor. *J Biol Chem* 1997;272:4663–4670.
19. Du J, Meng XP, Delafontaine P. Transcriptional regulation of the insulin-like growth factor-I receptor gene: evidence for protein kinase C dependent and independent pathways. *Endocrinology* 1996;138:1378.
20. Kato H, Faria TN, Stannard B, et al. Role of tyrosine activity in signal transduction by the insulin-like growth factor-I (IGF-I) receptor. Characterization of kinase-deficient IGF-I receptors and the action of an IGF-I-mimetic antibody (alpha IR-3). *J Biol Chem* 1993;268:2655–2661.
21. Soos MA, Field CE, Siddle K. Purified hybrid insulin/insulin-like growth factor-I receptors bind insulin-like growth factor-I but not insulin with high affinity. *Biochem J* 1993;290:419–426.
22. Sell C, Dumenil G, Deneaud C, et al. Effect of a null mutation of the insulin-like growth factor I receptor gene on growth and transformation of mouse embryo fibroblasts. *Mol Cell Biol* 1994;14:3604–3612.
23. Liu JP, Baker J, Perkins AS, et al. Mice carrying null mutations of the genes encoding insulin like growth

factor I (IGF-I) and type 1 IGF receptor (IGF/r). *Cell* 1993;75:73–82.

24. Rubin R, Baserga R. Biology of disease: insulin-like growth factor-I receptor: its role in cell proliferation, apoptosis, and tumorigenicity. *Lab Invest* 1995;13: 311–331.

25. Sun XJ, Rothenberg P, Kahn CR, et al. Structure of the insulin receptor substrate IRS-I defines a unique signal transduction protein. *Nature* 1991;351:73–77.

26. Sun XJ, Wang LM, Zhang Y, et al. Role of IRS-2 in insulin and cytokine signaling. *Nature* 1995;377:173.

27. Myers MJ, White MF. The IRS-1 signaling system. *Trends Biol Sci* 1994;19:289.

28. Takasu N, Takasu M, Komiya I, et al. Insulin-like growth factor-I stimulates inositol phosphate accumulation, a rise in cytosol free calcium, and proliferation in cultured thyroid cells. *J Biol Chem* 1989;264: 18485–18488.

29. Kojima I, Mogami H, Ogata E. Oscillation of cytoplasmic free calcium concentration induced by insulin-like growth factor-I. *Am J Physiol* 1992;262:E307–311.

30. Beitner-Johnson D, LeRoith D. Insulin like growth factor I stimulates tyrosine phosphorylation of endogenous c-Crk. *J Biol Chem* 1995;270:5187–5190.

31. Pillay TS, Sasoka T, Olefsky JM. Insulin stimulates tyrosine dephosphorylation of pp125 focal adhesion kinase. *J Biol Chem* 1995;270:991–994.

32. Stewart CS, Rotwein P. Growth, differentiation, and survival: multiple physiologic functions for insulin-like growth factors. *Physiol Rev* 1966;76:1005.

33. Flaument RS, Kojima S, Abe M, et al. Activation of latent transforming growth factor beta. *Adv Pharmacol* 1993;24:51.

34. Lau MM, Stewart CHE, Liu Z, et al. Loss of imprinted IGF-II cation independent mannose 6 phosphate receptor results in fetal overgrowth and perinatal lethality. *Gene Dev* 1994;8:2953.

35. Okomoto T, Katada T, Murayama Y, et al. A simple structure encodes G protein activity function of the IGF-I/mannose 6 phosphate receptor. *Cell* 1990;62: 709.

36. Clemmons DR. Insulin like growth factor binding proteins. In: Kostyo JL, ed. *Handbook of Physiology. Hormonal control of growth.* New York: Oxford University Press, 1999:1901.

37. Isgaard J, Nilsson A, Vikma A, et al. Growth hormone regulates the level of IGF-I mRNA in rat growth plate. *Endocrinology* 1988;122:1515.

38. Adamo ML. Regulation of insulin like growth factor I gene expression. *Diabetes Rev* 1995;3:2.

39. Bondy CA, Lee WH. Patterns of insulin-like growth factor gene expression in brain: functional implications. *Ann NY Acad Sci* 1993;692:33–43.

40. Edwall D, Schalling M, Jennische E, et al. Induction of insulin-like growth factor I messenger ribonucleic acid during regeneration of rat skeletal muscle. *Endocrinology* 1989;124:820–825.

41. Fath KA, Alexander RW, Delafontaine P. Abdominal coarctation increases insulin-like growth factor I mRNA levels in rat aorta. *Circ Res* 1993;72:271–277.

42. Cercek B, Fishbein MC, Forrester JS, et al. Induction of insulin-like growth factor I messenger RNA in rat

aorta after balloon denudation. *Circ Res* 1990;66: 1755–1760.

43. Adamo ML, Bach MA, Roberts CT, et al. Regulation of insulin IGF-I and IGF-II gene expression. In: LeRoith D, ed. *Insulin like growth factors: molecular and cellular aspects.* Boca Raton, FL: CRC Press, 1990: 271–303.

44. Fagin JA, Melmed S. Relative increase in insulin-like growth factor-I messenger ribonucleic acid levels in compensatory renal hypertrophy. *Endocrinology* 1987; 120:718.

45. Underwood LE, VanWyk JJ. Normal and aberrant growth. In: *Williams textbook of endocrinology,* 8th ed. Philadelphia: WB Saunders, 1991:1079–1104.

46. Hong Y, Pedesen NL, Brismar K, et al. Quantitative genetic analyses of insulin like growth factor I (IGF-I), IGF binding protein-1 and insulin levels in middle-aged and elderly twins. *J Clin Endocrinol Metab* 1996; 81:1791–1797.

47. Zapf J, Walter H, Froesch ER. Radioimmunological determinations of IGF-I and IGF-II in normal subjects and in patients with growth disorders and extrapancreatic tumor hypoglycemia. *J Clin Invest* 1981;68: 1321–1330.

48. Clemmons DR, Underwood LE, Ridgway EC. Evaluation of acromegaly by radioimmunoassay of somatomedin-C. *N Engl J Med* 1979;301:1138–1142.

49. Chernausek SD, Underwood LE, Utiger RD, et al. Growth hormone secretion and plasma somatomedin-C in primary hypothyroidism. *Clin Endocrinol (Oxf)* 1983;19:337–344.

50. Isley WL, Underwood LE, Clemmons DR. Dietary components that regulate serum somatomedin-C in humans. *J Clin Invest* 1983;71:175–182.

51. Merimee TJ, Zapf J, Froesch ER. Insulin-like growth factors in fed and fasted states. *J Clin Endocrinol Metab* 1982;55:999–1002.

52. Bereket A, Lang CH, Blethen SL, et al. Effect of insulin on the insulin-like growth factor system in children with new onset insulin-dependent diabetes mellitus. *J Clin Endocrinol Metab* 1995;80:1312–1317.

53. Blum WF, Albertsson-Wikland K, Rosberg S, et al. Serum levels of insulin-like growth factor I (IGF-I) and IGF binding protein-3 reflect spontaneous growth hormone secretion. *J Clin Endocrinol Metab* 1993;76: 1610–1616.

54. Boer H, Blok GJ, Popp-Snijders C, et al. Monitoring of growth hormone replacement therapy in adults, based on measurements of serum markers. *J Clin Endocrinol Metab* 1996;81:1371–1377.

55. Grinspoon S, Clemmons DR, Swearingen B, et al. Serum insulin-like growth factor-binding protein-3 levels in the diagnosis of acromegaly. *J Clin Endocrinol Metab* 1995;80:927–932.

56. Bang P. Serum proteolysis of IGFBP-3. *Prog Growth Fact Res* 1995;6:285–292.

57. Guidice LC, Farrell EM, Pham H, et al. Insulin like growth factor binding proteins in maternal serum throughout gestation and in the puerperium. *J Clin Endocrinol Metab* 1990;71:806–816.

58. Clemmons DR, Busby WH, Snyder DK. Variables controlling the secretion of insulin-like growth factor

binding protein-2 in normal human subjects. *J Clin Endocrinol Metab* 1991;73:727–733.

59. Ooi GT, Orlowski CC, Brown AL, et al. Different tissue distribution and hormonal regulation of messenger RNAs encoding rat insulin-like growth factor binding proteins-1 and 2. *Mol Endocrinol* 1990;4:321–328.

60. Suikkari A-M, Koivisto VA, Koistinen R, et al. Dose-response characteristics for suppression of low molecular weight plasma insulin-like growth factor binding protein by insulin. *J Clin Endocrinol Metab* 1989;68:135–140.

61. Ooi GT, Tseng LY, Tran MQ, et al. Insulin rapidly decreases insulin-like growth factor-binding protein-1 gene transcription in streptozotocin-diabetic rats. *Mol Endocrinol* 1992;6:2219–2228.

62. Powell DR, Lee PDK, DePaolis LA, et al. Dexamethasone stimulates expression of insulin-like growth factor-binding protein-1 gene expression in human hepatoma cells. *Growth Regul* 1993;3:11–13.

63. Unterman T, Oehler DT, Ngyuen H, et al. A novel DNA/protein complex interacts with the insulin-like growth factor binding protein-1 (IGFBP-1) insulin response sequence and is required for maximal effects of insulin and glucocorticoids on promoter function. *Prog Growth Fact Res* 1995;6:119–129.

64. Bar RS, Boes M, Clemmons DR, et al. Insulin differentially alters transcapillary movement of intravascular IGFBP-1, IGFBP-2 and endothelial cell IGF binding proteins in rat heart. *Endocrinology* 1990;127:497–499.

65. Westwood M, Gibson JM, Williams AC, et al. Hormonal regulation of circulating insulin-like growth factor-binding protein-1 phosphorylation status. *J Clin Endocrinol Metab* 1995;80:3520–3527.

66. Lewitt MS, Denyer GS, Cooney GJ, et al. Insulin-like growth factor binding protein-1 modulates blood glucose levels. *Endocrinology* 1991;129:2254–2256.

67. Scharla SH, Strong DD, Mohan S, et al. 1,25-Dihydroxyvitamin D3 differentially regulates the production of insulin-like growth factor I (IGF-I) and IGF-binding protein-4 in mouse osteoblasts. *Endocrinology* 1991;129:3139–3146.

68. Stiles CD, Capone GT, Scher CD, et al. Dual control of cell growth by somatomedin and platelet-derived growth factor. *Proc Natl Acad Sci USA* 1979;76:1279–1284.

69. Travali S, Reiss K, Ferber A, et al. Constitutively expressed c-myb abrogates the requirement for insulin-like growth factor-I in 3T3 fibroblasts. *Mol Cell Biol* 1991;11:731–736.

70. Lowe WL. Biologic actions of the insulin-like growth factors. In: LeRoith D, ed. *Insulin-like growth factors: molecular and cellular aspects.* Boca Raton, FL: CRC Press, 1991:49.

71. Vetter U, Zapf J, Heit W, et al. Human fetal and adult chondrocytes. Effect of insulin-like growth factors I and II, insulin, and growth hormone on clonal growth. *J Clin Invest* 1986;77:1903–1908.

72. Florini JR, Ewton DZ, Root SL. IGF-I stimulates terminal myogenic differentiation by induction of myogenin gene expression. *Mol Endocrinol* 1991;5:718–724.

73. Florini JR, Ewton DZ, Root SL. Insulin-like growth

factors, muscle growth and myogenesis. *Diabetes Rev* 1995;3:73.

74. Caroni P, Grandes P. Nerve sprouting in innervated adult skeletal muscle induced by exposure to high levels of insulin-like growth factor-I. *J Cell Biol* 1990;1110:1307–1317.

75. Guidice LC. Insulin like growth factors and ovarian follicular development. *Endocr Rev* 1992;13:641.

76. Penhoat A, Naville D, Jaillard L, et al. Hormonal regulation of insulin-like growth factor-I secretion by bovine adrenal cells. *J Biol Chem* 1989;264:6858–6862.

77. Satisteban P, Kohn DL, DiLauro R. Thyroglobulin gene expression is regulated by insulin and insulin-like growth factor I as well as thyrotropin in FRTL 5 cells. *J Biol Chem* 1987;262:4068.

78. Wolfe BL, Rich CB, Goud HD, et al. Insulin-like growth factor-I regulates transcription of the elastin gene. *J Biol Chem* 1993;268:12418–12426.

79. Alemany J, Borras T, dePablo F. Transcriptional stimulation of the delta 1-crystallin gene by insulin-like growth factor I and insulin requires DNA cis elements in chicken. *Proc Natl Acad Sci USA* 1990;87:3353–3357.

80. Urban RJ, Shupnik MA, Bodenburg YH. Insulin-like growth factor-I increases expression of the porcine P-450 cholesterol side chain cleavage gene through a GC-rich domain. *J Biol Chem* 1994;269:25761–25769.

81. Sell C, Rubini R, Rubin R, et al. Simian virus 40 large tumor antigen is unable to transform mouse embryo fibroblasts lacking type I insulin like growth factor receptor. *Proc Natl Acad Sci USA* 1993;90:11217–11221.

82. Resnicoff MD, Abraham W, Yutaboonchai HL, et al. The insulin-like growth factor-I receptor protects tumor cells from apoptosis *in vitro. Cancer Res* 1995;55:2463.

83. LeRoith D, Werner H, Beitner-Johnson D, et al. Molecular and cellular aspects of the insulin like growth factor I receptor. *Endocr Rev* 1995;16:143.

84. Lassare C, Binoux M. Insulin-like growth factor binding protein-3 is functionally altered in pregnancy plasma. *Endocrinology* 1994;134:1254–1262.

85. Fowlkes J, Enghild JJ, Suzuki N, et al. Matrix metalloproteases degrade insulin like growth factor binding protein-3 in dermal fibroblast cultures. *J Biol Chem* 1994;269:25742–25746.

86. Gockerman A, Clemmons DR. Porcine aortic smooth muscle cells secrete a serine protease for insulin like growth factor binding protein-2. *Circ Res* 1995;76:514–521.

87. Conover CA. A unique receptor independent mechanism by which insulin like growth factor I regulates the availability of insulin like growth factor binding protein in normal and transformed fibroblasts. *J Clin Invest* 1991;88:1354–1361.

88. Rees C, Clemmons DR, Horvitz GD, et al. A protease-resistant form of insulin-like growth factor binding protein-4 (IGFBP-4) inhibits IGF-I actions. *Endocrinology* 1998;139:4182–4188.

89. Ankrapp DP, Jones JI, Clemmons DR. Characterization of insulin like growth factor binding protein-1 kinases from human hepatoma cells. *J Cell Biochem* 1996;60:387–399.

90. Jones JI, D'Ercole AJ, Camacho-Hubner C, et al. Phosphorylation of insulin-like growth factor binding protein in cell culture and *in vivo:* effects on affinity for IGF-I. *Proc Natl Acad Sci USA* 1991;88:7481–7485.

91. Frost RA, Bereket A, Wilson TA, et al. Phosphorylation of insulin-like growth factor binding protein-1 in patients with insulin-dependent diabetes mellitus and severe trauma. *J Clin Endocrinol Metab* 1994;78: 1533–1535.

92. Coverley JA, Baxter RC. Regulation of insulin-like growth factor (IGF) binding protein-3 phosphorylation by IGF-I. *Endocrinology* 1995;136:5778–5781.

93. Jones JI, Gockerman A, Busby WH, et al. Extracellular matrix contains insulin-like growth factor binding protein-5: potentiation of the effects of IGF-I. *J Cell Biol* 1993;121:679–687.

94. Elgin RG, Busby WH, Clemmons DR. An insulin-like growth factor binding protein enhances the biologic response to IGF-I. *Proc Natl Acad Sci USA* 1987;84: 3254–3258.

95. Kratz G, Lake M, Ljungstrom K, et al. Effect of recombinant IGF binding protein-1 on primary cultures of human keratinocytes and fibroblasts: selective enhancement of IGF-I but not IGF-II induced cell proliferation. *Exp Cell Res* 1992;202:381–385.

96. Jones JI, Gockerman A, Busby WH Jr, et al. Insulin-like growth factor binding protein 1 stimulates cell migration and binds to the $\alpha 5\beta_1$ integrin by means of its Arg-Gly-Asp sequence. *Proc Natl Acad Sci USA* 1993; 90:10553–10557.

97. DeMellow JSM, Baxter RC. Growth hormone dependent insulin-like growth factor binding protein both inhibits and potentiates IGF-I stimulated DNA synthesis in skin fibroblasts. *Biochem Biophys Res Commun* 1988;156:199–204.

98. Conover CA. Potentiation of insulin-like growth factor (IGF) action by IGF-binding protein-3: studies of underlying mechanism. *Endocrinology* 1992;130:3191–3199.

99. Leal SM, Liu Q, Huang GS, et al. The type V transforming growth factor beta receptor is a putative insulin like growth factor binding protein 3 receptor. *J Biol Chem* 1997;272:20572–20576.

100. Oh Y, Muller HL, Ng L, et al. Transforming growth factor-beta–induced cell growth inhibition in human breast cancer cells is mediated through insulin-like growth factor-binding protein-3 action. *J Biol Chem* 1995;270:13589–13592.

101. Schoenle E, Zapf J, Humbel RE, et al. Insulin-like growth factor I stimulates growth in hypophysectomized rats. *Nature* 1982;296:252–253.

102. Douglas RG, Gluckman PD, Ball B, et al. The effects of infusion of insulin-like growth factor I (IGF-I), IGF-II and insulin on glucose and protein metabolism in fasted lambs. *J Clin Invest* 1991;88:614–622.

103. Olanrewaju H, Patel L, Seidel ER. Trophic action of local intraileal infusion of insulin like growth factor I: polyamine dependence. *Am J Physiol* 1992;263:E282–E286.

104. Jacob RJ, Sherwin RS, Bowen L, et al. Metabolic effects of IGF-I and insulin in spontaneously diabetic BB/w rats. *Am J Physiol* 1991;260:E262–E268.

105. Cox GN, McDermott MJ, Merkel E, et al. Recombinant human insulin-like growth factor binding protein-1 inhibits growth stimulated by IGF-I and growth hormone in hypophysectomized rats. *Endocrinology* 1994;35: 1913–1920.

106. Galiano RD, Zhao L, Clemmons DR, et al. Interaction between the insulin-like growth factor family and the integrin receptor family in tissue repair processes. *J Clin Invest* 1996;98:2462–2468.

107. Bagi CM, Brommage R, Adams SO, et al. Benefit of systemically administered rh IGF-I and rh IGF-I/IGBP-3 on cancellous bone in oophorectomized rats. *J Bone Miner Res* 1994;9:1301–1312.

108. Stewart CH, Bates DC, Calder TA, et al. Potentiation of insulin-like growth factor (IGF-I) activity by an antibody: supportive evidence for enhancement of IGF-I bioavailability *in vivo* by IGF binding proteins. *Endocrinology* 1993;133:1462–1465.

109. Behringer RR, Lewin TM, Quaife CJ, et al. Expression of insulin-like growth factor I stimulates normal somatic growth in growth hormone deficient transgenic mice. *Endocrinology* 1990;127:1033–1040.

110. Matthews LS, Hammer RE, Behringer RR, et al. Growth enhancement of transgenic mice expressing human insulin-like growth factor-I. *Endocrinology* 1988;123:2827–2833.

111. Rajkumar K, Barron D, Lewitt M, et al. Growth retardation and hyperglycemia in insulin-like growth factor binding protein-1 transgenic mice. *Endocrinology* 1995;136:4029.

112. Dai A, Xing Y, Boney CM, et al. Human insulin-like growth factor binding protein-1 (hIGFBP-1) transgenic mice: characterization and insights into the regulation of IGFBP-1 expression. *Endocrinology* 1994;135: 1316–1327.

113. Murphy LJ, Molnar P, Lu X, et al. Expression of human insulin-like growth factor–binding protein-3 in transgenic mice. *J Mol Endocrinol* 1995;15:293–303.

114. DeChiara RM, Efstratiadis A, Robertson EJ. A growth deficiency phenotype in heterozygous mice carrying an insulin-like growth factor II gene disruption. *Nature* 1990;345:78–80.

115. Pintar JE, Schuller A, Cerro JA, et al. Genetic ablation of IGFBP-2 suggests functional redundancy in the IGFBP family. *Prog Growth Fact Res* 1995;6:437.

116. Schuller AC, Pintar JE. Embryonic growth deficit in IGFBP-4 deficient mice. *Presented at the 80th Endocrine Society Meeting, New Orleans, LA, June 14–18, 1998:*OR6-1(abst).

117. Jennische E, Skottner A, Hansson HA. Dynamic changes in insulin-like growth factor I immunoreactivity correlate with repair events in rat ear after freeze-thaw injury. *Exp Mol Pathol* 1987;47:193–201.

118. Khorsondi MJ, Fagin JA, Ginnella-Neto et al. Regulation of insulin-like growth factor I and its receptor in rat aorta after balloon degradation: evidence for local bioactivity. *J Clin Invest* 1992;90:1926–1931.

119. Yakar S, Liu JU, Stannard B, et al. Normal growth and development in the absence of insulin-like growth factor-I. *Proc Natl Acad Sci USA* 1999;96:7324–7329.

120. Guler H-P, Zapf J, Froesch ER. Short-term metabolic effects of recombinant human insulin-like growth factor-I in healthy adults. *N Engl J Med* 1987;317:137–140.

121. Boulware S, Tamborlane W, Sherwin R. Diverse effects of insulin like growth factor I on glucose lipid-I amino acid metabolism. *Am J Physiol* 1992;262: 130–133.

122. Kupfer SR, Underwood LE, Baxter RC, et al. Enhancement of the anabolic effects of growth hormone and insulin like growth factor-I by the use of both agents simultaneously. *J Clin Invest* 1993;91:391–397.

123. Guler H-P, Schmid C, Zapf J, et al. Effects of recombinant insulin-like growth factor-I on insulin secretion and renal function in normal human subjects. *Proc Natl Acad Sci USA* 1989;86:2868–2872.

124. Moses AC, Young SCJ, Morrow LA, et al. Recombinant human insulin-like growth factor I increases insulin sensitivity and improves glycemic control in type II diabetes. *Diabetes* 1996;45:95–100.

125. Walker JL, Ginalska-Malinowska M, Romer TC, et al. Effects of infusion of insulin-like growth factor-I in a child with growth hormone insensitivity syndrome. *N Engl J Med* 1991;324:1483–1488.

126. Guevara-Aguirre J, Vasconez O, Martinez V, et al. A randomized double blind placebo controlled trial of safety and efficacy of recombinant human insulin like growth factor I in children with growth hormone receptor deficiency. *J Clin Endocrinol Metab* 1995;80: 1393–1398.

Skeletal Growth Factors,
edited by Ernesto Canalis.
Lippincott Williams & Wilkins, Philadelphia, © 2000.

7

Insulin-like Growth Factors and the Skeleton

Cheryl A. Conover

Department of Medicine, Mayo Clinic and Mayo Foundation, Rochester, Minnesota 55905

Insulin-like growth factors (IGFs) are key players in skeletal physiology. However, the precise roles they play in the various aspects of bone growth, remodeling, and repair continue to be defined. As discussed in the preceding chapter, the IGF regulatory system is immensely complex and to fully understand it depends on integrated knowledge of the peptides, receptors, binding proteins (IGFBPs), and IGFBP proteases involved. This chapter presents a brief overview of recent progress important to our understanding of the IGF system in bone, with particular emphasis on local control of bone remodeling. Potential clinical applications of this knowledge are explored in Chapter 8.

INSULIN-LIKE GROWTH FACTOR ACTION IN BONE

Bone remodeling consists of recruitment, proliferation, differentiation, and complex interactions of bone-forming osteoblastic cells and bone-resorbing osteoclastic cells. The IGFs appear to be involved in all aspects of the remodeling process.

The two major IGF peptides, IGF-I and IGF-II, are capable of stimulating bone formation *in vitro* and *in vivo* (1–3); however, assignment of distinct roles for IGF-I and IGF-II is still a matter of debate. As is discussed later, specific IGF actions in bone may depend on the animal species, bone cell type and stage of differentiation, relative IGF receptor number, presence of IGFBPs, and activity of IGFBP proteases. Recent data indicate that IGFs may also regulate

bone resorption, and this chapter reviews new developments with IGFs and osteoclasts.

It has been shown frequently and is generally accepted that the actions of IGF-I and IGF-II are mediated through type I IGF receptors present on osteoblastic and osteoclastic cells (4–7). Type I IGF receptors belong to the family of signaling tyrosine kinases (8). However, osteoblasts and osteoclasts also possess type II IGF/mannose-6-phosphate receptors (6,9,10), and recent data suggest that IGF-II may exert some of its effects in bone cells through type II IGF receptor–mediated changes in intracellular calcium ion flux (11). A physiological role for the type II IGF/mannose-6-phosphate receptor in bone remains to be determined.

Insulin-like Growth Factors and Bone Formation

The process of new bone formation includes recruitment, proliferation, differentiation, and maturation of cells into specialized matrix-producing osteoblasts. There is substantive evidence from both *in vitro* and *in vivo* studies for IGF involvement, but it remains an important goal to define the precise roles the IGFs play in driving and/or regulating the steps in this process.

Recruitment

The bone marrow stroma contains pluripotential cells that can be recruited and committed to the osteoblast, chondrocyte, or adipocyte lineage. This important source of new bone-forming cells plays a key role in skeletal physiology and pathology and, thus, offers a potential target for therapeutic agents; however, there are no published studies as yet on the potential role of IGFs in the initial recruitment/commitment of osteoprogenitor cells. In recent studies, Thomas et al. (12) employed a conditionally immortalized human marrow stromal (hMS) cell line which has the ability to differentiate into either mature osteoblasts or adipocytes (13). These hMS cells expressed functional receptors and responded to IGF-I and IGF-II with increased proliferation; however, treatment with IGFs did not induce expression of *Cbfa1*, the key transcription factor for commitment to the osteoblast lineage, or expression of alkaline phosphatase, type I collagen, and osteocalcin, markers of osteoblast differentiation. Thus, IGFs did not directly modulate commitment of hMS cells to the osteoblast pathway.

Proliferation/Differentiation

The IGFs are commonly cited as being important regulators of osteoprogenitor cell proliferation and maturation, although few studies directly address this issue. In murine TC-1 stromal cells grown under conditions that promote osteogenic differentiation, IGF-I stimulated ^{3}H-thymidine incorporation threefold (14). Tanaka and coworkers (15–17) reported that rat primary stromal cell cultures induced to differentiate with dexamethasone pretreatment respond to IGF with increased expression of bone matrix markers. Since IGF responsiveness may be species-specific (18), it was also important to determine the effects of the IGFs on human marrow stromal cells. Langdahl et al. (19) recently reported comparative effects of IGF-I and IGF-II in primary cultures of hMS cells. IGF-I was mitogenic for these cells; however, the data for effects on differentiated function showed considerable variability, most likely due to the heterogeneity of the primary cultures. As noted previously, clonal hMS cells responded to exogenous IGFs with increases in DNA synthesis and cell number, but IGFs alone failed to influence commitment; however, once these cells

were induced to differentiate toward the osteoblast lineage, IGF treatment significantly increased type I IGF collagen expression (12). Thus, IGFs appear to stimulate osteoblastic cell proliferation and differentiated function depending on the stage of cell maturation.

Extracellular Matrix Formation

IGF-I and IGF-II not only act to stimulate proliferation of osteoblast precursors and early-stage osteoblasts but they also promote bone matrix formation by the fully differentiated osteoblast (1–3,20,21). IGFs stimulate type I collagen and noncollagenous matrix protein synthesis in bone cultures independently of their mitogenic activity. In addition, IGFs inhibit collagen degradation via inhibition of collagenase expression by osteoblasts (22). Delany et al. (23) recently demonstrated that endogenous IGFs promote tonic inhibition of collagenase synthesis in cultured rat osteoblasts. Furthermore, endogenous and exogenous IGFs are associated with indices of active bone matrix production *in vivo* (24–26).

Other

IGF increased vascular endothelial growth factor (VEGF) expression in human osteosarcoma cells and in primary cultures of fetal murine calvarial osteoblasts (27). VEGF acts locally on endothelium to stimulate angiogenesis, an essential component of bone remodeling. IGF stimulated inorganic phosphate transport in osteogenic cells (28). Phosphate is necessary for the formation and mineralization of bone extracellular matrix.

Insulin-like Growth Factors and Bone Resorption

Compared to bone formation, much less is known about potential actions of IGFs on bone resorption.

Osteoclasts are derived from hematopoietic stem cells in the bone marrow, and there are now ample data to support a role for IGFs in osteoclast progenitor cell recruitment and differentiation. Type I IGF receptors are present on human preosteoclastic cells (29), and several studies have demonstrated that IGF-I can act directly to stimulate formation of tartrate-resistant acid phosphatase (TRAP)-positive multinucleated cells from hematopoietic precursors (7,30–32). IGF-I also mediates the migration of preosteoclastic cells toward bone-derived endothelial cells *in vitro* (33).

In addition, IGF can stimulate osteoclast activation. Mochizuki et al. (30) reported that IGF-I, but not IGF-II, stimulated bone resorption by preexisting osteoclasts. The studies of Hill et al. (34) suggested that osteoblasts mediate this IGF-I stimulation of osteoclast activation since they found no stimulation of isolated osteoclast activity unless osteoblasts were present. On the other hand, mature human, rat, and rabbit osteoclasts express type I IGF receptors (7,26,34); therefore, direct IGF bioeffects are possible in the modulation of osteoclast function. Indeed, IGF-I immunoreactivity (but not mRNA) is present in TRAP-positive osteoclasts *in vivo* (35).

Identification of the exact mechanism notwithstanding, it is clear that IGF-I can stimulate bone resorption by enhancing osteoclast recruitment and supporting the formation and activation of osteoclasts. It may be that IGF-I production by osteoblasts and its regulation by bone-resorbing agents such as parathyroid hormone (PTH, see below) constitute a major local factor coupling bone formation and resorption. Furthermore, if there truly is a selective effect of IGF-I versus IGF-II on osteoclast activity (30), then osteoblast activity and bone formation could be favored with IGF-II.

SKELETAL INSULIN-LIKE GROWTH FACTOR

IGF-I and IGF-II are available to bone through delivery from the circulation, local synthesis, and release from stores in the bone matrix. Since skeletal IGF may be more relevant to bone remodeling than serum (liver-derived) IGF, the focus here is on local IGF availability through *de novo* synthesis by bone cells and deposition/release from bone matrix.

TABLE 7.1. *Insulin-like growth factor (IGF) expression* in vitro: *rat osteoblastic cells*

	IGF-I	IGF-II	References
Basal expression	+ +	+	1
Hormonal regulation			
PTH (cAMP)	↑	∅	40,41
Estrogen	↑↓∅	∅	46,48
Glucocorticoid	↓	∅	49,51
Local regulation			
TGF-β	↓	↓	55
BMP-2	↑	↑	56
BMP-7	↑	↑	57
FGF	↓	↓	55
PDGF	↓	↓	55
IL-6	↑	∅	59
Prostaglandin	↑∅	↑	60,62

∅, no change; ↑, increased; ↓, decreased; BMP, bone morphogenetic protein; cAMP, cyclic adenosine monophosphate; FGF, fibroblast growth factor; IL-6, interleukin-6; PDGF, platelet-derived growth factor; PTH, parathyroid hormone; TGF-β, transforming growth factor-β.

Pattern of Insulin-like Growth Factor Expression in Bone

IGFs are expressed by primary cultures of osteoblasts as well as by transformed and osteosarcoma-derived osteoblastic cell lines. There is distinct species specificity in regard to gene expression, with rat osteoblasts primarily expressing IGF-I and human osteoblasts primarily expressing IGF-II (Tables 7.1, 7.2). It remains unclear whether IGF-I and IGF-II actually serve specific functions which differ in the different species or whether the functions are the same and the bone physiology differs among species (36).

TABLE 7.2. *Insulin-like growth factor (IGF) expression* in vitro: *human osteoblastic cells*

	IGF-I	IGF-II	References
Basal expression	+	+ +	54
Hormonal regulation			
PTH (cAMP)	↑	∅	42
Estrogen	↑	∅	47
Glucocorticoid	↓	∅	50
Local regulation			
TGF-β	↑	∅	42
BMP-7	∅	↑	45,58
CaCl₂	∅	↑	64

∅, no change; ↑, increased; ↓, decreased; BMP, bone morphogenetic protein; cAMP, cyclic adenosine monophosphate; PTH, parathyroid hormone; TGF-β, transforming growth factor-β.

In addition, the stage of osteoblast differentiation (i.e., whether preosteoblast, early-stage proliferating osteoblast, mature matrix-secreting osteoblast, or late-stage "osteocyte" embedded in mineralized matrix) appears to influence the pattern of IGF expression. For example, in fetal rat calvarial cultures, IGF-I secretion was shown to be biphasic. Early-stage IGF-I expression was associated with cell proliferation. As preosteoblasts differentiated, IGF-I secretion decreased, with a second increase late during mineralization (37).

As in vitro, the relative expression of IGF-I and IGF-II in bone in vivo varies with species and during development (25,26,38). Nevertheless, in both rodent and human models, IGF expression is found to be highest in the "plump" osteoblasts involved in active bone remodeling. Shinar et al. (24) demonstrated an association between IGF-I mRNA expression and the osteogenic regions of rat bone during postnatal development. Similarly, Middleton et al. (25) and Andrew et al. (26) showed in adult human osteophyte tissue and normally healing human fracture, respectively, that IGF-I and IGF-II expression was strongest in osteoblasts actively forming bone and weak or absent in quiescent flat bone lining cells and in osteocytes.

A study looking at the temporal aspects of IGF expression during rat bone formation, induced by implantation of demineralized bone matrix, indicated a transient increase in IGF-I mRNA occurring at day 3 associated with proliferation of osteoblastic cells as well as an increase in IGF-II that was highest by day 11 during osteoblast differentiation (39). The differential expression of IGF-I and IGF-II in this study implies specific roles for IGF-I and IGF-II in bone formation.

Regulation of Insulin-like Growth Factor Expression in Bone

Hormones and local growth factors regulate IGF expression in osteoblastic cells (Tables 7.1, 7.2), and, indeed, the IGFs have been implicated as mediating the skeletal effects of several of these agents in vitro and in vivo. In general, hormones appear to preferentially regulate IGF-I

expression, and these studies have been done primarily using rat bone cell models. There is little evidence for hormonal regulation of IGF-II expression in human or rodent bone cells. As is discussed later, local factors may be more important determinants of IGF-II expression.

Hormones

The major hormones that regulate the skeleton also regulate IGF-I expression (Tables 7.1, 7.2). Canalis et al. (40) first presented evidence that the anabolic effects of intermittent PTH on rat bone cells were largely through increased osteoblast IGF-I expression. PTH stimulated IGF-I transcription in fetal rat calvarial cells through increased cyclic adenosine monophosphate (cAMP) production and cAMP-activated protein kinase (41). There is evidence for similar PTH effects on IGF-I expression in human bone cells with the use of cAMP-elevating agents (42). These data lend support to in vivo studies whereby intermittent PTH administration to ovariectomized (OVX) rats increased osteoblast IGF-I gene expression in cancellous bone osteoblasts and restored bone mass (43). As noted above, PTH-induced expression of IGF-I by osteoblasts could also influence the formation and activation of osteoclasts (32).

Evidence for a direct effect of other hormones on IGF-I expression in bone cells is more controversial. Liver expression of IGF-I is growth hormone (GH)–dependent, but there are no consistent data supporting a direct effect of GH on bone IGF-I expression. A GH effect on cultured bone cells may be species-specific (18,44,45).

Estrogen treatment increased IGF-I expression in rodent and human osteoblasts transfected with estrogen receptors (46,47). On the other hand, McCarthy et al. (48) found that estrogen treatment decreased previously induced IGF-I mRNA but had no effect alone in primary fetal rat osteoblasts with human estrogen receptor transfection. There is no consensus estrogen-responsive element in the IGF-I promoter, and it may be that any estrogen effect is through an interaction in the cAMP-dependent pathway (positive or negative depending on the system and/or conditions) that normally enhances IGF-I expression in skeletal cells.

Glucocorticoids decrease IGF-I synthesis in primary rat and human osteoblast cultures (49,50). In rat osteoblastic cells, glucocorticoids decreased IGF-I expression by inhibiting its transcription (51). Cheng et al. (52) reported that dexamethasone-induced differentiation of bone marrow stromal cells into cells of the osteoblast phenotype was accompanied by decreases in IGF-I but increases in IGF-II. 1,25-Dihydroxyvitamin D_3 has been reported to inhibit IGF-I expression in mouse MC3T3-E1 cell cultures (53). However, as osteoblastic cells differentiate *in vitro* and *in vivo*, IGF-I secretion decreases and IGF-II increases (37,39). Therefore, hormones such as 1,25-dihydroxyvitamin D_3 and glucocorticoids which induce differentiation, may indirectly affect IGF expression.

Growth Factors

Growth factors and cytokines produced by bone cells or released from stores in the bone matrix may regulate IGF expression by osteoblasts. The list of these potential factors continues to grow, and there is still much work to be done (Tables 7.1, 7.2).

Transforming growth factor-β (TGF-β), a major local regulator of bone cell metabolism, has been shown to decrease IGF-I and IGF-II expression in rat osteoblasts (55) but to increase IGF-I expression (with no change in IGF-II mRNA) in human osteoblasts (42). Bone morphogenetic proteins (BMPs), members of the TGF-β superfamily, have produced more consistent results. There are multiple BMPs, and several of these have the unique ability to promote growth and differentiation of mesenchymal cells into matrix-producing osteoblasts. This multistep conversion appears to be mediated, in part, through the IGF system. BMP-2 increased IGF-I and IGF-II mRNA expression in rat osteoblastic cells (56). BMP-7 also increased IGF-I and IGF-II mRNA expression in primary cultures of fetal rat calvaria, and antisense oligonucleotides of IGF-I and IGF-II mRNA sequence decreased the BMP-7-induced increase in alkaline phosphatase activity (57). The mitogenic/differentiative effects of BMP-7 on human bone cells may also be mediated via IGF-II (45,58). So far, BMPs are the only growth factors identified that increase IGF-II expression. Other local growth factors, fibroblast growth factor (FGF) and platelet-derived growth factor (PDGF), decreased IGF expression in rat osteoblasts (55).

Interleukin-6 (IL-6) is a cytokine produced by skeletal cells that is mitogenic for bone cells *in vitro* and can increase bone resorption through recruitment of osteoclasts. These effects may be due to the ability of IL-6 and its soluble receptor to increase IGF-I expression in osteoblasts (59).

The prostaglandins are emerging as significant regulators of IGF expression in bone cells. In particular, prostaglandin E_2 (PGE$_2$) and prostacyclin (PGI$_2$) are synthesized locally in the skeleton following exposure to PTH, cytokines, and mechanical strain; and these prostaglandins, when added exogenously, stimulate IGF expression in osteoblasts *in vitro* (60–62). Extracellular CaCl$_2$-stimulated proliferation of osteoblasts and osteosarcoma cells *in vitro* was shown to be mediated by increased IGF (63,64).

Mechanical Loading and Insulin-like Growth Factor Expression in Bone

Bone remodels itself in response to physical forces so that bone structure and mass remain optimal to give strength and support to the body. The mechanism by which mechanical strain and loading stimulate bone formation is not clearly understood, but the IGFs have been implicated as important mediators of this adaptive property of bone.

An understanding of mechanosensors and response transduction in bone requires an appreciation of a little-studied osteoblast subtype, the osteocyte. Osteocytes do not replicate or produce new bone, but they form an intercommunicating network of cells embedded in the bone. Therefore, these cells are strategically situated to sense changes in mechanical strain and equipped to transmit signals to bone surfaces where formation and resorption occur.

Lean et al. (65,66) clearly demonstrated a role

for the osteocyte as a sensor of mechanical strain and for IGF expression as a tranducer of the osteogenic response to strain. Following a single acute episode of dynamic loading to rat bone, IGF-I mRNA expression was detected in osteocytes within 30 minutes and showed an intense hybridization signal by 6 hours. The focal pattern of osteocyte IGF-I mRNA hybridization was directly related to the local strain environment. Significantly, this increase in IGF-I expression in the osteocytes preceded the increase in matrix protein and IGF-I mRNA in bone surface cells. Thus, induction of IGF-I expression in osteocytes occurred before the onset of bone formation in response to mechanical strain. Studies by Mikuni-Takagaki et al. (67) provide *in vitro* demonstration of a specific role for osteocytes and IGF in mechanical response transduction, consistent with the *in situ* experiments.

Several *in vivo* and *in vitro* studies suggest that mechanical loads or the electrical potentials they generate stimulate immediate prostaglandin release from bone cells, which, in turn, stimulates IGF expression in osteocytes and osteoblasts (61,62,65,68). In perfusable cores of adult canine cancellous bone, strain-induced PGI_2 was immunolocalized to osteocytes and surface osteoblasts, whereas PGE_2 was localized to surface osteoblasts only (61). Furthermore, exogenous PGI_2 increased IGF-II release from osteocytes and surface osteoblasts. Studies by Zaman et al. (62) also indicate a role for IGF-II and PGI_2 in early strain response in load-related rat bone remodeling. In their studies, exogenous PGI_2 increased IGF-II with no change in IGF-I; exogenous PGE_2 increased IGF-I and IGF-II. These findings indicate an important relationship among mechanical strain, prostaglandin synthesis, and IGFs. Inconsistencies with regard to specific prostaglandin response and action may reflect different species and experimental conditions. In particular, Mikuni-Takagaki et al. (67) noted that strain affects preosteoblasts in a PGE_2-dependent manner but that physiological strain affects young osteocytes in a PGE_2-independent manner. Different species and experimental conditions may similarly explain seeming inconsistencies in IGF response. It is of note

that canine bone best resembles human bone (36) and that human and canine osteoblastic cells respond to mechanical and low-energy electromagnetic stimuli with increased IGF-II expression (61,69,70). Thus, IGF-II may be the primary form of IGF regulated by physical strain in human bone. IGF-II is a likely candidate to mediate load-related osteogenesis because IGF-II expression is not otherwise influenced by many of the normal osteotropic agents.

Insulin-like Growth Factors in Bone Matrix

IGFs are incorporated into mineralized bone matrix *in vivo* and retain activity when extracted (71). Thus, the skeletal IGF made available through osteoclastic activity may be consequential to bone physiology. The relative abundance of IGF-I and IGF-II stored in bone reflects species-specific osteoblast expression (72). In humans, IGF-II is not only more abundant than IGF-I in bone matrix, it is the most abundant of all of the growth factors stored in bone (73).

Recently, Seck et al. (74) measured IGF-I and IGF-II content of bone matrix in 533 human biopsies. IGF-I in cancellous bone had a negative association with age and a positive association with bone volume. The absolute concentration of IGF-II in these bone biopsies was eightfold greater than that of IGF-I, consistent with osteoblast expression data (Table 7.2). There was no significant relationship of IGF-II level with age or cancellous bone volume, but there was a positive association with osteoblast surface. Nicolas et al. (75) also showed that IGF-I, but not IGF-II, levels in human femoral cortical bone decreased with age.

IGF-I and IGF-II levels are increased in human bone matrix of patients with osteoarthritis and its associated increased bone density (76). It was speculated that the resistance to osteoporosis seen in patients with osteoarthritis may be directly related to the increased skeletal concentrations of IGF and the general increase in the biosynthetic activity of osteoblasts in this condition.

Rats exercised for 9 weeks on a treadmill, a form of mechanical stimulation of bone by muscle contraction, also show increased periosteal bone formation rate and increased IGF-I bone content (77).

Intermittent PTH treatment of rats resulted in increased bone mineral density of the lumbar spine and increased levels of matrix-associated IGF-I content; there was no effect of PTH on IGF-II content (78). PTH had no effect on serum IGF levels in these experiments, indicating that the increased skeletal concentrations were likely due to production and deposition by the bone cells themselves and consistent with the ability of PTH to stimulate IGF-I, but not IGF-II, expression in rat osteoblasts.

Supraphysiological estrogen therapy increased bone matrix IGF-I concentrations in OVX rats (79), lending *in vivo* evidence to a stimulatory effect of estrogen on skeletal concentrations of IGF-I. In contrast, other groups (80,81) demonstrated that estrogen treatment decreased bone IGF-I mRNA levels in OVX rats. Although there is no clear explanation, these seeming discrepancies may reflect differential effects of estrogen on osteoblast IGF-I expression and peptide deposition in the matrix. Slater et al. (82) have demonstrated that estrogen can increase the focal incorporation of IGF-I and IGF-II into extracellular matrix produced by fetal human osteoblasts *in vitro* independently of any effect on IGF synthesis. These findings suggest that synthesis of IGF and its deposition in matrix may be differentially regulated and, furthermore, that estrogen deficiency could alter the store of IGF available for bone remodeling.

SKELETAL INSULIN-LIKE GROWTH FACTOR BINDING PROTEIN

IGF bioavailability in bone is determined not only by bone cell expression and by release of the peptides from matrix, as discussed above, but also by the actions of IGFBPs. Six high-affinity IGFBPs have been characterized (83), and there are data to support roles for all six of the IGFBPs in bone.

Insulin-like Growth Factor Binding Protein Action in Bone

Although key players, it has not been possible as yet to assign a specific physiological role to any of the IGFBPs in any system. Sufficient amounts of purified or recombinantly expressed IGFBP have only recently been available to perform the biological studies. Moreover, the specific cell setting *in vitro* and, likely, *in vivo* appears to influence outcome. This is due, in large part, to the variety of posttranslational modifications that can occur which have profound effects on IGFBP structure/function and, hence, IGF action (84). Furthermore, there is increasing awareness that IGFBPs might have IGF-independent effects as well (85). This section summarizes studies examining IGFBP actions specifically in bone cell models.

IGFBP-1 has not been considered a major player in the bone IGF regulatory system since no IGFBP-1 expression was detected in any of the osteoblastic cell models. Indeed, IGFBP-1 expression has been considered relatively specific to liver and certain reproductive tissues (86); however, recent studies have demonstrated that high-dose glucocorticoids induce IGFBP-1 expression in normal human osteoblasts and that this expression is associated with suppressed type I collagen secretion (87,88).

IGFBP-2, at excess molar concentrations, can inhibit the actions of IGFs on osteoblast replication and matrix synthesis (89). At equimolar concentrations, IGF-II plus IGFBP-2 is as effective as IGF-II alone at stimulating the growth of normal human osteoblasts in culture (90). This appears to be due to the preferential ability of the IGFBP-2/IGF-II complex to bind to bone cell–derived extracellular matrix (90). This binding may bring about a conformational change resulting in reduced IGFBP-2 affinity and release of IGF-II for receptor activation.

IGFBP-3 has been shown to have both inhibitory and stimulatory effects on bone cells. In the intact form, exogenous IGFBP-3 is a potent inhibitor by virtue of an affinity for IGF that is tenfold greater than that of the IGF receptors; however, a truncated form of IGFBP-3 potentiated IGF-I action in osteoblasts (91). Furthermore, Ernst and Rodan (92) found that accumulation of endogenous IGFBP-3 correlated with enhanced IGF-I activity in osteoblastic cells. Presumably, posttranslational modifications are key to the biological effectiveness of IGFBP-3 and need to be explored further in the context of the bone microenvironment.

IGFBP-4 has been consistently shown to inhibit IGF-stimulated effects in a variety of bone cell models (93–96). Indeed, IGFBP-4 was originally isolated from human bone cell culture media by Mohan et al. (93) as "inhibitory IGFBP."

IGFBP-5, like IGFBP-3, has been shown to have both inhibitory and stimulatory effects on bone. When intact and in solution, endogenous or exogenous IGFBP-5 inhibits IGF-stimulated bone cell growth (5,95). However, IGFBP-5 is not normally intact or in solution in the bone cell environment due to an active IGFBP-5 protease secreted by bone cells (97) and to the strong affinity of IGFBP-5 for hydroxyapatite, which preferentially localizes it in the extracellular matrix, where it appears to be protected from proteolysis (98). IGFBP-5 in the extracellular matrix is associated with potentiation of IGF action (99). Also, in this form, IGFBP-5 serves to anchor IGF-II to human bone matrix (98). Andress and colleagues (100,101) further showed that a truncated form of IGFBP-5 will enhance the mitogenic potency of IGF-I or IGF-II in mouse osteoblastic cultures. Similarly, Mohan et al. (102) reported IGFBP-5 stimulation of IGF-induced proliferation of human osteoblasts. Interestingly, this truncated form of IGFBP-5 also pos-

sesses intrinsic mitogenic activity mediated by an IGFBP-5 "receptor" on osteoblasts (103). In a preliminary report, IGFBP-5 administration to mice for 10 days increased serum markers of bone formation (104). New data suggest that IGFBP-5 may act not only on osteoblasts but also on osteoclasts and their precursors (105).

IGFBP-6 is unique among the IGFBPs in its high affinity for IGF-II compared to IGF-I and, thus, is postulated to perform a key role in modulating IGF-II activity in bone. Addition of recombinant human IGFBP-6 preferentially blocked IGF-II-stimulated DNA synthesis in rat osteoblastic cells (106).

Insulin-like Growth Factor Binding Protein Expression in Bone

IGFBPs are present in the bone microenvironment. Normal and osteosarcoma-derived osteoblastic cells *in vitro* are capable of expressing IGFBP-1 through IGFBP-6 under varying conditions (Tables 7.3, 7.4). As found for IGF expression, these variables include species, stage of differentiation/transformation, culture conditions, and hormonal regulation. In general, IGFBP-4, IGFBP-5, and IGFBP-6 are the predominant forms in the different bone cell models, IGFBP-2 and IGFBP-3 expression is

TABLE 7.3. *Insulin-like growth factor binding protein (IGFBP) expression* in vitro: *rat osteoblastic cells*

	IGFBP-1	IGFBP-2	IGFBP-3	IGFBP-4	IGFBP-5	IGFBP-6	References
Basal expression	∅	+	+	+	+	+	119
Hormonal regulation							
PTH				↑	↑		32,111,112
Glucocorticoid	∅	↓	↓	↓	↓	↑	113,115,116
Vitamin D$_3$					↑		112
Local regulation							
TGF-β					↓		120
BMP-2					↓		121
BMP-7		∅	↑	↓	↓	↓	57
IGF		∅			↑		111,119,123
Prostaglandin		∅	↑	↑	↑	∅	119
FGF				↓	↓	↓	120
PDGF					↓		120
IL-6					↑		128
Retinoic acid					↑		123

∅, no change; ↑, increased; ↓, decreased; BMP, bone morphogenetic protein; FGF, fibroblast growth factor; IL-6, interleukin-6; PDGF, platelet-derived growth factor; PTH, parathyroid hormone; TGF-β, transforming growth factor-β.

TABLE 7.4. *Insulin-like growth factor binding protein (IGFBP) expression* in vitro: *human osteoblastic cells*

	IGFBP-1	IGFBP-2	IGFBP-3	IGFBP-4	IGFBP-5	IGFBP-6	References
Basal expression	Ø	+	+	+	+	+	87
Hormonal regulation							
PTH				↑	↑		94
Glucocorticoid	↑		↓	↓Ø	↓	Ø	87,114,117
Insulin	↓		Ø	Ø	Ø	Ø	117
Vitamin D$_3$		Ø	↑				118
Estrogen			Ø	↑			96
Androgen			↑	↓			141
Local regulation							
TGF-β				↓			137
BMP-7			↑	↓	↑		58,122
IGF			Ø	Ø	↑		125
Retinoic acid					↓	↑	124

Ø, no change; ↑, increased; ↓, decreased; BMP, bone morphogenetic protein; PTH, parathyroid hormone; TGF-β, transforming growth factor-β.

variable, and IGFBP-1 expression is relatively specific for normal human osteoblasts.

The *in situ* pattern of IGFBP expression in the rat and mouse shows IGFBPs 2, 4, 5, and 6 expressed in osteoblasts (107). There was no IGFBP-3 expression in bone cells; rather, IGFBP-3 mRNA was localized to capillaries invading the perichondrium and periosteum. Human bone cells from different skeletal sites express IGFBPs 3, 4, and 5 (108).

The developmental stage of the osteoblast is an important determinant of IGFBP secretion. *In vivo* and *in vitro,* osteoblasts progress through a developmental sequence from committed precursors to mature differentiated cells that form a mineralized matrix. In primary cultures of fetal rat calvaria, maximum levels of IGFBP-2 and IGFBP-5 mRNA are associated with proliferating preosteoblasts. IGFBPs 3, 4, and 6 are associated with mature, fully differentiated osteoblasts. Birnbaum and Wiren (109) showed that if differentiation was prematurely induced, the IGFBP pattern would be that of the mature osteoblast and that if differentiation was delayed, the pattern would be that of proliferating cells. Interestingly, osteocyte-like cells in mineralized matrix expressed primarily IGFBP-4 and IGFBP-6. It may be that this developmental regulation of IGFBP secretion in the osteoblast lineage results in specific targeting of IGFs to particular cell types and modification of IGF

bioactivity at appropriate times in the remodeling process.

Although among bone-derived cells, only osteoblasts have been extensively investigated for expression, production, and function of IGFBPs, recent reports suggest their importance in preosteoblasts and osteoclasts as well. Murine TC-1 stromal cells constitutively secrete IGFBPs 2 through 6, with IGFBPs 4, 5, and 6 being the most abundantly expressed (110). hMS cells express IGFBPs 3 through 6 (12). Preosteoclastic cells express IGFBP-2 and IGFBP-4 (29).

Regulation of Insulin-like Growth Factor Binding Protein Expression

Production of IGFBPs by osteoblastic cells is regulated by essentially the same hormones and growth factors that regulate IGF expression, suggesting an importance to their coordinate control in skeletal physiology. A summary of recent studies describing *in vitro* regulation of IGFBP expression is provided in Tables 7.3 and 7.4. Only a few of the findings are remarked upon here.

IGFBP-4 is the most abundantly expressed of the IGFBPs in bone *in vitro* and *in vivo*. PTH increases IGFBP-4 mRNA and protein expression in human and rat osteoblasts via a cAMP-dependent pathway (94,111). PTH also induces IGFBP-5 mRNA expression by a cAMP-dependent mechanism (111,112). PTH induction of IGFBP-5, in addition to IGF-I (32), in osteoblasts may play a role in PTH-stimulated osteoclast cell formation.

Glucocorticoid treatment of human and rat osteoblasts decreased expression of IGFBPs 2 through 5 (87,113–115). Glucocorticoids either increased or had no effect on IGFBP-6 expression, depending on whether rat or human osteoblasts, respectively, were treated (87,116). Glucocorticoids induced IGFBP-1 expression in normal human osteoblast cells, and this induction was effectively suppressed by insulin (117).

The vitamin D_3 analogue Ro24-5531 decreased proliferation, induced differentiation, and markedly increased IGFBP-3 expression in MG-63 human osteosarcoma cells (118). However, a direct antiproliferative effect of IGFBP-3 on these cells was not found. 1,25-Dihydroxyvitamin D_3 stimulated IGFBP-4 mRNA expression in UMR-106 rat osteosarcoma cells (112).

Regulation of IGFBPs by local skeletal factors varies considerably among the different osteoblastic cells (Tables 7.3, 7.4). Interestingly, IGFs themselves induce IGFBP-5 mRNA expression in human and rat osteoblasts (111, 119,123,125). IGF treatment also decreased IGFBP-4 levels in medium conditioned by normal human osteoblasts (125); however, it was later documented that this effect was independent of any change in IGFBP-4 gene expression and reflected the ability of IGFs to activate IGFBP-4 proteolysis (126,127).

Studies of *in vivo* regulation of IGFBP have primarily examined serum concentrations in different physiological and pathophysiological conditions, but serum levels may not reflect local bone IGFBP expression. Nicolas et al. (129) directly measured IGFBP-5 content of human femoral cortical bone; they found an age-related decrease in skeletal IGFBP-5 content which paralleled the decrease in IGF content.

SKELETAL INSULIN-LIKE GROWTH FACTOR BINDING PROTEIN PROTEASES

Proteolysis of IGFBP is as important as synthesis in determining IGFBP site-specific and condition-specific availability and action. Proteolytic activities have been described in serum and other biological fluids that can cleave IGFBP-1 through IGFBP-6 with varying specificities (130). Many of the responsible proteases are previously characterized enzymes that cleave multiple IGFBPs. Others are apparently novel proteases that are relatively specific for a single form of IGFBP. The importance of IGFBP regulation by proteases is indicated by resultant modification in IGFBP affinity for IGFs or complete destruction of IGF binding potential. In addition, IGFBP proteolysis may produce cleavage products with unique functions. IGFBP proteases have been identified in several bone cell systems (Table 7.5).

Normal human osteoblasts and MG-63 human osteosarcoma cells secrete an acid-activated IGFBP protease identified as cathepsin D (87,131). Activated cathepsin D is not IGFBP-specific and will proteolyze IGFBPs 1 through 5 (97). It is postulated that this enzyme is active in the acidic pericellular environment of tumors and/or in the acidic lacunae created by osteoclasts (131). Plasmin is another broad-spectrum IGFBP protease active in MG-63 osteosarcoma cells (132). Matrix metalloproteases degrade IGFBPs 3 and 5 and are regulated during MC3T3-E1 osteoblast differentiation in culture (133).

A novel IGFBP-4 protease has been identified in media conditioned by normal human osteoblasts (126,127) and, recently, in cultured hMS cells (12). Based on physiochemical similarities with the protease secreted by normal human fibroblasts and cleavage site analyses, this enzyme belongs to the astacin family of metalloproteases (134,135). IGFBP-4 is the only IGFBP substrate for this protease, which is active in a broad pH range of 5.5 to 9.0. The IGFBP-4 protease can be regulated at multiple levels. The unique feature of this enzyme is its absolute dependence on IGFs for functional activation. The mechanism is unclear, but in cell-free assay, no proteolysis of endogenous or exogenous IGFBP-4 in cell-conditioned medium occurs unless IGFs are present. In general, IGF-II is more effective than IGF-I at activating proteolysis (126), and overexpression of IGF-II in normal

TABLE 7.5. *Insulin-like growth factor binding protein (IGFBP) proteases in bone cell models*

Protease	Model	Specificity	References
Cathepsin D	MG-63, hOB	Broad	87,131
Plasmin	MG-63	Broad	132
MMP	MC3T3-E1	Broad	133
IGFBP-4 protease	hOB, hMS	IGFBP-4	126,127
IGFBP-5 protease	U2, hOB	IGFBP-5	97,127,139

hMS, human marrow stroma; hOB, human osteoblast; MMP, matrix metalloproteinase.

human osteoblasts can confer seemingly constitutive IGFBP-4 protease activity (136). TGF-β is another positive regulator of IGFBP-4 proteolysis in human osteoblasts. Unlike IGF-II, however, TGF-β does not directly activate proteolysis but rather appears to stimulate production/secretion of the enzyme (137). IGFBP-4 proteolysis can also be controlled by inhibitors produced by bone cells and associated with the early transformation process (138). In addition, estrogen treatment decreased IGF-dependent IGFBP-4 proteolysis in estrogen-responsive bone cells, but it was not determined whether estrogen acts to decrease protease expression or increase inhibition (96). IGF-II-dependent IGFBP-4 proteolysis has been shown to enhance IGF-I action in normal human osteoblasts (126).

Normal human osteoblasts and U2 human osteosarcoma cells secrete IGFBP-5-specific protease activity (97,127). This proteolytic activity is distinct from that regulating IGFBP-4 in that it appears to be a cation-dependent serine protease and IGFs attenuate rather than stimulate enzyme activity. Recently, a novel human serine protease with homology to a family of bacterial stress-response proteases was identified and cloned from a human osteoblast library (139). The recombinantly expressed protease was found to selectively cleave IGFBP-5. Interestingly, the cDNA for this protease encodes for an IGF binding motif at the amino terminus (140). Although high mRNA expression indicates that this enzyme may account for IGFBP-5 proteolysis in normal human osteoblasts, very low expression in U2 osteosarcoma cells suggests that there is more than one IGFBP-5 protease produced by bone cells. The physiological significance of IGFBP-5 proteolysis in bone is un-

known. However, the truncated form of IGFBP-5 purified from U2 cell-conditioned medium has been shown to potentiate IGF action in bone cells and to possess intrinsic mitogenic activity (100,101).

SUMMARY

The critical importance of IGFs to the skeleton is attested to by the scores of studies demonstrating the following:

- IGFs stimulate osteoblastic cell proliferation and matrix formation *in vitro* and *in vivo*.
- IGFs stimulate formation and activation of osteoclasts.
- IGFs are the most abundant of the growth factors produced by and stored in bone.
- IGF expression and deposition into matrix are regulated by local and systemic effectors of bone metabolism.
- IGFs transduce the osteogenic response to mechanical strain.
- IGFBPs are produced by bone cells and modulate IGF actions on bone; they also may have IGF-independent effects on bone cell physiology.
- IGFBP proteases are produced by bone cells and modify IGFBP structure/function.

The challenge now is to integrate and harness this knowledge.

REFERENCES

1. Canalis E. Insulin-like growth factor, an autocrine regulator of skeletal cells. In: *The insulin-like growth factors and their regulatory proteins.* Amsterdam: Elsevier, 1994:307–313.
2. Mohan S, Baylink DJ. Insulin-like growth factor sys-

tem components and the coupling of bone formation to resorption. *Horm Res* 1996;45[Suppl 1]:59–62.

3. Rosen CJ, Donahue LR. Insulin-like growth factors and bone: the osteoporosis connection revisited. *Proc Soc Exp Biol Med* 1998;219:1–7.

4. Centrella M, McCarthy TL, Canalis E. Receptors for insulin-like growth factors-I and -II in osteoblast-enriched cultures from fetal rat bone. *Endocrinology* 1990;126:39–44.

5. Conover CA, Kiefer MC. Regulation and biological effect of endogenous insulin-like growth factor binding protein-5 in human osteoblastic cells. *J Clin Endocrinol Metab* 1993;76:1153–1159.

6. Raile K, Hoflich A, Kessler U, et al. Human osteosarcoma (U-2 OS) cells express both insulin-like growth factor-I (IGF-I) receptors and insulin-like growth factor-II/mannose-6-phosphate (IGF-II/M6P) receptors and synthesize IGF-II: autocrine growth stimulation by IGF-II via the IGF-I receptor. *J Cell Physiol* 1994;159: 531–541.

7. Hou P, Sato T, Hofstetter W, et al. Identification and characterization of the insulin-like growth factor I receptor in mature rabbit osteoclasts. *J Bone Miner Res* 1997;12:534–540.

8. Nissley P, Lopaczynski W. Insulin-like growth factor receptors. *Growth Factors* 1991;5:29–43.

9. Mohan S, Linkhart T, Rosenfeld R, et al. Characterization of the receptor for insulin-like growth factor II in bone cells. *J Cell Physiol* 1989;140:169–176.

10. Ishibe M, Nojima T, Ishibashi T, et al. Comparison of the type-2 insulin-like growth factor receptor in normal osteoblasts and osteosarcoma-derived osteoblast-like cells. *J Orthop Res* 1995;13:643–648.

11. Martinez DA, Zuscik MJ, Ishibe M, et al. Identification of functional insulin-like growth factor-II/mannose-6-phosphate receptors in isolated bone cells. *J Cell Biochem* 1995;59:246–257.

12. Thomas T, Gori F, Conover CA, et al. Response of bipotential human marrow stromal cells to insulin-like growth factors: effects on binding protein production proliferation, and commitment to osteoblasts and adipocytes, endocrinology 1999;140:5036–5044.

13. Hicok KC, Thomas T, Gori F, et al. Development and characterization of conditionally immortalized osteoblast precursor cell lines from human bone marrow stroma. *J Bone Miner Res* 1998;13:205–217.

14. Grellier P, Feliers D, Yee D, et al. Interaction between insulin-like growth factor-I and insulin-like growth factor-binding proteins in TC-1 stromal cells. *J Endocrinol* 1996;149:519–529.

15. Tanaka H, Quarto R, Williams S, et al. *In vivo* and *in vitro* effects of insulin-like growth factor-I (IGF-I) on femoral mRNA expression in old rats. *Bone* 1994;15: 647–653.

16. Tanaka H, Liang CT. Effect of platelet-derived growth factor on DNA synthesis and gene expression in bone marrow stromal cells derived from adult and old rats. *J Cell Physiol* 1995;164:367–375.

17. Tanaka H, Liang CT. Mitogenic activity but not phenotype expression of rat osteoprogenitor cells in response to IGF-I is impaired in aged rats. *Mech Ageing Dev* 1996;92:1–10.

18. Denis I, Pointillart A, Lieberherr M. Effects of growth hormone and insulin-like growth factor-I on the prolif-

eration and differentiation of cultured pig bone cells and rat calvaria cells. *Growth Regul* 1994;4:123–130.

19. Langdahl BL, Kassem M, Moller MK, et al. The effects of IGF-I and IGF-II on proliferation and differentiation of human osteoblasts and interactions with growth hormone. *Eur J Clin Invest* 1998;28:176–183.

20. Jonsson KB, Ljunghall S, Karlstöm O, et al. Insulin-like growth factor I enhances the formation of type I collagen in hydrocortisone-treated human osteoblasts. *Biosci Rep* 1993;13:297–302.

21. Gangji V, Rydziel S, Gabbitas B, et al. Insulin-like growth factor II promoter expression in cultured rodent osteoblasts and adult rat bone. *Endocrinology* 1998; 139:2287–2292.

22. Canalis E, Rydziel S, Delany AM, et al. Insulin-like growth factors inhibit interstitial collagenase synthesis in bone cell cultures. *Endocrinology* 1995;136:1348–1354.

23. Delany AM, Rydziel S, Canalis E. Autocrine downregulation of collagenase-3 in rat bone cell cultures by insulin-like growth factors. *Endocrinology* 1996;137: 4665–4670.

24. Shinar DM, Endo N, Halperin D, et al. Differential expression of insulin-like growth factor-I (IGF-I) and IGF-II messenger ribonucleic acid in growing rat bone. *Endocrinology* 1993;132:1158–1167.

25. Middleton J, Arnott N, Walsh S, et al. Osteoblasts and osteoclasts in adult human osteophyte tissue express the mRNAs for insulin-like growth factors I and II and the type 1 IGF receptor. *Bone* 1995;16:287–293.

26. Andrew JG, Hoyland J, Freemont AJ, et al. Insulin-like growth factor gene expression in human fracture callus. *Calcif Tissue Int* 1993;53:97–102.

27. Goad DL, Rubin J, Wang H, et al. Enhanced expression of vascular endothelial growth factor in human SaOS-2 osteoblast-like cells and murine osteoblasts induced by insulin-like growth factor I. *Endocrinology* 1996; 137:2262–2268.

28. Palmer G, Bonjour J-P, Caverzasio J. Expression of a newly identified phosphate transporter/retrovirus receptor in human SaOS-2 osteoblast-like cells and its regulation by insulin-like growth factor I. *Endocrinology* 1997;138:5202–5209.

29. Fiorelli G, Formigli L, Orlandini SZ, et al. Characterization and function of the receptor for IGF-I in human preosteoclastic cells. *Bone* 1996;18:269–276.

30. Mochizuki H, Hakeda Y, Wakatsuki N, et al. Insulin-like growth factor-I supports formation and activation of osteoclasts. *Endocrinology* 1992;131:1075–1080.

31. Slootweg MC, Most WW, van Beek E, et al. Osteoclast formation together with interleukin-6 production in mouse long bones is increased by insulin-like growth factor-I. *J Endocrinol* 1992;132:433–438.

32. Kaji H, Sugimoto T, Kanatani M, et al. Insulin-like growth factor-I mediates osteoclast-like cell formation stimulated by parathyroid hormone. *J Cell Physiol* 1997;172:55–62.

33. Formigli L, Fiorelli G, Benvenuti S, et al. Insulin-like growth factor-I stimulates *in vitro* migration of preosteoclasts across bone endothelial cells. *Cell Tissue Res* 1997;288:101–110.

34. Hill PA, Reynolds JJ, Meikle MC. Osteoblasts mediate insulin-like growth factor-I and -II stimulation of osteoclast formation and function. *Endocrinology* 1995; 136:124–131.

35. Lazowski DA, Fraher LJ, Hodsman A, et al. Regional variation of insulin-like growth factor-I gene expression in mature rat bone and cartilage. *Bone* 1994;15: 563–576.

36. Aerssens J, Boonen S, Lowet G, et al. Interspecies differences in bone composition, density, and quality: potential implications for *in vivo* bone research. *Endocrinology* 1998;139:663–670.

37. Birnbaum RS, Bowsher RR, Wiren KM. Changes in IGF-I and -II expression and secretion during the proliferation and differentiation of normal rat osteoblasts. *J Endocrinol* 1995;144:251–259.

38. Bikle DD, Harris J, Halloran BP, et al. Expression of the genes for insulin-like growth factors and their receptors in bone during skeletal growth. *Am J Physiol* 1994;267:E278–E286.

39. Prisell PT, Edwall D, Lindblad JB, et al. Expression of insulin-like growth factors during bone induction in rat. *Calcif Tissue Int* 1993;53:201–205.

40. Canalis E, Centrella M, Burch W, et al. Insulin-like growth factor I mediates selective anabolic effects of parathyroid hormone in bone cultures. *J Clin Invest* 1989;83:60–65.

41. McCarthy TL, Thomas MJ, Centrella M, et al. Regulation of insulin-like growth factor I transcription by cyclic adenosine 3′,5′-monophosphate (cAMP) in fetal rat bone cells through an element with exon 1: protein kinase A–dependent control without a consensus AMP response element. *Endocrinology* 1995;136:3901–3908.

42. Okazaki R, Durham SK, Riggs BL, et al. Transforming growth factor-β and forskolin increase all classes of insulin-like growth factor-I transcripts in normal human osteoblast-like cells. *Biochem Biophys Res Commun* 1995;207:963–970.

43. Watson P, Lazowski D, Han V, et al. Parathyroid hormone restores bone mass and enhances osteoblast insulin-like growth factor I gene expression in ovariectomized rats. *Bone* 1995;16:357–365.

44. Ohlsson C, Vidal O. Effects of growth hormone and insulin-like growth factors on human osteoblasts. *Eur J Clin Invest* 1998;28:184–186.

45. Kanzaki S, Baxter RC, Knutsen R, et al. Evidence that human bone cells in culture secrete insulin-like growth factor (IGF)-II and IGF binding protein-3 but not acid-labile subunit both under basal and regulated conditions. *J Bone Miner Res* 1995;10:854–858.

46. Ernst M, Rodan GA. Estradiol regulation of insulin-like growth factor-I expression in osteoblastic cells: evidence for transcriptional control. *Mol Endocrinol* 1991;5:1081–1089.

47. Kassem M, Okazaki R, Harris SA, et al. Estrogen effects on insulin-like growth factor gene expression in a human osteoblastic cell line with high levels of estrogen receptor. *Calcif Tissue Int* 1998;62:60–66.

48. McCarthy TL, Shu H, Casinghino S, et al. 17β-Estradiol potently suppresses cAMP-induced insulin-like growth factor-I gene activation in primary rat osteoblast cultures. *J Biol Chem* 1997;272:18132–18139.

49. McCarthy TL, Centrella M, Canalis E. Cortisol inhibits the synthesis of insulin-like growth factor-I in skeletal cells. *Endocrinology* 1990;126:1569–1575.

50. Swolin D, Brantsing C, Matejka G, et al. Cortisol decreases IGF-I mRNA levels in human osteoblast-like cells. *J Endocrinol* 1996;149:397–403.

51. Delany AM, Canalis E. Transcriptional repression of insulin-like growth factor I by glucocorticoids in rat bone cells. *Endocrinology* 1995;136:4776–4781.

52. Cheng S-L, Zhang S-F, Mohan S, et al. Regulation of insulin-like growth factors I and II and their binding proteins in human bone marrow stromal cells by dexamethasone. *J Cell Biochem* 1998;71:449–458.

53. Scharla SH, Strong DD, Mohan S, et al. 1,25-Dihydroxyvitamin D_3 differentially regulates the production of insulin-like growth factor I (IGF-I) and IGF-binding protein-4 in mouse osteoblasts. *Endocrinology* 1991; 129:3139–3146.

54. Okazaki R, Conover CA, Harris SA, et al. Normal human osteoblast-like cells consistently express genes for insulin-like growth factors I and II but transformed human osteoblast cell lines do not. *J Bone Miner Res* 1995;10:788–793.

55. Canalis E, Pash J, Gabbitas B, et al. Effects of prostaglandin E_2 on bone formation in cultured fetal rat calvariae: role of insulin-like growth factor-I. *Endocrinology* 1993;133:33–38.

56. Canalis E, Gabbitas B. Bone morphogenetic protein 2 increases insulin-like growth factor I and II transcripts and polypeptide levels in bone cell cultures. *J Bone Miner Res* 1994;9:1999–2005.

57. Yeh L-CC, Adamo ML, Kitten AM, et al. Osteogenic protein-1 mediated insulin-like growth factor gene expression in primary cultures of rat osteoblastic cells. *Endocrinology* 1996;137:1921–1931.

58. Knutsen R, Honda Y, Strong DD, et al. Regulation of insulin-like growth factor system components by osteogenic protein-1 in human bone cells. *Endocrinology* 1995;136:857–865.

59. Franchimont N, Gangji V, Durant D, et al. Interleukin-6 with its soluble receptor enhances the expression of insulin-like growth factor-I in osteoblasts. *Endocrinology* 1997;138:5248–5255.

60. Pash JM, Delany AM, Adamo ML, et al. Regulation of insulin-like growth factor I transcription by prostaglandin E_2 in osteoblast cells. *Endocrinology* 1995; 136:33–38.

61. Rawlinson SCF, Mohan S, Baylink DJ, et al. Exogenous prostacyclin, but not prostaglandin E_2, produces similar response in both G6PD activity and RNA production as mechanical loading, and increases IGF-II release, in adult cancellous bone in culture. *Calcif Tissue Int* 1993;53:324–329.

62. Zaman G, Suswillo RFL, Cheng MZ, et al. Early responses to dynamic strain change and prostaglandins in bone-derived cells in culture. *J Bone Miner Res* 1997;12:769–777.

63. Sugimoto T, Kanatani M, Kano J, et al. IGF-I mediates the stimulatory effect of high calcium concentration on osteoblastic cell proliferation. *Am J Physiol* 1994; 266:E709–E716.

64. Honda Y, Fitzsimmons RJ, Baylink DJ, et al. Effects of extracellular calcium on insulin-like growth factor II in human bone cells. *J Bone Miner Res* 1995;10: 1660–1665.

65. Lean JM, Jagger CJ, Chambers TJ, et al. Increased insulin-like growth factor I mRNA expression in rat osteocytes in response to mechanical stimulation. *Am J Physiol* 1995;268:E318–E327.

66. Lean JM, MacKay AG, Chow JWM, et al. Osteocytic expression of mRNA for c-fos and IGF-I: an immediate

early gene response to an osteogenic stimulus. *Am J Physiol* 1996;270:E937–E945.

67. Mikuni-Takagaki Y, Suzuki Y, Kawase T, et al. Distinct responses of different populations of bone cells to mechanical stress. *Endocrinology* 1996;137:2028–2035.

68. Raab-Cullen DM, Thiede MA, Petersen DN, et al. Mechanical loading stimulates rapid changes in periosteal gene expression. *Calcif Tissue Int* 1994;55:473–478.

69. Fitzsimmons RJ, Strong DD, Mohan S, et al. Low-litude, low-frequency electric field-stimulated bone cell proliferation may in part be mediated by increased IGF-II release. *J Cell Physiol* 1992;150:84–89.

70. Fitzsimmons RJ, Ryaby JT, Mohan S, et al. Combined magnetic fields increase insulin-like growth factor-II in TE-85 human osteosarcoma bone cell cultures. *Endocrinology* 1995;136:3100–3106.

71. Farley JR, Tarbaux N, Murphy LA, et al. *In vitro* evidence that bone formation may be coupled to bone resorption by release of mitogen(s) from resorbing bone. *Metabolism* 1987;36:314–321.

72. Bautista CM, Mohan S, Baylink DJ. Insulin-like growth factors I and II are present in the skeletal tissues of ten vertebrates. *Metabolism* 1990;39:96–100.

73. Mohan S, Linkhart TA, Jennings JC, et al. Identification and quantification of four distinct growth factors stored in human bone matrix. *J Bone Miner Res* 1987; 2:44–47.

74. Seck T, Scheppach B, Scharla S, et al. Concentration of insulin-like growth factor (IGF)-I and -II in iliac crest bone matrix from pre- and postmenopausal women: relationship to age, menopause, bone turnover, bone volume, and circulating IGFs. *J Clin Endocrinol Metab* 1998;83:2331–2337.

75. Nicolas V, Prewett A, Bettica P, et al. Age-related decreases in insulin-like growth factor-I and transforming growth factor-β in femoral cortical bone from both men and women: implications for bone loss with aging. *J Clin Endocrinol Metab* 1994;78:1011–1016.

76. Dequeker J, Mohan S, Finkelman RD, et al. Generalized osteoarthritis associated with increased insulin-like growth factor types I and II and transforming growth factor β in cortical bone from the iliac crest: possible mechanism of increased bone density and protection against osteoporosis. *Arthritis Rheum* 1993;36: 1702–1708.

77. Yeh JK, Aloia JF, Chen M, et al. Effect of growth hormone administration and treadmill exercise on serum and skeletal IGF-I in rats. *Am J Physiol* 1994; 266:E129–E135.

78. Pfeilschifter J, Laukhuf F, Müller-Beckmann B, et al. Parathyroid hormone increases the concentration of insulin-like growth factor-I and transforming growth factor beta 1 in rat bone. *J Clin Invest* 1995;96:767–774.

79. Erdmann J, Storch S, Pfeilschifter J, et al. Effects of estrogen on the concentration of insulin-like growth factor-I in rat bone matrix. *Bone* 1998;22:503–507.

80. Barengolts EI, Kouznetsova T, Segalene A, et al. Effects of progesterone on serum levels of IGF-1 and on femur IGF-1 mRNA in ovariectomized rats. *J Bone Miner Res* 1996;11:1406–1412.

81. Turner RT, Backup P, Sherman PJ, et al. Mechanism of action of estrogen on intramembranous bone formation: regulation of osteoblast differentiation and activity. *Endocrinology* 1992;131:883–889.

82. Slater M, Patava J, Kingham K, et al. Modulation of growth factor incorporation into ECM of human osteoblast-like cells in vitro by 17β-estradiol. *Am J Physiol* 1994;267:E990–E1001.

83. Shimasaki S, Ling N. Identification and molecular characterization of insulin-like growth factor binding proteins (IGFBP-1, -2, -3, -4, -5, and -6). *Prog Growth Factor Res* 1991;3:243–266.

84. Conover CA. Post-translational modification of the IGFBPs in the IGF system. In: Rosenfeld RG, Roberts CT, eds. *The IGF system.* Totowa: Humana Press, 1999.

85. Oh Y, Yamanaka Y, Kim H-S, et al. IGF-independent actions of IGFBPs. In: Takano K, Hizuka N, Takahashi S-I, eds. *Molecular mechanisms to regulate the activities of insulin-like growth factors.* New York: Elsevier, 1998:125–133.

86. Lee PDK, Giudice LC, Conover CA, et al. Insulin-like growth factor binding protein-1: recent findings and new directions. *Proc Soc Exp Biol Med* 1997;216: 319–357.

87. Okazaki R, Riggs BL, Conover CA. Glucocorticoid regulation of insulin-like growth factor-binding protein expression in normal human osteoblast-like cells. *Endocrinology* 1994;134:126–132.

88. Conover CA. Insulin-like growth factor binding proteins and bone: new findings. In: *Proceedings of the 3rd annual DSL International Scientific Meetings, Feldafing, Germany, September 30–October 4,* 1995: 20–21.

89. Feyen JHM, Evans DB, Binkert C, et al. Recombinant human [Cys^{281}] insulin-like growth factor-binding protein 2 inhibits both basal and insulin-like growth factor I-stimulated proliferation and collagen synthesis in fetal rat calvariae. *J Biol Chem* 1991;66:19469–19474.

90. Khosla S, Hassoun AAK, Baker BK, et al. Insulin-like growth factor system abnormalities in hepatitis C-associated osteosclerosis: potential insights into increasing bone mass in adults. *J Clin Invest* 1998;101: 2165–2173.

91. Schmid C, Rutishauser J, Schlapfer I, et al. Intact but not truncated insulin-like growth factor binding protein-3 (IGFBP-3) blocks IGF-I-induced stimulation of osteoblasts: control of IGF signalling to bone cells by IGFBP-3-specific proteolysis? *Biochem Biophys Res Commun* 1991;179:579–585.

92. Ernst M, Rodan GA. Increased activity of insulin-like growth factor (IGF) in osteoblastic cells in the presence of growth hormone (GH): positive correlation with the presence of the GH-induced IGF-binding protein BP-3. *Endocrinology* 1990;127:807–814.

93. Mohan S, Bautista CM, Wergedal J, et al. Isolation of an inhibitory insulin-like growth factor (IGF) binding protein from bone cell-conditioned medium: a potential local regulator of IGF action. *Proc Natl Acad Sci USA* 1989;86:8338–8342.

94. LaTour D, Mohan S, Linkhart TA, et al. Inhibitory insulin-like growth factor-binding protein: cloning, complete sequence, and physiological regulation. *Mol Endocrinol* 1990;4:1806–1814.

95. Kiefer MC, Schmid C, Waldvogel M, et al. Characterization of recombinant human insulin-like growth factor binding proteins 4, 5, and 6 produced in yeast. *J Biol Chem* 1992;18:12692–12699.

96. Kassem M, Okazaki R, DeLeon D, et al. Potential

mechanism of estrogen-mediated decrease in bone formation: estrogen increases production of inhibitory insulin-like growth factor-binding protein-4. *Proc Assoc Am Physicians* 1996;108:156–164.

97. Conover CA. Insulin-like growth factor binding protein proteolysis in bone cell models. *Prog Growth Factor Res* 1995;6:301–309.

98. Bautista CM, Baylink DJ, Mohan S. Isolation of a novel insulin-like growth factor (IGF) binding protein from human bone: a potential candidate for fixing IGF-II in human bone. *Biochem Biophys Res Commun* 1991;176:756–763.

99. Jones JI, Gockerman A, Busby WH Jr, et al. Extracellular matrix contains insulin-like growth factor binding protein-5: potentiation of the effects of IGF-I. *J Cell Biol* 1993;121:679–687.

100. Andress DL, Birnbaum RS. Human osteoblast-derived insulin-like growth factor (IGF) binding protein-5 stimulates osteoblast mitogenesis and potentiates IGF action. *J Biol Chem* 1992;267:22467–22472.

101. Andress DL, Loop SM, Zapf J, et al. Carboxy-truncated insulin-like growth factor binding protein-5 stimulates mitogenesis in osteoblast-like cells. *Biochem Biophys Res Commun* 1993;195:25–30.

102. Mohan S, Nakao Y, Honda Y, et al. Studies on the mechanism by which insulin-like growth factor (IGF) binding protein-4 (IGFBP-4) and IGFBP-5 modulate IGF actions in bone cells. *J Biol Chem* 1995;35:20424–20431.

103. Andress DL. Insulin-like growth factor-binding protein-5 (IGFBP-5) stimulates phosphorylation of the IGFBP-5 receptor. *Am J Physiol* 1998;274:E744–E750.

104. Richman C, Baylink DJ, Lang K, et al. Evidence that recombinant human insulin-like growth factor-5 (rhIGFBP-5) is a potential new therapy to increase bone formation. *J Bone Miner Res* 1998;23[Suppl]:S585 (abst).

105. Chihara K, Sugimoto T. The action of GH/IGF-I/IGFBP in osteoblasts and osteoclasts. *Horm Res* 1997;48[Suppl 5]:45–49.

106. Schmid C, Schlapfer I, Keller A, et al. Effects of insulin-like growth factor (IGF) binding proteins (Bps) -3 and -6 on DNA synthesis of rat osteoblasts: further evidence for a role of auto-paracrine IGF I but not IGF II in stimulating osteoblast growth. *Biochem Biophys Res Commun* 1995;212:242–248.

107. Wang E, Wang J, Chin E, et al. Cellular patterns of insulin-like growth factor system gene expression in murine chondrogenesis and osteogenesis. *Endocrinology* 1995;136:2741–2751.

108. Malpe R, Baylink DJ, Linkhart TA, et al. Insulin-like growth factor (IGF)-I, -II, IGF binding proteins (IGFBP)-3, -4, and -5 levels in the conditioned media of normal human bone cells are skeletal site-dependent. *J Bone Miner Res* 1997;12:423–430.

109. Birnbaum RS, Wiren KM. Changes in insulin-like growth factor-binding protein expression and secretion during the proliferation, differentiation, and mineralization of primary cultures of rat osteoblasts. *Endocrinology* 1994;135:223–230.

110. Grellier P, Yee D, Gonzalez M, et al. Characterization of insulin-like growth factor binding proteins (IGFBP) and regulation of IGFBP-4 in bone marrow stromal cells. *Br J Haematol* 1995;90:249–257.

111. Conover CA, Bale LK, Clarkson JT, et al. Regulation of insulin-like growth factor binding protein-5 messenger ribonucleic acid expression and protein availability in rat osteoblast-like cells. *Endocrinology* 1993;132:2525–2530.

112. Nasu M, Sugimoto T, Chihara K. Stimulatory effects of parathyroid hormone and 1,25-dihydroxyvitamin D$_3$ on insulin-like growth factor-binding protein-5 mRNA expression in osteoblastic UMR-106 cells: the difference between transient and continuous treatments. *FEBS Lett* 1997;409:63–66.

113. Delany AM, Dong Y, Canalis E. Mechanisms of glucocorticoid action in bone cells. *J Cell Biochem* 1994;56:295–302.

114. Chevalley T, Strong DD, Mohan S, et al. Evidence for a role for insulin-like growth factor binding proteins in glucocorticoid inhibition of normal human osteoblast-like cell proliferation. *Eur J Endocrinol* 1996;134:591–601.

115. Gabbitas B, Pash JM, Delany AM, et al. Cortisol inhibits the synthesis of insulin-like growth factor-binding protein-5 in bone cell cultures by transcriptional mechanisms. *J Biol Chem* 1996;271:9033–9038.

116. Gabbitas B, Canalis E. Cortisol enhances the transcription of insulin-like growth factor-binding protein-6 in cultured osteoblasts. *Endocrinology* 1996;137:1687–1692.

117. Conover CA, Lee PDK, Riggs BL, et al. Insulin-like growth factor-binding protein-1 expression in cultured human bone cells: regulation by insulin and glucocorticoid. *Endocrinology* 1996;137:3295–3301.

118. Velez-Yanguas MC, Kalebic T, Maggi M, et al. 1α,25-Dihydroxy-16-ene-23-yne-26,27-hexafluorocholecalciferol (Ro24-5531) modulation of insulin-like growth factor-binding protein-3 and induction of differentiation and growth arrest in a human osteosarcoma cell line. *J Clin Endocrinol Metab* 1996;81:93–99.

119. McCarthy TL, Casinghino S, Centrella M, et al. Complex pattern of insulin-like growth factor binding protein expression in primary rat osteoblast enriched cultures: regulation by prostaglandin E$_2$, growth hormone, and the insulin-like growth factors. *J Cell Physiol* 1994;160:163–175.

120. Canalis E, Gabbitas B. Skeletal growth factors regulate the synthesis of insulin-like growth factor binding protein-5 in bone cell cultures. *J Biol Chem* 1995;270:10771–10776.

121. Gabbitas B, Canalis E. Bone morphogenetic protein-2 inhibits the synthesis of insulin-like growth factor-binding protein-5 in bone cell cultures. *Endocrinology* 1995;136:2397–2403.

122. Hayden JM, Strong DD, Baylink DJ, et al. Osteogenic protein-1 stimulates production of insulin-like growth factor binding protein-3 nuclear transcripts in human osteosarcoma cells. *Endocrinology* 1997;138:4240–4247.

123. Dong Y, Canalis E. Insulin-like growth factor (IGF) I and retinoic acid induce the synthesis of IGF-binding protein 5 in rat osteoblastic cells. *Endocrinology* 1995;136:2000–2006.

124. Zhou Y, Mohan S, Linkhart TA, et al. Retinoic acid regulates insulin-like growth factor-binding protein expression in human osteoblast cells. *Endocrinology* 1996;137:975–983.

125. Hassager C, Fitzpatrick LA, Spencer EM, et al. Basal

and regulated secretion of insulin-like growth factor binding proteins in osteoblast-like cells is cell line specific. *J Clin Endocrinol Metab* 1992;75:228–233.

126. Durham SK, Kiefer MC, Riggs BL, et al. Regulation of insulin-like growth factor binding protein 4 by a specific insulin-like growth factor binding protein 4 proteinase in normal human osteoblast-like cells: implications in bone cell physiology. *J Bone Miner Res* 1994;9:111–117.

127. Kanzaki S, Hilliker S, Baylink DJ, et al. Evidence that human bone cells in culture produce insulin-like growth factor-binding protein-4 and -5 proteases. *Endocrinology* 1994;134:383–392.

128. Franchimont N, Durant D, Canalis E. Interleukin-6 and its soluble receptor regulate the expression of insulin-like growth factor binding protein-5 in osteoblast cultures. *Endocrinology* 1997;138:3380–3356.

129. Nicolas V, Mohan S, Honda Y, et al. An age-related decrease in the concentration of insulin-like growth factor binding protein-5 in human cortical bone. *Calcif Tissue Int* 1995;57:206–212.

130. Conover CA. IGFBP regulation by proteases. In: Takano K, Hizuka N, Takahashi S-I, eds. *Molecular mechanisms to regulate the activities of insulin-like growth factors. Proceedings of the 4th International Symposium on Insulin-Like Growth Factors, Tokyo, Japan, October 21–24, 1997.* Amsterdam: Elsevier, Excerpta Medica International Congress Series, 1998:107–114.

131. Conover CA, DeLeon DD. Acid-activated insulin-like growth factor-binding protein-3 proteolysis in normal and transformed cells: role of cathepsin D. *J Biol Chem* 1994;269:7076–7080.

132. Lalou C, Silve C, Rosato R, et al. Interactions between insulin-like growth factor-I (IGF-I) and the system of plasminogen activators and their inhibitors in the control of IGF-binding protein-3 production and proteolysis in human osteosarcoma cells. *Endocrinology* 1994;135:2318–2326.

133. Thrailkill KM, Quarles LD, Nagase H, et al. Characterization of insulin-like growth factor-binding protein

5-degrading proteases produced throughout murine osteoblast differentiation. *Endocrinology* 1995;136:3527–3533.

134. Conover CA, Durham SK, Zapf J, et al. Cleavage analysis of insulin-like growth factor (IGF)-dependent IGF-binding protein-4 proteolysis and expression of protease-resistant IGF-binding protein-4 mutants. *J Biol Chem* 1995;270:4395–4400.

135. Lawrence JB, Bale LK, Haddad TC, et al. Characterization and partial purification of the insulin-like growth factor (IGF)-dependent IGF binding protein-4 specific protease from human fibroblast conditioned media. *Growth Horm IGF Res* 1999;9:25–34.

136. Durham SK, DeLeon DD, Okazaki R, et al. Regulation of insulin-like growth factor (IGF)-binding protein-4 availability in normal human osteoblast-like cells: role of endogenous IGFs. *J Clin Endocrinol Metab* 1995;80:104–110.

137. Durham SK, Riggs BL, Conover CA. The insulin-like growth factor-binding protein-4 (IGFBP-4)–IGFBP-4 protease system in normal human osteoblast-like cells: regulation by transforming growth factor-β. *J Clin Endocrinol Metab* 1994;79:1752–1758.

138. Durham SK, Riggs BL, Harris SA, et al. Alterations in insulin-like growth factor (IGF)-dependent IGF-binding protein-4 proteolysis in transformed osteoblastic cells. *Endocrinology* 1995;136:1374–1380.

139. Hou J, Conover CA, Smeekens SP. Selective cleavage of insulin-like growth factor binding protein-5 by a novel human stress response pathway serine protease: identification, expression, and functional characterization. *Presented at the 80th annual meeting of the Endocrine Society, June 24–27, 1998. New Orleans, LA.*

140. Zumbrunn J, Trueb B. Primary structure of a putative serine protease specific for IGF-binding proteins. *FEBS Lett* 1996;398:187–192.

141. Gori F, Hofbauer LC, Conover CA, et al. Effects of androgens on the insulin-like growth factor/insulin-like growth factor binding protein system in a novel androgen-responsive human osteoblastic cell line. *Presented at the 80th annual meeting of the Endocrine Society, June 24–27, 1998, New Orleans, LA.*

Skeletal Growth Factors,
edited by Ernesto Canalis.
Lippincott Williams & Wilkins, Philadelphia, © 2000.

8

Clinical Aspects of the Insulin-like Growth Factors

Clifford J. Rosen

*Maine Center for Osteoporosis Research and Education, St. Joseph Hospital,
Bangor, Maine 04401*

It has been more than four decades since Salmon and Daughaday (1) made the seminal observation that the action of growth hormone (GH) on cartilage is mediated through a circulating factor absent in hypophysectomized animals. Over the ensuing years, discoveries concerning the identity of insulin-like growth factors (IGFs), their receptors, various IGF binding proteins (IGFBPs), and a host of tissue-specific IGFBP proteases were made by investigators in several areas of endocrinology (2). The advent of recombinant peptide technology made possible preclinical research and clinical trials of GH as well as IGF-I not only for various GH-deficiency states but also for heart failure, neurological conditions, diabetes mellitus, muscle disorders, various catabolic states, stress syndromes, sarcopenia, and osteoporosis (3). Likewise, improved assay methodology has led to more widespread use of serum IGF-I as an indicator of GH status in both adults and children. More recently, serum IGF-I measurements have been studied in relation to the development and manifestation of chronic disease states.

The advances of the last decade are important for researchers and clinicians. GH replacement is now an approved and widely accepted therapy for GH deficiency (GHD) states. Use of serum IGF-I to monitor responsiveness in this condition is now commonplace. The diagnosis of severe GHD is clinically straightforward, but uncertainty remains regarding interpretation of serum IGF-I levels after midlife, when distin-

guishing between normal age-related decline in IGF-I levels and GHD is more controversial. Whereas therapeutic trials with GH and/or IGF-I have been undertaken in a number of therapeutic venues, there is growing concern about possible adverse effects of these agents with respect to neoplasia, particularly if superphysiological IGF-I serum levels are achieved and maintained over decades. In this chapter, I examine the clinical utility of IGF-I as both a diagnostic and a therapeutic technique in respect to skeletal disorders. Most of the discussion and overview focuses on circulating IGF-I; other chapters in this book cover the skeletal IGF regulatory system, and the clinical aspects of IGF-I center on circulatory levels with their relationship to tissue activity. Throughout this chapter, the conundrum surrounding extrapolation of serum levels to tissue action will be examined. Long-term issues relating to side effects and pathogenesis of specific diseases in relation to circulating IGF-I will be discussed because this is becoming a leading area of study. IGF-II is not examined in depth, in part because there are no clinical investigations using this peptide and because serum IGF-II levels in normal and skeletal disease states remain unexplored.

IGF-I and IGF-II are found in high concentrations in serum; nearly every mammalian cell type can synthesize and export both growth factors. The IGF regulatory system in each organ is tissue-specific, but all share certain components. IGFs circulate in a molar ratio of 2:1 (IGF-

II:IGF-I) (5,6). The IGF-I gene is expressed in many tissues, but liver is the primary source of circulating IGF-I (7). In extracellular tissues, IGF-I is bound to a family of IGFBPs. More than 75% of circulating IGF-I is carried in a trimeric complex composed of IGFBP-3, the largest-molecular-weight IGFBP, and a liver-derived glycoprotein known as the acid-labile subunit (ALS) (8). ALS is a member of a leucine-rich repeat family of proteins that is important for binding to the carboxy-terminal domain of IGFBP-3 (8). All three components of the trimeric complex are induced by GH and, therefore, are affected by states of GH deficiency or excess (9). Recently, it has been reported that IGFBP-5 can form ternary circulating complexes with ALS and IGF-I (10).

The other IGFBPs are considerably smaller than IGFBP-3 and can traverse the capillary membrane. In serum, IGFBPs provide binding capacity for IGFs in excess of their usual serum concentrations. This extends their half-life and forms a circulating reservoir. A very small proportion of serum IGF-I is unbound in healthy individuals, although the physiological role of ''free'' IGF-I has not been defined. The binding proteins share about 50% sequence homology and contain highly conserved cysteine residues (11). In serum, their concentrations range from 100 to 5,000 ng/ml, and except for IGFBP 3, which has the highest circulating concentration, IGFBPs are relatively unsaturated. Recently, a family of IGF-specific, low-affinity IGFBP-related proteins has been identified (IGFBPrP-1–4) (11). Their precise physiological role has not been defined, although they possess the capacity to act on target cells independently of IGFs.

Although both IGFs are mitogens, IGF-II is more active during *prenatal* life than IGF-I; IGF-I is the principal regulator of *postnatal* linear growth. Changes in serum IGF-I with puberty are associated with linear growth, although the predictive value of IGF-I in terms of final height is not as strong as might be predicted. The effects of circulating IGF-I on peak bone mass, cross-sectional area of the femur, and mineral content are currently under intense investigation. Much less is known about IGF-II in relation to bone mass, despite its relative abundance in the circulation and skeleton. IGFs enhance bone functions, and each can be regulated by hormones and cytokines.

A unique component of the IGF regulatory system is comprised of the IGFBP-specific proteases, which cleave intact IGFBPs, thereby altering binding of the IGFs to IGFBPs (12–19). These proteases, some of which act only on certain tissues and others of which may function within the circulation or extracellular space, are under the control of autocrine, paracrine, and hormonal influences. In particular, IGFBP tissue-specific proteases can act as comitogens by cleaving intact binding proteins into lower-molecular-weight fragments that bind the IGFs less avidly (13). In addition, IGFBP fragments may act as agonists and enhance IGF bioactivity (14). Some of these proteases act on extracellular components, thereby permitting cells to penetrate organic matrices (15). One of the more familiar IGFBP-specific proteases which circulate and arise from the prostate is prostate-specific antigen (PSA), which cleaves IGFBP-3, is upregulated by testosterone, and is likely to be critical in skeletal and distant neoplastic metastases. The activities of the IGFBP-specific proteases add another layer of complexity to the circulating IGF regulatory system.

DETERMINANTS OF SERUM INSULIN-LIKE GROWTH FACTOR-I CONCENTRATIONS

Growth

There is a dynamic equilibrium between circulating levels of IGF-I and tissue production of this peptide. However, caution must be exercised when interpreting changes in serum IGF-I as alterations in local tissue production. Table 8.1 lists the factors which can control serum levels of IGF-I, but specific regulatory factors may diverge, affecting hepatic synthesis, versus those factors controlling extrahepatic tissue production, including bone. Since its discovery as a sulfation factor more than 40 years ago, IGF-I

TABLE 8.1. *Factors which affect circulating insulin-like growth factor-I (IGF-I) concentrations*

Major direct determinants of circulating IGF-I levels
GH
Protein–calorie intake
Catabolic stressors
  Illnesses
  Sepsis
  Trauma
  Anorexia/bulimia nervosa
Thyroxine
Insulin
Binding affinity of the acid-labile subunit for IGFBP-3/IGF-I

Indirect determinants operating through the GH/IGF-I axis
Aging
Body fat (leptin?)
Estrogens
Androgens
Adrenal androgens (e.g., DHEA)?
Inflammatory cytokines?
Exercise

Other determinants which could directly affect circulating IGF-I
Zinc
PTH
PTH-related peptide
Estrogens
Androgens
Adrenal androgens
Platelet-derived growth factor
Inflammatory cytokines

DHEA, dehydroepiandrosterone; GH, growth hormone; IGFBP-3, IGF binding protein 3; PTH, parathyroid hormone.

has been considered a mediator of GH activity in bone (1). In the skeleton, GH stimulates osteoblast and chondrocyte production of IGF-I, IGFBP-3, and possibly IGFBP-4 (16–18). Serum levels of IGF-I reflect GH secretion to a certain degree and therefore have been used clinically as a surrogate indicator of GH status. Indeed, low serum IGF-I is found in GH deficiency states of children and adults, whereas high levels of IGF-I are found in acromegaly (19). The interpretation of serum IGF-I levels that fall within the normal range and their relation to disease states is the subject of much controversy. In terms of GHD, serum levels likely reflect skeletal content and activity. In rats and mice, alterations in serum IGF-I also reflect cortical bone content of IGF-I and *in vitro* synthesis of IGF-I by bone cells (20).

Nutrition

Although GH represents the principal regulator of circulating IGF-I, other determinants affect IGF-I concentrations. The nutrient status of an individual can profoundly affect serum IGF-I (21). For example, protein–calorie malnutrition severely limits IGF-I synthesis in the liver and leads to a 50% reduction in circulating concentrations even among healthy volunteers (22). Starvation also is associated with reduced bone formation and increased bone resorption. These changes are due to declining skeletal IGF-I concentrations as well as alterations in postreceptor GH action, a decreased number of GH receptors, and alterations in IGFBPs (22). Yet these effects occur despite a marked increase in GH production. Thus, in protein–calorie malnutrition, there is peripheral resistance to GH, leading to dissociation between GH and IGF-I concentrations. The bioactivity of IGF-I is also markedly reduced by malnutrition (22). In part, this may be related to a marked increase in IGFBP-1. Both nutrient intake and insulin status determine serum IGFBP-1 concentrations and the extent of phosphorylation of IGFBP-1, which in turn determines IGF binding affinity (23). With starvation, IGFBP-1 increases and binds IGF-I more avidly. This occurs because of a decline in substrate availability and suppressed insulin levels. Since IGFBP-1 is also synthesized by osteoblasts, it is conceivable that this IGFBP contributes to the marked impairment in bone formation noted with starvation. Similarly, during chronic insulin deficiency, serum IGFBP-1 concentrations are increased, potentially leading to growth retardation in poorly controlled type I, insulin-dependent, diabetes mellitus (IDDM) (24). Moreover, osteopenia and reduced bone formation have been noted in IDDM, and this might be a function of high skeletal production of IGFBP-1.

Another inhibitory IGFBP which is increased in some chronic diseases and could have an impact on bone formation is IGFBP-4. This binding protein is principally regulated by parathyroid hormone (PTH) (25). However, in one study, the highest levels of IGFBP-4 were found in elderly persons who sustained a hip fracture and had undergone significant weight loss prior to their injury (26). This implies that there may be other regulatory factors associated with poor nutrition (e.g., cytokines) which could trigger local production of inhibitory IGFBPs. A marked change in the bioactivity of IGF-I due to IGFBP perturbations may be responsible for growth retardation in malnourished children. In addition to IGFBP changes, there is evidence that zinc deficiency, a common accompaniment of protein–calorie malnutrition, results in a decline in IGF-I synthesis in liver and bone. In experimental animals, zinc repletion leads to increased hepatic IGF-I expression, although longitudinal studies in humans have not shown a rise in serum IGF-I following zinc supplementation alone (22).

Aging

Advanced age is associated with a progressive decrease in serum IGF-I concentrations, as GH secretion declines approximately 14% per decade of life (27–28). Thus, over a lifetime, GH production is reduced substantially. This decrement is due to increased somatostatinergic tone and a generalized reduction in the pulses of GH-releasing hormone and GH-releasing peptides (29). Declining sex steroid production may also have a negative impact on the GH–IGF-I axis (30). One cause for age-associated decline in serum IGF-I is reduced sex steroid production. Alterations in body composition and, specifically, increases in visceral body fat can negatively affect the hypothalamic GH–GHRH axis, possibly acting via leptin (31). The altered GH secretion in the elderly results in low serum concentrations of IGF-I and IGFBP-3.

Aging affects circulating IGFBPs in both men and women. The inhibitory IGFBP-4 increases dramatically with advancing age in both men and women (32), and serum IGFBP-1 concentrations are higher in the elderly than in younger people (33). On the other hand, IGFBP-3 and IGFBP-5 are lower in older individuals (34).

These changes in stimulatory and inhibitory IGFBPs are consistent with *in vitro* evidence that senescent cells have impaired cellular responsiveness to the IGFs, and osteoblasts from older patients are resistant to IGF-I stimulation (35). Although age-associated changes in IGFs could lead to osteoporosis, there is still much debate about the role IGFs and IGFBPs play in determining overall bone mineral density (BMD) and fracture risk.

Sex Steroids

One consistent finding in serum IGF-I concentrations, whether they are measured during puberty or advanced age, is a gender difference. Men exhibit 10% to 15% higher serum IGF-I concentrations than women across all ages following puberty (36). The cause for this difference is not clear, but several attempts have been made to link high or low serum levels of IGF-I to the pathogenesis of chronic diseases including osteoporosis, breast cancer, prostate cancer, and Alzheimer's disease. The picture is complex, in part because both estrogen and testosterone can affect pituitary GH release as well as tissue IGF-I expression. There is strong evidence that total and free testosterone concentrations in serum correlate with GH secretory bursts in pubertal boys (37). Furthermore, administration of testosterone to young hypogonadal men and boys with isolated gonadotropin-releasing hormone (GnRH) deficiency increases serum levels of IGF-I (38). However, the precise mechanism and site of action of androgens are not defined, in part because androgens are converted to estrogens via aromatization, resulting in delays in GH secretion. This mechanism may be extremely important regarding the aging skeleton, since new cross-sectional and longitudinal data demonstrate that total estradiol levels are a better predictor of BMD in the elderly man than serum testosterone (39). Furthermore, osteoblasts possess the capacity to aromatize androgens to estrogens, thereby providing a local site for steroid regulation (40). Case reports of men with osteoporosis and deficient aromatase activity indicate that exogenous estrogens, not androgens, partially restore bone mass (41,42).

Several lines of evidence suggest that there may be a causal relationship between endogenous estrogens and serum IGF-I. First, cross-sectional studies have demonstrated that serum estradiol levels correlate with IGF-I in both men and women (43). Second, both cross-sectional and longitudinal studies have demonstrated that serum IGF-I declines during the early menopausal years (44,45). Third, preliminary studies suggest that low serum IGF-I levels in elderly women correlate more closely to years since menopause than to chronological age (46). Finally, percutaneous, but not oral, estrogen administration to postmenopausal women results in an increase in serum IGF-I concentrations (47).

Adrenal androgens may also affect circulating IGF-I. For example, dehydroepiandrosterone sulfate (DHEA-S) levels decline with age, and their absolute concentrations in postmenopausal women correlate with serum IGF-I (48). Similarly in premenopausal women with adrenal androgen excess and insulin resistance, serum IGF-I concentrations are relatively high, and in a randomized placebo-controlled trial of DHEA, serum IGF-I levels rose in both elderly men and women (48–49). There is some preliminary evidence that, in a subset of adolescent women with eating disorders, DHEA-S increases serum IGF-I (Leboff, personal communication; 50). These studies support the thesis that weak adrenal androgens have a positive impact on serum and, possibly, skeletal IGF-I. There are no data on adrenal androgen action on IGFBPs. However, appropriate trials can determine whether these compounds prevent bone resorption, stimulate bone formation, or affect both phases of bone remodeling.

Gonadal steroids regulate IGFBPs. Estrogen and progesterone stimulate the production of IGFBP-4, while estrogen inhibits osteoblastic IGFBP-3 synthesis (51,52). On the other hand, testosterone stimulates IGFBP-3 synthesis and activates a critical IGFBP-3 protease, PSA (62).

Genetic Control

There is tremendous heterogeneity in serum IGF-I concentrations among healthy adults. Nor-

mal levels can range from 100 to 300 ng/ml, and although GH remains the major regulatory factor controlling serum levels, it is clear that there are other determinants (54). Indeed, it is likely that the IGF-I phenotype is a continuous variable representing a complex polygenic trait. Hence, there should be some element of heritability for IGF-I expression, which may or may not be controlled at the pituitary level. Several lines of evidence have emerged which support that tenet:

1. Twin and general population studies have demonstrated that serum IGF-I is a heritable phenotype (55,56).
2. Serum IGF-I levels differed by nearly 30% among healthy inbred strains of mice of the same body weight and length and similar GH levels (20).
3. A polymorphic microsatellite within the IGF-I gene is associated with differences in serum IGF-I levels in several cohorts even after correction for age and sex (57).

These lines of evidence suggest that there are strong heritable determinants of the IGF-I phenotype and that these unknown factors may be critical in defining adult levels of IGF-I independent of growth hormone. Apart from polymorphic variations in the IGF-I gene itself, there are a number of candidate genes that might be subject to subtle polymorphic variation between individuals (with respect to function or level of expression) and could influence IGF-I serum concentrations. These include genes encoding somatostatin, GH-releasing hormone, GH, and their receptors.

Other Regulatory Factors

In addition to factors previously described, adequate insulin is a prerequisite for IGF-I expression in the liver (58–60). Thyroxine was recently shown to upregulate IGF-I expression in rat femorae, and this may explain the stimulatory effect of thyroid hormone on bone turnover (59). PTH is a major stimulator of skeletal IGF-I expression (61,62), and IGF-I mediates collagen biosynthesis and other anabolic properties induced by PTH (63). Studies of the IGF-I gene in rat osteoblast have demonstrated that there is a cyclic adenosine monophosphate (cAMP) response region in the exon 1 promoter, which may be the site of PTH regulation of IGF-I expression (64). Interestingly, there is an estrogen response element in that region which is responsible for downregulating IGF-I expression (65). Whether there is a gender difference in skeletal PTH responsiveness remains to be determined, although several preliminary studies suggest that male inbred strains of mice as well as male GH-deficient mice have a more vigorous bone density response to PTH than female mice (LR Donahue, personal communication, 1999). In humans, there are no gender studies with PTH to determine if this effect also occurs, although the most vigorous skeletal response to PTH has been reported in men (66).

INSULIN-LIKE GROWTH FACTOR-I IN SKELETAL DISEASE

Relationship to Bone Mass

Serum concentrations of IGF-I peak during puberty at about the same time as acquisition of peak bone mass; serum IGF-I declines with aging, with a slope similar to age-related bone loss (67,68). Hence, it is not surprising that the role of circulating IGF-I in bone cell metabolism and bone turnover has been the subject of tremendous research interest. Intuitively, it appears that alterations in circulating IGF-I could play a role in modulating bone remodeling and thereby affect bone mass and fracture risk. For example, GHD individuals with low serum IGF-I and IGFBP-3 concentrations have reduced BMD and a significantly greater risk of osteoporotic fractures (69). In adults with acquired GHD, serum IGF-I as well as IGFBP-3 correlate closely with femoral and spine BMD. However, attempts to correlate BMD with serum IGF-I in older individuals have produced conflicting results, thereby making a true ''cause-and-effect'' relationship more difficult to establish. In part, this may relate to tissue-specific expression of IGF-I, and factors determining its regulation in the liver may differ from factors regulating IGF-I in the skeleton. It also may be related to the multiple factors regulating serum IGF-I, GH, nutri-

tional status, physical activity, and insulin production.

Two recent studies in large cohorts of men and women have suggested a more powerful relationship between IGF-I and bone. Langlois and colleagues (70) measured serum IGF-I and BMD in 425 women and 257 men, aged 72 to 94 years, from the Framingham Heart Study. The investigators corrected for several confounding variables, including weight, height, protein intake, smoking, mobility, weight change, and body mass index. Serum IGF-I was positively associated with BMD at all sites of the hip, radius, and lumbar spine in women after adjustment for all factors. A threshold effect of higher BMD was evident at each of three femoral sites and the spine for women in the highest quintile of serum IGF-I (i.e., serum levels > 180 ng/ml) versus those in the lower four quintiles. These data suggest that IGF-I levels are associated with BMD in older women.

Recently, Bauer and colleagues (71) reported on the relationship of IGF-I and IGFBP-3 concentrations to hip fractures in 9,704 women from the Study of Osteoporotic Fractures (SOF). In this prospective study, serum was measured for IGF components in 148 women who subsequently sustained hip fractures after 4 years of follow-up and 349 women selected randomly from the cohort. Women in the lowest quartile of IGF-I concentrations (<80 ng/ml) had a 60% greater risk of hip fracture and incidence of vertebral fracture than did other women. Moreover, adjustment for calcaneal BMD did not change those associations and IGFBP-3 was not associated with a greater risk of fractures. This is the first prospective study to identify IGF-I as a potential risk factor for fracture in older individuals, but the finding is not totally surprising since IGF-I levels fall with protein–calorie undernutrition and catabolic states, and older women with recent or past weight loss are at higher risk for hip fractures (72). Hence, it is unclear if this risk factor has pathogenic implications. Indeed, low IGF-I levels can be induced in mice or humans simply by reducing protein intake. Whether this is sufficient to cause suppression in bone turnover and bone loss remains to be defined.

Studies of individuals who have osteoporosis

at a young age also point toward a pathogenic role for IGF-I in the development of low bone mass. Idiopathic osteoporosis in men is a condition characterized by low serum IGF-I levels, a family history of osteoporosis, low bone turnover with decreased bone formation, hypercalciuria in some patients, and very low bone mass with fractures before the age of 60 (73,74). In a cohort of male subjects with idiopathic osteoporosis, Kurland and colleagues (83) noted that serum IGF-I levels correlate with lumbar BMD and that men with this condition have levels of circulating IGF-I almost 1 standard deviation below age-matched controls despite normal GH dynamics. Recently, it was noted that the same men with idiopathic osteoporosis have a higher frequency of a recessive polymorphism in the IGF-I gene which, independent of GH, accounts for nearly 20% lower serum IGF-I concentrations than in men or women without that specific genotype (57). These data suggest that serum IGF-I levels may reflect skeletal activity, especially bone formation, and that this correlation may be independent of GH secretion.

Peak Bone Mass Acquisition

Adult bone mass is determined by the rate of bone acquisition and the rate of bone loss. Most of the variance in BMD at any site in adults and elders is determined by the peak bone mass. In an effort to define the relationship between IGF-I and peak bone acquisition, Rosen and colleagues (20,76) have been studying inbred strains of mice whose BMD is almost exclusively (>80%) determined by genetic determinants of acquisition. This group reported that serum IGF-I levels in various inbred strains of mice are closely linked to BMD; that is, the highest bone density strains have the highest serum IGF-I levels. In addition, serum IGF-I could be related to skeletal content of IGF-I as well as *in vitro* production of IGF-I from cortical and trabecular osteoblasts. Moreover, serum IGF-I cosegregates with the femoral BMD phenotype and accounts for more than 20% of the variance in bone mass in mice obtained from intercrosses between two strains with widely divergent bone densities (20,76). These data suggest that serum

IGF-I levels, at least partially, reflect skeletal content and may be important in peak bone acquisition.

Further support for this hypothesis comes from preliminary studies in rats. Weaver and colleagues (C. Weaver, personal communication, 1999) have detected peak bone mass determined by dual-energy x-ray absorptiometry (DEXA) and quantitative computerized tomography (QCT) in Sprague-Dawley rats at approximately 9 to 11 weeks of age. Coincidentally, peak serum IGF-I levels occur between 5 and 8 weeks of age. Furthermore, a strong correlation between cross-sectional area of the femur and serum IGF-I was noted, suggesting that IGF-I plays an important role in determining final size of the adult bone. This may have major implications in humans in terms of fracture risk since it is a widely held tenet that larger bones fracture less.

Experimental studies in adolescents are less developed, but recent work by Gilsanz and colleagues (V. Gilsanz, personal communication, 1999) sheds some light on the relationship between serum IGF-I and BMD. This group has previously shown that volumetric BMD may be a better determinant of true bone mass than two-dimensional studies by DEXA. In two separate studies, they examined adolescent boys and girls using QCT measurements of the femur and vertebrae, as well as serum IGF-I. In the first study, 197 normal-health white children (aged 8 to 18 years) were evaluated in a cross-sectional manner. Serum IGF-I correlated significantly with both mid-shaft cross-sectional area of the femur and cortical bone area ($r = 0.50$, $p < 0.0001$) but did not correlate with the material density of bone. Serum IGF-I remained a significant contributor to femoral cross-sectional area even after correction for age, gender, weight, and femoral length. In a second study, black and white adolescent boys and girls were studied longitudinally over 2 years from Tanner II to Tanner V. There were 41 black and 44 white boys and girls in the cohort who completed the study. Serum IGF-I was measured by radioimmunoassay (RIA), and the same IGF-I polymorphism reported by Rosen et al. (27) was examined. Serum IGF-I levels were significantly higher in blacks than whites (526 $\pm$ 44 ng/ml versus 476 $\pm$ 36 ng/ml, $p < 0.01$), as was the femoral cross-sectional area (FCSA) as measured by QCT (5.20 $\pm$ 0.43 versus 4.96 $\pm$ 0.19 cm^2, $p = 0.01$). IGF-I levels correlated with FCSA in both boys and girls ($r = 0.31, p = 0.03$ in girls; $r = 0.16, p = 0.05$ in boys). The frequency of the IGF-I 192/192 genotype was 0.31 for all children, and it did not differ by gender or race; this frequency was identical to the previous reports by Rosen et al. However, for those boys and girls with the 192/192 genotype, serum levels of IGF-I were 13% lower than in boys or girls with any other genotype (547 $\pm$ 30 ng/ml versus 618 $\pm$ 34 ng/ml, $p = 0.05$). Of note in this study was the finding that the IGF-I genotype (192/192) was not associated with differences in final height or BMD of the spine or hip but was associated with a 5.5% lower FCSA than those with any other genotype.

In sum, these preliminary studies suggest the following:

1. Serum IGF-I can be related to bone mass acquisition in humans and other species.
2. Differences in IGF-I among individuals may be related to heritable factors.
3. Effects of IGF-I on bone mass may be timed to coincide with the acceleration of pubertal growth and maximum calcium accretion.
4. IGF-I may act directly on bone to increase cross-sectional area, thereby enhancing bone mass and strength in humans and other species.

Clearly, additional studies are needed with a shift in focus toward bone acquisition rather than bone loss.

Treatment of Osteoporosis

Most studies have shown that subcutaneous administration of recombinant human (rh) GH or rhIGF-I to various animals can enhance linear growth, stimulate new bone formation, and increase bone turnover (77,78). Some of the most compelling evidence to date about the use of GH in low bone mass states comes from studies of adult GHD patients. In several trials, rhGH replacement therapy increases BMD in the spine approximately 3% to 4% over a 2-year period (79). The effect is greater in men than women,

irrespective of hormonal replacement, but long-term studies have not been completed to assess its efficacy on fracture prevention. Hence, it is difficult to determine whether marked increases in bone mass persist and whether these changes result in stronger bones.

More disappointing are studies using rhGH in osteoporotic elderly individuals. Although early work by Rudman and colleagues (80) suggested a marked increase in BMD after short-term rhGH, this promise has not materialized. Indeed, several studies of osteoporotic patients receiving rhGH have shown that the increase in BMD during treatment is relatively similar in magnitude to that obtained with conventional antiresorptive therapy (81–84). For the most part, this can be traced to rather marked increases in bone resorption which accompany changes in bone formation. However, even employing the combination of GH and an antiresorptive agent such as calcitonin, little additional benefit on bone mass beyond that of an antiresorptive alone is noted.

Human trials with rhIGF-I to prevent bone loss or enhance bone formation have only recently been undertaken; these will be discussed only briefly here and are discussed in greater detail in Chapter 32. Ebeling et al. (85) treated postmenopausal women with varying doses of subcutaneous rhIGF-I for 6 days. All patients showed a dose-dependent increase in markers of bone formation and bone resorption; a similar effect was demonstrated in 24 men with idiopathic osteoporosis treated for 6 weeks and in elderly women treated for 4 weeks (84,86). The maximum rise in bone formation occurred after 3 weeks, and IGF-I at low doses did not change parameters of bone resorption.

In these trials, hypoglycemia was not a consistent complication; however, to circumvent the hazard of hypoglycemia and to capitalize on the possibility that delivery of IGF-I complexed to IGFBP-3 could enhance the effects of IGF-I alone, several studies have used combination therapy. In ovariectomized rats, IGF-I and IGFBP-3 were more effective on bone formation than IGF-I alone, and higher doses of IGF-I were deliverable without significant hypoglycemia (87). Early phase I trials employing IGF-I/IGFBP-3 complex in young and elderly volunteers have been promising and have shown that hypoglycemia does not occur even though the serum concentrations of IGF-I achieved can be quite high (approaching 1,000 ng/ml) (D. Rosen, personal communication 1998). In addition, short-term increases in markers of bone formation and bone resorption were noted. In a small, phase II, placebo-controlled clinical trial, the IGF-I/IGFBP-3 complex was administered to patients who had sustained hip fractures. After 3 months, grip strength and BMD in the contralateral hip were greater in those women who received complex versus those who received placebo. Larger studies are needed, however, before the usefulness of this compound can be fully realized.

There is cause for cautious optimism for the use of rhIGF-I to augment bone mass in older individuals and patients with specific metabolic disorders. However, in contrast to trials with rhGH, there have been no long-term placebo-controlled trials with rhIGF-I in which BMD is a primary outcome. Determination of fracture prevention efficacy will have to await longer studies. Finally, there are no data on long-term safety of the IGFs in respect to cellular processes such as apoptosis or neoplastic transformation. However, an alternative to long-term rhIGF-I might be short-term therapy for specific catabolic states. rhGH and certain GH-releasing peptides are already undergoing trials in Europe to reduce the catabolic stress of burns, major surgery, and hip fractures. It is not inconceivable that rhIGF-I may actually prove to be efficacious and safe.

INSULIN-LIKE GROWTH FACTOR-I AND NEOPLASMS

Acromegalics are at increased risk for colonic neoplasms. Interest in the association between serum IGF-I concentrations and cancer risk has increased with reports that individuals with higher IGF-I levels (or lower IGFBP-3 levels) within the broad normal range between acromegaly and GHD have increased risk of prostate, colon, and breast cancers (88–92). Chan et al. (98) demonstrated that, among a nested cohort of men in the Physician's Health Study, the

highest quartile of plasma IGF-I levels was associated with a 4.3-fold relative risk of prostate cancer compared to the lowest quartile (88). This association was independent of baseline PSA concentrations and suggested that IGF-I might be an independent predictor of prostate cancer risk. The major findings of this study were subsequently confirmed by Wolk et al. (91). In a separate study of similar design utilizing women in the Nurses Health Study, Hankinson et al. (99) noted that among premenopausal women less than age 50 years there was a 4.5-fold relative risk of breast cancer in the highest quartile of plasma IGF-I compared to the lowest quartile. Adjustment for IGFBP-3 increased the predictive value of IGF-I in two of these studies (88,89). Indeed, IGFBP-3 was shown to be inversely related to risk, whereas IGF-I was positively related to risk. This relationship was particularly strong in a study concerning predictive value of IGF-I and IGFBP-3 with respect to colon cancer (91).

The inverse relationship of IGF-I to IGFBP-3 with respect to risk of neoplasia deserves comment. Normally, both IGFBP-3 and IGF-I are regulated by GH and, therefore, these two peptides exhibit a strong and direct correlation in the serum. Conceivably, certain individuals may have polymorphic variations in the promoter regions of the genes encoding IGF-I or IGFBP-3 that lead to lack of coordinated expression of IGF-I and IGFBP-3, and such variants might be linked to high IGF-I: IGFBP-3 ratios, increased cellular proliferation, and hence increased accumulation of somatic cell mutations and cancer risk. Acromegalics may have subtle, rather than extreme, increased cancer risk because in this condition both IGF-I and IGFBP-3 are elevated and changes in the IGF-I: IGFBP-3 ratio are subtle (92).

Other studies, some of which have utilized antineoplastic drugs, have provided further indirect evidence that the IGF regulatory system is involved in the pathobiology of neoplasia, in terms of both risk of cancer and behavior of cancers. Only a few of many examples are listed here. With respect to risk, it is highly relevant that a positive correlation between GH level (or IGF-I level) and breast epithelial cell proliferation was seen in an aged rhesus monkey model (93). With respect to neoplastic behavior, tumor growth in IGF-I–deficient mice has been shown to be reduced relative to control mice (104). Furthermore, it has recently been shown that fenretinide, a synthetic retinoid with antitumor activity, reduced plasma IGF-I levels and increased IGFBP-3 concentrations, especially among premenopausal women (95). Also, tamoxifen has been shown to decrease IGF-I serum concentrations and to downregulate IGF-I induction of tyrosine phosphorylation of the IGF-I receptor and inhibit signaling in MCF-7 cells (96). Dunn et al. (107), utilizing a p53-deficient mouse model, demonstrated that, as expected, dietary restriction lowered serum IGF-I and that this was associated with increased apoptosis and decreased tumor progression (97). Furthermore, IGF-I administration to these diet-restricted mice increased cell proliferation and blocked the inhibitory effect of dietary restriction to tumor growth. Taken together, these and other experimental data suggest that the IGF-I system must be involved in tumor development and progression. However, there are many unanswered questions. For example, it has not been established that the relationship between IGF-I levels and cancer risk is causal. More work is also needed to reconcile some of the observations (98).

CONCLUSIONS

IGF-I is a potent stimulator of bone formation. Circulating levels of this peptide are relatively high but are not necessarily biologically active due to the presence of IGFBPs in serum. Changes in skeletal and circulating IGF-I concentrations are similar in several model systems, suggesting that serum IGF-I correlates with bone mass and may provide an indirect indicator of skeletal status. Early results correlating IGF-I with bone mass have been conflicting, although recent studies focusing on peak bone mass acquisition are illuminating. Use of rhGH or rhIGF-I to treat individuals with low bone mass or osteoporosis is still in its infancy. Many questions need to be addressed about this therapeutic approach and its ultimate cost–benefit ratios.

REFERENCES

1. Salmon WD, Duaghaday WH. A hormonally controlled serum factor which stimulates sulphate incorporation by cartilage in vitro. J Lab Clin Med 1957;49:825–836.
2. Jones JI, Clemmons DR. Insulin-like growth factors and their binding proteins: biological actions. Endocr Rev 1995;1:3–34.
3. Rudman D, Feller AG, Nelgrag HS. Effect of human GH in men over age 60. N Engl J Med 1990;323:52–60.
4. Zapf J, Schmid C, Froesche ER. Biological and immunological properties of IGF-I and IGF-II. J Clin Endocrinol Metab 1984;13:7–12.
5. Zapf J, Froesch ER. IGFs/somatomedins: structure, secretion, biological actions and physiological roles. Horm Res 1986;24:121–130.
6. Mohan S, Baylink DJ. Autocrine and paracrine aspects of bone metabolism. Growth Gen Horm 1990;6:1–9.
7. Rajaram S, Baylink DJ, Mohan S. IGFBPs in serum and other biological fluids. Endocr Rev 1997;18:801–831.
8. Blum WF, Alberttson K, Roseberg S, et al. Serum levels of IGF-I and IGFBP-3 reflect spontaneous GH secretion. J Clin Endocrinol Metab 1993;76:1610–1630.
9. Twigg SM, Baxter RC. IGF binding protein 5 forms an alternative ternary complex with IGFs and the acid-labile subunit. J Biol Chem 1998;273:6074–6079.
10. Binoux M. IGF-binding protein-3 and acid-labile subunit: what is the pecking order? Eur J Endocrinol 1997; 137:605–609.
11. Oh Y. IGFBPs and neoplastic models: new concepts for roles of IGFBPs in regulation of cancer cell growth. Endocrine 1997;7:115–117.
12. Campbell PG, Novak TF, Yanoscik TB, et al. Involvement of the plasmin system in dissociation of IGFBP complex. Endocrinology 1992;130:1401–1402.
13. Kanzaki S, Hilliker S, Baylink DJ, et al. Evidence that human bone cells in culture produce IGFBP-4 and IGFBP-5 proteases. Endocrinology 1994;134:383–392.
14. Fowlkes J, Enghild J, Suzuki K, et al. Matrix metalloproteinases degrade IGFBP-3 in dermal fibroblast cultures. J Biol Chem 1994;269:25742–25746.
15. Thraillkill K, Quarles LD, Nagase H, et al. Characterization of IGFBP-5 degrading proteases produced throughout murine osteoblast differentiation. Endocrinology 1995;136:3527–3533.
16. Canalis E, McCarthy TL, Centrella M. Growth factors and bone remodeling. J Clin Invest 1988;81:277–281.
17. Mohan S. IGF binding proteins in bone cell regulation. Growth Regul 1993;3:65–68.
18. Mohan S, Baylink DJ. Serum IGFBP-4 and IGFBP-5 in aging and age-associated diseases. Endocrine 1997; 7:87–91.
19. Chan K, Spencer EM. General aspects of the IGFBPs. Endocrine 1997;7:95–97.
20. Rosen CJ, Dimai HP, Vereault D, et al. Circulating and skeletal insulin-like growth factor-1 (IGF-I) concentrations in two inbred strains of mice with different bone mineral densities. Bone 1997;21:217–223.
21. Rosen CJ, Conover C. Growth insulin like growth factor-I axis in aging: a summary of an NIA sponsored symposium. J Clin Endocrinol Metab 1997;82:3919–3922.
22. Estivarez CE, Ziegler TR. Nutrition and the IGF system. Endocrine 1997;7:65–71.

23. Coverley JA, Baxter RC. Phosphorylation of IGFBPs. *Mol Cell Endocrinol* 1997;128:1–5.
24. Conover CA. The role of IGFs and IGFBPs in bone cell biology. In: Bilezikian JP, Raisz LR, Rodan G, eds. *Principles of bone biology.* San Diego: Academic Press, 1996:607–618.
25. Mohan S, Farley JR, Baylink DJ. Age-related changes in IGFBP-4 and IGFBP-5 in human serum and bone: implications for bone loss with aging. *Prog Growth Factor Res* 1995;6:465–473.
26. Cook F, Rosen CJ, Vereault D, et al. Major changes in the circulatory IGF regulatory system after hip fracture surgery. *J Bone Miner Res* 1996;11:S327.
27. Veldhuis JD, Iranmanesh A, Weltman A. Elements in the pathophysiology of diminished GH secretion in aging humans. *Endocrine* 1997;7:41–48.
28. Toogood AA, O'Neil PA, Shalet SA. Beyond the somatopause: GHD in adults over age 60. *J Clin Endocrinol Metab* 1996;81:460–465.
29. Hoffman AR, Lieberman SA, Butterfield G, et al. Functional consequences of the somatopause and its treatment. *Endocrine* 1997;7:73–76.
30. Ho KY, Evans WS, Blizzard R, et al. Effects of sex and age on twenty four hour profiles of GH secretion in men. *J Clin Endocrinol Metab* 1987;64:51–58.
31. Ahren B, Larsson H, Wilhemsson C, et al. Regulation of circulating leptin in humans. *Endocrine* 1997;7:1–8.
32. Donahue LR, Hunter SJ, Sherblom AP, et al. Age-related changes in serum IGFBPs in women. *J Clin Endocrinol Metab* 1990;71:575–579.
33. Gelato MC, Frost RA. IGFBP-3 functional and structural implications in aging and wasting syndromes. *Endocrine* 1997;7:81–85.
34. Clemmons DR, Elgin RG, Han VKM, et al. Cultured fibroblast monolayers secrete a protein that alters the cellular binding of somatomedin C/IGF I. *J Clin Invest* 1986;77:1548–1556.
35. Davis PY, Frazier CR, Shapiro JR, et al. Age-related changes in effects of IGF-I on human osteoblast like cells. *Biochem J* 1997;324:753–760.
36. Grogean T, Vereault D, Millard PS, et al. A comparative analysis of methods to measure IGF-I in human serum. *Endocr Metab* 1997;4:109–114.
37. Martha PM, Gooman KM, Blizzard RM, et al. Endogenous GH secretion and clearance in normal boys as determined by deconvolution analysis. *J Clin Endocrinol Metab* 1992;74:336–344.
38. Hobbs CJ, Plymate SR, Rosen CJ, et al. Testosterone administration increases IGF-I in normal men. *J Clin Endocrinol Metab* 1993;77:776–780.
39. Andersen GH, Francis RM, Silly PL, et al. Sex hormones and osteopenia in men. *Calcif Tissue Int* 1998; 62:185–188.
40. Burich HB, Wolf L, Budde R, et al. Androstenedione metabolism in cultured human osteoblast like cells. *J Clin Endocrinol Metab* 1992;75:101–105.
41. Smith EP, Boyd F, Frank G, et al. Estrogen resistance caused by a mutation in the ER gene in a man. *N Engl J Med* 1994;331:1056–1061.
42. Carani C, Quirk C, Sinai M, et al. Effect of testosterone and estradiol in a male with aromatase deficiency. *N Engl J Med* 1997;337:91–95.
43. Greendale GA, Delstein S, Barrett Connor E. Endogenous sex steroids and bone mineral density in older men and women. *J Bone Miner Res* 1997;12:1833–1843.
44. Poehlman ET, Toth MJ, Ades PA, et al. Menopause associated changes in plasma lipids, insulin-like growth factor-I and blood pressure: a longitudinal study. *Eur J Clin Invest* 1997;27:322–326.
45. Ravn P, Overgaard K, Spencer EM, et al. IGF-I and IGF-II in healthy females. *Eur J Endocrinol* 1995;132: 313–319.
46. LeBoff MS, Rosen CJ, Glowacki J. Changes in growth factors and cytokines in postmenopausal women. *J Bone Miner Res* 1995;10:241–261.
47. Shewmon DA, Stock JL, Rosen CJ, et al. Effects of estrogen and tamoxifen on Lp(a) and IGF-I in healthy postmenopausal women. *Art Thromb* 1995;14:1586–1592.
48. DePugola G, Lespite L, Grizzulli VA, et al. IGF-I and DHEA-S in obese females. *Int J Obes Relat Metab Disord* 1993;11:481–483.
49. Morales AJ, Nolan JJ, Lukes CC, et al. Effects of replacement doses of DHEA in men and women. *J Clin Endocrinol Metab* 1994;78:1360–1361.
50. Labrie F, Belanger A, Cusan L, et al. Physiological changes in DHEA are not reflected by serum levels of active androgens and estrogens but their metabolites. *J Clin Endocrinol Metab* 1997;82:2403–2409.
51. Rosen CJ, Vereault D, Steffens C, et al. Effect of age and estrogen status on the skeletal IGF regulatory system. *Endocrine* 1997;7:77–80.
52. Tremollieres FA, Strong DD, Baylin D, et al. Progesterone and promogesterone stimulate human bone cell proliferation and IGF-II production. *Acta Endocrinol (Copenh)* 1992;126:329–337.
53. Koperak C, Fittsimmons R, Stein D, et al. Studies of the mechanisms by which androgens enhance mitogenesis and differentiation of bone cells. *J Clin Endocrinol Metab* 1990;71:329–337.
54. Commuzie G, Blangero J, Mahaney MC, et al. Genetic and environmental correlates among hormone levels and means of body fat accumulation and topography. *J Clin Endocrinol Metab* 1996;81:597–600.
55. Kao PC, Matheny AP, Lang CA. IGF-I comparisons in healthy twin children. *J Clin Endocrinol Metab* 1994; 78:310–312.
56. Kurland E, Rackoff PJ, Adler RA, et al. Heritability of serum IGF-I and its relationship to bone density. *Presented at the Endocrine Society Meeting, New Orleans,* 1998:S156.
57. Rosen CJ, Kurland ES, Vereault D, et al. Association between serum insulin growth factor-I (IGF-1) and a simple sequence repeat in IGF-1 gene: implications for genetic studies of bone mineral density. *J Clin Endocrinol Metab* 1998;83:2286–2290.
58. Rosen CJ, Donahue LR, Hunter SJ. IGFs and bone: the osteoporosis connection. *Proc Soc Exp Biol Med* 1994; 206:83–102.
59. Milne M, Kang M, Wuail JM, et al. Thyroid hormone excess increases IGF-I transcripts in bone marrow cell cultures: divergent effects on vertebral and femoral cell cultures. *Endocrinology* 1998;139(5):2527–2534.
60. Hayden J, Mohan S, Baylink DJ. The IGF system and the coupling of formation to resorption. *Bone* 1995;17: 93S–98S.
61. Linkhart TA, Mohan S. PTH stimulates relase of IGF-I and IGF-II from neonatal mouse calvariae. *Endocrinology* 1989;125:1484–1491.
62. McCarthy TL, Centrella M, Canalis E. PTH enhances

the transcript and polypeptide levels of IGF-I in osteo-blast enriched cultures from fetal rat calvariae. *Endocrinology* 1989;124:1247–1253.

63. Canalis E, Centrella M, Bach W, et al. IGF-I mediates selective anabolic effects of PTH in bone cell cultures. *J Clin Invest* 1989;63:60–65.

64. McCarthy TL, Centrella M, Canalis E. Regulatory effects of IGF-I and IGF-II on bone collagen synthesis in rat calvarial cells. *Endocrinology* 1989;124:301–308.

65. McCarthy TL, Ji C, Slu H, et al. 17 Beta estradiol suppresses cyclic AMP induced IGF-I gene transcription in primary rat osteoblast cultures. *J Biol Chem* 1997;272:18132–18139.

66. Slowik DM, Rosenthal DI, Doppelt SH, et al. Restoration of spinal bone mass in osteoporotic males by treatment with human PTH and 1,25 dihydroxyvitamin D. *J Bone Miner Res* 1986;1:377–388.

67. Rosen CJ, Conover C. Growth hormone/insulin-like growth factor-I axis in aging: a summary of a National Institutes of Health aging-sponsored symposium. *J Clin Endocrinol Metab* 1997;82:3919–3922.

68. Slootwigh MC. Growth hormone and bone. *Horm Metab Res* 1998;25:335–345.

69. Bing-you RG, Denis MG, Rosen CJ. Low bone mineral density in adults with previous hypothalamic pituitary tumors. *Calcif Tissue Int* 1993;52:183–187.

70. Langlois JA, Rosen CJ, Visser M, et al. Association between insulin-like growth factor 1 and bone mineral density in older women and men: the Framingham Heart Study. *J Clin Endocrinol Metab* 1998;83:4257–4262.

71. Bauer DC, Rosen C, Cauley J, et al. Low serum IGF-1 but not IGFBP-3 predicts hip and spine fracture: the study of osteoporotic fracture. *J Bone Miner Res* 1998:s561.

72. Ensrud KE, Cauley J, Lipschutz R, et al. Weight change and fractures in older women. Study of osteoporotic fracture. *Arch Intern Med* 1997;157:857–863.

73. Reed BY, Zerwekh JE, Sakhaee K, et al. Serum IGF 1 is low and correlated with osteoblastic surface in idiopathic osteoporosis. *J Bone Miner Res* 1995;10:1218–1224.

74. Kurland ES, Rosen CJ, Cosman F, et al. IGF-I in men with idiopathic osteoporosis. *J Clin Endocrinol Metab* 1997;82:2799–2805.

75. Kurland ES, Chan F, Vereault D, et al. Growth hormone IGF-I axis in men with idiopathic osteoporosis and reduced circulating levels of IGF-I. *J Bone Miner Res* 1996;11:S1323.

76. Beamer WG, Donahue LR, Rosen CJ, et al. Genetic variability in adult bone density among inbred strains of mice. *Bone* 1996;18:397–403.

77. Isakson OGP, Lendahl A, Nelson A, et al. Mechanisms of stimulating effect of GH on long bone growth. *Endocr Rev* 1987;8:426–438.

78. Inzuchki SE, Robbins RJ. Effect of GH on human bone biology. *J Clin Endocrinol Metab* 1994;79:691–694.

79. Beshyah SA, Kyd P, Thomas E, et al. The effects of prolonged GH replacement on bone turnover and bone mineral density in hypopituitary adults. *Clin Endocrinol (Oxf)* 1995;42:249–254.

80. Rudman D, Feller AG, Nelgrag HS. Effect of human GH in men over age 60. *N Engl J Med* 1990;323:52–60.

81. Rudman D, Feller AG, Chohn L. Effect of rhGH on body composition in elderly men. *Horm Res* 1991;36:73–81.

82. Papadakis MA, Grady D, Black D, et al. GH replacement in healthy older men improves body composition but not functional activity. *Ann Intern Med* 1996;124:708–716.

83. Thompson JL, Butterfield GE, Marcus R. The effects of recombinant rhIGF-I and GH on body composition in elderly women. *J Clin Endocrinol Metab* 1995;80:1845–1852.

84. Ghiron L, Thompson J, Halloway L, et al. Effects of rhIGF-I and GH on bone turnover in elderly women. *J Bone Miner Res* 1995;10:1844–1877.

85. Ebeling P, Jones J, O'Fallon W, et al. Short term effects of recombinant IGF-I on bone turnover in normal women. *J Clin Endocrinol Metab* 1993;77:1384–1387.

86. Johansson AG, Lindh E, Ljunghall S. IGF-I stimulates bone turnover in osteoporosis. *Lancet* 1992;339:1619.

87. Bagi CM, Brommage R, DeLeon L, et al. Benefit of systemically administered rh IGF-I/IGFBP-3 on cancellous bone in ovariectomized rats. *J Bone Miner Res* 1994;9:1301–1312.

88. Chan JM, Stampfer MJ, Giovannucci E, et al. Plasma insulin-like growth factor-1 and prostate cancer risk: a prospective study. *Cell* 1998;297:563–566.

89. Hankinson SE, Willett WC, Colditz GA, et al. Circulating concentrations of insulin-like growth factor-1 and risk of breast cancer. *Lancet* 1998;351:1393–1396.

90. Ma J, Pollak M, Giovannucci E, et al. A prospective study of plasma levels of IGF-I, IGFBP-3 and colon cancer risk among men. *J Natl Cancer Inst* 1999 *(in press)*.

91. Wolk A, Mantzoros CS, Andersson S-O, et al. Insulin-like growth factor 1 and prostate cancer risk: a population-based, case-control study. *J Natl Cancer Inst* 1998;90:911–915.

92. Juul A, Main K, Blum WF, et al. The ratio between serum levels of insulin-like growth factor (IGF)-1 and the IGF binding proteins (IGFBP)-1, 2 and 3 decreases with age in healthy adults and is increased in acromegalic patients. *Clin Endocrinol (Oxf)* 1994;41:85–93.

93. Ng ST, Zhou J, Adesanya OO, et al. Growth hormone treatment induces mammary gland hyperplasia in aging primates. *Nat Med* 1997;3:1141–1144.

94. Yang XF, Beamer W, Huynh HT, et al. Reduced growth of human breast cancer xenografts in hosts homozygous for the ''lit'' mutation. *Cancer Res* 1996;56:1509–1511.

95. Torrisi R, Paradi S, Fontana V, et al. Effect of fenretinide on plasma IGF-I and IGFBP-3 in early breast cancer patients. *Int J Cancer* 1998;76:787–790.

96. Guvakova MA, Surmacz E. Tamoxifen interferes with the IGF-I receptor signaling pathway in breast cancer cells. *Cancer Res* 1997;57:2606–2610.

97. Dunn SE, Kari FW, French J, et al. Dietary restriction reduces IGF-I levels which modulates apoptosis, cell proliferation and tumor progression in p53 deficient mice. *Cancer Res* 1997;57:4667–4672.

98. Zhang L, Zhou W, Velculescu VE, et al. Gene expression profiles in normal and cancer cells. *Science* 1997;276:1268–1272.

Skeletal Growth Factors,
edited by Ernesto Canalis.
Lippincott Williams & Wilkins, Philadelphia, © 2000.

9

Biology of Platelet-Derived Growth Factor

Harry C. Lowe, Louise A. Rafty,* Tucker Collins, Levon M. Khachigian

*Centre for Thrombosis and Vascular Research, University of New South Wales, Sydney, NSW 2052, Australia; and *Vascular Research Division, Department of Pathology, Brigham and Women's Hospital and Harvard Medical School, Boston, Massachusetts 02115.*

Platelet-derived growth factor (PDGF) was first identified as a product of human platelets based on its ability to stimulate the growth of fibroblasts (1), vascular smooth muscle cells (2), and glial cells (3). Despite its early discovery and nomenclature as a platelet product, it is now recognized to be a ubiquitous mitogenic and chemotactic factor secreted by many cell types with diverse roles in a number of physiological and pathological processes.

PLATELET-DERIVED GROWTH FACTOR LIGANDS AND RECEPTORS

Platelet-derived Growth Factor

PDGF is a dimer composed of an A and/or a B chain, each encoded by separate genes and regulated independently (4–6). Somatic cell hybrid chromosome segregation analysis (7) and *in situ* hybridization (8) localized the PDGF-A-chain gene to the distal portion of the short arm of chromosome 7 (7p21–p22). Restriction endonuclease analysis further identified that PDGF-A is composed of seven exons spanning approximately 24 kb of genomic DNA (9). Exon 1 contains an unusually long 5'-untranslated region (UTR) and signal peptide. Exons 2 and 3 encode the amino-terminal propeptide. Exons 4 and 5 encode most of the mature PDGF-A protein. Exon 6, which is alternatively spliced, encodes a highly basic 15–amino acid carboxyl-terminal region. Exon 7 encodes three amino acids located at the carboxyl terminus of the shorter

chain, as well as the 3'-UTR (8). S1 nuclease mapping and polymerase chain reaction analyses revealed that both short (lacking exon 6) and long A-chain transcripts are expressed in several normal and transformed cells (10). Three PDGF-A-chain transcripts, of 1.8, 2.3, and 2.8 kb, have been detected in human umbilical vein endothelial cells and in other normal and transformed cells in culture (7,8,11). RNase H studies have mapped these mRNA species to the same promoter and initiation site (12). Primer extension analysis has mapped the transcription start site to 36 bp downstream of a consensus TATAA sequence in both human endothelial and hepatoblastoma cells (8).

The human PDGF-B gene is located on chromosome 22 (22q12.3-q13.1) (13,14) and spans approximately 24 kb of DNA. The PDGF-B gene is virtually identical to the transforming protein of the simian sarcoma virus (SSV) p28[sis] (15,16). Both PDGF-B chain and the homologous gene product of simian virus (p[v-sis]) are capable of transformation (15). This provided the first structural and functional link between an oncogene and a cellular growth factor.

Like the A chain, PDGF-B is composed of seven exons. Exon 1 contains a long 5'-UTR and the signal sequence. The second and third exons encode the propeptide and the first two amino acids of the mature protein. Exons 4 and 5 encode the mature protein and the start of the carboxyl-terminal propeptide. Exon 6 encodes for the remainder of the propeptide. Exon 7 encodes the 3'-UTR (17). The size of the predominant

PDGF-B transcript detected in human umbilical vein endothelial cells is 3.5 to 3.7 kb (18).

Dimeric PDGF protein has a molecular mass between 28 and 35 kDa and occurs naturally in one of three biologically active isoforms (AA, BB, AB) (19). The A and B chains are synthesized as precursor molecules that undergo proteolytic processing. These precursor chains share 40% sequence homology, whereas the mature chains each consist of about 100 amino acids and share approximately 60% homology (7). PDGF is a glycoprotein with carbohydrate content of less than 10% (20).

Platelet-derived Growth Factor Receptors

PDGF isoforms exert their effects on target cells by binding with different specificities to two structurally related protein tyrosine kinase receptors (21). Two receptors for PDGF, denoted the PDGF α and β receptors, were subsequently cloned from human cells (22,23). The genes for the α and β receptors have been mapped to human chromosomes 4 (4q11-q12) (24) and 5 (5q23-31) (25), respectively. These receptors are structurally related transmembrane glycoproteins with five extracellular immunoglobulin-type domains and an intracellular split tyrosine kinase domain (26). The three outermost immunoglobulin domains are involved in ligand binding (27,28).

The PDGF α and β receptors bind the PDGF isoforms with different affinities. The β receptor binds to PDGF-BB with high affinity (0.1 nM) and PDGF-AB with lower affinity (1 nM) (29,30). The α receptor binds to all three PDGF isoforms with a dissociation constant of approximately 0.1 nM. PDGF binding induces noncovalent receptor dimerization, whose combination is dependent on the PDGF isoform. PDGF-AA induces α–α heterodimers, whereas PDGF-BB stimulates the formation of all three dimeric types (α–α, α–β, and β–β). Dimerization is accompanied by receptor autophosphorylation. The number of autophosphorylation sites in the PDGF α and β receptors is three and nine, respectively (31). Receptor autophosphorylation facilitates the interaction of signaling molecules directly with the receptor tyrosine kinase and the initiation of phosphorylation-dependent signal transduction (26). Signaling pathways triggered by PDGF are discussed later.

EXPRESSION PATTERN

Normal Development

Embryogenesis

PDGF and its receptors are expressed in the developing human embryo as well as that of other species (reviewed in 32). In general, PDGF-A and the PDGF α receptor are expressed earlier and more widely during embryogenesis than PDGF-B or the PDGF β receptor. PDGF-A or -B is expressed in epithelial layers, whereas the α and β receptors are found predominantly in adjacent mesenchymal layers. The patterns of ligand and receptor expression vary within the same tissue during the course of development. Coexpression of PDGF ligand and receptor suggests the existence of autocrine and paracrine signaling and that switching between the two may occur as development proceeds (32).

Embryonic PDGF-A and PDGF α-receptor expression is similar in *Xenopus* and mice (32–34). In early embryogenesis, PDGF-A is expressed in the animal pole ectoderm while the PDGF α receptor is expressed in the mesoderm, except for the notochord (35). With somite development, the PDGF α receptor is also expressed in the neural crest, which is of ectodermal origin. As this migrates, the adjacent pharyngeal endoderm expresses PDGF-A. Later in embryogenesis, PDGF-A is produced at the surface ectoderm and muscle of the mouse limb, whereas the PDGF α receptor is expressed in the mesenchymal limb bud and perichondrium (36).

PDGF-B and PDGF β-receptor expression in development is less well documented. PDGF-B has been localized in only a few cases, all within the second half of gestation (37). In the rat, PDGF-B is expressed in lung and kidney epithelium (32,38). The PDGF β receptor has also been localized to lung epithelium and mesenchymal tissue adjacent to glomerular epithelium (39).

The importance of PDGF in development is

supported by studies of knockout mice for PDGF-A, PDGF-B, and the PDGF β receptor (reviewed in 40,47). The study of PDGF lends itself to the application of knockout technology in that there are only loci to target two ligand and two receptor genes, and the ligand–receptor interaction is already well characterized (41). Knockouts for all four loci have been studied: PDGF-A (42), PDGF-B (43), PDGF β receptor (44), and PDGF α receptor (45).

Knockout mice for PDGF-B and PDGF β receptor are embryonically lethal and appear similar (43,44). Generalized hemorrhaging and edema occur by embryonic day 17 (E17) to E19. Many mice die before birth; those surviving to birth often have beating hearts and motor reflexes but do not breathe spontaneously (43,44). Mature microvascular pericytes, contractile cells similar to smooth muscle cells, which are formed in a number of tissues (48), are absent in PDGF-B knockouts. The PDGF β receptor is expressed on progenitor pericytes, but without PDGF-B these may fail to migrate or proliferate, and further development is not achieved (47). Pericyte function is unclear, although a role in the support of capillary structure is suggested (48). This is consistent with the abnormal capillaries in PDGF-B knockouts and the generalized hemorrhage which occurs (47). The kidney glomerulus shows a striking lack of mesangial cells, resulting in a lack of capillary tuft formation (49). This absence of mesangial cells is associated with an absence of basement membrane folding, mesangial matrix, and capillary network, suggesting that mesangial cells are important in the formation of these structures (49). Mesangial cells are related to microvascular pericytes (50), consistent with a role for PDGF-B in mesangial cell development.

PDGF-A knockout mice are phenotypically distinct (42). Fifty percent are lost before E10; most of the remaining survive to a few weeks following birth but are invariably severely growth-retarded (42). There is widespread severe emphysema, associated with absence of α smooth muscle actin–positive cells in the alveolar septa, reduced extracellular elastin, and reduced elastin mRNA–positive cells in the alveo-

lar smooth muscle cells (SMCs) or precursor cells (49).

The ontogeny of pericytes, mesangial cells, and alveolar SMCs has led to the proposal of a common theme of PDGF-dependent SMC development, whereby PDGF receptor–positive SMC progenitors progress from proximal to distal sites along PDGF-expressing epithelial or endothelial tubes (40).

The analysis of the PDGF ligand and receptor knockout mice has provided some insights into the importance of PDGF in development; however, these gene inactivation studies resulted in embryonic lethality, and the mice are not usable for evaluations of gene function in adult disease processes. To address this issue, chimeric mice were generated, composed of an unmarked wild-type strain and another embryo from a marked strain carrying a targeted allele for the PDGF β receptor. If the disrupted allele is important, the two genotypes participate unequally during development, and the magnitude of this difference is a measure of the role of the gene in development. Chimera analysis revealed surprising information about the role of PDGF β-receptor function during development: first, PDGF β-receptor expression is important for the development of all muscle lineages (vascular and intestinal, smooth muscle cardiac and skeletal); second, PDGF β-receptor expression is not important for the development of fibroblast lineages; third, PDGF β-receptor function is not important for the development of endothelial cells or leukocytes. This approach should allow the function of PDGF β receptors to be elucidated in adult mouse disease models (51).

Sites at which PDGF has been localized during human development are listed in Table 9.1.

Nervous System

PDGF expression is early and widespread in the developing nervous system. In mice, PDGF-A transcripts are expressed in the spinal cord as early as day 12 and in the brain by day 15, albeit at lower levels. PDGF-A protein has also been localized to the spinal cord by day 18 using immunohistochemistry (52). In rats, PDGF-B immunoreactivity has been detected within devel-

TABLE 9.1. *Platelet-derived growth factor (PDGF) ligand*
and receptor expression during human development

Ligand/receptor	Tissue	Cell type
Preorganogenesis		
PDGF-A	Placenta	Vascular smooth muscle cells
PDGF α	Placenta	Mesenchyme
PDGF-B	Placenta, blood vessel	Cytotrophoblasts, endothelial cells
PDGF β	Blood vessel	Vascular smooth muscle cells, mesenchyme
During organogenesis		
PDGF-B	Kidney	Glomerular epithelium
PDGFβ	Kidney	Metanephric blastema, interstitial cells, vascular cells
PDGF-B	Kidney	Mesangial cells

From refs. 32, 39, 73, 259.

oping olfactory neurons in all stages of embryonic development and in adults (53). PDGF-B transcripts have also been detected within widespread locations in the adult nonhuman primate, including neurons, principal dendrites, the dorsal horn of the spinal cord, and the posterior pituitary (54). This early, widespread pattern of PDGF expression is consistent with a role for PDGF in glial and neuronal cell development (52).

Glial cell development may be profoundly influenced by PDGF. In normal development, oligodendrocyte precursor type 2 (O-2A) cells proliferate and then differentiate into oligodendrocytes (55). This process begins soon after birth and is driven by PDGF derived from type 1 astrocytes (56,57). PDGF-A causes O-2A cells to proliferate but blocks differentiation (55). PDGF-driven proliferation is also influenced by surrounding axonal activity; one hypothesis is that axonal activity may, at least in part, control the release and/or synthesis of PDGF (58).

Neuronal development appears to be specifically dependent on the PDGF α receptor (55,59). A role for PDGF-A, PDGF-B, or the PDGF β receptor in this process is less well defined. Knockout mice for the PDGF α receptor have deformed neural plates and disorganized or absent mesoderm and usually die by day 11 *in utero* (45). The neural tube is kinked or waved, suggesting a growth imbalance (59). Mice surviving up to the sixteenth day of gestation have a variety of brain defects, including absent olfac-

tory bulbs, abnormal choroid, and deformed ventricles (45). This is in contrast with mice lacking PDGF-A, PDGF-B, or the PDGF β receptor, which have severe multisystem abnormalities with no apparent neuronal abnormalities (45). Overall, these studies suggest a necessary role for the PDGF α receptor in neurological development but do not exclude a role for PDGF-A, PDGF-B, or the PDGF β receptor.

Normal Adult Tissues

PDGF is expressed in a wide variety of normal adult human cell types of mesenchymal origin (Table 9.2). PDGF is expressed in developing and adult bone and in new bone formation as part of fracture healing. Most is known about PDGF-A, which is expressed in osteoblasts, osteoclasts, and fibrous cells (43,60). PDGF induces osteoblasts to undergo proliferation, chemotaxis, and matrix apposition (60–63). The AA and BB isoforms appear to be equally effective at this induction in humans (64), although their relative effectiveness is apparently species-dependent (65). The role of PDGF in adult and developing bone is discussed in detail in chapter 10.

Endothelial Cells

That cultured vascular endothelial cells express mRNA for PDGF-A and -B and secrete PDGF protein has been recognized for over a decade (18,66–68). Curiously, PDGF is not ex-

TABLE 9.2. *Expression of platelet-derived growth factor (PDGF) by adult human cell types*

Tissue/organ	Cell type	Reference
Hemopoietic	Platelet, megakaryocyte, monocyte, macrophage	254
		78
		255
Vascular	Endothelial, smooth muscle	66
		76
Neural	Neuron, astrocyte	52
		256
Reproductive	Mammary, epithelial, uterine endometrium,	257
	myometrium, placental cytotrophoblast	258
		259
Other	Fibroblast, kidney, mesangial	260
		261

pressed in aortic endothelial cells of the normal rat artery wall unless this cell type is activated by stresses such as mechanical injury (69). Microvascular endothelial cells in culture and in endothelium after injury express β and α receptors, respectively, suggesting that PDGF may act in an autocrine manner in certain endothelial cell subtypes and conditions (70,71). Endothelial PDGF expression is also influenced by a large number of soluble factors and physical stresses (see following and Table 9.3).

Smooth Muscle Cells

PDGF is expressed in vascular SMCs. PDGF-A mRNA is expressed in the tunica media of the rat artery, whereas PDGF-B is expressed in the adventitia (67,72). The β receptor is also expressed in this cell type (73,74). Expression is developmentally regulated; rat pup SMCs secrete 60 times the amount of PDGF secreted by adult cells (75,76). Recently, this has been found to be due, at least in part, to differences in the

TABLE 9.3. *Factors modulating endothelial cell platelet-derived growth factor (PDGF) expression*

Factor(s)	Effect		Reference
Physical			
Shear stress	A/B	+	262
			263
Cyclic strain	B	+	196
Hypoxia	B	+	264
Culturing	B	+	18
Differentiation	B	−	265
Cytokine			
IL-1, IL-6	PDGF	+	266
			267
IFN	PDGF	−	267
TNF	PDGF	−	268
Growth factor			
FGF-1	A	+	269
FGF-2	PDGF	−	270
TGF-β	A, B	+	206
			271
Drug			
Phorbol ester	A, B	+	271
ACE inhibitor	A	−	272
Other			
Thrombin	B	+	273
			271
LDL	PDGF	−	274
H_2O_2	A	+	275

ACE, angiotensin-converting enzyme; FGF, fibroblast growth factor; IFN, interferon; IL, interleukin; LDL, low-density lipoprotein; TGF, transforming growth factor; TNF, tumor necrosis factor.

TABLE 9.4. *Factors modulating vascular smooth muscle cell platelet-derived growth factor (PDGF) expression*

Factor(s)	Effect		Reference
Physical			
Age	B	−	75
	A or B	−	76
Culturing	B	+	75
	A	+	74
External stenting	A or B	−	276
Injury	A, B	+	70
			123
Cytokine			
TNF-α	A	+	269
Growth factor			
PDGF	A	+	74
TGF-β	A	+	277
FGF-1	A	+	269
FGF-2	A	+	69
Angiotensin II	A	−	278
Drug			
Dexamethasone	A	−	279
Phorbol ester	A	+	269
			204
4-Hydroxy-2-nonenal	A	+	280
Cyclosporin A	A	−	281
Other			
Thrombin	A	+	282
LDL	A	+	123

FGF, fibroblast growth factor; LDL, low density lipoprotein; TGF, transforming growth factor; TNF, tumor necrosis factor.

nuclear content of certain transcription factors (77). PDGF expression in SMCs, like that in endothelial cells, is modulated by a number of physical and biological factors (see following and Table 9.4).

Hemopoietic Cells

In platelets, PDGF is stored within α granules and released upon platelet activation (78). In human platelets, the composition of PDGF is 70% AB, 25% BB, and 5% AA (79). This ratio is species-specific, being, for example, almost entirely PDGF-BB in the pig (80). Since platelets lack the capacity to direct transcription, α-granular PDGF is derived from platelet precursors, megakaryocytes. Megakaryocytes express mRNA for PDGF-A and PDGF-B (75,81). The cultured human stem cell line K562, when treated with phorbol ester, induces megakaryocytic differentiation, PDGF-A and PDGF-B expression, and secretion of PDGF (19,79). PDGF is also expressed in a number of other hemopoietic cell types in normal and pathological settings (see following and Table 9.2; reviewed in 67).

Normal Processes

Inflammation

PDGF has been implicated to play an important role during the inflammatory process via its effects on interstitial cells and blood elements (reviewed in 82). For example, PDGF stimulates vascular SMC proliferation and promotes migration of fibroblasts to inflammatory sites (83,84). PDGF promotes superoxide anion production by eosinophils (85), while the PDGF α receptor on platelets can mediate inhibition of platelet aggregation (86).

Wound Healing

Wound healing is the process of connective tissue formation and organization which follows the coagulative process at the site of epidermal injury. PDGF is involved at an early stage, being released from activated platelets and macrophages during coagulation. This, in concert with other growth factors, such as fibroblast growth factor-2 (FGF-2), promotes proliferation and migration of SMCs, fibroblasts, and leukocytes (84).

PDGF is expressed in a time-dependent manner during this process. PDGF β-receptor expression has been documented in human and pig wounds. PDGF α- and β-receptor expression has been observed following surgical treatment of perigenital acne inversa in humans. The α and β subunits were expressed at 6, 12, and 19 days after incision and were not present in normal subjects. At 47 days, coincident with complete reepithelialization, there was no receptor expression (87). Similar patterns of receptor expression have been demonstrated in a number of models of acute and chronic wound healing (reviewed in 88). Exogenous PDGF-BB, administered in picomolar amounts, has been shown to shorten wound-healing time and to increase wound tensile strength in a number of models of incisional and excisional wounds, consistent with PDGF playing a role in this reparative response to injury (89,90).

Angiogenesis

Angiogenesis involves the outgrowth and formation of new capillary blood vessels from existing vessels by sprouting. As such, it is distinct from vasculogenesis, or the formation of new vessels from blood islands of committed stem cells in early embryogenesis (91). Angiogenesis is important in a variety of settings, including inflammation, wound healing, cardiovascular disease, and oncogenesis. PDGF has been implicated in this process (reviewed in 91). PDGF is not generally considered in the same light as vascular endothelial growth factor (VEGF) and FGF-2 as a direct agonist of angiogenesis since it does stimulate macrovascular endothelial proliferation (92,93). However, the expression of PDGF receptors on microvascular endothelial cells *in vitro* (71,94,95) and on a strain of bovine aortic endothelial cells which spontaneously

undergo cord and tube formation during development (96) suggests that PDGF is an angiogeneic factor. Using video lapse microscopy to directly view cell movement, PDGF-BB has been shown to increase endothelial cell migration into regions of tissue injury, thus contributing directly to the angiogenic process (97).

Apoptosis

PDGF-BB added to rat vascular SMCs in culture induces apoptosis in a dose- and time-dependent manner, as measured by DNA fragmentation following gel electrophoresis. In contrast, PDGF-AA has no effect (93). The mechanism by which PDGF can induce apoptosis is, at least in part, mediated via the bcl-2 family of regulatory proteins, which inhibit apoptosis (98). A related protein, bcl-x, exists in two forms as a result of alternative splicing. Overexpression of the long form, bcl-xl, suppresses apoptosis, whereas the short form, bcl-xs, induces apoptosis. PDGF-BB downregulates bcl-2 and bcl-xl and increases bcl-xs (99).

Coordinated and localized apoptosis appears to be important in normal wound healing and is part of a process of initial inflammation, followed by a reduction in inflammation associated with reepithelialization. Apoptosis is, at least in part, thought to facilitate inflammatory cell infiltration (100). Diabetic wounds show reduced rates of apoptosis and slower rates of reepithelialization. PDGF applied locally has no effect on this rate of apoptosis, but in combination with insulin-like growth factor II (IGF-II) increases the rate of apoptosis and wound healing to rates approaching controls (100).

Pathological States

Neoplasia

Evidence linking PDGF to neoplasia is well documented following demonstration of the structural homology between the PDGF B-chain and p^{v-sis} (16,101) and the expression of PDGF-A and PDGF-B mRNA, protein, and receptors in a variety of solid tumors and leukemic cell lines (30,102). More recent data have implicated

PDGF in malignant processes of transformation, proliferation, invasion, angiogenesis, and metastasis. Autocrine and paracrine mechanisms involving PDGF have been proposed. Autocrine mechanisms support the notion of clonal selection and loss of growth regulation key to malignant change (reviewed in 103).

An autocrine role for PDGF in tumor proliferation has been recognized for over a decade. PDGF stimulates DNA synthesis and cell proliferation in malignant gliomas *in vivo* and *in vitro* (104–106). Gliomas secrete a PDGF-like mitogenic factor and express receptors for PDGF (106). The PDGF isoforms responsible and the importance of PDGF in relation to other growth factors remain unclear (107).

Tumor invasion and migration is a highly complex process, dependent not only on PDGF but also on epidermal growth factor, FGF-2, transforming growth factor-β (TGF-β), matrix metalloproteinases, and gangliosides in several *in vitro* models (108). PDGF plays a number of roles, including directly increasing metalloproteinase activity (109) or stimulating angiogenesis through interleukin-1 (IL-1) (110) (reviewed in 103). There is also evidence linking PDGF to metastasis (111).

These initial insights may be important in the assessment and treatment of malignancy. For example, PDGF-A expression in gastric carcinoma has been found to provide prognostic value (112). Greater understanding of the role(s) of PDGF in malignancy should determine whether PDGF is an appropriate therapeutic target in the management of neoplasia (107).

Atherosclerosis

Atherosclerosis involves a complex series of cellular and molecular changes in response to some form of arterial injury culminating in the formation of intraarterial lesions. It involves SMC and macrophage proliferation, matrix formation, lipid accumulation, and an inflammatory response (113,114). Endothelial activation leads to surface molecule expression, monocyte/macrophage adhesion, and migration of these inflammatory cells toward the media. PDGF is secreted from activated macrophages,

activated endothelial cells, SMCs, and platelets during thrombus formation. This leads to migration of SMCs to the intima and proliferation. The plaque develops as a consequence of matrix formation and lipid accumulation. Several lines of evidence indicate that PDGF and its receptors are produced by different cell types in the developing atherosclerotic lesion.

In early human atherosclerotic lesions, PDGF A- and B-chain transcripts have been demonstrated in plaque intimal cells (115). In advanced carotid artery lesions, the PDGF-B chain is expressed at five times the rate found in normal vessels (116). Cells cultured from atheromatous lesions provide additional evidence for the involvement of PDGF in the plaque. SMCs cultured from these lesions express mRNA for PDGF-A but not PDGF-B (117). These cultured cells stimulate SMC growth, and this is decreased, although not abolished, by PDGF antibodies (117).

A large body of evidence for the involvement of PDGF in neointima formation comes from work performed using rat models of vascular injury. Three models of injury have been described. The first, and most widely used, model is balloon angioplasty to the rat carotid artery, which mimics human coronary angioplasty in that it relies on an inflated balloon catheter to stretch intima and media (118). The second model uses the same balloon, though uninflated and simply drawn through the artery, to denude endothelium without vessel stretch (70). The third model uses a filament loop to denude endothelial cells without causing subendothelial trauma in a similar manner to the uninflated balloon (119). A major limitation in the extrapolation of data from these models to human atherosclerosis is that injury in rats is applied to vessels free of disease.

There is evidence for the involvement of PDGF in all of these models. In the inflation model, balloon deendothelialization leads initially to platelet adherence, followed by SMC migration from the medium to the intima within 2 to 7 days and neointima formation from 4 to 14 days (118,120,121). PDGF antibodies recognizing all three PDGF ligand isoforms reduce intimal thickening after injury, without altering the thymidine labeling index (83), suggesting inhibition of migration but not proliferation. This contrasts with findings using FGF-2 antibodies, which inhibit replication and migration (119). PDGF-BB increases SMC migration from medium to intima and leads to intimal thickening in the first 7 days after injury (122). Expression of PDGF β receptor increases twofold 1 week after injury (123), whereas α-receptor expression is not altered from its basal level of expression. Neointima formation following injury is decreased by infusion with PDGF antibody (83). Following endothelial denudation, PDGF-A, PDGF-B, and the α receptor are inducibly expressed in endothelium (69). PDGF-A is also expressed by SMCs as they migrate to the intima in this model (124).

PDGF-B is expressed at low or undetectable levels in the uninjured rat vessel wall and was initially thought not to be influenced by injury, as detected by Northern blotting (123). However, more recently, using *in situ* hybridization of en face prepared, balloon-injured arteries, a subpopulation of SMCs was shown to express PDGF-B, which further increased when subcultured (125).

Evidence for the role of PDGF-A in neointima formation is incomplete and conflicting. PDGF-A mRNA increases markedly after balloon injury (123). However, since PDGF-AA has only a modest influence on SMC migration *in vitro* (123) and can even inhibit this process (126,127), the significance of injury-induced PDGF-A expression is unclear. These data contrast with findings using antisense oligonucleotides targeting PDGF-A, which reduce SMC proliferation in spontaneously hypertensive rats but not in normotensive animals (128). In response to mechanical injury, PDGF-A may be biologically active after it has combined with PDGF-B.

SMC proliferation and migration are also key processes in restenosis following therapeutic coronary dilation procedures, by either angioplasty or stenting. Renarrowing of the vessel wall occurs in 30% to 50% of patients undergoing angioplasty (129) and 30% following stenting within 6 months (130). Clinical studies provide evidence for the importance of PDGF in this process. Restenotic lesions are associated with significant intimal hyperplasia, consisting mainly of SMCs (131). The PDGF antagonist trapidil (5-methyl-7-diethylamino-S-triazolo-1, 5-pyrimidine) has been found to reduce restenosis after angioplasty from 39.7% to 24.2% compared to an aspirin control group (132) and is currently under further investigation; however, trapidil has a number of other effects, such as direct activation of protein kinase A (PKA) (133), phosphodiesterase inhibition (134), and coronary vasodilatory activity (135). Hence, its effects on SMC proliferation and migration may be independent of PDGF antagonism. Indeed, trapidil inhibits PDGF- and phorbol myristate acetate (PMA)–induced SMC mitogenesis in a dose-dependent manner, but this has been shown to be due to direct activation of PKA rather than PDGF receptor antagonism (133). Tranilast (*N*-(3,4-dimethoxycinnamoyl) anthranilic acid) is another agent shown to inhibit PDGF-induced SMC migration and proliferation (136). It has recently been found to be effective at reducing the incidence of restenosis (137). This agent also has a number of additional effects, including inhibition of VEGF (138), TGF-β (139), cyclooxygenase 2 (COX-2) (140), angiotensin II (141), and c-myc (142). The contribution of PDGF inhibition to the clinical effects of both agents remains unclear at present.

Other Pathological States

Inflammatory Disease

PDGF expression also occurs in a number of inflammatory disease states. Most investigation has focused on renal inflammatory disease, specifically glomerulonephritis. The PDGF B-chain is expressed only in low amounts in the adult kidney, but PDGF protein and receptor expression is upregulated in renal disease (reviewed in 143). In health, the main sources of PDGF in the kidney are mesangial and glomerular cells, microvascular endothelial cells, collecting duct cells, and vascular SMCs (144). In disease, the PDGF β receptor shows increased expression in proliferative glomerulonephritis, as demonstrated by immunohistochemistry in the glomerular mesangium, intimal SMCs, and interstitium

(143,145). PDGF-B mRNA, protein, and β receptor have been demonstrated in a number of other forms of glomerulonephritis, including membranoproliferative glomerulonephritis and immunoglobulin A nephropathy (146–148). PDGF expression does not occur in minimal-change nephropathy, and in general, the intensity of expression correlates with the degree of histological change (143).

PDGF may also be significant in inflammatory lung disease. PDGF-B is expressed in mononuclear cells from bronchioalveolar lavage in patients with sarcoidosis (149). Idiopathic pulmonary fibrosis is associated with macrophages expressing increased levels of PDGF-A mRNA compared to normal controls (150). In temporal or giant cell arteritis, PDGF-A and PDGF-B protein levels are elevated in macrophages, SMCs, and multinucleated giant cells (151). Likewise, in rheumatoid arthritis, synovial tissues express higher levels of PDGF-AA and PDGF-BB protein, as well as the α and β receptors (152).

Other Disease

There is evidence for the involvement of PDGF in the pathogenesis of diabetes. *In vitro*, elevated glucose increases PDGF-BB binding, PDGF β-receptor mRNA and protein expression, and PDGF-B protein levels in human monocyte-derived macrophages (153,154). In experimental animal models of induced diabetes, PDGF-B, though not PDGF-A, expression increases at 3 weeks relative to controls (155).

Since PDGF plays a role in the developing nervous system, interest has focused on its role in degenerative neurological disease, particularly in the demyelinating disease multiple sclerosis (reviewed in 156). In tissue culture, PDGF promotes oligodendroglial maturation (157,158) and ameliorates myelin-like membrane damage caused by the addition of lysophosphatidylcholine to cultured oligodendroglia (159). In a rat model of Huntington's disease, the number of PDGF-immunoreactive astrocytes increased, though PDGF-A and PDGF-B mRNA and protein did not alter significantly (160). These data suggest a role for PDGF in the repair of the neurodegenerative process in general and in the repair of myelin in particular.

PLATELET-DERIVED GROWTH FACTOR REGULATION

Transcription

In the same way that early work on the structure and mechanism of action of PDGF in the 1980s led to increased understanding of growth factors and cytokines in general (reviewed in 161,162), recent insights into the transcriptional mechanisms controlling PDGF expression suggest that certain regulatory pathways may be a common theme in the inducible expression of other pathophysiologically relevant genes (reviewed in 164). Elucidation of the molecular mechanisms controlling PDGF transcription have been made possible by the isolation and study of genomic clones for the PDGF ligand genes.

The minimal promoter region for PDGF-A in human vascular endothelial cells consists of a region containing approximately 100 bp (164). This region of the promoter is highly GC-rich and contains multiple consensus binding sites for the zinc-finger transcription factor Sp1 (151), activating protein (AP-2) (165), and the immediate-early gene product Egr-1 (166,167). Sp1 binds to a specific region of the proximal PDGF-A promoter, between -71 and -55 bp, and directs basal expression of the gene in vascular endothelial cells (164,168). Other sites playing regulatory roles within the promoter have been identified, such as a site at -102 to -82 bp which interacts with nuclear proteins from human mesangial cells exposed to PMA (169).

The minimal promoter for the human PDGF-B gene is also comprised of around 100 bp in a number of cell types (170–172). Two positive regulatory sites have been identified by linker scanning mutational analysis and named the SIS distal and SIS proximal elements (170). *In vivo* footprinting demonstrated that the sequence 5'-CCACCCAC-3' within the SIS proximal element is occupied in intact cells (173). A number of functionally important transcription factors have also been shown to interact with the PDGF-B promoter, among them Sp1, Sp3, and Egr-1 (163,171,174). Sp1 was the first endogenous nuclear factor found to bind to the PDGF promoter (171) via the 5'-CCACCCAC-3' motif in the SIS proximal element. This binding is required for basal expression of PDGF-B in vascular endothelial cells (171). Interaction of Sp1 with the PDGF-B promoter occurs in a number of cell types, including vascular SMCs (124), human umbilical vein endothelial cells (175), Jurkat T cells (176), and U2-OS cells (174).

Sp3, a member of the zinc-finger transcription factor family, binds to the same motif within the proximal PDGF-B promoter (174). In contrast with reports demonstrating repression of gene transcription by Sp3 (177,178), Sp3 appears to upregulate PDGF-B promoter–dependent expression in vascular SMCs (124) and U2-OS cells (174).

Egr-1 has recently been found to play an important role in the transcriptional regulation of both chains of PDGF (reviewed in 47, 163). Egr-1 (also known as TIS8, krox-24, and NGFI-A) is a 60-kDa protein containing three zinc-finger DNA-binding domains located toward the carboxyl-terminal end of the molecule (179). These zinc-finger domains facilitate the interaction of Egr-1 with its consensus binding site, GCG(T/G)GGGGG (179,180).

Egr-1/Sp1 Interplay as a Regulator of Inducible Platelet-derived Growth Factor Gene Expression

A paradigm has emerged in recent years in which inducible PDGF expression involves the displacement of Sp1 by Egr-1 from common binding sites in the PDGF promoter (69,163). This model is based on initial observations from work using the PDGF-A promoter, which contains consensus binding sites for Sp1 and Egr-1, and the positive transcriptional response of the PDGF-A gene to PMA (164).

The proximal PDGF-B promoter does not contain a consensus binding site for Egr-1, yet Egr-1/Sp1 interplay also appears to be a regulatory feature of inducible PDGF-B expression

(69). The PDGF-B promoter contains a functional binding element for Sp1 (171,175,176) which is protected from partial *in vitro* DNase I digestion by Egr-1. Using footprinting, Egr-1 binds to this element in a specific manner. Mutations that no longer facilitate the interaction of Egr-1 compromise PMA-inducible promoter activity (163).

Egr-1 activity is itself also under negative regulation. Two corepressors have been identified: nerve growth factor inhibitor-A (NGF-A)–binding protein-1 (NAB-1) and NAB-2 (181–183). The exact mechanism of these inhibitors is unclear, but NAB-1 has been shown to bind to a 34–amino acid domain of Egr-1 called R1 (183). NAB-1 is expressed constitutively, whereas NAB-2 is rapidly and transiently expressed by many of the same stimuli that induce Egr-1 (47).

Transcriptional Regulation in Response to Pathophysiological Processes

PDGF transcription and its regulation have been investigated in a number of experimental vascular pathological settings. These include the response to mechanical injury, exposure to fluid shear stress, cyclic strain, and various growth factors.

In the rat endothelial denudation model, Egr-1 is not expressed in unmanipulated arteries but is rapidly induced at the wound edge within minutes of injury (69). Injury-induced Egr-1 binds to the PDGF-A and PDGF-B promoters prior to expression of these genes at the wound edge. These findings provided the first functional link between a transcription factor and the inducible expression of a pathophysiologically relevant gene in endothelial cells following injury (69). Egr-1 has also been shown to interact with and displace Sp1 from the proximal promoters of several other genes induced at the endothelial wound edge following injury in the rat aorta (69), including tissue factor (184,185), TGF-β (186), and urokinase plasminogen activator (u-PA) (187). This raises the possibility that Egr-1 and Sp1 interplay is a common regulatory theme in the inducible expression of many other genes whose products influence cell movement, proliferation, and thrombosis in the vessel wall (69).

Fluid shear stress, the tangential force exerted on endothelium by flowing blood, has received considerable attention as a modulator of endothelial structure and function and as a contributor to the process of atherogenesis (reviewed in (188). Alterations in shear stress result in elevated PDGF-A mRNA and protein levels *in vivo* (189). Endothelial cells exposed to physiological levels of shear stress *in vitro* demonstrate elevated PDGF-A mRNA expression (190). Egr-1 transcription is increased in response to shear stress, whereas levels of Sp1 remain unaltered. Upon synthesis, Egr-1 protein translocates to the nucleus, binds to a PDGF-A shear stress–response element (SSRE) by displacing Sp1, and drives the expression of this gene. The SSRE confers shear inducibility onto a promoter–reporter construct, which is otherwise unresponsive to shear stress (190). Portability is supported by additional work demonstrating that shear stress induction of the tissue factor promoter is mediated by Egr-1 (191,192). Induced expression of Egr-1 and tissue factor in response to shear stress has also recently been demonstrated in a rat model of partial carotid occlusion (191).

PDGF-B expression is also elevated in endothelial cells following exposure to shear stress, and this is, at least in part, due to an SSRE in the proximal region (193). The ubiquitous transcription factor NF-κB p50-p65 is activated by shear stress (194) and interacts with the PDGF-B SSRE in a transient manner (195). PDGF-B is also induced in cells exposed to another type of fluid biomechanical force. Cyclic strain, the repetitive distension of the blood vessel wall during the cardiac cycle, also modulates PDGF-B expression, although the mechanism appears to be distinct from that of the SSRE (196). PDGF-B mRNA and protein increase when endothelial cells are exposed to a 10% (though not to a 6%) cyclic strain independently of the SSRE and dependent on a region residing farther upstream (196). PDGF-A mRNA and protein also increase after exposure to cyclic strain (197). Recent studies indicate that cyclic strain-induced PDGF-A expression is mediated by Egr-1 (197).

Recent studies have delineated the mechanism by which Egr-1 is activated in endothelial cells following mechanical injury. FGF-2 lacks a classic signal peptide for exocytic secretion, and since it is basally expressed, it is found preformed in endothelial cells and SMCs. Endothelial cells repond to the presence of FGF-2 by increased expression and nuclear accumulation of Egr-1, which then interacts with the proximal PDGF-A promoter (198). Endothelial monolayers preincubated with neutralizing antibodies to FGF-2 show marked inhibition of the induction of Egr-1 and its upstream mitogen-activated protein kinases (MAPKs) after injury and interaction with the PDGF-A promoter (198). That FGF-2 is locally released following balloon angioplasty of atherosclerotic lesions in humans without significant platelet activation (Lowe and Khachigian, unpublished data) suggests that paracrine activation by endogenous FGF-2 may be among the earliest events triggering the development of intravascular lesions (198,199).

Alternative Transcription Start Sites

There is evidence for an alternative transcription start site in PDGF-A (67); this is located 470 bp downstream of the original transcription start site. This distal alternative promoter includes a TATA element and a proximal region consisting largely of GC elements (200). The alternative PDGF-A transcript is expressed in fetal, newborn, and adult brain and kidney but not in macrophages (201). Several smaller PDGF-B mRNA species have been detected as a result of alternative transcription start sites. These include 2.8- and 3.0-kb transcripts from vascular endothelial cells exposed to cycloheximide and TGF-β (202) and a 2.5-kb transcript in WM115 melanoma cells in response to cycloheximide (203).

Other Regulatory Pathways

mRNA Stability

PDGF mRNA stability is altered upon exposure to PMA and PDGF-BB. In human mesangial cells, the half-lives of PDGF-A and PDGF-B mRNA are each around 100 min. These are both reduced to around 70 min in the presence of PMA (204,205). Conversely, PDGF-BB increases PDGF-B mRNA stability by 1.5-fold in the same cell line, with no effect on PDGF-A stability (205).

PDGF mRNA half-life varies about threefold across a wide spectrum of cell types, including endothelial, smooth muscle, neoplastic, and phorbol ester–treated megakaryocyte cell lines, suggesting that mRNA stability may not play a significant regulatory role (75,173,206,207).

Alternative Splicing

Studies in human umbilical vein endothelial cells and U343 glioma cells determined that PDGF-A undergoes alternative splicing in exon 6 (8,9,208,209). Several distinct PDGF-A transcripts have been identified in these and U2-OS osteosarcoma cells, in which exons 2 and 6 are absent or present (200). Splicing of exon 2 is not expected to result in the formation of a functional protein (210). The two PDGF-A-chain isoforms, A_L and A_S, resulting from alternative exon 6 splicing, have also been identified in a number of mammalian-cell types, including rabbit and mouse (210–212). The functional significance of PDGF-A-chain exon 6 splicing has received considerable attention (reviewed in 213). PDGF-A_s, in general, is at least as abundant as PDGF-A_L, depending on the tissue and species studied (34,214). PDGF-A_L is retained at the cell surface and extracellular matrix of producing cells, whereas PDGF-A_s is released (215). Alternative splicing of exon 6 thus plays an important regulatory role in the secretion of the PDGF-A chain. Other functions that have been ascribed to the longer form of PDGF-A include nuclear transport signaling (216,217), glycosaminoglycan binding (218,219), mitogenesis (220), and migration (221).

Exon 1 of the 3.5-kb PDGF-B transcript contains a 1-kb long untranslated region (5′-UTR). This UTR, is well conserved and a strong translational inhibitor, as shown by cell-free translational systems and reporter gene and transient transfection analyses (222–225). It is a highly G + C-rich region and contains multiple open reading frames upstream of the translational start site (226). The region harbors an internal ribosomal entry site, which relieves translational inhibition during megakaryocyte differentiation in a 5′-end-independent manner (227).

Expression of a shorter, 2.8-kb, transcript lacking the 5′-UTR has been described in human umbilical vein endothelial cells (202). More recently, a 2.6-kb form, also lacking the 5′-UTR, has been demonstrated in the developing rat brain. Levels of expression of this shorter mRNA appear to correlate with PDGF-B protein immunoreactivity, suggesting that this shorter form results in increased translational efficiency (228).

PDGF translational control has also been conferred using antisense oligodeoxynucleotides *in vitro*. A 15-bp oligodeoxynucleotide, complementary to the region spanning the initiation codon of rat PDGF-A-chain mRNA, inhibited the production of PDGF-A-chain protein in SMCs derived from spontaneously hypertensive rats, without affecting levels of PDGF-A mRNA (128).

Post-translational Regulation

PDGF activity may be regulated at the post-translational level by glycosylation and binding proteins. The molecular mass range of naturally occuring PDGF is due, in large part, to glycosylation (5,229). At least two proteins bind to PDGF and regulate its activity. α_2-Macroglobulin binds PDGF in a reversible manner, leaving only an unbound PDGF fraction biologically active (230–233). The SPARC (secreted protein, acidic and rich in cysteine) glycoprotein specifically binds PDGF-AB and PDGF-BB and inhibits its interaction with the PDGF receptor (234). It does not appear to have effects on PDGF-AA binding (67).

SIGNAL TRANSDUCTION

Mitogen-activated Protein Kinases

PDGF initiates a multitude of biological effects through the activation of intracellular signal-transduction pathways. These include phosphatidylinositol turnover, calcium mobilization, and activation of signaling pathways involving MAPKs (235). MAPK activation mediates two processes typifying vascular lesion formation and SMC proliferation and migration (236).

When activated by ligand binding, the intracellular portion of the PDGF β receptor interacts with several molecules involved in signal-transduction pathways (26). These proteins bind to the phosphorylated receptor via a well-conserved 100–amino acid src homology (SH2) domain (237). Such proteins include phospholipase C-γ1 (PLCγ1), phosphatidylinositol 3-kinase (PI3K), Src, and molecular adapters such as Shc, Grb2, and Nck (238). Upon stimulation by PDGF, Ras activation is achieved via signal tranducers such as shc, Grb2, and Sos (239). Activated Ras triggers a kinase cascade with sequential activation of Raf-1 and MAPK/extracellular signal–regulated kinase (ERK). ERK then translocates to the nucleus, where it phosphorylates certain transcription factors (238). Substrates of ERK also include nonnuclear serine/threonine kinase p90srk, cytoskeletal proteins, and cytosolic phospholipase A_2 (240). Evidence that MAPK activation following PDGF stimulation results in cell proliferation and migration was demonstrated upon overexpression of a dominant negative form of MAPKK (241,242). Conversely, overexpression of a constitutively active form of MAPKK stimulated cell proliferation and transformation (241,243).

Protein Kinase C

The protein kinase C (PKC) family comprises a large group of serine/threonine kinases mediating PDGF-stimulated signal transduction (244). PDGF activates PLCγ1, which catalyzes the breakdown of phosphatidylinositol bisphosphate, triggering cytosolic calcium increase, PKC activation, and PKC translocation to the cell membrane (238). In hematopoietic 32D and NIH 3T3 cells, PKC-δ undergoes ligand-dependent translocation from the cytosol to the membrane, tyrosine phosphorylation, and activation in response to PDGF (245). In vascular SMCs, PKC translocates from the cytosol to the plasma membrane in response to PDGF-AA and PDGF-BB stimulation (246).

Other PKC isoforms appear to mediate PDGF-induced differentiation. In Rat-1 fibroblasts, PDGF activates PKC-ζ, which mediates PDGF activation of MAPK (247). In NIH 3T3 fibroblasts, PKC-δ overexpression does not alter the ability of PDGF to induce a mitogenic response, suggesting that PKC-δ may not mediate PDGF-induced DNA synthesis (245). Moreover, PKC-δ overexpression in 32D cells transfected with PDGF-B receptors caused monocytic differentiation in response to PDGF stimulation (21).

Immediate-Early Genes

A large number of immediate-early genes are activated by PDGF. These genes, which are defined by induction without prerequisite protein synthesis (248), include c-*fos*, c-*jun* (28), *jun*B, c-*myc* (249), and Egr-1 (250). PDGF induction of c-*fos*, c-*jun*, and *jun*B is blocked by genistein, which interferes with receptor autophosphorylation, demonstrating that receptor autophosphorylation is essential for immediate-early gene induction (251,286). PDGF induction of Egr-1, however, was not inhibited by genistein or the oncogenes v-*ras* (252) and v-*mos* (253), suggesting that PDGF signaling is not necessarily dependent on receptor tyrosine autophosphorylation (248).

PDGF has been strongly implicated in a diverse array of normal and pathological settings. Some of these processes appear to involve autocrine and/or paracrine growth loops. PDGF binds to specific cell surface receptors and activates signaling and transcriptional pathways, which in turn stimulate cellular changes and/or the expression of other genes. The production of PDGF is controlled at multiple levels, including transcription, mRNA stability, translation, and secretion, as well as by binding proteins. A greater understanding of the mechanisms involved in the synthesis of PDGF and how it elicits its many biological effects will facilitate more specific therapeutic approaches in the management of diseases in which it plays a role.

REFERENCES

1. Kohler N, Lipton A. Platelets as a source of fibroblast growth promoting activity. *Exp Cell Res* 1974;87:297–301.
2. Ross R, Glomset J, Kariya B, et al. A platelet dependent serum factor that stimulates the proliferation of arterial smooth muscle cells *in vitro. Proc Natl Acad Sci USA* 1974;30:1207–1210.
3. Westermark B, Wasteson A. A platelet factor stimulating human normal glial cells. *Exp Cell Res* 1976;98:170–174.
4. Antoniades HN, Scher CD, Stiles CD. Purification of platelet-derived growth factor. *Proc Natl Acad Sci USA* 1979;76:1809–1813.
5. Deuel TF, Huang JS, Proffit RT, et al. Human platelet-derived growth factor: purification and resolution into two active protein fractions. *J Biol Chem* 1981;256:8896–8899.
6. Heldin CH, Westermark B, Wasteson A. Platelet derived growth factor: purification and partial characterisation. *Proc Natl Acad Sci USA* 1979;76:3722–3726.
7. Betsholtz C, Johnsson A, Heldin CH, et al. cDNA sequence and chromosomal localization of human platelet-derived growth factor A-chain and its expression in tumor cell lines. *Nature* 1986;320:695–699.
8. Bonthron DT, Morton CC, Orkin SH, et al. Platelet-derived growth factor A chain: gene structure, chromosomal location, and basis for alternative mRNA splicing. *Proc Natl Acad Sci USA* 1988;85:1492–1496.
9. Rorsman F, Bywater M, Knott TJ. et al. Structural characterization of the human platelet-derived growth factor A-chain cDNA and gene: alternative exon usage predicts two different precursor proteins. *Mol Cell Biol* 1988;8:571–577.
10. Young RM, Mendoza AE, Collins T, et al. Alternatively spliced platelet-derived growth factor A-chain transcripts are not tumor specific but encode normal cellular proteins. *Mol Cell Biol* 1990;10:6051–6054.
11. Collins T, Pober JS, Gimbrone MA Jr. et al. Cultured human endothelial cells express platelet-derived growth factor A chain. *Am J Pathol* 1987;127:7–12.
12. Takimoto Y, Wang ZY, Kobler K, et al. Promoter region of the human platelet-derived growth factor A-chain gene. *Proc Natl Acad Sci USA* 1991;88:1686–1690.
13. Bartram CR, de Klein A, Hagenmeijer A, et al. Localisation of the human c-sis oncogene in ph-negative chronic myelocytic leukemia by *in situ* hybridization. *Blood* 1984;63:223–225.
14. Dalla-Favera R, Gallo RC. Giallongo A, et al. Chromosomal localisation of the human homologue (c-sis) of the simian sarcoma virus onc gene. *Science* 1982;219:686–688.
15. Devare SG, Reddy EP, Law DJ, et al. Nucleotide sequence of the simian sarcoma virus genome: demonstration that its acquired cellular sequences encode the transforming gene product p28sis. *Proc Natl Acad Sci USA* 1983;30:731–735.
16. Doolittle RF, Hunkapiller MW, Hood IE, et al. Simian sarcoma virus onc gene, v-sis, is derived from the gene (or genes) encoding a platelet-derived growth factor. *Science* 1983;221:275–277.
17. Johnsson A, Betsholtz C. Heldin CH, et al. The C-SIS gene encodes a precursor of the B chain of platelet derived growth factor. *EMBO J* 1984;3:921–928.
18. Barrett TB, Gajdusek CM, Schwartz SM, et al. Expression of the sis gene by endothelial cells in culture and *in vivo. Proc Natl Acad Sci USA* 1984;81:6772–6774.
19. Hammacher A, Nister M, Westermark B, et al. A human glioma cell line secretes three structurally and functionally different dimeric forms of platelet-derived growth factor. *Eur J Biochem* 1988;176:179–186.
20. Deuel TF, Huang JS. Platelet-derived growth factor: purification, properties, and biological activities. In: Brown EB, ed. *Progress in hematology,* vol 8. New York: Grune and Stratton, 1983:201–221.
21. Heldin CH, Ostman A, Ronnstrand L. Signal transduction via platelet derived growth factor receptors. *Biochim Biophys Acta* 1998;1378:F79–F113.
22. Claesson-Welsh L, Eriksson A, Moren A, et al. cDNA cloning and expression of a human platelet-derived growth factor (PDGF) receptor specific for a B-chain-containing PDGF molecule. *Mol Cell Biol* 1988;8:3476–3486.
23. Claesson-Welsh L, Eriksson A, Westermark B, et al. cDNA cloning and expression of the human A-type platelet derived growth factor (PDGF) receptor establishes structural similarity to the B-type receptor. *Proc Natl Acad Sci USA* 1989;86:4917–4921.
24. Matsui T, Heidaran M, Miki T, et al. Isolation of a novel receptor cDNA establishes the existence of two PDGF receptor genes. *Science* 1989;243:1532–1535.
25. Yarden Y, Escobedo JA, Kuang WJ, et al. Structure of the receptor for platelet-derived growth factor helps define a family of closely related growth factor receptors. *Nature* 1986;323:226–232.
26. Claesson-Welsh L. Platelet-derived growth factor receptor signals. *J Biol Chem* 1994;269:32023–32026.
27. Heidaran MA, Pierce JH, Jensen RA, et al. Chimeric alpha- and beta-platelet-derived growth factor (PDGF) receptors define three immunoglobulin-like domains of the alpha-PDGF receptor that determine PDGF-AA binding specificity. *J Biol Chem* 1990;265:18741–18744.
28. Yu JC, Mahadevan D, LaRochelle WJ, et al. Structural coincidence of alpha PDGFR epitopes binding to platelet-derived growth factor-AA and a potent neutralizing monoclonal antibody. *J Biol Chem* 1994;269:10668–10674.
29. Hammacher A, Mellstrom K, Heldin CH, et al. Isoform-specific induction of actin reorganization by platelet-derived growth factor suggests that the functionally active receptor is a dimer. *EMBO J* 1989;8:2489–2495.
30. Heldin NE, Gustavsson B, Claesson-Welsh L. et al. Aberrant expression of receptors for platelet-derived growth factor in an anaplastic thyroid carcinoma cell line. *Proc Natl Acad Sci USA* 1988;85:9302–9306.
31. Yoyote K, Mori S, Siegbahn A, et al. Structural determinants in the platelet-derived growth factor alpha-receptor implicated in modulation of chemotaxis. *J Biol Chem* 1996;271:5101–5111.
32. Ataliotis P, Mercola M. Distribution and functions of platelet-derived growth factors and their receptors during embryogenesis. *Int Rev Cytol* 1997;172:95–127.
33. Jones SD, Ho L, Smith JC, et al. The *Xenopus* platelet-derived growth factor alpha receptor cDNA cloning and demonstration that mesoderm induction estab-

lishes the lineage-specific pattern of ligand and receptor gene expression. *Dev Genet* 1993;14:185–193.

34. Mercola M, Melton DA, Stiles CD. Platelet-derived growth factor A chain is maternally encoded in *Xenopus* embryos. *Science* 1988;241:1223–1225.

35. Palmieri SL, Stiles CD, Mercola M. PDGF in the developing embryo. *Cytokines* 1993;5:115–128.

36. Ho L, Symes K, Yordan C. et al. Localization of PDGF A and PDGFR alpha mRNA in *Xenopus* embryos suggests signalling from neural ectoderm and pharyngeal endoderm to neural crest cells. *Mech Dev* 1994;48: 165–174.

37. Orr-Urtreger A, Lonai P. Platelet-derived growth factor-A and its receptor are expressed in separate, but adjacent cell layers of the mouse embryo. *Development* 1992;115:1045–1058.

38. Han RNN, Liu J, Tanswell AK, et al. Ontogeny of platelet-derived growth factor receptor (PDGFR) in fetal lung. *Microsc Res Tech* 1993;26:381–388.

39. Alpers CE, Seifert RA, Hudkins KL, et al. Development patterns of PDGF B-chain, PDGF-receptor, and alpha-actin expression in human glomerulogenesis. *Kidney Int* 1992;42:390–399.

40. Lindahl P, Betsholtz C. Not all myofibroblasts are alike: revisiting the role of PDGF-A and PDGF-B using PDGF-targeted mice. *Curr Opin Nephrol Hypertens* 1998;7:21–26.

41. Claesson-Welsh L. PDGF receptors: structure and mechanism of action. In: Westermark B, Sorg C, eds. *Cytokines. Biology of platelet-derived growth factor.* Basel: Karger, vol. 5, 1993:31–43.

42. Bostrom H, Willetts K, Pekny M, et al. PDGF-A signalling is a critical event in lung alveolar myofibroblast development and alveogenesis. *Cell* 1996;85:863–873.

43. Leveen P, Pekny M, Gebre-Medhin S, et al. Mice deficient for PDGF B show renal, cardiovascular and hematological abnormalities. *Genes Dev* 1994;8:1875–1887.

44. Soriano P. Abnormal kidney development and hematogical disorders in PDGF β receptor mutant mice. *Genes Dev* 1994;8:1888–1896.

45. Schatteman GC, Morrison-Graham K, Van Koppen A, et al. Regulation and role of PDGF receptor alpha subunit expression during embryogenesis. *Development* 1992;115:123–131.

46. Lindahl P, Johansson BR, Leveen P, et al. Pericyte loss and microaneurysm formation in PGDF-B-deficient mice. *Science* 1997;277:242–245.

47. Silverman ES, Collins T. Pathways of Egr-1 mediated gene transcription in vascular biology. *Am J Pathol* 1999;154:665–670.

48. Sims DE. The pericyte—a review. *Tissue Cell* 1986; 18:153–174.

49. Betsholtz C, Raines EW. Platelet-derived growth factor: a key regulator of connective tissue cells in embyogenesis and pathogenesis. *Kidney Int* 1997;51: 1361–1369.

50. Schlondorff D. The glomerular mesangial cell: an expanding role for a specialized pericyte. *FASEB J* 1987; 1:272–281.

51. Crosby JR, Seifert RA, Soriano P, et al. Chimaeric analysis reveals role of PDGF receptors in all muscle lineages *Nat Genet* 1998;18:385–388.

52. Yeh HJ, Ruit K, Wang YX, et al. PDGF A chain is expressed in mammalian neurons during development and maturity. *Cell* 1991;64:209–216.

53. Sasahara A, Kott JN, Sasahara M, et al. Platelet-derived growth factor B-chain-like immunoreactivity in the developing and adult rat brain. *Dev Brain Res* 1992; 68:41–53.

54. Sasahara M, Fries JW, Raines EW, et al. PDGF B-chain in neurons of the central nervous system, posterior pituitary, and in a transgenic model. *Cell* 1991;64: 217–227.

55. Valenzuela CF, Kazlauskas A, Weiner JL. Roles of platelet-derived growth factor in the developing and mature nervous systems. *Brain Res Brain Res Rev* 1997;24:77–89.

56. Engel U, Wolswijk G. Oligodendrocyte type 2 astrocyte (O-2A) progenitor cells derived from adult rat spinal cord: *in vitro* characteristics and response to PDGF, bFGF and NT-3. *Glia* 1996;16:16–26.

57. Raff MC. Glial cell diversification in the rat optic nerve. *Science* 1989;243:1450–1455.

58. McKinnon RD, Matsui T, Dubois-Dalcq M, et al. FGF modulates the PDGF-driven pathway of oligodendrocyte development. *Neuron* 1990;5:603–614.

59. Morrison-Graham K, Schatteman GC, Bork T, et al. A PDGF receptor mutation in the mouse (patch) perturbs the development of a non-neuronal subset of neural crest-derived cells. *Development* 1992;115:133–142.

60. Horner A, Bord S, Kemp P, et al. Distribution of platelet-derived growth factor (PDGF) A chain mRNA, protein, and PDGF-alpha receptor in rapidly forming human bone. *Bone* 1996;19:353–362.

61. Centrella MT, McCarthy ML, Canalis E. Platelet-derived growth factor enhances deoxyribonucleic acid and collagen synthesis in osteoblast-enriched cultures from fetal rat parietal bone. *Endocrinology* 1989;125: 13–19.

62. Cochran DL, Rouse CA, Lynch SE, et al. Effects of platelet-derived growth factor isoforms on calcium release from neonatal mouse calvariae. *Bone* 1993;14: 53–58.

63. Pfeilschifter J, Oechsner M, Naumann A, et al. Stimulation of bone matrix apposition *in vitro* by local growth factors: a comparison between insulin-like growth factor I platelet-derived growth factor, and transforming growth factor beta. *Endocrinology* 1990; 127:69–75.

64. Piche JE, Graves DT. Study of the growth factor requirements of human bone-derived cells: a comparison with human fibroblasts. *Bone* 1989;10:131–138.

65. Gilardetti RS, Chaibi MS, Stroumza J, et al. High-affinity binding of PDGF-AA and PDGF-BB to normal human osteoblastic cells and modulation by interleukin-1. *Am J Physiol* 1991;261:C980–C985.

66. DiCorleto PE, Bowen-Pope DF. Cultured endothelial cells produce a platelet-derived growth factor-like protein. *Proc Natl Acad Sci USA* 1983;80:1919–1923.

67. Dirks RPH, Bloemers HP. Signals controlling the expression of PDGF. *Mol Biol Rep* 1996;22:1–24.

68. Sitaras NM, Sariban E, Pantazis P, et al. Human iliac artery endothelial cells express both genes encoding the chains of platelet-derived growth factor (PDGF) and synthesize PDGF-like mitogen. *J Cell Physiol* 1987;132:376–380.

69. Khachigian LM, Lindner V, Williams AJ, et al. Egr-1-induced endothelial gene expression: a common

theme in vascular injury. *Science* 1996;271:1427–1431.

70. Lindner V, Reidy MA. Platelet-derived growth factor ligand and receptor expression by large vessel endothelium *in vivo*. *Am J Pathol* 1995;146:1488–1497.

71. Smits A, Hermansson M, Nister M, et al. Rat brain capillary endothelial cells express functional PDGF B-type receptors. *Growth Factors* 1989;2:1–8.

72. Beitz JG, Kim IS, Calabresi P, et al. Human microvascular endothelial cells express receptors for platelet-derived growth factor. *Proc Natl Acad Sci USA* 1991; 88:2021–2025.

73. Holmgren L, Glaser A, Pfeifer-Ohlsson S, et al. Angiogenesis during human extraembryonic development involves the spatiotemporal control of PDGF ligand and receptor gene expression. *Development* 1991;113: 749–754.

74. Sjolund M, Hedin U, Sejersen T, et al. Arterial smooth muscle cells express platelet-derived growth factor (PDGF) A chain mRNA, secrete a PDGF-like mitogen, and bind exogenous PDGF in a phenotype- and growth state–dependent manner. *J Cell Biol* 1988;106:403–413.

75. Majesky MW, Benditt EP, Schwartz SM. Expression and developmental control of platelet-derived growth factor A-chain and B-chain/Sis genes in rat aortic smooth muscle cells. *Proc Natl Acad Sci USA* 1988; 85:1524–1528.

76. Seifert RA, Schwartz SM, Bowen-Pope DF. Developmentally regulated production of platelet-derived growth factor-like molecules. *Nature* 1984;311:669–671.

77. Rafty LA, Khachigian LM. Zinc finger transcription factors mediate high constitutive platelet-derived growth factor-B expression in smooth muscle cells derived from aortae of newborn rats. *J Biol Chem* 1998; 273:5758–5764.

78. Kaplan DR, Chao FC, Stiles FC, et al. Platelet alpha granules contain a growth factor for fibroblasts. *Blood* 1979;53:1043–1052.

79. Hart CE, Bailey M, Curtis DA, et al. Purification of PDGF-AB and PDGF-BB from human platelet extracts and identification of all PDGF dimers in human platelets. *Biochemistry* 1990;29:166–172.

80. Stroobant P, Waterfield MD. Purification and properties of porcine platelet-derived growth factor. *EMBO J* 1984;3:2963–2967.

81. Gladwin AM, Carrier MJ, Beesley JE, et al. Identification of mRNA for PDGF B-chain in human megakaryocytes isolated using a novel immunomagnetic separation method. *Br J Haematol* 1990;76:333–339.

82. Mannaioni PF, Di Bello MG, Masini E. Platelets and inflammation: role of platelet-derived growth factor, adhesion molecules and histamine. *Inflamm Res* 1997; 46:4–18.

83. Ferns GA, Raines EW, Sprugel KH, et al. Inhibition of neointimal smooth muscle accumulation after angioplasty by an antibody to PDGF. *Science* 1991;253: 1129–1132.

84. Soma Y, Takehara K, Ishibashi Y. Alteration of the chemotactic response of human skin fibroblasts to PDGF by growth factors. *Exp Cell Res* 1994;212: 274–277.

85. Bach MK, Brashler JR, Stout BK, et al. Platelet-derived growth factor can activate purified primate, phorbol myristate acetate-primed eosinophils. *Int Arch Allergy Appl Immunol* 1991;94:167–168.

86. Vassbotn FS, Havnen OK, Heldin CH, et al. Negative feedback regulation of human platelets via autocrine activation of the platelet-derived growth factor alpha-receptor. *J Biol Chem* 1994;269:13874–13879.

87. Meyer-Ingold W, Eichner W. Platelet derived growth factor. *Cell Biol Int* 1995;19:389–398.

88. Hosgood G. Wound healing. The role of platelet-derived growth factor and transforming growth factor beta. *Vet Surg* 1993;22:490–495.

89. Pierce GF, Mustoe TA, Altrock BW, et al. Role of platelet-derived growth factor in wound healing. *J Cell Biochem* 1991;45:319–326.

90. Pierce GF, Tarpley JE, Allman RM, et al. Tissue repair processes in healing chronic pressure ulcers treated with recombinant platelet-derived growth factor BB. *Am J Pathol* 1994;145:1399–1410.

91. Battegay EJ. Angiogenesis: mechanistic insights, neovascular diseases, and therapeutic prospects. *J Mol Med* 1995;73:333–346.

92. Krane J, Murphy DP, Gottlieb AB. Increased dermal expression of platelet derived growth factor receptors in growth activated skin wounds and psoriasis. *J Invest Dermatol* 1991;96:983–986.

93. Olerud J, Usui ML, Hart CE. Localization of PDGF and PDGF receptor in human cutaneous wounds. *J Invest Dermatol* 1991;96:563(abst).

94. Plate KH, Breier G, Farrell CL, et al. Platelet-derived growth factor receptor-beta is induced during tumor development and upregulated during tumor progression in endothelial cells in human gliomas. *Lab Invest* 1992;67:529–534.

95. Risau W, Drexler H, Mironov V. et al. Platelet-derived growth factor is angiogenic *in vivo*. *Growth Factors* 1992;7:261–266.

96. Battegay EJ, Rupp J, Iruela-Arispe L, et al. PDGF-BB modulates endothelial proliferation and angiogenesis *in vitro* via PDGF beta-receptors. *J Cell Biol* 1994; 125:917–928.

97. Thommen R, Humar R, Misevic G, et al. PDGF BB increases endothelial migration and cord movements during angiogenesis *in vitro*. *J Cell Biochem* 1997;64: 403–413.

98. Williams GT, Smith CA. Molecular regulation of apoptosis: genetic controls on cell death. *Cell* 1993; 74:777–779.

99. Okura T, Igase M. Kitami Y, et al. Platelet-derived growth factor induces apoptosis in vascular smooth muscle cells: roles of the Bcl-2 family. *Biochim Biophys Acta* 1998;1403:245–253.

100. Brown DL, Kao WW, Greenhalgh DG. Apoptosis down-regulates inflammation under the advancing epithelial wound edge: delayed patterns in diabetes and improvement with topical growth factors. *Surgery* 1997;121:372–380.

101. Waterfield MD, Scrace GT, Whittle N, et al. Platelet-derived growth factor is structurally related to the putative transforming protein p28sis of simian sarcoma virus. *Nature* 1983;304:35–39.

102. Pantazis P, Sariban E. Bohan CA, et al. Synthesis of PDGF by cultured human T cells transformed with HTLV-I and II. *Oncogene* 1987;1:285–289.

103. Silver BJ. Platelet-derived growth factor in human malignancy. *Biofactors* 1992;3:217–227.

104. Frappaz D, Singletary SE, Spitzer G, et al. Enhancement of growth of primary metastatic fresh human tumors of the nervous system by epidermal growth factor in serum-free short term culture. *Neurosurgery* 1988; 23:355–359.

105. Pollack IF, Randall MS, Kristofik MP, et al. Response of low-passage human malignant gliomas *in vitro* to stimulation and selective inhibition of growth factor-mediated pathways. *J Neurosurg* 1991;75:284–293.

106. Westphal M, Brunken M, Rohde E, et al. Growth factors in cultured human glioma cells: differential effects of FGF, EGF and PDGF. *Cancer Lett* 1988;38: 283–296.

107. Finn PE, Bjerkvig R, Pilkington GJ. The role of growth factors in the malignant and invasive progression of intrinsic brain tumours. *Anticancer Res* 1997;17: 4163–4172.

108. Engebraaten O, Bjerkvig R, Pedersen PH, et al. Effects of EGF, bFGF, NGF and PDGF(bb) on cell proliferative migratory and invasive capacities of human brain-tumour biopsies *in vitro*. *Int J Cancer* 1993;53: 209–214.

109. Di Stefano JF, Kirchner M, Dagenhardt K, et al. Activation of cancer cell proteases and cytotoxicity by EGF and PDGF growth factors. *Am J Med Sci* 1990;300: 9–15.

110. Smith RJ, Justen JM, Sam LM, et al. Platelet-derived growth factor potentiates cellular responses of articular chondrocytes to interleukin-1. *Arthritis Rheum* 1991; 34:697–706.

111. Poggi A, Vicenzi E, Cioce V, et al. Platelet contribution to cancer cell growth and migration: the role of platelet growth factors. *Haemostasis* 1988;18:18–28.

112. Katano M, Nakamura M. Fujimoto K, et al. Prognostic value of platelet-derived growth factor-A (PDGF-A) in gastric carcinoma. *Ann Surg* 1998;227:365–371.

113. Ross R. The pathogenesis of atherosclerosis: a perspective for the 1990's. *Nature* 1993;362:801–808.

114. Ross R. Atherosclerosis—an inflammatory disease. *N Engl J Med* 1999;340:115–126.

115. Wilcox JN, Smith KM, Williams LT, et al. Platelet-derived growth factor mRNA detection in human atherosclerotic plaques by *in-situ* hybridization. *J Clin Invest* 1988;82:1134–1143.

116. Barrett TB, Benditt EP. sis (platelet-derived growth factor B chain) gene transcript levels are elevated in human atherosclerotic lesions compared to normal artery. *Proc Natl Acad Sci USA* 1987;84:1099–1103.

117. Libby P, Warner SJC, Salomon RN, et al. Production of platelet derived growth factor like mitogen by smooth muscle cells from human atheroma. *N Engl J Med* 1988;318:1493–1498.

118. Clowes AW, Reidy MA. Clowes MM. Kinetics of cellular proliferation after arterial injury. I. Smooth muscle growth in the absence of endothelium. *Lab Invest* 1983;49:327–333.

119. Lindner V, Reidy MA, Fingerle J. Regrowth of arterial endothelium. Denudation with minimal trauma leads to complete endothelial cell regrowth. *Lab Invest* 1989; 6:556–563.

120. Clowes AW, Clowes MM. Kinetics of cellular proliferation after arterial injury. IV. Heparin inhibits rat smooth muscle mitogenesis and migration. *Circ Res* 1986;58:839–845.

121. Lindner V, Reidy MA. Role of basic fibroblast growth factor in proliferation of endothelium and smooth muscle after denuding injury *in vivo*. *EXS* 1992;61: 386–368.

122. Jawien A, Bowen-Pope DF, Lindner V, et al. Platelet-derived growth factor promotes smooth muscle migration and intimal thickening in a rat model of balloon angioplasty. *J Clin Invest* 1992;89:507–511.

123. Majesky M, Reidy MW, Bowen-Pope DF, et al. PDGF ligand and receptor gene expression during repair of arterial injury. *J Cell Biol* 1990;111:2149–2158.

124. Silverman ES, Khachigian LM, Lindner V, et al. Inducible PDGF A-chain transcription in smooth muscle cells is mediated by Egr-1 displacement of Sp1 and Sp3. *Am J Physiol* 1997;273:H1415–H126.

125. Lindner V. Role of basic fibroblast growth factor and platelet-derived growth factor (B-chain) in neointima formation after arterial injury. *Z Kardiol* 1995;84: 137–144.

126. Koyama N, Hart CE, Clowes AW. Different functions of the platelet-derived growth factor-alpha and -beta receptors for the migration and proliferation of cultured baboon smooth muscle cells. *Circ Res* 1994;75: 682–691.

127. Koyama N, Morisaki N, Saito Y, et al. Regulatory effects of platelet-derived growth factor-AA homodimer on migration of vascular smooth muscle cells. *J Biol Chem* 1992;267:22806–22812.

128. Fukuda N, Kubo A, Watanabe Y, et al. Antisense oligodeoxynucleotide complementary to platelet-derived growth factor A-chain messenger RNA inhibits the arterial proliferation in spontaneously hypertensive rats without altering their blood pressures. *J Hypertens* 1997;15:1123–1136.

129. Dangas G, Fuster V. Management of restenosis after coronary intervention. *Am Heart J* 1996;132:428–436.

130. Kastrati A, Schuhlen H, Hausleiter J, et al. Restenosis after coronary stent placement and randomization to a 4-week combined antiplatelet or anticoagulant therapy: six-month angiographic follow-up of the Intracoronary Stenting and Antithrombotic Regimen (ISAR) Trial [see comments]. *Circulation* 1997;96:462–467.

131. Cercek B, Sharifi B, Barath P, et al. Growth factors in pathogenesis of coronary arterial restenosis. *Am J Cardiol* 1991;68:24C-33C.

132. Maresta A, Balducelli M, Cantini L, et al. Trapidil (triazolopyrimidine), a platelet-derived growth factor antagonist, reduces restenosis after percutaneous transluminal coronary angioplasty. Results of the randomized, double-blind STARC study. *Circulation* 1994;90: 2710–2715.

133. Bonisch D, Weber AA, Wittpoth M, et al. Antimitogenic effects of trapidil in coronary artery smooth muscle cells by direct activation of protein kinase A. *Mol Pharmacol* 1998;54:241–248.

134. Bartel SH, Tenor H, Krause EG. Trapidil derivatives as potent inhibitors of cyclic AMP phosphodiesterase from heart and coronary arteries. *Biochim Biophys Acta* 1985;44:K31–K35.

135. Noguchi K, Tomoike II, Kawachi Y, et al. Effects of trapidil and nitroglycerin on coronary circulation in conscious dogs. *Arzneimittelforschung* 1984;34:872–876.

136. Miyazawa K, Kikuchi S. Fukuyama J, et al. Inhibition of PDGF- and TGF-β1-induced collagen synthesis, migration and proliferation by tranilast in vascular

smooth muscle cells from spontaneously hypertensive rats. *Atherosclerosis* 1995;118:213–221.

137. Kosuga K, Tamai H, Ueda K, et al. Effectiveness of tranilast on restenosis after directional coronary atherectomy. *Am Heart J* 1997;134:712–718.

138. Isaji M, Miyata H, Ajisawa Y, et al. Inhibition by tranilast of vascular endothelial growth factor (VEGF)/ vascular permeability factor (VPF)-induced increase in vascular permeability in rats. *Life Sci* 1998;63:PL71– PL74.

139. Ward MR. Sasahara T, Agrotis A, et al. Inhibitory effects of tranilast on expression of transforming growth factor-beta isoforms and receptors in injured arteries. *Atherosclerosis* 1998;137:267–275.

140. Inoue H, Ohshima H, Kono H, et al. Suppressive effects of tranilast on the expression of inducible cyclooxygenase (COX2) in interleukin-1beta-stimulated fibroblasts. *Biochem Pharmacol* 1997;53:1941– 1944.

141. Miyazawa K, Fukuyama J, Misawa K, et al. Tranilast antagonizes angiotensin II and inhibits its biological effects in vascular smooth muscle cells. *Atherosclerosis* 1996;121:167–173.

142. Miyazawa K, Hamano S, Ujiie A. Antiproliferative and c-myc mRNA suppressive effect of tranilast on newborn human vascular smooth muscle cells in culture. *Br J Pharmacol* 1996;118:915–922.

143. Abboud HE. Role of platelet derived growth factor in renal injury. *Annu Rev Physiol* 1995;57:297–309.

144. Floege J, Johnson RJ, Alpers CE, et al. Visceral glomerular epithelial cells can proliferate *in vivo* and synthesize PDGF-B chain. *Am J Pathol* 1993;142: 637–650.

145. Couser WG, Johnson RJ. Mechanisms of progressive renal disease in glomerulonephritis. *Am J Kidney Dis* 1994;23:193–195.

146. Jaffer FE, Knauss TC, Poptic E, et al. Endothelin stimulates DNA synthesis and PDGF secretion in mesangial cells. *Kidney Int* 1990;38:1193–1198.

147. Johnson RJ. The glomerular response to injury: progression or resolution? *Kidney Int* 1994;45:1769– 1782.

148. Johnson RJ, Raines EW, Floege J, et al. Inhibition of mesangial cell proliferation and matrix expansion in glomerulonephritis in the rat by antibody to platelet-derived growth factor. *J Exp Med* 1992;175:1413– 1416.

149. Deguchi Y, Kishimoto S. Enhancement of c-sis proto-oncogene transcription in bronchoalveolar mononuclear cells from patients with pulmonary sarcoidosis. *J Clin Pathol* 1990;43:295–297.

150. Nagaoka I, Trapnell BC, Crystal RG. Upregulation of platelet-derived growth factor -A and -B expression in alveolar macrophages of individuals with idiopathic pulmonary fibrosis. *J Clin Invest* 1990;85:2023–2027.

151. Kaiser M, Weyand CM, Bjornsson J, et al. Platelet-derived growth factor, intimal hyperplasia, and ischemic complications in giant cell arteritis. *Arthritis Rheum* 1998;41:623–633.

152. Ohba T, Takase Y, Ohbara M, et al. Thrombin in the synovial fluid of patients with rheumatoid arthritis mediates proliferation of synovial fibroblast-like cells by induction of platelet derived growth factor. *J Rheumatol* 1996;23:1505–1511.

153. Inaba T, Ishibashi S, Gotoda T, et al. Enhanced expression of platelet-derived growth factor-beta receptor by high glucose. Involvement of platelet-derived growth factor in diabetic angiopathy. *Diabetes* 1996;45: 507–512.

154. Mizutani M, Okuda Y, Yamaoka T, et al. High glucose and hyperosmolarity increase platelet-derived growth factor mRNA levels in cultured human vascular endothelial cells. *Biochem Biophys Res Commun* 1992;187: 664–669.

155. Nakamura T, Fukui M, Ebihara I, et al. mRNA expression of growth factors in glomeruli from diabetic rats. *Diabetes* 1993;42:450–456.

156. Webster HD. Growth factors and myelin regeneration in multiple sclerosis. *Multi Scler* 1997;3:113–120.

157. Grinspan J, Wrabetz L, Kamholz J. Oligodendrocyte maturation and myelin gene expression in PDGF-treated cultures from rat cerebral white matter. *J Neurocytol* 1993;22:322–333.

158. Honegger P, Tenot-Sparti M. Developmental effects of basic fibroblast growth factor and platelet-derived growth factor on glial cells in a three-dimensional cell culture system. *J Neuroimmunol* 1992;40:295–303.

159. Fressinaud C, Vallat JM, Pouplard-Barthelaix A. Platelet-derived growth factor partly prevents chemically induced oligodendrocyte death and improves myelin-like membrane repair *in vitro*. *Glia* 1996;16:40–50.

160. Sjoborg M, Pietz K, Ahgren A, et al. Expression of platelet-derived growth factor after intrastriatal ibotenic acid injury. *Exp Brain Res* 1998;119:245–250.

161. Khachigian LM, Chesterman CN. Platelet derived growth factor and its receptor: structure and roles in normal growth and pathology. *Platelets* 1993;4: 304–315.

162. Ross R, Raines EW. Platelet-derived growth factor—its role in health and disease. *Adv Exp Med Biol* 1988;234:9–21.

163. Khachigian LM, Collins T. Inducible expression of Egr-1-dependent genes. A paradigm of transcriptional activation in vascular endothelium. *Circ Res* 1997;81: 457–461.

164. Khachigian LM, Williams AJ, Collins T. Interplay of Sp1 and Egr-1 in the proximal platelet-derived growth factor A-chain promoter in cultured vascular endothelial cells. *J Biol Chem* 1995;270:27679–27686.

165. Imagawa M, Chiu R, Karin M. Transcription factor AP-2 mediates induction by two different signal-transduction pathways: protein kinase C and cAMP. *Cell* 1987;51:251–260.

166. Sukhatme VP, Cao XM, Chang LC. et al. A zinc finger-encoding gene coregulated with c-fos during growth and differentiation, and after cellular depolarization. *Cell* 1988;53:37–43.

167. Tsai-Morris CH, Cao XM, Sukhatme VP. 5′ Flanking sequence and genomic structure of Egr-1, a murine mitogen inducible zinc finger encoding gene. *Nucleic Acids Res* 1988;16:8835–8846.

168. Lin X, Wang Z, Gu L, et al. Functional analysis of the human platelet-derived growth factor A-chain promoter region. *J Biol Chem* 1992;267:25614–25619.

169. Bhandari B, Wenzel UO, Marra F, et al. A nuclear protein in mesangial cells that binds to the promoter region of the platelet-derived growth factor-A chain gene. Induction by phorbol ester. *J Biol Chem* 1995; 270:5541–5548.

170. Jin HM, Robinson DF, Liang Y, et al. SIS/PDGF-B promoter isolation and characterization of regulatory

elements necessary for basal expression of the SIS/PDGF-B gene in U2-OS osteosarcoma cells. *J Biol Chem* 1994;269:28648–28654.

171. Khachigian LM, Fries JW, Benz MW. et al. Novel cis-acting elements in the human platelet-derived growth factor B-chain core promoter that mediate gene expression in cultured vascular endothelial cells. *J Biol Chem* 1994;269:22647–22656.

172. Pech M, Rao CD, Robbins KC, et al. Functional identification of regulatory elements within the promoter region of platelet-derived growth factor 2. *Mol Cell Biol* 1989;9:396–405.

173. Dirks RPH, Jansen HJ, Gerritsma J, et al. Localization and functional analysis of DNase-1-hypersensitive sites in the human c-sis/PDGF-B gene transcription unit and its flanking regions. *Eur J Biochem* 1993;211: 509–519.

174. Liang Y, Robinson DF, Dennig J, et al. Transcriptional regulation of the SIS/PDGF-B gene in human osteosarcoma cells by the Sp family of transcription factors. *J Biol Chem* 1996;271:11792–11797.

175. Scarpati EM, DiCorleto PE. Identification of a thrombin response element in the human platelet-derived growth factor B-chain (c-sis) promoter. *J Biol Chem* 1996;271:3025–3032.

176. Trejo SR, Fahl WE, Ratner L. c-sis/PDGF-B promoter transactivation by the Yax protein of human T-cell leukemia virus type 1. *J Biol Chem* 1996;271:14584–14590.

177. Hagen G, Muller S, Beato M, et al. Sp1-mediated transcriptional activation is repressed by Sp3. *EMBO J* 1994;13:3843–3851.

178. Majello B, De Luca P, Hagen G, et al. Different members of the Sp1 multigene family exert opposite transcriptional regulation of the long terminal repeat of HIV-1. *Nucleic Acids Res* 1994;22:4914–4921.

179. Gashler A, Sukhatme VP. Early growth response protein 1 (Egr-1): prototype of a zinc-finger family of transcription factors. *Prog Nucleic Acid Res Mol Biol* 1995;50:191–224.

180. Christy B, Nathans D. Functional serum response elements upstream of the growth factor-inducible gene zif268. *Mol Cell Biol* 1989;9:4889–4895.

181. Russo MW, Sevetson BR. Milbrandt J. Identification of NAB1, a repressor of NGFI-A- and Krox20-mediated transcription. *Proc Natl Acad Sci USA* 1995;92: 6873–6877.

182. Svaren J, Sevetson BR, Apel ED, et al. NAB2, a corepressor of NGFI-A (Egr-1) and Krox20, is induced by proliferative and differentiative stimuli. *Mol Cell Biol* 1996;16:3545–3553.

183. Swirnoff AH, Apel ED, Svaren J, et al. NAB1, a corepressor of NGFI-A (Egr-1), contains an active transcriptional repression domain. *Mol Cell Biol* 1998;18: 512–524.

184. Cui MZ, Parry GC, Oeth P, et al. Transcriptional regulation of the tissue factor gene in human epithelial cells is mediated by Sp1 and EGR-1. *J Biol Chem* 1996; 271:2731–2739.

185. Mackman N, Morrissey JH, Fowler B, et al. Complete sequence of the human tissue factor gene, a highly regulated cellular receptor that initiates the coagulation protease cascade. *Biochemistry* 1989;28:1755–1762.

186. Kim SJ, Glick A, Sporn MB, et al. Characterization of the promoter region of the human transforming growth factor-beta 1 gene. *J Biol Chem* 1989;264:402–408.

187. Riccio A, Grimaldi G, Verde P, et al. The human urokinase-plasminogen activator gene and its promoter. *Nucleic Acids Res* 1985;13:2759–2771.

188. Topper JN, Gimbrone MA Jr. Blood flow and vascular gene expression: fluid shear stress as a modulator of endothelial phenotype. *Mol Med Today* 1999;5:40–46.

189. Kraiss LW, Geary RL, Mattesson EJ, et al. Acute reductions in blood flow and shear stress induce platelet-derived growth factor-A expression in baboon prosthetic grafts. *Circ Res* 1996;79:45–53.

190. Khachigian LM, Anderson KR, Halnon NJ, et al. Egr-1 is activated in endothelial cells exposed to fluid shear stress and interacts with a novel shear-stress-response element in the PDGF A-chain promoter. *Arterioscler Thromb Vasc Biol* 1997;17:2280–2286.

191. Houston P, Dickson MC, Ludbrook V, et al. Fluid shear stress induction of the tissue factor promoter *in vitro* and *in vivo* is mediated by Egr-1. *Arterioscler Thromb Vasc Biol* 1999;19:281–289.

192. Schwachtgen JL, Houston P, Campbell C, et al. Fluid shear stress activation of egr-1 transcription in cultured human endothelial and epithelial cells is mediated via the extracellular signal-related kinase 1/2 mitogen-activated protein kinase pathway. *J Clin Invest* 1998;101: 2540–2549.

193. Resnick N, Collins T, Atkinson W, et al. Platelet-derived growth factor B chain promoter contains a cis-acting fluid shear-stress-responsive element. *Proc Natl Acad Sci USA* 1993;90:4591–4595.

194. Lan Q, Mercurius KO, Davies PF. Stimulation of transcription factors NF kappa B and AP1 in endothelial cells subjected to shear stress. *Biochem Biophys Res Commun* 1994;201:950–956.

195. Khachigian LM, Resnick N, Gimbrone MA Jr, et al. Nuclear factor-kappa B interacts functionally with the platelet-derived growth factor B-chain shear-stress response element in vascular endothelial cells exposed to fluid shear stress. *J Clin Invest* 1995;96:1169–1175.

196. Sumpio BE, Du W, Galagher G, et al. Regulation of PDGF-B in endothelial cells exposed to cyclic strain. *Arterioscler Thromb Vasc Biol* 1998;18:349–355.

197. Wilson E, Sudhir K, Ives HE. Mechanical strain of rat vascular smooth muscle cells is sensed by specific extracellular matrix/integrin interactions. *J Clin Invest* 1995;96:2364–2372.

198. Santiago FS, Lowe HC, Day FL, et al. Egr-1 induction by injury is triggered by release and paracrine activation by fibroblast growth factor 2. *Am J Pathol* 1999; 154:937–944.

199. Lowe HC, Chesterman CN, Khachigian LM. Left main coronary artery stenosis after percutaneous transluminal coronary angioplasty: importance of remaining minimally invasive. *Cathet Cardiovasc Intervent* 1999; 46:254–255.

200. Rorsman F, Leveen P, Betsholtz C. Platelet-derived growth factor (PDGF) A-chain mRNA heterogeneity generated by the use of alternative promoters and alternative polyadenylation sites. *Growth Factors* 1992;7: 241–251.

201. Feng L, Xia Y, Tang WW, et al. Cloning a novel form of rat PDGF A-chain with a unique 5′-UT: regulation during development and in glomerulonephritis. *Biochem Biophys Res Commun* 1993;194:1453–1459.

202. Fen Z, Daniel TO. 5′ Untranslated sequences determine degradative pathway for alternate PDGF B/c-sis mRNA's. *Oncogene* 1991;6:953–959.

203. Leveen P, Betsholtz C, Westermark B. Negative transacting mechanisms controlling expression of platelet-derived growth factor A and B MRNA in somatic cell hybrids. *Exp Cell Res* 1993;207:283–289.

204. Bhandari B, Abboud HE. Platelet derived growth factor-A chain gene expression in cultured mesangial cells: regulation by phorbol ester at the level of mRNA abundance, transcription and mRNA stability. *Mol Cell Endocrinol* 1993;91:185–191.

205. Bhandari B, Woodruff K, Abboud HE. Platelet-derived growth factor B-chain gene expression in mesangial cells: effect of phorbol ester on gene transcription and mRNA stability. *Mol Cell Endocrinol* 1994;140:31–36.

206. Daniel TO, Fen Z. Distinct pathways mediate transcriptional regulation of platelet-derived growth factor B/c-sis expression. *J Biol Chem* 1988;263:19815–19820.

207. Press RD, Samols D, Goldthwait DA. Expression and stability of c-sis mRNA in human glioblastoma cells. *Biochemistry* 1988;27:5736–5741.

208. Collins T, Bonthron DT, Orkin SH. Alternative RNA splicing affects function of encoded platelet-derived growth factor A chain. *Nature* 1987;328:621–624.

209. Tong BD, Auer DE, Jaye M, et al. cDNA clones reveal differences between human glial and endothelial cell platelet-derived growth factor A-chains. *Nature* 1987;328:619–621.

210. Sanchez A, Chesterman CN, Sleigh MJ. Novel human PDGF-A gene transcripts derived by alternative mRNA splicing. *Gene* 1991;98:295–298.

211. Nakahara K, Nishimura H, Kuro-o M, et al. Identification of three types of PDGF-A chain gene transcripts in rabbit vascular smooth muscle and their regulated expression during development and by angiotensin II. *Biochem Biophys Res Commun* 1992;184:811–818.

212. Rorsman F, Leveen P, Betsholtz C. Characterization of the mouse PDGF A-chain gene. Evolutionary conservation of gene structure, nucleotide sequence and alternative splicing. *Growth Factors* 1992;6:303–313.

213. Khachigian LM, Chesterman CN. Platelet-derived growth factor and alternative splicing: a review. *Pathology* 1992;24:280–290.

214. Matoskova BF, Rorsman F, Svensson V. et al. Alternative splicing of the platelet-derived growth factor A-chain transcript occurs in normal as well as tumor cells and is conserved among mammalian species. *Mol Cell Biol* 1989;9:3148–3150.

215. Kelly JL, Sanchez A, Brown G, et al. Accumulation of PDGF isoforms in the extracellular matrix. *J Cell Biol* 1993;121:1153–1163.

216. Maher DW, Lee BA, Donoghue DJ. The alternatively spliced exon of the platelet-derived growth factor A chain encodes a nuclear targeting signal. *Mol Cell Biol* 1989;9:2251–2253.

217. Rakowicz-Szulczynska EM, Rodeck Herlyn MU, et al. Chromatin binding of epidermal growth factor, nerve growth factor, and platelet-derived growth factor in cells bearing the appropriate surface receptors. *Proc Natl Acad Sci USA* 1986;83:3728–3732.

218. Khachigian LM, Owensby DA, Chesterman CN. A tyrosinated peptide representing the alternatively spliced exon of the platelet-derived growth factor A-chain binds specifically to cultured cells and interferes with binding of several growth factors. *J Biol Chem* 1992;267:1660–1666.

219. Ostman A, Backstrom G, Fong N, et al. Expression of three recombinant homodimeric isoforms of PDGF in *Saccharomyces cerevisiae:* evidence for difference in receptor binding and functional activities. *Growth Factors* 1989;1:271–281.

220. Bywater MF, Rorsman F, Bongcam-Rudolff E, et al. Expression of recombinant platelet-derived growth factor A- and B-chain homodimers in rat-1 cells and human fibroblasts reveals differences in protein processing and autocrine effects. *Mol Cell Biol* 1988;8:2753–2762.

221. Fukuda N, Kishioka H, Satoh C, et al. Role of long-form PDGF A-chain in the growth of vascular smooth muscle cells from spontaneously hypertensive rats. *Am J Hypertens* 1997;10:1117–1124.

222. Kozak M. Influences of mRNA secondary structure on initiation by eukaryotic ribosomes. *Proc Natl Acad Sci USA* 1986;83:2580–2584.

223. Rao CD, Pech M, Robbins KC. et al. The 5′ untranslated sequence of the c-sis/platelet-derived growth factor 2 transcript is a potent translational inhibitor. *Mol Cell Biol* 1988;8:284–292.

224. Ratner L. Regulation of expression of the c-sis proto-oncogene. *Nucleic Acids Res* 1989;17:4101–4115.

225. Ratner LB, Thielan B, Collins T. Sequences of the 5′ portion of the human c-sis gene: characterization of the transcriptional promoter and regulation of expression of the protein product by 5′ untranslated mRNA sequences. *Nucleic Acids Res* 1987;15:6017–6036.

226. Rao CD, Igarashi H, Chiu I-M. et al. Structure and sequence of the human c-sis/platelet-derived growth factor 2 (sis/PDGF-2) transcriptional unit. *Proc Natl Acad Sci USA* 1986;83:2392–2396.

227. Bernstein J, Shefler I, Elroy-Stein O. The translational repression mediated by the platelet-derived growth factor 2/c-sis mRNA leader is relieved during megakaryocyte differentiation. *J Biol Chem* 1995;270:10559–10565.

228. Sasahara M, Amano S, Sato H. et al. Normal developing rat brain expresses a platelet-derived growth factor B chain (c-sis) mRNA truncated at the 5′ end. *Oncogene* 1998;16:1571–1578.

229. Antoniades HN. Human platelet-derived growth factor (PDGF): purification of PDGF-I and PDGF-II and separation of their reduced subunits. *Proc Natl Acad Sci USA* 1981;78:7314–7317.

230. Bonner JC, Goodell AL, Lasky JA, et al. Reversible binding of platelet-derived growth factor-AA, -AB, and -BB isoforms to a similar site on the ''slow'' and ''fast'' conformations of alpha 2-macroglobulin. *J Biol Chem* 1992;267:12837–12844.

231. Huang JS, Huang SS, Deuel TF. Specific covalent binding of platelet-derived growth factor to human plasma alpha 2-macroglobulin. *Proc Natl Acad Sci USA* 1984;81:342–346.

232. Raines EW, Bowen-Pope DF, Ross R. Plasma binding proteins for platelet-derived growth factor that inhibit its binding to cell-surface receptors. *Proc Natl Acad Sci USA* 1984;81:3424–3428.

233. Singh JP, Chaikin MA, Stiles CD. Phylogenetic analy-

sis of platelet-derived growth factor by radio-receptor assay. *J Cell Biol* 1982;95:667–671.

234. Raines EW, Lane TF, Iruela-Arisp ML, et al. The extracellular glycoprotein SPARC interacts with platelet-derived growth factor (PDGF)-AB and -BB and inhibits the binding of PDGF to its receptors. *Proc Natl Acad Sci USA* 1992;89:1281–1285.

235. Pazin MJ, Williams LT. Triggering signaling cascades by receptor tyrosine kinases. *Trends Biochem Sci* 1992; 17:374–378.

236. Bornfeldt KE, Raines EW, Nakano T, et al. Insulin-like growth factor-1 and platelet-derived growth factor-BB induce directed migration of human arterial smooth muscle cells via signaling pathways that are distinct from those of proliferation. *J Clin Invest* 1994;93: 1266–1274.

237. Pawson T, Gish GD. SH2 and SH3 domains: from structure to function. *Cell* 1992;71:359–362.

238. Chiarugi P, Cirri P, Marra F, et al. The Src and signal transducers and activators of transcription pathways as specific targets for low molecular weight phosphotyrosine-protein phosphatase in platelet-derived growth factor signaling. *J Biol Chem* 1998;273:6776–6785.

239. Bonfini L, Migliaccio E, Pellicci G, et al. Not all Shc's roads lead to ras. *Trends Biochem Sci* 1996;21:258–261.

240. Davis RJ. The mitogen-activated protein kinase signal transduction pathway. *J Biol Chem* 1993;268:14553–14556.

241. Cowley SP, Paterson H, Kemp P, et al. Activation of MAP kinase is necessary and sufficient for PC12 differentiation and for transformation of NIH 3T3 cells. *Cell* 1994;77:841–852.

242. Seger R, Seger D, Reszka AA, et al. Overexpression of mitogen activated protein kinase kinase (MAPKK) and its mutant in NIH3T3 cells. Evidence that MAPKK involvement in cellular proliferation is regulated by phosphorylation of serine residues in its kinase subdomains VII and VIII. *J Biol Chem* 1994;269:25699–25709.

243. Mansour SJ, Matten WT, Hermann AS, et al. Transformation of mammalian cells by constitutively active MAP kinase. *Science* 1994;265:966–970.

244. Heidaran MA, Beeler JF. Yu JC, et al. Differences in substrate specificities of alpha and beta platelet-derived growth factor (PDGF) receptors. Correlation with their ability to mediate PDGF transforming functions. *J Biol Chem* 1993;268:9287–9295.

245. Li W, Yu JC, Michieli P. Stimulation of the platelet-derived growth factor b receptor signaling pathway activates protein kinase C-δ. *Mol Cell Biol* 1994;14: 6727–6735.

246. Inui H, Kitami Y, Tani M, et al. Differences in signal transduction between platelet-derived growth factor (PDGF) α and β receptors in vascular smooth muscle cells. *J Biol Chem* 1994;269:30546–30552.

247. van Dijk MCM, Hilkmann H, van Blitterswijk WJ. Platelet derived growth factor activation of mitogen-activated protein kinase depends on the sequential activation of phosphatidylcholine-specific phospholipase C, protein kinase C-z and Raf-1. *Biochem J* 1997;325: 303–307.

248. Mundschau LJ, Forman LW, Weng H. et al. Platelet-derived growth factor (PDGF) induction of egr-1 is

independent of PDGF receptor autophosphorylation on tyrosine. *J Biol Chem* 1994;23:16137–16142.

249. Kelly K, Cochran BH, Stiles CD, et al. Cell-specific regulation of the c-myc gene by lymphocyte mitogens and platelet-derived growth factor. *Cell* 1983;35: 603–610.

250. Rupprecht HD, Dann P, Sukhatme VP. et al. Effect of vasoactive agents on induction of Egr-1 in rat mesangial cells: correlation with mitogenicity. *Am J Physiol* 1992;263:F623–F636.

251. Hill TD, Dean NM, Mordan LJ, et al. PDGF-induced activation of phospholipase C is not required for induction of DNA synthesis. *Science* 1990;248:1660–1663.

252. Rake JB, Quinones MA, Faller DV. Inhibition of platelet-derived growth factor-mediated signal transduction transforming ras. Suppression of receptor autophosphorylation. *J Biol Chem* 1991;266:5348–5352.

253. Faller DV, Mundschau LJ, Forman LW, et al. v-mos suppresses platelet-derived growth factor (PDGF) type-beta receptor autophosphorylation and inhibits PDGF-BB-mediated signal transduction. *J Biol Chem* 1994;269:5022–5029.

254. Vinci G, Tabilio A, Deschamps JF, et al. Immunological study of *in vitro* maturation of human megakaryocytes. *Br J Haematol* 1984;56:589–605.

255. Martinet Y, Bitterman PB, Mornex JF, et al. Activated human monocytes express the c-sis proto-oncogene and release a mediator showing PDGF-like activity. *Nature* 1986;19:158–160.

256. Noble M, Murray K, Stroobant P. et al. Platelet-derived growth factor promotes division and motility and inhibits premature differentiation of the oligodendrocyte/type-2 astrocyte progenitor cell. *Nature* 1989;333: 560–562.

257. Bronzert DA, Bates SE, Sheridan JP, et al. Transforming growth factor-beta induces platelet-derived growth factor (PDGF) messenger RNA and PDGF secretion while inhibiting growth in normal human mammary epithelial cells. *Mol Endocrinol* 1990;4:981–989.

258. Boehm KD, Daimon M, Gorodeski IG, et al. Expression of the insulin-like and platelet-derived growth factor genes in human uterine tissues. *Mol Reprod Dev* 1990;27:93–101.

259. Goustin AS, Betsholtz C, Pfeifer-Ohlsson S, et al. Coexpression of the sis and mye proto-oncogenes in developing human placenta suggests autocrine control of trophoblast growth. *Cell* 1985;41:301–312.

260. Paulsson Y, Hammacher A, Heldin CH, et al. Possible positive autocrine feedback in the prereplicative phase of human fibroblasts. *Nature* 1987;328:715–717.

261. Abboud HE, Poptic E, DiCorleto PE. Production of platelet-derived growth factor-like protein by rat mesangial cells in culture. *J Clin Invest* 1987;80:675–683.

262. Hsieh HJ, Li NQ, Frangos JA. Shear stress increases endothelial platelet-derived growth factor mRNA levels. *Am J Physiol* 1991;260:H642–646.

263. Hsieh HJ, Li NQ, Frangos JA. Shear-induced platelet-derived growth factor gene expression in human endothelial cells is mediated by protein kinase C. *J Cell Physiol* 1992;150:552–558.

264. Kourembanas S, Hannan RL, Faller DV. Oxygen tension regulates the expression of the platelet-derived growth factor-β chain gene in human endothelial cells. *J Clin Invest* 1990;86:670–674.

265. Jaye M, McConathy E. Drohan W, et al. Modulation

of the sis gene transcript during endothelial cell differentiation *in vitro*. *Science* 1985;228:882–885.

266. Calderon TM, Sherman J, Wilkerson H, et al. Interleukin 6 modulates c-sis gene expression in cultured human endothelial cells. *Cell Immunol* 1992;143: 118–126.

267. Suzuki H, Shibano K, Okane M, et al. Interferon-gamma modulates messenger RNA levels of c-sis (PDGF-B chain), PDGF-A chain, and IL-1 beta genes in human vascular endothelial cells. *Am J Pathol* 1989; 134:35–43.

268. Hajjar KA, Hajjar DP, Silverstein RL, et al. Tumor necrosis factor-mediated release of platelet-derived growth factor from cultured endothelial cells. *J Exp Med* 1987;166:235–245.

269. Winkles JA, Gay CG. Regulated expression of PDGF A-chain mRNA in human saphenous vein smooth muscle cells. *Biochem Biophys Res Commun* 1991;180: 519–524.

270. Kourembanas S, Faller D. Platelet-derived growth factor production by human umbilical vein endothelial cells is regulated by basic fibroblast growth factor. *J Biol Chem* 1989;264:4456–4459.

271. Starksen NF, Harsh GR, Gibbs VC, et al. Regulated expression of the platelet-derived growth factor A chain gene in microvascular endothelial cells. *J Biol Chem* 1987;262:14381–14384.

272. Yamaguci M, Gallati H, Baur W, et al. Both lisinopril and verapamil reduced platelet-derived growth factor-A chain in RNA levels in human saphenous vein endothelical cells stimulated by thrombin. *Surgery* 1994; 115:492–502.

273. Harlan JM, Thompson PJ, Ross RR, et al. Alpha-thrombin induces release of platelet-derived growth factor-like molecule(s) by cultured human endothelial cells. *J Cell Biol* 1986;103:1129–1133.

274. Fox PL, DiCorleto PE. Modified low density lipoproteins suppress production of a platelet-derived growth factor-like protein by cultured endothelial cells. *Proc Natl Acad Sci USA* 1986;83::4774–4778.

275. Montisano DF, Mann T, Spragg RG. H_2O_2 increases expression of pulmonary artery endothelial cell platelet-derived growth factor mRNA. *J Appl Physiol* 1992; 73:2255–2262.

276. Mehta D, George SJ, Jeremy JY, et al. External stenting reduces long-term medial and neointimal thickening and platelet derived growth factor expression in a pig model of arteriovenous bypass grafting. *Nat Med* 1998; 4:235–239.

277. Majack RA, Majesky MW, Goodman LV. Role of PDGF-A expression in the control of vascular smooth muscle cell growth by transforming growth factor-beta. *J Cell Biol* 1990;111:239–247.

278. Naftilan AJ, Pratt RE, Dzau VJ. Induction of platelet-derived growth factor A-chain and c-myc gene expressions by angiotensin II in cultured rat vascular smooth muscle cells. *J Clin Invest* 1989;83:1419–1424.

279. Nakano T, Raines EW, Abraham JA, et al. Glucocorticoid inhibits thrombin-induced expression of platelet-derived growth factor A-chain and heparin-binding epidermal growth factor-like growth factor in human aortic smooth muscle cells. *J Biol Chem* 1993;268: 22941–22947.

280. Ruef J, Rao GN, Li F, et al. Induction of rat aortic smooth muscle cell growth by the lipid peroxidation product 4-hydroxy-2-nonenal. *Circulation* 1998;97: 1071–1078.

281. Nares S, Ng MC, Dill RE, et al. Cyclosporine A upregulates platelet-derived growth factor B chain in hyperplastic human gingiva. *J Periodontol* 1996;67: 271–278.

282. Kanthou C, Benzakour O, Patel G, et al. Thrombin receptor activating peptide (TRAP) stimulates mitogenesis, c-fos and PDGF-A gene expression in human vascular smooth muscle cells. *Thromb Haemost* 1995; 74:1340–1347.

Skeletal Growth Factors,
edited by Ernesto Canalis.
Lippincott Williams & Wilkins, Philadelphia, © 2000.

10

Platelet-Derived Growth Factor

Skeletal Actions and Regulation

Ernesto Canalis and *David M. Ornitz

*Departments of Research and Medicine, Saint Francis Hospital and Medical Center, Hartford,
Connecticut 06105-1299; and University of Connecticut School of Medicine,
Farmington, Connecticut 06030; *Department of Molecular Biology and Pharmacology,
Washington University Medical School, St. Louis, Missouri 63110*

Platelet-derived growth factor (PDGF) is a polypeptide formed by two amino acid chains, which are the product of two related genes, the PDGF A and the PDGF B genes. The chains may form either homodimers or heterodimers, and PDGF can be expressed as PDGF AA, BB, or AB. PDGF BB is the most potent form of the growth factor and frequently has been used to characterize its effects in skeletal and nonskeletal cells. Although PDGF was initially isolated from platelets, it was subsequently found to be expressed by skeletal and a variety of nonskeletal tissues. The PDGF A and B genes are expressed by both normal and malignant cells and are believed to act as autocrine and paracrine regulators of cell growth; however, platelets are the largest source of the growth factor, which is released following platelet aggregation. This would indicate a role for the growth factor in conditions of platelet aggregation, such as wound and fracture healing. Although the PDGF A and B genes are expressed by skeletal cells, the basal level of expression in skeletal tissue is relatively limited. This may suggest that the systemic form of the growth factor is more relevant to changes in bone cell function (1,2).

EFFECTS OF PLATELET-DERIVED GROWTH FACTOR ON SKELETAL TISSUE

PDGF has important actions on bone remodeling and regulatory effects on bone formation and bone resorption. PDGF is a potent mitogen for cells of the osteoblastic lineage, and as a consequence, it increases the number of cells expressing the osteoblastic phenotype (3,4). The effects of PDGF on cell replication are observed in cultures of intact calvariae and of cells of the osteoblastic lineage. In intact calvariae, the mitogenic effect of PDGF is for the most part observed in cells of the periosteal layer, a layer rich in fibroblasts and preosteoblastic cells. PDGF is one of the most potent mitogens for skeletal cells in culture and increases DNA labeling with [^{3}H]thymidine by five- to tenfold depending on the culture model and conditions used. Bone histomorphometric analysis of cultured calvariae treated with PDGF revealed a substantial increase in the number of preosteoblastic cells (Fig. 10.1) (5). Radiolabeling experiments with [^{3}H]thymidine revealed that PDGF BB caused an increase in the number of radiolabeled cells present in the osteoprogenitor zone and an increase in the number of skeletal fibroblasts. Acutely, PDGF did not increase the number of differentiated osteoblasts, although it is presumed that the preosteoblastic cells, replicating under the influence of PDGF, eventually differentiate into mature osteoblasts. Intact calvariae exposed to PDGF did not display an immediate increase in osteoblastic function. In fact, acutely, PDGF causes only modest increases in collagen synthesis, which are proportional to the in-

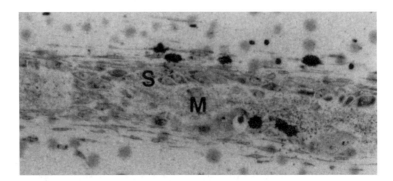

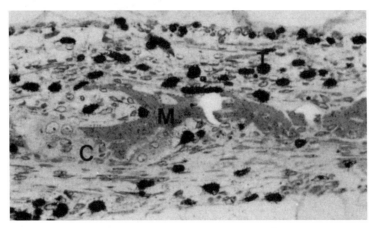

FIG. 10.1. Effect of platelet-derived growth factor (PDGF) BB on [³H]thymidine incorporation in control cultured rat calvariae *(top)* and cultures treated with PDGF BB for 24 hours *(bottom)*. (From ref. 5, with permission.)

creased cell number, and, on a cell-to-cell basis, does not increase or decrease the synthesis of collagen (3). Bone histomorphometric analysis of calvariae labeled with [³H]proline confirm the biochemical findings. Following acute exposure to PDGF, there is a decrease in matrix apposition rates, indicating that PDGF does not increase and tends to decrease the differentiated function of the osteoblast (5). Studies in long-term cultures of cells of the osteoblastic lineage revealed that PDGF inhibits the formation of fully differentiated osteoblasts. In a model normally characterized by osteoblastic cell layering, nodule formation, and mineralization, PDGF prevented these events (6). In accordance with this effect, PDGF suppressed osteoblastic differentiated function and decreased alkaline phosphatase activity and type I collagen expression. The mitogenic effects of PDGF are noted in less

differentiated cells of the osteoblastic lineage and in cultures of bone marrow stromal cells. Similar to the effects observed in cultures of long-term osteoblasts and intact calvariae, PDGF partially inhibits the differentiation of stromal cells into cells of the osteoblastic lineage and decreases the differentiated function of mature cells (7). This would suggest that although preosteoblastic cells that replicate under the influence of PDGF may mature and form osteoblasts, they do so at the expense of other factors present in the bone microenvironment, and PDGF itself may impair this process.

The marked effects of PDGF on cell replication suggest a role in osteogenesis and repair, roles that are confirmed by the active expression of PDGF A and its α receptor in models of rapid bone formation, such as heterotopic and osteophytic bone formation (8). This observation also suggests an autocrine or paracrine function for PDGF in the process of osteogenesis. PDGF modifies the expression of various skeletal matrix proteins, including osteocalcin, osteopontin, and osteonectin, although the effect is somewhat dependent on the cell type studied. In cultures of cells of the osteoblastic lineage, PDGF decreases osteocalcin expression, an effect that is in accordance with the acute inhibitory actions of PDGF on the differentiated function of the osteoblast (6). In chondrocytes, PDGF increases osteonectin expression, whereas in osteoblasts PDGF BB and basic fibroblast growth factor (FGF) decrease the expression of this matrix protein (9,10). Basic FGF acts by destabilizing osteonectin transcripts, but the mechanisms involved in the action of PDGF have not been explored. Osteonectin binds PDGF B chains and appears to play a role in wound repair, which may or may not involve PDGF. The growth factor also increases osteopontin expression in osteoblasts, but the exact function of this matrix protein is not clear (11).

In addition to its effects on bone formation, PDGF enhances bone resorption, indicating a role in increasing bone remodeling (12). The mechanism of increased bone resorption has not been elucidated, but PDGF increases the number of osteoclasts and the osteoclastic-eroded surface, suggesting that it may enhance bone resorption by increasing the replication or recruitment of osteoclast precursors (5). In agreement with its effects on bone resorption, PDGF induces the expression of matrix metalloproteinases by the osteoblast (Fig. 10.2) (13,14). These proteases are considered active participants in the degradation of the osteoid and play a role in bone resorption. Matrix metalloproteinases comprise a family of related proteolytic enzymes including collagenases, gelatinases, and strome-

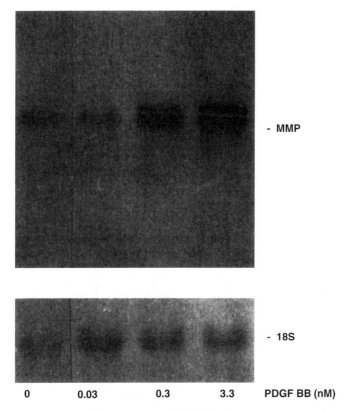

FIG. 10.2. Effect of platelet-derived growth factor *(PDGF)* BB on collagenase 3 (matrix metalloproteinase, *MMP*) expression in osteoblastic cells. (From ref. 13, with permission.)

lysins (15,16). There are three collagenases: collagenase 1, expressed by human osteoblasts, fibroblasts, and chondrocytes; collagenase 2, expressed by neutrophils; and collagenase 3, expressed by rat and human osteoblasts, human chondrocytes, and cells present in breast cancer (16–18). Collagenases 1, 2, and 3 degrade type I collagen with similar efficiency, whereas collagenase 3 degrades type II collagen more efficiently than does collagenase 1 (19). PDGF has been shown to induce collagenase 1 expression in human skin fibroblasts and collagenase 3 expression in rat osteoblasts (13,20). PDGF increases collagenase 3 mRNA and protease levels by transcriptional and posttranscriptional mechanisms. PDGF increases the rate of transcription of the collagenase 3 gene as determined by nuclear run-on assays, and stabilizes collagenase 3 mRNA in transcriptionally arrested osteoblasts so that the half-life of collagenase 3 mRNA is prolonged significantly following exposure to PDGF. Through these two mechanisms, PDGF increases collagenase 3 mRNA and protease levels in bone. PDGF acts on the collagenase 3 gene by protein kinase C (PKC)-dependent pathways since the effect is blocked by PKC inhibitors. Furthermore, PDGF induces the transcription factors c-*fos* and c-*jun,* members of the activator protein-1 (AP-1) complex that can be activated by PKC-dependent pathways. The effect of PDGF on c-*fos* and c-*jun* expression is observed in osteoblasts, and the collagenase 3 gene contains AP-1 binding sites, which are activated by PDGF and responsible for the stimulatory effect of PDGF on this gene (21,22). Currently, there is no information about elements responsible for the stabilization of collagenase 3 transcripts by PDGF. It is possible that PDGF suppresses the binding or expression of cytoplasmic or nuclear proteins that interact with specific RNA sequences and destabilize the collagenase transcript. In cultures of intact rat calvariae, PDGF increases the degradation of newly synthesized collagen, an effect probably due to the induction of collagenase by the osteoblast. This may cause an increase in matrix degradation and bone turnover in skeletal tissue following exposure to PDGF.

PLATELET-DERIVED GROWTH FACTOR RECEPTORS

Cells of the osteoblastic lineage, like nonskeletal cells, express two distinct classes of PDGF receptors, the PDGF α receptor, which binds PDGF A and B chains, and the PDGF β receptor, which binds PDGF B chains with high affinity and does not bind PDGF A chains (23). The two PDGF receptors are structurally and functionally related, and their extracellular binding regions contain five immunoglobulin-like domains. The PDGF β receptor has a molecular mass of 180 kDa, whereas the α receptor has a molecular mass of 140 kDa (24,25). PDGF binding to its receptor results in receptor dimerization and activation of intrinsic tyrosine kinase activity, leading to autophosphorylation (26). Ligand-activated PDGF receptors can stimulate various signal-transduction pathways, including those dependent on PKC, protein kinase A, and intracellular calcium changes (27). The signal-transduction pathways involved in the response to PDGF are cell type–dependent, and different genes respond to different pathways. In skeletal cells, PDGF appears to act by calcium-dependent and PKC-dependent mechanisms since it does not induce cyclic adenosine monophosphate (cAMP) in osteoblastic cells. PDGF BB induces and upregulates PDGF α and β receptor transcript and protein levels, indicating a positive feedback mechanism that may potentiate the biological actions of PDGF (28).

Experiments in cultured osteoblasts have revealed that these cells contain approximately 40,000 to 50,000 high-affinity PDGF AA and BB binding sites per cell with a K_d of 0.1 to 0.2 nM in human osteoblasts (29). This would suggest a similar number of PDGF α and β receptors in human bone cells, although studies in rat osteoblasts indicate a higher number of PDGF α than β receptors and different dissociation constants (30). PDGF binding and activity in osteoblasts can be modified by various cytokines present in the bone microenvironment. Interleukin-1 (IL-1) increases the response to PDGF through specific regulation of the α receptor in the murine osteoblast-like cell line

MC3T3-E1 and in primary cultures of rat osteo-blasts (30,31). In rodent cells, IL-1 increases PDGF α transcripts and PDGF AA binding to the α receptor but does not modify the binding of PDGF BB. Similarly, another inflammatory cytokine, tumor necrosis factor α, increases the binding of PDGF AA, but not PDGF BB, to these cells. PDGF AA is biologically weaker than PDGF BB, and the enhancement of its bind-ing results in a significant increase in activity. Treatment of cells of the osteoblastic lineage with IL-1 enhances the mitogenic effects of PDGF AA, which becomes equipotent with PDGF BB. The stimulatory effects of IL-1 on PDGF AA binding are selected in rodent cells and not observed in human osteoblasts (29). The reason for the discrepancy is not clear. In addi-tion to inflammatory cytokines, transforming growth factor (TGF) β regulates PDGF AA binding in human and rodent osteoblasts (30). In contrast to IL-1, TGF-β decreases PDGF AA binding in human and rodent osteoblastic cells, as well as in 3T3 fibroblasts, and limits the mito-genic actions of PDGF (32,33). TGF-β also in-hibits the binding of PDGF BB but to a much lesser extent than the binding of PDGF AA. It is important to note that cytokines modulate pri-marily the binding of PDGF AA to its receptors, and the effect on PDGF BB is quite modest. The reason for this selectivity is not apparent, but PDGF A chains bind to α, and not to β, recep-tors, suggesting selective regulation at the level of the α receptor. Decreases in PDGF AA bind-ing are usually secondary to decreases in PDGF α receptor transcripts, and result in reduced ty-rosyl kinase phosphorylation (33). The regula-tion of PDGF binding to its receptor appears to be limited to TGF-β1, basic FGE, and inflamma-tory cytokines since hormones and other growth factors with important effects on osteoblastic cell function, such as parathyroid hormone (PTH), 1,25 dihydroxyvitamin D_3, cortisol, prostaglandin E_2, and insulin-like growth factor (IGF)-I have no effect on PDGF binding in os-teoblastic cells (34).

PDGF binding also can be modified by altera-tions in PDGF binding proteins. PDGF BB binds to α_2 macroglobulin and to osteonectin or SPARC (secreted protein acidic and rich in cys-teine) (35,36). Since the bone matrix contains significant amounts of osteonectin, and osteone-ctin binds and prevents the activity of PDGF B chains, a mechanism to regulate PDGF BB ac-tions in osteoblasts involves modifying the lev-els of osteonectin in the bone microenvironment. Selected growth factors with biological actions in bone cells, such as basic FGF and PDGF BB itself, inhibit osteonectin expression in osteo-blasts, and this may be a way utilized by PDGF BB to enhance its activity in cells of the osteo-blastic lineage (10).

INTERACTIONS OF PLATELET-DERIVED GROWTH FACTORS WITH OTHER GROWTH FACTORS SECRETED BY SKELETAL CELLS

In addition to direct effects on genes ex-pressed by cells of the osteoblastic lineage, PDGF has important actions on the expression and activity of other cytokines secreted by skele-tal cells. Skeletal cells synthesize IGF-I and IGF-II, and the two isoforms of the growth factor have important effects on bone formation and enhance the differentiated function of the osteo-blast. IGF-I and IGF-II stimulate the synthesis of type I collagen and decrease bone collagen degradation by inhibiting collagenase expres-sion (37). These effects are opposite to those of PDGF in osteoblasts, and it is not surprising that PDGF inhibits IGF-I and IGF-II expression in these cells. PDGF BB decreases IGF-I and IGF-II mRNA and polypeptide levels in primary cul-tures of osteoblasts (Fig. 10.3) (38,39). The in-hibitory effect of PDGF on IGF-I and IGF-II expression is independent of its mitogenic prop-erties since it is not modified by hydroxyurea. IGF-II is one of the most abundant growth fac-tors present in bone, and although it is develop-mentally regulated and the serum levels of IGF-II decline after birth, selected adult tissues, such as brain, heart, and bone, continue to synthesize this growth factor. To characterize the mecha-nisms involved in IGF-II gene regulation in ro-dent osteoblasts, recent studies from our labora-tory examined the expression of IGF-II and IGF-

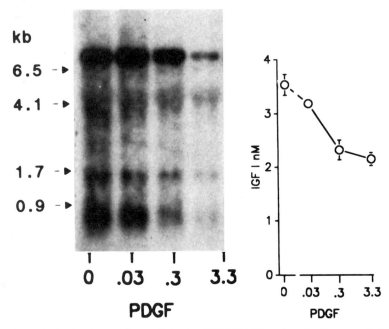

FIG. 10.3. Effect of platelet-derived growth factor *(PDGF)* BB on insulin-like growth factor I mRNA and protein levels in osteoblastic cells. (From ref. 38, with permission.)

II gene promoters in adult rat bone and in cultured osteoblasts. The rodent IGF-II gene is complex, and its transcription is initiated by three distinct promoters termed P1, P2, and P3 (40). The expression of IGF-II in osteoblasts and adult rat calvariae is driven by the IGF-II promoter P3. PDGF BB inhibited IGF-II transcription as determined by nuclear run-on assays and did not modify the half-life of IGF-II mRNA in transcriptionally arrested osteoblastic cells. IGF-II downregulation by PDGF BB occurred through repression of P3, the IGF-II promoter that initiates the transcription of IGF-II transcripts of 3.6 and 1.2 kb (41).

The activity of IGF-I and IGF-II in osteoblasts is regulated by six IGF binding proteins (IGFBPs) termed IGFBP-1 through IGFBP-6. These IGFBPs are regulated by different mechanisms and appear to have different functions in osteoblasts. IGFBP-5 is unique since, under certain circumstances, it enhances the effects of IGF-I on bone cell growth (42). PDGF BB decreases IGFBP-5 mRNA and protein levels in osteoblast cultures by transcriptional mechanisms and does not alter the stability of IGFBP-

5 mRNA in transcriptionally arrested cells (43). Reduced levels of IGFBP-5 in the bone microenvironment may be an additional level of control of IGF function in bone. In addition, PDGF induction of matrix metalloproteinases, such as collagenase, results in fragmentation of IGFBP-5. The function of IGFBP-5 fragments in osteoblasts is not known and is currently under study.

PDGF regulates the expression of other skeletal cytokines. This is not surprising since PDGF increases bone resorption and cytokines play a critical role in this process. PDGF BB increases IL-6 mRNA and protein levels in cells of the osteoblastic lineage, and IL-6 stimulates bone resorption by increasing osteoclast formation and recruitment (Fig. 10.4) (44). These effects are analogous to those observed with PDGF in intact calvariae, and PDGF BB causes rapid induction of IL-6 mRNA in osteoblast cultures. The effect is transcriptional and involves PKC- and calcium-dependent pathways. The stimulation of IL-6 expression by PDGF BB is mimicked by phorbol esters and by ionomycin, known to activate PKC- and calcium-dependent

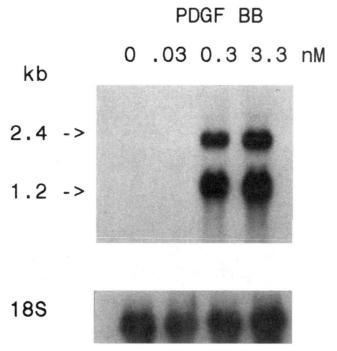

FIG. 10.4. Effect of platelet-derived growth factor *(PDGF)* BB on interleukin (IL)-6 expression in osteoblastic cells. (From ref. 44, with permission.)

pathways, respectively; and it is decreased by the PKC inhibitor sangivamycin and by the intracellular calcium chelator 1,2-bis(*o*-aminophenoxy)ethane-*N, N, N′, N′*-tetraacetic acid acetoxymethylester (BAPTA-AM) (44). In agreement with the activation of PKC- and calcium-dependent pathways, the effect of PDGF BB on IL-6 transcription appears to be due to induction or activation of nuclear proteins that interact with an AP-1 site and a cAMP response element, within the multiple response element, present in the promoter region of the IL-6 gene. The induction of IL-6 by PDGF BB is likely to result in a cascade of events occurring in the bone microenvironment. IL-6 itself is autoregulated in osteoblasts and, like PDGF, causes a marked induction of collagenase 3 transcription in osteoblast cultures (Fig. 10.5) (45,46). These observations indicate that there are redundant mechanisms ensuring the effects of PDGF in bone. It is possible that IL-6 mediates selected actions of PDGF on the replication of cells of the osteoblastic lineage and on bone remodeling.

This is the case in cultures of human fibroblasts, where PDGF-dependent cell proliferation is secondary to increased IL-6 (47). However, the mitogenic effects of IL-6 on cells of the osteoblastic lineage are more modest than those observed with PDGF BB, suggesting either direct actions of PDGF BB on these cells or the involvement of additional cytokines present in the bone microenvironment. In fibroblast cultures, PDGF enhances IL-1 receptor expression, but at the present time it is not known if similar effects occur in cells of the osteoblastic lineage (48).

ACTIONS OF PLATELET-DERIVED GROWTH FACTOR *IN VIVO*

Although there is considerable knowledge about the actions of PDGF BB *in vitro,* information about its effects *in vivo* is more limited. Systemic administration of PDGF BB to ovariectomized rats prevents bone loss and maintains bone mineral density of the spine (49). Bone histomorphometric analysis revealed that PDGF

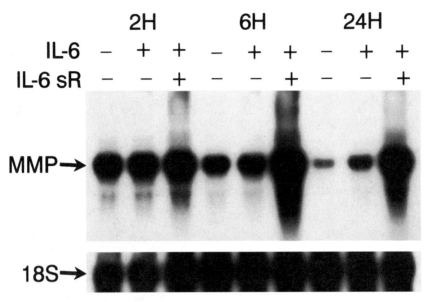

FIG. 10.5. Effect of interleukin *(IL)*-6 and its soluble receptor *(IL-6sR)* on collagenase 3 (MMP) expression in osteoblastic cells. (From ref. 46, with permission.)

increases the number of osteoblasts and increases bone formation. These results are consistent with the effects of PDGF BB *in vitro*. It is likely that the mitogenic effects of PDGF on preosteoblasts result in an increased number of osteoblastic cells, which are capable of forming bone. Surprisingly, PDGF does not change osteoclast number when administered systemically to ovariectomized rats. This may be due to the model chosen since estrogen-deficient rats display a substantial increase in bone resorption and remodeling that may preclude an additional effect by PDGF. However, changes in osteoclast number might occur if PDGF is administered to intact animals. Topical application of PDGF to rat craniotomy defects results in stimulated soft tissue repair and a wound phenotype but not in increased osteogenesis (50). These results are not surprising since the effects of PDGF are not specific to cells of the osteoblastic lineage, and its effects on extraskeletal cells may determine the prevalent phenotype. Similarly, when PDGF BB is administered systemically, fibroblast replication and fibrosis develop in extraskeletal tissues (49). At present, there are no reports of transgenic mice overexpressing PDGF AA or BB in cells of the osteoblastic lineage. Mice with

mutations introduced into either the PDGF B or PDGF β receptor genes do not develop a skeletal phenotype and do display renal and cardiovascular abnormalities (51,52). Glomerular tufts do not develop because of absent mesangial cells. The animals display large arteries, dilated hearts, anemia, and thrombocytopenia. These observations suggest that PDGF does not play a role in skeletal development. It is possible that the animals do not display a skeletal phenotype because they do not survive past birth, and a bone phenotype may require a prolonged absence of the growth factor. It is also possible that PDGF is not necessary for the maintenance of a bone phenotype and it is needed only in conditions of acute remodeling and repair, whereas other growth factors are required for the basal maintenance of the skeletal phenotype.

PDGF may accelerate wound and possibly fracture healing (53). Normal wound healing occurs in three stages: a first stage directed to the migration of neutrophils, monocytes, and fibroblasts into the wound; a second involving the activation of wound macrophages and fibroblasts, resulting in the synthesis of growth factors and extracellular matrix proteins; and a third involving tissue remodeling with active collagen turnover. Topical application of PDGF to experimental wounds results in a transiently accelerated healing response. Histologically, there is an initial increase in cellularity and in the formation of granulation tissue in wounds treated with PDGF BB; IGF I seems to have a synergistic effect with PDGF (53,54). The effects of PDGF on endothelial cell proliferation and angiogenesis are likely beneficial to the process of wound and fracture repair since appropriate vascularization is required for healing (55). Although PDGF enhances the early process of wound healing, 3 months past wounding there is no difference between control and PDGF-exposed wounds, which achieve similar strength. This indicates an early, but not a delayed, effect of PDGF on wound healing. There is less information regarding the possible role of PDGF in fracture than in wound healing. Its effects on bone cell replication and collagenase expression suggest a function in this process since repair requires an additional number of cells as well as active remodeling. In support of this hypothesis, PDGF A and B genes are expressed in cells present in healing fractures. The PDGF A gene is expressed by multiple cell types present in the fracture, whereas PDGF B gene expression is more restricted, detected primarily in osteoblasts (56). These findings suggest that PDGF can play a dual role in fracture healing, a systemic one when released by aggregating platelets and a local one when expressed by cells present at the fracture site; however, more definitive information is required about the specific actions of PDGF on fracture repair. It is possible that PDGF acts directly on skeletal cells, or its actions could be mediated by other factors known to play a role in tissue repair, such as hepatocyte growth factor or scatter factor. Inflammatory cytokines present at the fracture site might play a role in modulating the binding of PDGF to specific cell surface receptors and regulating PDGF activity.

EXPRESSION OF PLATELET-DERIVED GROWTH FACTOR A AND B GENES BY SKELETAL CELLS

Although the major source of PDGF is the systemic circulation, and skeletal cells are likely exposed to significant concentrations of PDGF following platelet aggregation, skeletal cells also express the PDGF A and B genes. There appears to be widespread expression of PDGF A and PDGF α receptor in developing human bone, confirming its role in osteogenesis and possibly bone repair. Since normal osteoblasts and osteosarcoma cells express and respond to PDGF, it is likely that under certain circumstances PDGF acts as an autocrine regulator of osteoblastic cell replication and function (57–61). Similarly, bone marrow stromal cells express both the PDGF A and B genes and respond to PDGF, indicating that PDGF may act as an autocrine regulator of early cells of the osteoblastic lineage (62). The synthesis of PDGF AA in osteoblast cultures as well as in stromal cells is enhanced by TGF-β1, but this effect is not specific to skeletal cells; TGF-β1 also upregulates PDGF A gene expression in endothelial cells (58,62,63). The expression of the PDGF A gene is also enhanced by PDGF AA and PDGF BB so that following an initial induction of PDGF A, this autoregulatory mechanism may serve to allow sustained levels of the growth factor in bone (Fig. 10.6). The effects of PDGF on PDGF A gene expression are mimicked by phorbol esters, but inhibitors of PKC activity do not prevent the induction of PDGF A transcripts by PDGF. The exact gene elements responsible for the effects of PDGF on the PDGF A gene have not been examined in osteoblastic cultures, although a serum response element present in the PDGF A promoter is responsible for the autoregulation of PDGF in extraskeletal cells and could also be responsible for the autoinduction of PDGF A in osteoblasts (64). Since both TGF-β and PDGF itself are released by platelets following platelet aggregation, the subsequent induction of PDGF AA by skeletal cells may be a mechanism to ensure adequate levels of PDGF AA in the bone microenvironment in conditions that follow platelet aggregation, such as fracture repair. However, under basal conditions, there is probably no need for normal skeletal cells to be exposed to large concentrations of PDGF, and the levels of PDGF in cultured osteoblasts are about 1,000 times lower than those of more abundant skeletal growth factors, such as IGF-I and IGF-

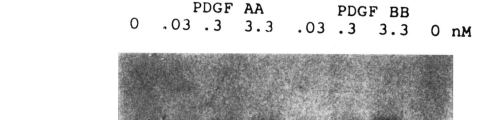

FIG. 10.6. Effect of platelet-derived growth factor *(PDGF)* AA and BB on PDGF A expression in osteoblastic cells. (From ref. 59, with permission.)

II. In contrast to normal osteoblasts, osteosarcoma cell lines appear to express higher levels of PDGF A and B transcripts. This may be due to the availability of necessary transcription factors for the basal expression of the PDGF A and B genes (65). Primary cultures of normal osteoblasts express virtually undetectable levels of PDGF B transcripts, and TGF-β increases its expression (Fig. 10.7). This effect is transcriptional, and TGF-β does not modify PDGF B mRNA decay in transcriptionally arrested cells but increases the rate of PDGF B transcription in osteoblasts (66). This effect also is observed in endothelial cells (67). In contrast to the effect

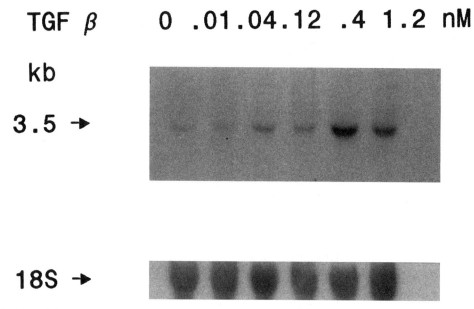

FIG. 10.7. Effect of transforming growth factor β1 *(TGF-β)* on platelet-derived growth factor (PDGF) BB expression in osteoblastic cells. (From ref. 66, with permission.)

of TGF-β, other growth factors secreted by skeletal cells, such as PDGF BB itself, basic FGF, and IGF-I, do not modify the expression of the PDGF B gene in osteoblastic cultures. These observations suggest that PDGF BB may act not only as a systemic but also as a local regulator of bone cell function following induction by TGF-β. Furthermore, PDGF BB may cause a secondary increase in PDGF AA, a dual mechanism used to ensure adequate levels of PDGF in the bone microenvironment in conditions of bone remodeling and repair.

In summary, PDGF has important effects on bone cell replication, and it increases the replication of cells of the osteoblastic and osteoclastic lineages. As such, it increases the number of osteoblasts capable of forming bone and plays an important role in bone remodeling but does not increase the differentiated function of the osteoblast. PDGF has interactions with other growth factors secreted by skeletal cells, and although PDGF is expressed by osteoblasts, its systemic form probably plays a more significant function in bone. At the local level, TGF-β induces both PDGF genes, and PDGF A is autoregulated. The effects of PDGF on cell mitogenesis and bone remodeling and the fact that platelets release the factor following aggregation suggest a role in fracture repair.

ACKNOWLEDGMENTS

This work was supported in part by grant AR 21707 from the National Institute of Arthritis and Musculoskeletal and Skin Diseases. The author thanks Ms. Charlene Gobeli for secretarial assistance.

REFERENCES

1. Heldin C-H, Westermark B. Platelet-derived growth factors: a family of isoforms that bind to two distinct receptors. *Br Med Bull* 1989;45:453–464.
2. Westermark B, Heldin C-H. Platelet-derived growth factors. Structure, function and implications in normal and malignant cell growth. *Acta Oncol* 1993;32:101–105.
3. Canalis E, McCarthy TL, Centrella M. Effects of platelet-derived growth factor on bone formation *in vitro*. *J Cell Physiol* 1989;140:530–537.
4. Centrella M, McCarthy TL, Canalis E. Platelet-derived growth factor enhances deoxyribonucleic acid and collagen synthesis in osteoblast-enriched cultures from fetal rat parietal bone. *Endocrinology* 1989;125:13–19.
5. Hock JM, Canalis E. Platelet-derived growth factor enhances bone cell replication, but not differentiated function of osteoblasts. *Endocrinology* 1994;134:1423–1428.
6. Yu X, Hsieh SC, Bao W, et al. Temporal expression of PDGF receptors and PDGF regulatory effects on osteoblastic cells in mineralizing cultures. *Am J Physiol* 1997; 272:1709–1716.
7. Tanaka H, Liang CT. Effect of platelet-derived growth factor on DNA synthesis and gene expression in bone marrow stromal cells derived from adult and old rats. *J Cell Physiol* 1995;164:367–375.
8. Horner A, Bord S, Kemp P, et al. Distribution of platelet-derived growth factor (PDGF) A chain mRNA, protein, and PDGF-alpha receptor in rapidly forming human bone. *Bone* 1996;19:353–362.
9. Chandrasekhar S, Harvey AK, Johnson MG, et al. Osteonectin/SPARC is a product of articular chondrocytes/cartilage and is regulated by cytokines and growth factors. *Biochim Biophys Acta* 1994;1221:7–14.
10. Delany AM, Canalis E. Basic fibroblast growth factor destabilizes osteonectin mRNA in osteoblasts. *Am J Physiol* 1998;274:C734–C740.
11. Sodek J, Chen J, Nagata T, et al. Regulation of osteopontin expression in osteoblasts. *Ann NY Acad Sci* 1995; 760:223–241.
12. Cochran DL, Rouse CA, Lynch SE, et al. Effects of platelet-derived growth factor isoforms on calcium release from neonatal mouse calvariae. *Bone* 1993;14: 53–58.
13. Varghese S, Delany AM, Liang L, et al. Transcriptional and posttranscriptional regulation of interstitial collagenase by platelet-derived growth factor BB in bone cell cultures. *Endocrinology* 1996;137:431–437.
14. Holliday LS, Welgus HG, Fliszar CJ, et al. Initiation of osteoclast bone resorption by interstitial collagenase. *J Biol Chem* 1997;272:22053–22058.
15. Freije JMP, Diez-Itza I, Balbin M, et al. Molecular cloning and expression of collagenase 3, a novel human matrix metalloproteinase produced by breast carcinomas. *J Biol Chem* 1994;269:16766–16773.
16. Matrisian LM, Hogan BLM. Growth factor regulated proteases and extracellular matrix remodeling during mammalian development. *Curr Top Dev Biol* 1990;24: 219–259.
17. Rifas L, Fausto A, Scott MJ, et al. Expression of metalloproteinases and tissue inhibitors of metalloproteinases in human osteoblast-like cells: differentiation is associated with repression of metalloproteinase biosynthesis. *Endocrinology* 1994;134:213–221.
18. Quinn CO, Scott DK, Brinckerhoff CE, et al. Rat collagenase. Cloning, amino acid sequence comparison, and parathyroid hormone regulation in osteoblastic cells. *J Biol Chem* 1990;265:22342–22347.
19. Knäuper V, Lopez-Otin C, Smith B, et al. Biochemical characterization of human collagenase-3. *J Biol Chem* 1996;271:1544–1550.
20. Bauer EA, Cooper TW, Huang JS, et al. Stimulation of *in vitro* human skin collagenase expression by platelet-derived growth factor. *Proc Natl Acad Sci USA* 1985; 82:4132–4136.
21. Rajakumar RA, Quinn CO. Parathyroid hormone induc-

tion of rat interstitial collagenase mRNA in osteosarcoma cells is mediated through an AP-1 binding site. *Mol Endocrinol* 1996;10:867–878.

22. Okazaki R, Ikeda K, Sakamoto A, et al. Transcriptional activation of c-*fos* and c-*jun* protooncogenes by serum growth factors in osteoblast-like MC3T3-E1 cells. *J Bone Miner Res* 1992;7:1149–1155.

23. Hart CE, Forstrom JW, Kelly JD, et al. Two classes of PDGF receptor recognize different isoforms of PDGF. *Science* 1988;240:1529–1531.

24. Yarden Y, Escobedo JA, Kuang W-J, et al. Structure of the receptor for platelet-derived growth factor helps define a family of closely related growth factor receptors. *Nature* 1986;323:226–232.

25. Claesson-Welsh L, Erikkson A, Morjn A, et al. cDNA cloning and expression of a human platelet-derived growth factor (PDGF) receptor specific for B-chain-containing PDGF molecules. *Mol Cell Biol* 1988;8:3476–3486.

26. Heldin C-H, Ernlund A, Rorsman C, et al. Dimerization of B-type platelet-derived growth factor receptors occurs after ligand binding and is closely associated with receptor kinase activation. *J Biol Chem* 1989;264:8905–8912.

27. Claesson-Welsh L. Platelet-derived growth factor receptor signals. *J Biol Chem* 1994;269:32023–32026.

28. Erikkson A, Nister M, Levjen P, et al. Induction of platelet-derived growth factor α- and β-receptor mRNA and protein by platelet-derived growth factor BB. *J Biol Chem* 1991;266:21138–21144.

29. Gilardetti RS, Chaibi MS, Stroumza J, et al. High-affinity binding of PDGF-AA and PDGF-BB to normal human osteoblastic cells and modulation by interleukin-1. *Am J Physiol* 1991;261:980–985.

30. Centrella M, McCarthy TL, Kusmik WF, et al. Isoform-specific regulation of platelet-derived growth factor activity and binding in osteoblast-enriched cultures from fetal rat bone. *J Clin Invest* 1992;89:1076–1084.

31. Tsukamoto T, Matsui T, Nakata H, et al. Interleukin-1 enhances the response of osteoblasts to platelet-derived growth factor through the α receptor-specific up-regulation. *J Biol Chem* 1991;266:10143–10147.

32. Gronwald RGK, Seifert RA, Bowen-Pope DF. Differential regulation of expression of two platelet-derived growth factor receptor subunits by transforming growth factor-β. *J Biol Chem* 1989;264:8120–8125.

33. Yeh YL, Kang YM, Chaibi MS, et al. IL-1 and transforming growth factor-beta inhibit platelet-derived growth factor-AA binding to osteoblastic cells by reducing platelet-derived growth factor-alpha receptor expression. *J Immunol* 1993;150:5625–5632.

34. Kose KN, Xie JF, Carnes DL, et al. Pro-inflammatory cytokines downregulate platelet derived growth factor-alpha receptor gene expression in human osteoblastic cells. *J Cell Physiol* 1996;166:188–197.

35. Crookston KP, Webb DJ, LaMaree J, et al. Binding of platelet-derived growth factor-BB and transforming growth factor-β1 to α_2-macroglobulin *in vitro* and *in vivo:* Comparison of receptor-recognized and non-recognized α_2-macroglobulin conformations. *Biochem J* 1993;293:443–450.

36. Raines EW, Lane TF, Iruela-Arispe ML, et al. The extracellular glycoprotein SPARC interacts with platelet-derived growth factor (PDGF)-AB and -BB and inhibits the binding of PDGF to its receptors. *Proc Natl Acad Sci USA* 1992;89:1281–1285.

37. McCarthy TL, Centrella M, Canalis E. Regulatory effects of insulin-like growth factor I and II on bone collagen synthesis in rat calvarial cultures. *Endocrinology* 1989;124:301–309.

38. Canalis E, Pash J, Gabbitas B, et al. Growth factors regulate the synthesis of insulin-like growth factor-I in bone cell cultures. *Endocrinology* 1993;133:33–38.

39. Gabbitas B, Pash J, Canalis E. Regulation of insulin-like growth factor-II synthesis in bone cell cultures by skeletal growth factors. *Endocrinology* 1994;135:284–289.

40. Holthuizen PE, Cleutjens CBJM, Veenstra GJC, et al. Differential expression of the human, mouse, and rat IGF II genes. *Regul Pept* 1993;48:77–89.

41. Gangji V, Rydziel S, Gabbitas B, et al. Insulin-like growth factor II promoter expression in cultured rodent osteoblasts and adult rat bone. *Endocrinology* 1998;139:2287–2292.

42. Andress DL, Birnbaum RS. Human osteoblast-derived insulin-like growth factor (IGF) binding protein-5 stimulates osteoblast mitogenesis and potentiates IGF action. *J Biol Chem* 1992;267:22467–22472.

43. Canalis E, Gabbitas B. Skeletal growth factors regulate the synthesis of insulin-like growth factor binding protein-5 in bone cell cultures. *J Biol Chem* 1995;270:10771–10776.

44. Franchimont N, Canalis E. Platelet-derived growth factor stimulates the synthesis of interleukin-6 in cells of the osteoblast lineage. *Endocrinology* 1995;136:5469–5475.

45. Franchimont N, Rydziel S, Canalis E. Interleukin 6 is autoregulated by transcriptional mechanisms in cultures of rat osteoblastic cells. *J Clin Invest* 1997;100:1797–1803.

46. Franchimont N, Rydziel S, Delany AM, et al. Interleukin-6 and its soluble receptor cause a marked induction of collagenase 3 expression in rat osteoblast cultures. *J Biol Chem* 1997;272:12144–12150.

47. Roth M, Nauck M, Tamm M, et al. Intracellular interleukin 6 mediates platelet-derived growth factor induced proliferation of nontransformed cells. *Proc Natl Acad Sci USA* 1995;92:1312–1316.

48. Bonin PD, Singh JP. Modulation of interleukin-1 receptor expression and interleukin-1 response in fibroblasts by platelet-derived growth factor. *J Biol Chem* 1988;263:11052–11055.

49. Mitlak BH, Finkelman RD, Hill EL, et al. The effect of systemically administered PDGF-BB on the rodent skeleton. *J Bone Miner Res* 1996;11:238–247.

50. Marden LJ, Fan RSP, Pierce GF, et al. Platelet-derived growth factor inhibits bone regeneration induced by osteogenin, a bone morphogenetic protein, in rat craniotomy defects. *J Clin Invest* 1993;92:2897–2905.

51. Leveen P, Pekny M, Gebre-Medhin S, et al. Mice deficient for PDGF B show renal, cardiovascular, and hematological abnormalities. *Genes Dev* 1994;8:1875–1887.

52. Soriano P. Abnormal kidney development and hematological disorders in PDGF β-receptor mutant mice. *Genes Dev* 1994;8:1888–1896.

53. Deuel TF, Kawahara RS, Mustoe TA, et al. Growth factors and wound healing: platelet-derived growth fac-

tor as a model cytokine. *Annu Rev Med* 1991;42:567–584.

54. Pierce GF, Tarpley JE, Yanagihara D, et al. Platelet-derived growth factor (BB homodimer), transforming growth factor-β1, and basic fibroblast growth factor in dermal wound healing. *Am J Pathol* 1992;140:1375–1388.

55. Battegay EJ, Rupp J, Iruela-Arispe L, et al. PDGF-BB modulates endothelial proliferation and angiogenesis *in vitro* via PDGF β-receptors. *J Cell Biol* 1994;125:917–928.

56. Andrew JG, Hoyland JA, Freemont AJ, et al. Platelet-derived growth factor expression in normally healing human fractures. *Bone* 1995;16:455–460.

57. Zhang L, Leeman E, Carnes DC, et al. Human osteoblasts synthesize and respond to platelet-derived growth factor. *Am J Physiol* 1991;261:C348–C354.

58. Rydziel S, Ladd C, McCarthy TL, et al. Determination and expression of platelet-derived growth factor-AA in bone cell cultures. *Endocrinology* 1992;130:1916–1922.

59. Rydziel S, Shaikh S, Canalis E. Platelet-derived growth factor-AA and -BB (PDGF-AA and -BB) enhance the synthesis of PDGF-AA in bone cell cultures. *Endocrinology* 1994;134:2541–2546.

60. Betsholtz C, Johnsson A, Heldin C-H, et al. cDNA sequence and chromosomal localization of human plate-let-derived growth factor A-chain and its expression in tumour cell lines. *Nature* 1986;320:695–699.

61. Graves DT, Owen AJ, Barth RK, et al. Detection of c-*sis* transcripts and synthesis of PDGF-like proteins by human osteosarcoma cells. *Science* 1984;226:972–974.

62. Abboud SL. Regulation of platelet-derived growth factor A and B chain gene expression in bone marrow stromal cells. *J Cell Physiol* 1995;164:434–440.

63. Starksen NF, Harsh GR, Gibbs VC, et al. Regulated expression of the platelet-derived growth factor A chain gene in microvascular endothelial cells. *J Biol Chem* 1987;262:14381–14384.

64. Lin X, Wangz Z, Gu L, et al. Functional analysis of the human platelet-derived growth factor A-chain promoter region. *J Biol Chem* 1992;267:25614–25619.

65. Jin H-M, Robinson DF, Liang Y, et al. *SIS/PDGF-B* promoter isolation and characterization of regulatory elements necessary for basal expression of the *SIS/PDGF-B* gene in U2-OS osteosarcoma cells. *J Biol Chem* 1994;269:28648–28654.

66. Rydziel S, Canalis E. Expression and growth factor regulation of platelet-derived growth factor B transcripts in primary osteoblast cell cultures. *Endocrinology* 1996;137:4115–4119.

67. Daniel TO, Fen Z. Distinct pathways mediate transcriptional regulation of platelet-derived growth factor B/c-*sis* expression. *J Biol Chem* 1988;263:19815–19820.

Skeletal Growth Factors,
edited by Ernesto Canalis.
Lippincott Williams & Wilkins, Philadelphia, © 2000.

11

Fibroblast Growth Factors and Their Receptors

Andrew Baird and *David M. Ornitz

Ciblex Corporation, San Diego, California 92121 and °Department of Molecular Biology and Pharmacology, Washington University Medical School, St. Louis, Missouri 63110

Fibroblast growth factors (FGFs) represent a large family of polypeptides that are potent regulators of cell growth and differentiation (1–3). They play a major role in normal embryonic development and in tissue repair and regeneration and have been implicated in numerous pathologies, including the development and progression of several malignancies. FGFs act on cells that are primarily of mesodermal origin but have broader effects on cells derived from the ectoderm and endoderm. Depending on the target cell, the conditions of cell culture, and the presence or absence of other trophic agents, FGFs alter migration, morphology, differentiation, and proliferation (4). While first discovered for their action on fibroblasts, hence their name, their activities and physiological roles are considerably more extensive than is implied by their name. In fact, some members of the FGF family are not even mitogens for fibroblasts at all and would be better represented if thought of as epithelial growth factors.

To date, the family of FGFs consists of over 18 genes that encode proteins with 30% to 80% structural homology at the amino acid level (Fig. 11.1). More may still be identified as the human genome is fully characterized. Interleukin 1β, which has 20% homology with FGF1 and FGF2, is not usually considered a member of the FGF family, though it has a number of features in common with the FGFs, including a similar tertiary structure. While the members of the FGF family are designated FGF1 through FGF18, the

names of acidic FGF (FGF1), basic FGF (FGF2), and KGF (keratinocyte growth factor, FGF7) are also commonly used in the literature. Other names for the FGFs, like int2 (FGF3), hst1/ksFGF/kFGF (FGF4), hst2 (FGF6), androgen-induced growth factor (FGF8), and glial activating factor (FGF8), are in rare use as the nomenclature describing the FGF family becomes standardized (2–5).

There are four distinct genes that encode for high-affinity receptors for FGFs. Called FGFR1, FGFR2, FGFR3, and FGFR4, these genes encode a multitude of structural variants that result from alternative splicing of their mRNAs (1). As a result, the specificity of ligand binding can be drastically modified by the generation of one or another alternatively spliced form. The best example is FGF7, also known as KGF, which does not cross-react with any FGFR except a variant of FGFR2. Accordingly, it is very specific (6,7).

The basic structure of the FGFRs is the same; they belong to the immunoglobulin (Ig)-like family of tyrosine kinases. All possess three Ig-like domains, which can be processed to isoforms that contain two Ig-like domains connected to an intracellular tyrosine kinase domain activated by ligand binding. In some instances, genetic mutations in the transmembrane domain result in constitutive activation and, in humans, various forms of dwarfism (8,9).

The FGF ligand–FGFR interaction is further complicated by the role played by proteoglycans

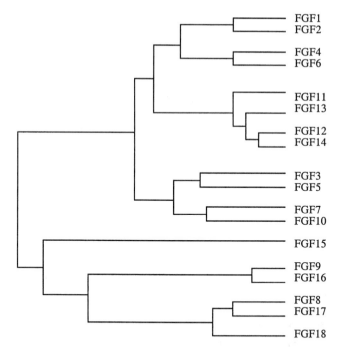

FIG. 11.1. Homologies of the fibroblast growth factor (FGF) family. Based on the sequences of rat FGFs 1, 2, 5, 7, 9, 10, 16, 17, and 18 and mouse FGFs 3, 4, 6, 8, 11, 12, 13, 14, and 15.

in FGF action. Specifically, FGFs have an unusually high affinity for heparin sulfates, which translates into an ability to interact with glycosaminoglycans like heparin. This binding causes conformational changes in the FGFs that result in altered receptor binding and protect the ligand from proteolysis and acid denaturation (10,11). Most importantly, this interaction appears to be required for significant ligand–receptor binding. Extracellular FGF binds to heparin sulfate proteoglycans in the matrix and at the cell surface; this binding is thought to protect the FGFs and serve as a reservoir of FGFs available after trauma, injury, or any pathophysiological event that might require a rapid mobilization of FGF activity (like angiogenesis). In this model, the release of matrix-degrading enzymes during embryonic development or tissue injury or after cell transformation to the cancer phenotype can serve to generate free, biologically active FGFs from these sites of sequestration (12,13). As some of the most powerful mitogens known, the FGFs appear to play key roles in significant human disease, like cancer.

THE FIBROBLAST GROWTH FACTOR FAMILY

The number of ligands identified in the FGF family is increasing, and as sequencing of the human genome has accelerated, the discovery of new, structurally related proteins is likely to continue. They are thought to derive from a common ancestral gene (Fig. 11.1), and they all share a common structure of three exons separated by two short introns. They are located on different chromosomes (Table 11.1) and appear to be highly regulated, presumably to control malignancy. In normal adult tissues, the predominant FGF gene products are FGF1 and FGF2. While the functional roles played by FGFs are currently under active investigation, significantly less is known about the more recently characterized molecules.

Fibroblast Growth Factors 1 and 2

Acidic and basic FGFs (now called FGF1 and FGF2, respectively) are the prototypic members

TABLE 11.1. *Chromosome location of fibroblast growth factors (FGFs) and their receptors and ligand specificity of binding*

Protein	Receptor specificity	Chromosome (human)	Locus	Reference
FGF1	All	5	q31–33	61
FGF2	1b,1c,2c,3c,4	4	q25–27	62
FGF3	1b,2b	11	q13	63
FGF4	1c,2c,3c,4	11	q13	63
FGF5	1c,2c	4	q21	64
FGF6	1c,2c,4	12	p13	65
FGF7	2b	15	q15–21	66
FGF8	2c,3c,4	10	q24–26	35
FGF9	2c,3b,3c	13	q11–12	66
FGF10	2b	5	p13–12	39
FGF11	?	17	q21	67
FGF12	?	3	q28	67
FGF13	?	X	q26	68
FGF14	?	13	Q34	43
FGF15	?	—	—	—
FGF16	?	—	—	—
FGF17	2c,3c,4	—	—	—
FGF18	?	—	—	—
FGFR1	—	8	p11.2–11.1	69
FGFR2	—	10	q26	70
FGFR3	—	4	p16.3	71
FGFR4	—	5	q35.1-qter	72

of the FGF family. First named for their different isoelectric points when first detected in, and purified from, tissue extracts, they have similar molecular weights and over 50% structural homology. Both have been isolated from numerous tissues and have been the subject of extensive reviews (1–4).

The gene for FGF1 is located on chromosome 5 and results in several mRNAs that differ in their 5′-untranslated region and not in their coding sequence (14). It is therefore likely that differential elements control mRNA translation in different tissues. In contrast, the mRNA encoding human FGF2 derives from a gene on chromosome 4 and encodes four proteins that contain an identical core of the FGF2 protein sequence (15,16). The three amino-terminally extended forms of FGF2 extend the 18-kDa molecule of 155 amino acids to proteins of 21, 22, and 25 kDa. These isoforms translocate to the nucleus, where they are thought to play a role in controlling transcription. The lowest molecular weight FGF2 is cytoplasmic, and while it can be released from cells, it appears to follow an unconventional release pathway (17,18). Unlike many of the other FGFs and all classically secreted proteins, both FGF1 and FGF2 lack a classical leader sequence and do not exit the cell through the endoplasmic reticular (ER) Golgi apparatus complex.

Both FGF1 and FGF2 stimulate the proliferation of mesodermal cells and many cells of neuroectodermal, ectodermal, and endodermal origin. They are also characterized by the wide array of activities that they can stimulate on different cell types (19). While they are perhaps best known as powerful angiogenic factors (because of their effects on endothelial cells), they also modulate differentiated function, delay senescence, inhibit apopotosis, and are chemotactic depending on the *in vitro* cell system used, the conditions of cell culture, and the target cell evaluated. *In vivo,* these FGFs are active in angiogenesis, nerve regeneration, cartilage repair, and wound healing, and are thought to play normal functions in tissue repair and homeostasis. The observations that inappropriate expression of FGFs can result in tumor growth and development (see below) also suggest that they participate in the production of a large variety of pathogenic conditions that result in cell proliferation or that are angiogenesis-dependent.

Fibroblast Growth Factor 3

With the structural characterization of FGF1 and FGF2, various databases could be evaluated for the presence of homologous proteins. The first of these FGFs so identified was int-2 (20). Int-2 (now FGF3) was first recognized as a cellular gene that was activated after integration of the mouse mammary tumor virus into the mouse genome. The gene is located on chromosome 11 (Table 11.1) and encodes a protein of 240 amino acids that has about 40% homology to FGFs 1 and 2. An extension at the amino terminus includes a classical leader sequence that allows it to be secreted through the ER Golgi, but interestingly, alternative forms of its mRNA encode an FGF3 that have no leader sequence. These isoforms remain inside the cell, where they are translocated to the nucleus to play a role in regulating gene transcription. The elements that control the production of one over another form of FGF3 have not been defined. The secreted form of FGF3 derives from a classical AUG codon, while the cellular form is derived when this AUG is overridden by the use of an alternative start site at a CUG codon.

The regulation of FGF3 transcription appears to be coordinated by three distinct promoters and two alternative polyadenylation sites. The gene generates six different RNA species, all with the same coding capacity, but FGF3 has two alternative upstream initiation codons in which a CUG is the major start site for FGF3. A downstream AUG codon initiates translation of the shorter 30.5-kDa protein. A number of replacement and deletion mutations have shown that the amino-terminal extension is crucial for nuclear import, although the nuclear targeting signals are located elsewhere in the protein. The decision to enter the secretory pathway or nucleus appears to depend on a balance of competing signals involving the amino terminus, a signal peptide, and the nuclear localization sequence. The relative position of the signaling motifs is also an important factor in establishing the proportion of FGF3 destined for the different intracellular compartments. Unfortunately, the physiological activities of FGF3 are ill-defined, but it is thought to play a role in embryonic development (21,22).

Fibroblast Growth Factor 4

When the genomic fragments of the human tumor-derived oncogene *hst1* were sequenced and the oncogene derived from a Kaposi's sarcoma cell line was characterized, they were found to encode the same 206–amino acid protein that had 40% homology to FGF1, FGF2, and FGF3. First called K-FGF and hst1, it is now commonly known as FGF4 (20,23) and locates on human chromosome 11 in close proximity to FGF3 (Table 11.1). The amino terminus of FGF4 is extended when compared to FGF1 and FGF2, and the extension includes a leader sequence for secretion through the ER Golgi. The mature protein is glycosylated, secreted, and transforming. It occurs with high frequency in some tumors, such as the stomach, and is found during normal embryonic development. Like FGF1 and FGF2, it is a highly angiogenic molecule, but unlike the prototypic FGFs, it is rare in adult tissues; it is thought to play a role in limb development (24) and somite patterning (25).

Fibroblast Growth Factor 5

The fifth member of the FGF family was identified from a cDNA library prepared from bladder cancer that was screened for transforming oncogenes (26). The protein encoded by the DNA isolated was found to have 40% homology to FGF1 and FGF2, hence making it FGF5. The 267–amino acid protein has a leader sequence and, as such, is secreted from cells through the ER Golgi like FGFs 3 and 4. For this reason, it is a transforming molecule that is found in many human tumor cell lines. It is a highly angiogenic protein that is normally found in embryonic development of brain, muscle, and heart. The amount of this protein found in adult tissues, however, is low when compared to FGF1 and FGF2 but detectable.

The human FGF5 gene has alternative polyadenylation sites which transcribe two main RNA species of 1.6 and 1.4 kb (26). The regulatory elements of transcription have yet to be identified, but there is evidence for translational control of FGF5 expression. The FGF5 mRNA contains a short out-of-frame open reading frame (ORF) upstream of the ORF coding for the growth factor. Deletion of the upstream ORF enhances FGF5 translation and transforming ability, supporting the observation that FGF5 is mitogenic and overexpressed in some human cancers.

Fibroblast Growth Factor 6

The sixth FGF was first detected as hst2 and as a cDNA that hybridized with probes encoding FGF4 (27,28). As a result, an FGF was sequenced that has 70% homology with FGF4 and about 30% with FGFs 1 and 2. While relatively little is known regarding the activities of FGF6 *in vivo*, it is angiogenic *in vivo*, transforming when expressed in cells and normally found during embryonic development, where it presumably mediates many of the activities first ascribed to FGF1 and FGF2. However, while FGF6 exhibits a restricted expression profile that is dominantly in the myogenic lineage (29), important functions have been suggested in wound healing and tissue regeneration (30). Like the FGFs with oncogenic potential, FGF6 has a leader sequence at its amino terminus that enables ER Golgi–dependent secretion.

Fibroblast Growth Factor 7

One of the most studied FGFs, FGF7 is unlike the other FGF mitogens in that it shows significant specificity for epithelial cells (6). First identified as keratinocyte growth factor (KGF), it has no effect on many target cells considered the usual targets for FGFs (i.e., endothelial cells). Because of its cell and receptor (FGFR2) specificity, KGF/FGF7 has no angiogenic activity. Its gene encodes an FGF7 with an amino terminus that has a leader sequence for secretion and a 22-kDa protein that has 35% homology to the other FGFs. Its mRNA is found in a number of stromal fibroblast cell lines derived from embryonic and adult tissues but is absent from epithelial cells. Of all the FGFs, FGF7 is the one with the clearest paracrine function, as it is always produced in stromal cells but acts only on target epithelial cells (31). If it is produced in cells that have the receptor expressed (see below), it is transforming. The specific isoform of FGFR that binds FGF7, however, is highly restricted in distribution and found almost exclusively on epithelial cells. Aberrant expression leads to proliferative disease.

There is a canonical TATA box 30 nucleotides upstream of its transcription-initiation site. Physiological FGF7 transcription is regulated developmentally by an enhancer element located in the 3′-untranslated region of exon 3. This enhancer contains a series of consensus binding sites for a number of known transcription factors, including SP1 and AP1. Although it is probable that the specific *trans* factors that control the FGF-7 gene will belong to the family of octamer-binding proteins (some known to be developmentally regulated), there is no evidence to date for posttranscriptional or even posttranslational control of FGF7.

Fibroblast Growth Factor 8

When the activity induced by androgen-treated Shionogi carcinoma cells was isolated and characterized, the molecule was found to have 30% to 40% homology with the other members of the FGF family and it was called FGF8 (32,33). The gene, located on human chromosome 10 (Table 11.1), encodes a protein that has a leader peptide, and for this reason, the molecule is found in conditioned media of FGF8-producing cells. While relatively little is known about FGF8, it is found during embryonic development and appears to play a key role in pattern development. Because of the spaciotemporal pattern of gene expression and the distribution of FGF8 protein immunoreactivity during development, it is likely that FGF8 is the true natural growth factor that is responsible for some of the activities first ascribed to FGF1 and FGF2 in embryonic development. Its distribution and expression patterns suggest a role in outgrowth and patterning of limb development (34,35).

Fibroblast Growth Factor 9

First identified in cell culture supernatants as a glial activating factor (36), FGF9 has 30% homology with the other FGFs and, with the exception that it stimulates the proliferation and activation of glial cells and other cells which express FGFRs, relatively little is known regarding its physiological function. Because FGF9 has relatively higher specificity for FGFR3 than do the other FGFs (37), it is likely to be the ligand responsible for the numerous skeletal disorders associated with the FGF axis. It ability to transform cells when overexpressed (38) supports the hypothesis that it may also be involved in the development of human malignancies.

Fibroblast Growth Factor 10

Emoto et al. (39) isolated a cDNA encoding a novel member of the FGF family that is most related to FGF7 (KGF). Like FGF7, FGF10 is mitogenic for keratinizing epidermal cells and essentially inactive on fibroblasts. Located on chromosome 5p13-p12, little is known regarding its activities, but recent studies have established that, like FGF7, it is involved in wound healing (40) and embryonic development (41) but appears to be differentially regulated and, like other FGFs, spacially restricted in its expression (42).

Fibroblast Growth Factors 11–14

Using degenerate polymerase chain reaction (PCR) and random DNA sequencing, Smallwood et al. (43) identified four additional members of the FGF family, referred to as fibroblast growth factor homologous factors (FHFs). The genes encoded proteins that were 30% homologous to other FGFs, although they have as much as 70% homology between themselves. Their physiological functions are not known, but they all lack signal peptides and contain nuclear localization sequences. They are expressed primarily in the nervous system, although a comprehensive analysis of protein distribution and gene expression has not been reported. It is assumed that they play a role in nervous system development and function, but their presence in heart and connective tissue implies a broader, possibly intracellular, function (44).

Fibroblast Growth Factor 15

When McWirter et al. (45) characterized the downstream targets of the homeodomain oncoprotein E2A-Pbx1, they identified a new member of the FGF family, FGF15. When the deduced sequence of FGF15 was compared to the other FGF family members, 30% homology was observed, with the greatest similarity being between FGF15 and FGF7 and the least between FGF15 and FGF8. FGF15 has a common FGF gene structure: three exons separated by two introns located at the exact same homologous sequence. Like many of the other FGFs, but unlike FGF1, FGF2, and the FHFs, FGF15 has a signal sequence for targeting to the ER Golgi and secretion. Remarkably, FGF15 is not transforming under these circumstances, suggesting that it does not mediate the effects of E2A-Pbx1 on 3T3 cells. In view of its similarity to FGF7 and the fact that 3T3 cells have no receptor that cross-reacts with FGF7, the findings also suggest that 3T3 cells do not possess a receptor for FGF15, which perhaps shares the same FGF7 receptor, FGFR2.

Although little is known regarding the physiological functions of FGF15, E2A-Pbx1 binds directly to a site proximal to its promoter, and the Pbx1 homeodomain is required for induction. The expression pattern of FGF15 suggests that it may play a specialized role in the nervous system. It first appears in the neuroectoderm soon after neurulation and remains restricted throughout development but never overlaps with the two other FGFs that are similarly restricted, FGFs 3 and 8.

Fibroblast Growth Factor 16

A cDNA encoding a novel member (207 amino acids) of the FGF family from rat heart was identified by homology-based PCR (46). FGF16 is most similar (73% amino acid identity) to FGF9 and, like FGF9, it lacks a typical signal sequence yet is efficiently secreted by Sf9 insect cells infected with recombinant baculovirus containing the FGF16 cDNA. FGF16 mRNA is predominantly expressed in the adult rat heart. In rat embryos, FGF16 mRNA is predominantly expressed in the brown adipose tissue, but expression decreases greatly after birth. Whether FGF16 might be a novel secreted FGF that plays a role in the development of brown adipose tissue is unknown.

Fibroblast Growth Factor 17

A cDNA encoding a novel member (216 amino acids) of the FGF family was identified from rat embryos by Hoshikawa et al. (47) soon after their characterization of FGF16. Among FGF family members, FGF17 is most similar (53.7% amino acid identity) to FGF8. FGF17 has a typical signal sequence at its amino terminus. FGF17 mRNA of approximately 2.1 kb has been detected in rat embryos at day 14.5 but not at days 10.5 and 19.5, and mRNA is found to be preferentially expressed in the neuroepithelia of the isthmus and septum of the rat embryonic brain at day 14. Whether FGF17 might be a novel secreted molecule in the induction and patterning of the embryonic brain is unknown.

Fibroblast Growth Factor 18

Using homology cloning strategies, Hoshikawa et al. (47) has also characterized the eighteenth member of the FGF family. It has a typical signal sequence and, as such, is a secreted protein. When the growth factor is expressed in insect cells and tested on FGF target cells, it is also biologically active. In this instance, FGF18 has neurite-promoting activity on PC12 cells. No information is available as to whether it is angiogenic. It is most homologous to FGFs 8 and 17, with which it has almost 53% amino acid identity. Like most FGFs, its physiological function remains largely unknown. Northern blotting and *in situ* hybridization point to gene expression in adult lungs but not in brain, heart, liver, or kidney. In spite of homology to FGF8, its localization is very distinct. Hence, in tissues like gonads, where FGF8 is found, there is no FGF18. The temporal and spatial patterns of expression of FGF18 are also dramatically different from FGFs 8 and 17.

HIGH-AFFINITY RECEPTORS

The FGFR family is one of several subclasses of tyrosine kinase receptors that are represented by four distinct genes: FGFR1 (sometimes called flg, or fms-like gene), FGFR2 (sometimes called bek, or bacterial-expressed kinase), FGFR3, and FGFR4 (1).

The FGFRs contain a single membrane-spanning domain, an extracellular domain, and an intracellular domain that has tyrosine kinase activity and is itself phosphorylated. The extracellular domain is characterized by three Ig-like domains, although each receptor gene can produce mRNA encoding smaller receptors with two or even one Ig domain (Fig. 11.2). The ligand-binding domains of the three and two Ig loop proteins appear to be similar.

The complexity of the receptor family is increased by a differential RNA splicing that is dictated by the exon structures of each gene. For example, no fewer than six different classes of FGFR1s can be produced from the FGFR1 gene. They either have no secretory signal sequence, deletion of the first Ig loop, alternative splicing into the third Ig loop, deletions prior to the third Ig loop, or truncation of the transmembrane domain to generate a soluble FGFR1. Together with the isoforms generated by FGFR2 and FGFR3 genes, there are over 100 different combinations possible at the cell surface.

The various isoforms of FGFRs have different binding affinities for different FGF ligands (18–30). Even the secreted form of FGFR1 is capable of binding FGF2 but not FGF1. Because the third Ig loop appears to confer selectivity, FGF1 or FGF2 or sometimes both will interact with FGFR1. When FGFR2 is spliced into the third Ig loop, it generates a receptor that recognizes FGF7 and FGF1 but not FGFs 2–6, 8, or 9. Similarly, FGF8 and FGF9 appear to have increased selectivity for FGFR3 (31). The isoforms of receptors that are truncated can act as binding proteins that are secreted from cells in the absence of a transmembrane domain or as dominant negative receptors when trapped at the cell surface. Data are only beginning to surface that suggest that different FGFRs might have different signaling roles. FGFR1 is often associ-

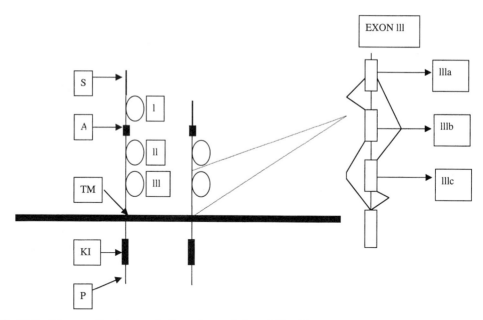

FIG. 11.2. Primary structure and alternative splicing of fibroblast growth factor receptors (FGFRs). A full-length FGFR exists with three immunoglobulin (Ig)-like domains, but the major alternative splicing pathways will express either Ig-like domain IIIb or IIIc. The indicated region of Ig-like domain III is the sequence subject to alternative splicing, but there are short forms of the receptor having only Ig-like domains II and III. Alternative splicing of FGFR in the Ig-like domain III region are from spliced exons IIIa, IIIb, and IIIc, yielding isoforms that differ only in their third Ig loop. Ligand specificity is outlined in Table 11.1. *SP,* signal peptide; *A,* acidic region; *I, II, III,* Ig-like domains; *TM,* transmembrane domain; *KI,* kinase insert; *P,* putative site of autophosphorylation.

ated with malignancies and transformation, while the other receptors are somewhat less associated with these. In any event, because signaling requires receptor dimerization, the complexity of the FGF–FGFR response is compounded by the possibility that heterogeneous dimers have different ligand specificity and altered intracellular substrates for tyrosine phosphorylation than do the homodimers.

LOW-AFFINITY RECEPTORS

If the number of FGF ligands and the number of high-affinity receptor isoforms were not enough to create significant complexity, the low-affinity receptors that interact with FGFs at the cell surface add yet more. First, the low-affinity receptors bind the FGFs with relatively high affinity (1 to 20 nM), so they are thought to play an important role in controlling their activities (1). It is only when they are compared to the

very-high-affinity FGF receptors (kda 1 to 10 pM) that FGF binding to all heparin sulfate proteoglycans (HSPGs) can be considered low. These HSPGs can be at the cell surface, in the extracellular matrix, or soluble in biological fluids. They consist of a core protein to which a variable number of glycosaminoglycan chains are linked. Depending on the core protein, HSPGs can be syndecans, glypicans, perlecans, or betaglycans, each having its own particular spectrum of FGF binding, localization in tissues, developmental expression pattern, and ability to control FGF activity. Located in biological fluids, on the cell surface, and in the extracellular matrix, they can sequester FGFs so that they either block interactions with their receptors, deliver FGFs to their high-affinity receptors to form a receptor complex, or simply stabilize the mitogens so that they are protease-resistant and acid-stable in a wound-healing milieu.

The sequestering function of HSPGs is probably best described for FGF2. Analyses of cells in culture, tissue sections of developing and adult tissues, and biochemical studies have all pointed to the localization of FGF2 in basement membranes, where it is bound to HSPGs (52). Here there are a large number of binding sites that serve to restrict the diffusion off FGF2 to other tissues and cellular compartments. There may also be a regulatory role for the HSPG interaction since the depot of mitogen allows a slow and gradual release to the high-affinity receptor. Accordingly, degradation of basement membranes during wound healing and tissue repair, embryonic development, tumor growth, and metastasis results in the release of FGFs from the basement membranes and their availability to cells expressing high-affinity receptors (12,13). Because the binding of FGFs to HSPGs is se-

quence-specific, their interaction is also independently controlled from other heparin-binding proteins like hepatocyte growth factor, antithrombin, and TGF-βs, to name a few.

In addition to the storage and sequestration functions of HSPGs in the control of FGF activities, there is compelling evidence that the HSPGs play a role, with the high-affinity receptor, in the signal-transduction cascade (53). When cells are chemically, enzymatically, or genetically stripped of their cell surface HSPGs, they are no longer responsive to FGFs unless the heparin GAG is added with FGFs to cells. Accordingly, the formation of a heteromultimeric receptor complex that consists of possibly several high- and low-affinity receptors and ligands appears to be responsible for binding, internalization, and cell responsiveness to FGFs.

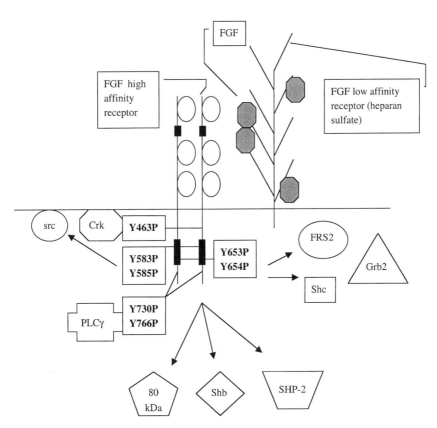

FIG. 11.3. Signal propagation from fibroblast growth factor receptor (FGFR)-1 to downstream signaling molecules depends on their tyrosine phosphorylation by molecules activated by the receptor or, in most cases, directly by the FGFR.

Based on the need for high-affinity receptors to dimerize to elicit a mitogenic response, the signaling complex most likely includes at least two high-affinity receptors, two HSPGs, and two ligands. Moreover, with the possibility of hetero-dimerization, specificity and responsiveness could be altered when FGFR1 dimerizes with another receptor, FGFR3 for example, at the cell surface. The generation of numerous molecular isoforms of each gene product underscores the complexity of the FGF–FGFR axis.

RECEPTOR ACTIVATION AND SIGNALING

Binding of FGF leads to dimerization of FGFR in a complex that includes heparin sulfate. Dimerization can occur between FGFRs of the same type or different types. As with many ligands, dimerization of the receptor tyrosine kinases appears to be a prerequisite for activation of the receptor's enzymatic activity. FGFR1 phosphorylation has been studied in considerable detail (Fig. 11.3). There are four phosphorylation sites in the kinase domain (Y653, Y654, Y730, Y766). A number of SH2 domain-containing enzymes and adaptors participate in FGFR signal tranduction. These domains are roughly 100 amino acids in length, conserved, and found in many different enzymes. Their activities are modified, usually activated, by interactions with phosphorylated receptors that alter their function to propagate signaling. For example, phosphorylation of Y766 in FGFR1 allows binding and subsequently tyrosine phosphorylation of phospholipase C (PLC)-γ, and Crk tyrosine phosphorylation and downstream signal transduction depend on Tyr^{463} in FGFR1. The activated FGFR1 dimer strongly binds PLC-γ (Tyr^{766}). The other signal-transduction molecules shown in Fig. 11.3 do not necessarily interact with any one single tyrosine phosphorylation site in the receptor. For example, FRS2 and the Src family tyrosine kinases are anchored in the membrane, whereas Crk, PLC-γ, Shc, SHP-2, Shb, and 80 KH are not. Signal propagation from FGFR1 to these downstream signaling molecules depends on their tyrosine phosphorylation,

which may be indirect but in most cases is probably direct via the enzymatic activity of FGFRs.

SUMMARY AND CONCLUSIONS

The bulk of the evidence surrounding FGFs implicates them in a role in tumor cell development and growth (54,55–60). Yet this complex family of 18 (and probably more) ligands also appears to play important roles in normal cell homeostasis. As their identities have been uncovered, attention has turned to understanding their function. The use of genetically altered mice with knocked out genes points to subtle roles for these FGFs and pivotal functions for their receptors. Clearly, research over the next few years will point to a better understanding of what role these molecules play in such processes as angiogenesis in adult and developing tissues.

REFERENCES

1. Galzie Z, Kinsella AR, Smith JA. Fibroblast growth factors and their receptors. *Biochem Cell Biol* 1997;75:669–685.
2. Coulier F, Pontarotti P, Roubin R, et al. Of worms and men: an evolutionary perspective on the fibroblast growth factor (FGF) and FGF receptor families. *J Mol Evol* 1997;44:43–56.
3. Burgess WH, Maciag T. The heparin-binding (fibroblast) growth factor family of proteins. *Annu Rev Biochem* 1989;58:575–606.
4. Baird A, Klagsbrun M. The fibroblast growth factor family. *Cancer Cells* 1991;3:239–243.
5. Baird A, Klagsbrun M. The fibroblast growth factor family: an overview. *Ann NY Acad Sci* 1991;638:xi–xii.
6. Finch PW, Rubin JS, Miki T, et al. Human KGF is FGF-related with properties of a paracrine effector of epithelial cell growth. *Science* 1989;245:752–755.
7. Miki T, Fleming TP, Bottaro DP, et al. Expression cDNA cloning of the KGF receptor by creation of a transforming autocrine loop. *Science* 1991;251:72–75.
8. Shiang R, Thompson LM, Zhu Y-Z, et al. Mutations in the transmembrane domain of FGFR3 cause the most common genetic form of dwarfism, achondroplasia. *Cell* 1994;78:335–342.
9. Bonaventure J, Rousseau F, Legeai-Mallet L, et al. Common mutations in the fibroblast growth factor receptor 3 (FGFR 3) gene account for achondroplasia, hypochondroplasia, and thanatophoric dwarfism. *Am J Med Genet* 1996;63:148–154.
10. Prestrelski SJ, Fox GM, Arakawa T. Binding of heparin to basic fibroblast growth factor induces a conformational change. *Arch Biochem Biophys* 1992;293:314–319.
11. Gospodarowicz D, Cheng J. Heparin protects basic and acidic FGF from inactivation. *J Cell Physiol* 1986;128:475–484.

12. Vlodavsky I, Bar-Shavit R, Ishai-Michaeli R, et al. Extracellular sequestration and release of fibroblast growth factor: a regulatory mechanism? *Trends Biochem Sci* 1991;16:268–271.

13. Bashkin P, Doctrow S, Klagsbrun M, et al. Basic fibroblast growth factor binds to subendothelial extracellular matrix and is released by heparitinase and heparin-like molecules. *Biochemistry* 1989;28:1737–1743.

14. Renaud F, el Yazidi I, Boilly-Marer Y, et al. Expression and regulation by serum of multiple FGF1 mRNA in normal transformed, and malignant human mammary epithelial cells. *Biochem Biophys Res Commun* 1996; 219:679–685.

15. Abraham JA, Mergia A, Whang JL, et al. Nucleotide sequence of a bovine clone encoding the angiogenic protein, basic fibroblast growth factor. *Science* 1986; 233:545–548.

16. Florkiewicz RZ, Sommer A. Human basic fibroblast growth factor gene encodes four polypeptides: three initiate translation from non-AUG codons. *Proc Natl Acad Sci USA* 1989;86:3978–3981.

17. Florkiewicz RZ, Majack RA, Buechler RD, et al. Quantitative export of FGF-2 occurs through an alternative, energy-dependent, non-ER/Golgi pathway. *J Cell Physiol* 1995;162:388–399.

18. Mignatti P, Rifkin DB. Release of basic fibroblast growth factor, an angiogenic factor devoid of secretory signal sequence: a trivial phenomenon or a novel secretion mechanism? *J Cell Biochem* 1991;47:201–207.

19. Baird A. Fibroblast growth factors: what's in a name? *Endocrinology* 1993;132:487–488.

20. Yoshida T, Miyagawa K, Odagiri H, et al. Genomic sequence of hst, a transforming gene encoding a protein homologous to fibroblast growth factors and the int-2-encoded protein. *Proc Natl Acad Sci USA* 1987;84: 7305–7309.

21. Wilkinson DG, Peters G, Dickson C, et al. Expression of the FGF-related proto-oncogene int-2 during gastrulation and neurulation in the mouse. *EMBO J* 1988;7: 691–695.

22. Wilkinson DG, Bhatt S, McMahon AP. Expression pattern of the FGF-related protooncogene *int*-2 suggests multiple roles in fetal development. *Development* 1989; 105:131–136.

23. Delli Bovi P, Curatola AM, Kern FG, et al. An oncogene isolated by transfection of Kaposi's sarcoma DNA encodes a growth factor that is a member of the FGF family. *Cell* 1987;50:729–737.

24. Niswander L, Tickle C, Vogel A, et al. Function of FGF-4 in limb development. *Mol Reprod Dev* 1994;39: 83–89.

25. Grass S, Arnold HH, Braun T. Alterations in somite patterning of *Myf-5*-deficient mice: a possible role for FGF-4 and FGF-6. *Development* 1996;122:141–150.

26. Zhan X, Bates B, Hu X, et al. The human FGF-5 oncogene encodes a novel protein related to fibroblast growth factors. *Mol Cell Biol* 1988;8:3487–3497.

27. Iida S, Yoshida T, Naito K, et al. Human *hst*-2 (FGF-6) oncogene: cDNA cloning and characterization. *Oncogene* 1992;7:303–309.

28. Marics I, Adelaide J, Raybaud F, et al. Characterization of the *HST*-related *FGF*.6 gene, a new member of the fibroblast growth factor gene family. *Oncogene* 1989; 4:335–340.

29. Han J-K, Martin GR. Embryonic expression of *Fgf-6* is restricted to the skeletal muscle lineage. *Dev Biol* 1993; 158:549–554.

30. Floss T, Arnold HH, Braun T. A role for FGF-6 in skeletal muscle regeneration. *Genes Dev* 1997;11:2040–2051.

31. Aaronson SA, Bottaro DP, Miki T, et al. Keratinocyte growth factor: a fibroblast growth factor family member with unusual target cell specificity. *Ann NY Acad Sci* 1991;638:62–77.

32. Gemel J, Gorry M, Ehrlich GD, et al. Structure and sequence of human *FGF8*. *Genomics* 1996;35:253–257.

33. Tanaka A, Miyamoto K, Minamino N, et al. Cloning and characterization of an androgen-induced growth factor essential for the androgen-dependent growth of mouse mammary carcinoma cells. *Proc Natl Acad Sci USA* 1992;89:8928–8932.

34. Vogel A, Rodriguez C, Izpisúa-Belmonte JC. Involvement of FGF-8 in initiation, outgrowth and patterning of the vertebrate limb. *Development* 1996;122:1737–1750.

35. White RA, Dowler LL, Angeloni SV, et al. Assignment of *FGF8* to human chromosome 10q25-q26: mutations in *FGF8* may be responsible for some types of acrocephalosyndactyly linked to this region. *Genomics* 1995;30: 109–111.

36. Miyamoto M, Naruo K-I, Seko C, et al. Molecular cloning of a novel cytokine cDNA encoding the ninth member of the fibroblast growth factor family, which has a unique secretion property. *Mol Cell Biol* 1993;13:4251–4259.

37. Hecht D, Zimmerman N, Bedford M, et al. Identification of fibroblast growth factor 9 (FGF9) as a high affinity, heparin dependent ligand for FGF receptors 3 and 2 but not for FGF receptors 1 and 4. *Growth Factors* 1995; 12:223–233.

38. Matsumoto-Yoshitomi S, Habashita J, Nomura C, et al. Autocrine transformation by fibroblast growth factor 9 (FGF-9) and its possible participation in human oncogenesis. *Int J Cancer* 1997;71:442–450.

39. Emoto H, Tagashira S, Mattei MG, et al. Structure and expression of human fibroblast growth factor-10. *J Biol Chem* 1997;272:23191–23194.

40. Tagashira S, Harada H, Katsumata T, et al. Cloning of mouse FGF10 and up-regulation of its gene expression during wound healing. *Gene* 1997;197:399–404.

41. Beer HD, Florence C, Dammeier J, et al. Mouse fibroblast growth factor 10: cDNA cloning, protein characterization, and regulation of mRNA expression. *Oncogene* 1997;15:221–2218.

42. Hattori Y, Yamasaki M, Konishi M, et al. Spatially restricted expression of fibroblast growth factor-10 mRNA in the rat brain. *Mol Brain Res* 1997;47:139–146.

43. Smallwood PM, Munoz-Sanjuan I, Tong P, et al. Fibroblast growth factor (FGF) homologous factors: new members of the FGF family implicated in nervous system development. *Proc Natl Acad Sci USA* 1996;93: 9850–9857.

44. Hartung H, Feldman B, Lovec H, et al. Murine FGF-12 and FGF-13: expression in embryonic nervous system, connective tissue and heart. *Mech Dev* 1997;64:31–39.

45. McWhirter JR, Goulding M, Weiner JA, et al. A novel fibroblast growth factor gene expressed in the developing nervous system is a downstream target of the chimeric homeodomain oncoprotein E2A-Pbx1. *Development* 1997;124:3221–3232.

46. Miyake A, Konishi M, Martin FH, et al. Structure and expression of a novel member, FGF-16, of the fibroblast growth factor family. *Biochem Biophys Res Commun* 1998;243:148–152.

47. Hoshikawa M, Ohbayashi N, Yonamine A, et al. Structure and expression of a novel fibroblast growth factor, FGF17, preferentially expressed in the embryonic brain. *Biochem Biophys Res Commun* 1998;244:187–191.

48. Ornitz DM, Leder P. Ligand specificity and heparin dependence of fibroblast growth factor receptors 1 and 3. *J Biol Chem* 1992;267:16305–16311.

49. Ornitz DM, Xu JS, Colvin JS, et al. Receptor specificity of the fibroblast growth factor family. *J Biol Chem* 1996; 271:15292–15297.

50. Blunt AG, Lawshé A, Cunningham ML, et al. Overlapping expression and redundant activation of mesenchymal fibroblast growth factor (FGF) receptors by alternatively spliced FGF-8 ligands. *J Biol Chem* 1997;272: 3733–3738.

51. Chellaiah AT, McEwen DG, Werner S, et al. Fibroblast growth factor receptor (FGFR) 3. Alternative splicing in immunoglobulin-like domain III creates a receptor highly specific for acidic FGF/FGF-1. *J Biol Chem* 1994;269:11620–11627.

52. Vlodavsky I, Folkman J, Sullivan R, et al. Endothelial cell-derived basic fibroblast growth factor: synthesis and deposition into subendothelial extracellular matrix. *Proc Natl Acad Sci USA* 1987;84:2292–2296.

53. Klagsbrun M, Baird A. A dual receptor system is required for basic fibroblast growth factor activity. *Cell* 1991;67:229–231.

54. Halaban R, Kwon B, Ghosh S, et al. bFGF as an autocrine growth factor in human melanomas. *Mol Cell Biol* 1988;8:2933–2941.

55. Peters G, Brookes S, Smith R, et al. The mouse homolog of the hst/k-FGF gene is adjacent to int-2 and is activated by proviral insertion in some virally induced mammary tumors. *Proc Natl Acad Sci USA* 1989;86:5678–5682.

56. Clausse N, Baines D, Moore R, et al. Activation of both *Wnt-1* and *Fgf-3* by insertion of mouse mammary tumor virus downstream in the reverse orientation: a reappraisal of the enhancer insertion model. *Virology* 1993; 194:157–165.

57. Rosen A, Sevelda P, Klein M, et al. First experience with FGF-3 (INT-2) amplification in women with epithelial ovarian cancer. *Br J Cancer* 1993;67:1122–1125.

58. Galdemard C, Brison O, Lavialle C. The proto-oncogene *FGF-3* is constitutively expressed in tumorigenic, but not in non-tumorigenic, clones of a human colon carcinoma cell line. *Oncogene* 1995;10:2331–2342.

59. Schmitt JF, Susil BJ, Hearn MTW. Aberrant FGF-2, FGF-3, FGF-4 and C-ERB-B2 gene copy number in human ovarian, breast and endometrial tumours. *Growth Factors* 1996;13:19–35.

60. Talarico D, Ittmann M, Balsari A, et al. Protection of mice against tumor growth by immunization with an oncogene-encoded growth factor. *Proc Natl Acad Sci USA* 1990;87:4222–4225.

61. Jaye M, Howk R, Burgess W, et al. Human endothelial cell growth factor: cloning, nucleotide sequence, and chromosome localization. *Science* 1986;233:541–545.

62. Mergia A, Eddy R, Abraham JA, et al. The genes for basic and acidic fibroblast growth factors are on different human chromosomes. *Biochem Biophys Res Commun* 1986;138:644–651.

63. Nguyen C, Roux D, Mattei MG, et al. The FGF-related oncogenes *hst* and *int.2*, and the *bcl.*1 locus are contained within one megabase in band q13 of chromosome 11, while the *fgf.*5 oncogene maps to 4q21. *Oncogene* 1988;3:703–708.

64. Dionne CA, Kaplan R, Seuánez H, et al. Chromosome assignment by polymerase chain reaction techniques: assignment of the oncogene FGF-5 to human chromosome 4. *Biotechniques* 1990;8:190–194.

65. De Lapeyriere O, Rosnet O, Benharroch D, et al. Structure, chromosome mapping and expression of the murine *Fgf*-6 gene. *Oncogene* 1990;5:823–832.

66. Mattei MG, DeLapeyriere O, Bresnick J, et al. Mouse Fgf7 (fibroblast growth factor 7) and Fgf8 (fibroblast growth factor 8) genes map to chromosomes 2 and 19 respectively. *Mamm Genome* 1995;6:196–197.

67. Verdier AS, Mattei MG, Lovec H, et al. Chromosomal mapping of two novel human FGF genes, *FGF11* and *FGF12*. *Genomics* 1997;40:151–154.

68. Lovec H, Hartung H, Verdier AS, et al. Assignment of FGF13 to human chromosome band Xq21 by *in situ* hybridization. *Cytogenet Cell Genet* 1997;76:183–184.

69. Wood S, Schertzer M, Yaremko ML. Sequence identity locates CEBPD and FGFR1 to mapped human loci within proximal 8p. *Cytogenet Cell Genet* 1995;70: 188–191.

70. Dionne CA, Modi WS, Crumley G, et al. BEK, a receptor for multiple members of the fibroblast growth factor (FGF) family, maps to human chromosome 10q25.3→ q26. *Cytogenet Cell Genet* 1992;60:34–36.

71. Keegan K, Rooke L, Hayman M, et al. The fibroblast growth factor receptor 3 gene (FGFR3) is assigned to human chromosome 4. *Cytogenet Cell Genet* 1993;62: 172–175.

72. Warrington JA, Bailey SK, Armstrong E, et al. A radiation hybrid map of 18 growth factor, growth factor receptor, hormone receptor, or neurotransmitter receptor genes on the distal region of the long arm of chromosome 5. *Genomics* 1992;13:803–808.

73. Ohbayashi N, Hoshikawa M, Kimura S, et al. Structure and expression of the mRNA encoding a novel fibroblast growth factor, FGF-18. *J Biol Chem* 1998;273:18161–18164.

Skeletal Growth Factors,
edited by Ernesto Canalis.
Lippincott Williams & Wilkins, Philadelphia, © 2000.

12

Fibroblast Growth Factors and Osteogenesis

Pierre J. Marie, Abderrahim Lomri, Françoise Debiais,
and Jérome Lemonnier

*INSERM U349, Cell and Molecular Biology of Bone and Cartilage Lariboisiere Hospital,
75475 Paris, France*

Bone formation results from complex events, which include the commitment of osteoprogenitor cells, the proliferation of preosteoblasts, and the differentiation of preosteoblasts into mature osteoblasts synthesizing a new bone matrix (1,2). A variety of factors can control the bone-formation process by acting on the commitment and recruitment of undifferentiated cells and by influencing the expression or repression of phenotypic markers (3–6). The most important factors regulating bone cell proliferation and differentiation are probably those that are expressed locally or released from the matrix, such as insulin-like growth factors (IGFs), members of the transforming growth factor-β (TGF-β) family, and fibroblast growth factors (FGFs).

FGFs comprise a family of 15 polypeptides which are involved in the control of a variety of processes (7,8). In the skeletal tissue, FGFs have important direct and indirect effects on the recruitment, differentiation, and probably survival of skeletal cells during development, postnatal growth, and bone remodeling and repair, which makes the skeleton an important target tissue for the effects of FGFs. The cellular effects of FGFs are largely dependent on the expression and function of FGF receptors (FGFRs) and on interactions with low-affinity coreceptors, whose expression is temporally and spatially regulated during skeletal development. The recent evidence that several FGFR mutations engender abnormalities in skeletal development emphasizes the importance of FGFR signaling in the control of skeletal formation. This review summarizes the present knowledge of FGF and FGFR expression and function in bone cells *in vitro* and *in vivo*.

EXPRESSION OF FIBROBLAST GROWTH FACTORS AND FGF RECEPTORS IN BONE

Expression of Fibroblast Growth Factors

Genes for the FGF family are expressed in early embryonic life, suggesting an important role in development. During early stages of mammalian development, FGF-3, FGF-4, and FGF-5 transcripts are expressed and implicated in mesoderm induction in concert with other factors, such as TGF-β and the bone morphogenetic proteins (BMPs) (9–12). FGF-8 and FGF-10 are expressed in the limb, and limb bud development is under the control of FGFs 2, 4, 8, and 10 (12–14). In addition, FGF-4 is involved in the formation of the mesenchyme, leading to the formation of the teeth (15). During late stages of skeletal development, FGF-1 or FGF-2 is found in undifferentiated mesenchymal cells and then in osteoblasts and chondroblasts, suggesting that FGF expression is inversely related to cell differentiation (16,17). In cartilage, FGF-2 is produced in the resting and proliferating zones of the epiphyseal growth plate, and its distribution might account for the distinct functional roles of cartilage cells (18,19). In bone cells, FGF-2 is produced in larger amounts than FGF-

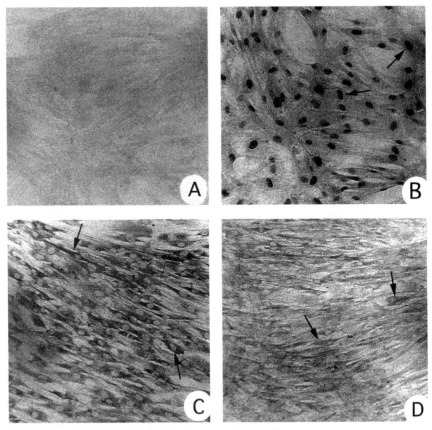

FIG. 12.1. Immunocytochemical analysis of FGF-2 **(B)**, FGFR-1 **(C)** and FGFR-2 **(D)** in human neonatal calvaria osteoblastic cells, compared to control cells incubated with the control peptide **(A)**. The cells show nuclear staining for FGF-2, strong FGFR-1 and weak FGFR-2 immunoreactivity (*arrows*). Original magnification: ×250. (Reproduced from Debiais et al., *J Bone Miner Res* 1998; 13:645–654 with permission of the American Society for Bone and Mineral Research).

1 and is stored in an active form in the extracellular matrix (20,21), presumably associated with heparin sulfate proteoglycans. Among the FGF-2 isoforms described, a short cytoplasmic isoform can be excreted and three larger forms are transferred into the nucleus, where they can interact directly with nuclear proteins (8). Although nuclear FGF-2 is found in human neonatal calvaria osteoblasts (Fig. 12.1) (22), its function remains unknown. However, endogenous FGF-2 appears to be regulated in osteoblastic cells (23). Indeed, FGF-2 and TGF-β increase FGF-2 transcripts, and TGF-β increases cytoplasmic and nuclear FGF-2 in the mouse calvaria-derived MC3T3-E1 cells (23). In addition, recent data indicate that prostaglandins and para-thyroid hormone increase FGF-2 and FGFR mRNA in bone cells (24,25). Thus, anabolic factors for bone may act in part by stimulating endogenous FGF-2 peptides in osteoblasts, suggesting that endogenous FGF-2 plays a role in the control of osteoblastic cell proliferation or differentiation during skeletal formation.

Expression of Fibroblast Growth Factor Receptors

The biological functions of FGFs are mediated by binding to high-affinity FGFRs. FGFRs comprise a family of four receptors with tyrosine kinase activity (26). Ligand binding leads to FGFR dimerization, phosphorylation of intrinsic tyrosine residues, initiation of down-stream kinase cascades, and activation of transcription factors. Multiple receptor isoforms of FGFRs have been described as a result of alternative mRNA splicing and polyadenylation (27,28). The tissue distribution of FGFRs 1 through 4 differs during development, which may be due to distinct temporal receptor expression and to species differences (29). A distinct spatiotemporal pattern of expression was found for FGFRs 1 through 3 during skeletal development in mouse, rat, chicken, and human (30–38) as well as during dental tissue development (39). FGFR-1 transcripts are diffusely expressed in mesenchyme and are found later in hypertrophic cartilage and osteoblasts. In the developing mouse, the FGFR-2 IIIc splice variant (bek) is strongly expressed in the sites of endochondral ossification in long bones as well as in facial and skull bones, and the gene is expressed later

in cartilage, perichondrium, and periosteum (30,32). In the developing human skeleton, FGFR-1 and FGFR-2 transcripts are expressed in the mesenchyme and later in the perichondrium and osteoblasts in long bones and calvaria (38) (Fig. 12.2). In postnatal life, rat calvaria osteoblasts mainly express FGFR-1 and FGFR-2 peptides (40). Interestingly, the pattern of FGFR-3 expression differs from that of FGFR-1 and FGFR-2 during skeletal development (34,35,38,40). FGFR-3 transcripts are found in cartilage rudiment, then in cartilage (Fig. 12.2) and not in mesenchymal cells or perichondral or periosteal cells until late stages of development.

The expression of FGFRs during development indicates that FGFR signaling is essential for the control of skeletal formation. The important role of FGFR-2 for initiation of limb bud development is shown in FGFR-2 −/− mice, which do not exhibit limb formation (41). Addi-

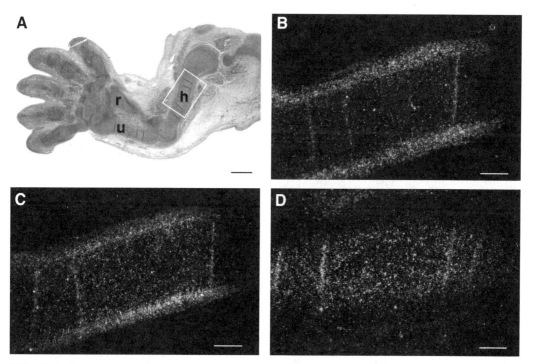

FIG. 12.2. Expression of transcripts for FGFRs in a 50–52 day human embryo upper limb. **A:** shows the HES staining and **B–D** shows details of the rectangle shown in **(A)** (h, humerus; u, ulna; r, radius). Sections hybridized with FGFR-1 **(B),** FGFR-2 **(C)** and FGFR-3 **(D)** probes show distinct expression of FGFRs in the primary osseus collar **(B, D)** and hypertrophic chondrocytes **(D)** of the humeral diaphysis. Scale bars: **A,** 600 μm; **B–D,** 200 μm. (Reprinted with permission from A–L Delezoide et al., 1998, INSERM U 393, AP-HP).

tionally, mutations in FGFR-1 and FGFR-2 in humans induce abnormal ossification of the cranial sutures (craniosynostosis) and formation of fused digits (42–44), showing the important role of these FGFRs during skeletal development. The role of FGFR-3 in endochondral growth is emphasized by the finding that FGFR-3 −/− mice show excessive long bone growth (45,46). Point mutations in FGFR-3 cause constitutive activation of FGFR-3, resulting in abnormal endochondral bone formation and achondroplasia, the most common form of dwarfism (47,48), which demonstrates the important role of FGFR-3 in the control of long bone cartilage growth.

Specific interactions between FGFs and FGFRs may occur at various stages of bone formation. For example, during the early stages of limb development, FGF-8 and FGF-10 can act on limb formation by binding to distinct FGFR-2 splice variants expressed locally (41). This provides a mechanism by which members of the FGF family can bind a specific FGFR isoform at a particular time and location to control the developmental process (14). During later stages of skeletogenesis, FGFR expression is also regulated in a cell-specific and temporal manner. FGFR-1 and FGFR-2 expression is high in chondrocytes and then decreases, while FGFR-3 expression in these cells increases (38,40). These changes in the expression of FGFRs in the developing cartilage are associated with distinct stages of chondrogenesis *in vivo* (38) and *in vitro* (40,49), suggesting that FGFs may control skeletal cells by binding to distinct FGFRs during skeletal development. This variation in FGFR expression together with the variable expression of FGFs is likely to be essential for the coordinated regulation of the effects of FGFs in the control of bone cell proliferation and differentiation during skeletal development and postnatal formation.

The expression of FGFRs during intramembranous bone formation also suggests an important role of FGFs and FGFRs in the control of the developing cranial vault. Calvarial bones are formed by the direct apposition of a bone matrix formed by osteoblasts originating from the differentiation of mesenchymal cells (50). The two edges of calvarial bones, or osteogenic fronts,

are separated by a suture composed of mesenchymal cells, a fraction of which differentiate into preosteoblasts and then osteoblasts, depositing a new bone matrix at the margins of the suture (Fig. 12.3). Studies in the developing mouse suture showed that FGFR-2 transcripts are present at the osteogenic fronts (51,52). In addition, endogenous FGF-2 expression was found to be elevated in mouse and rat fusing sutures (53,54). This may induce the proliferation of mesenchymal cells and downregulation of FGFR-2 transcripts in differential osteoblasts, leading to terminal differentiation of these cells (51). Recent data in the human developing cranial suture showed that suture cells express transcripts for FGFR-1, FGFR-2, and FGFR-3 (38). Our recent immunohistochemical analysis of the fetal human cranial suture demonstrated that FGFR-1 is diffusely localized in proliferating mesenchymal cells, preosteoblasts, and postmitotic osteoblasts whereas FGFR-2 and FGFR-3 are strongly expressed together with FGF-2 in preosteoblasts and osteoblasts (Fig. 12.3) (55). We also found that neonatal rat (40) and human calvarial osteoblastic cells (Fig. 12.1) show strong immunostaining for FGFR-1 and weaker staining for FGFR-2, suggesting that they are target cells for FGF-2. Collectively, these studies suggest that FGF–FGFR interactions are involved in the controlled balance between cell proliferation and differentiation in the fetal suture. However, other agents, such as BMP-2, BMP-4, TGF-βs, IGF-I, and IGF-II, may also be involved in the suture fusion since they are expressed in mouse, rat, and human sutures (53,54,56,57). In addition, TGF-βs 1, 2, and 3 released from the dura mater may play a role in rat suture fusion (58,59). The maintenance and development of the cranial suture may thus result from autocrine effects of FGF-2 as well as complex paracrine effects of other factors acting on proliferating and differentiating osteoblasts.

FIBROBLAST GROWTH FACTORS AND FGF RECEPTOR INTERACTIONS WITH HEPARIN SULFATE PROTEOGLYCANS

In addition to FGFRs, FGFs bind heparin sulfate proteoglycans (HSPGs), which are essential

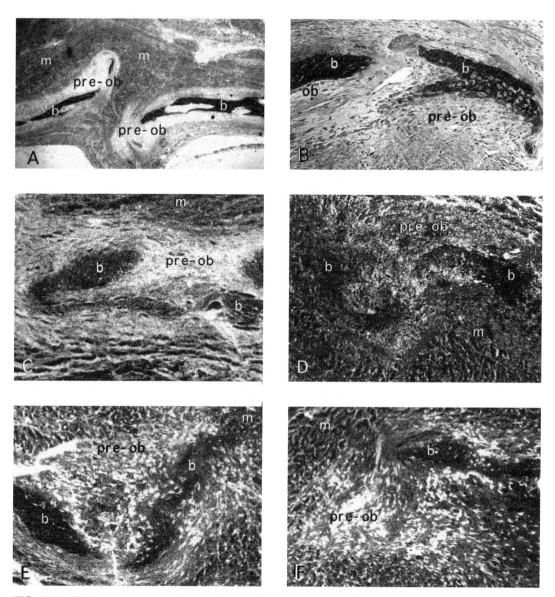

FIG. 12.3. Distinct immunoreactivity for FGF-2, FGFR-1, -2 and -3 in the normal human fetal coronal suture at 27 weeks of age. The normal suture, shown at low **(A)** and high **(B)** magnification, is composed of mesenchymal cells (*m*) that differentiate into pre-osteoblasts (*pre-ob*) and osteoblasts (*ob*) depositing a new bone (*b*) matrix along the suture edges. FGF-2 immunostaining is weak in mesenchymal cells and strong in pre-osteoblasts **(C)**. FGFR-1 is diffusely expressed in pre-osteoblasts **(D)** whereas FGFR-2 **(E)** and FGFR-3 **(F)** are strongly expressed in pre-osteoblasts and osteoblasts. Original magnification: × 125. (from Lemonnier et al., 1999, and unpublished data).

for FGF cellular actions (60). Heparin modulates the mitogenic activity of FGF-1 but not FGF-2 and enhances the inductive effects of FGF-1 and FGF-2 on bone resorption and the inhibitory effect of FGF-2 on collagen synthesis (61–63).

Recent data indicate that syndecans may control the effects of FGFs on skeletal cell proliferation and differentiation. Syndecans are cell surface transmembrane HSPGs which interact with FGF binding and signaling (64–67) and are expressed during skeletal development (68,69). Syndecan-1 is initially expressed in mesenchymal cells (68) and limb bud (69) and affects bone cell differentiation (70). Syndecan-2 is abundant in prechondrogenic cells but is low in differentiating chondrocytes and is present in the perichondrium and periosteum at the onset of osteogenesis (40,65). Syndecan-3 is expressed in mesenchymal cells during limb bud formation, and its expression is regulated by FGFs (71). At this stage, syndecan-3 mediates the ability of FGFs to promote the outgrowth and proliferation of limb mesoderm (72). At later stages, syndecan-3 is expressed in precartilage cells, in immature chondrocytes of the growth plate, and in the perichondrium, and may control chondrocyte proliferation during endochondral ossification (71,73). Syndecan-4 is highly expressed in chondrocytes (74) and osteoblasts (40). Recently, we found that syndecans are associated with FGFs during osteogenesis (40,55). In the human cranial suture, syndecan-1 and FGFR-1 are co-expressed diffusely, whereas syndecans 2 and 4 are colocalized with FGFR-2 and FGFR-3 in preosteoblasts and osteoblasts, revealing a specific common pattern of expression (55). During *in vitro* chondrogenic and osteogenic differentiation, rat chondrocytes coexpress FGFR-3, syndecan-2, and syndecan-4, and their expression decreases during differentiation (40), whereas rat calvarial osteoblasts express syndecans 1, 2, and 4 with FGFR-1 and FGFR-2 (40), indicating that syndecans can interact with FGFRs to control FGF actions during bone formation. This is supported by the finding that alterations of matrix- and cell-associated proteoglycan sulfation or synthesis inhibit the growth response to FGF-2 in cultured rat mandibular condyle (75). Thus, syndecans appear to be important coreceptors, modulating the actions of FGFs in skeletal cells to control endochondral and intramembranous formation in a spatiotemporal manner. Syndecans may also interact with other factors in bone since syndecan-2 modulates the mitogenic effects of granulocyte-macrophage colony-stimulating factor (GM-CSF) on human trabecular osteoblastic cells (76,77). Interestingly, FGF-2 and TGF-β were found to modulate the expression of syndecans

in several cell types (66,73,78,79). This may provide a local mechanism to regulate FGF–FGFR interactions in bone cells.

FIBROBLAST GROWTH FACTORS AND BONE FORMATION

In Vitro Effects of Fibroblast Growth Factors

In various systems *in vitro,* FGF-1 and FGF-2 were found to control osteoblastic cell proliferation and differentiation. FGF-1 and FGF-2 stimulate the proliferation of rat calvarial cells (80–82) and stromal bone cells (83–86). The mitogenic activity of FGF-2 is stronger than that of FGF-1 in the absence of heparin (87), and the growth response to FGF-2 appears to decrease with age (88). In addition, FGF-2 exerts complex effects on osteoblastic cell differentiation. In short-term culture, FGF-1 and FGF-2 inhibit alkaline phosphatase (ALP) activity and reduce collagen type I and osteocalcin expression (81,89,90). This dual effect of FGF-2 is not specific for osteoblastic cells since FGF-2 also stimulates cell proliferation and inhibits the odontoblast phenotype of human pulp cells that expresses FGFR-1 (91). In osteoblastic cells, the inhibitory effect of FGF-2 on type I collagen is mediated by a transcriptional mechanism and is independent of cell replication (89). Additionally, FGF-2 stimulates osteopontin, modulates osteonectin, and inhibits the parathormone-responsive adenylate cyclase activity in rat osteosarcoma cells (90,92,93). In these cells, FGF-2 acts in part via a pertussis toxin–sensitive G protein (93). Although FGF-1 and FGF-2 inhibit osteocalcin expression in rat calvarial cells (87,94), FGF-2 enhances osteocalcin in bovine bone cells (95) and directly affects osteocalcin transcription in mouse calvarial cells (96–98). In these cells, FGF-2 and cyclic adenosine monophosphate (cAMP) have synergistic effects on osteocalcin expression (96), and osteocalcin promoter elements conferring FGF-2 responsiveness have been identified (97). In addition to modulating osteoblast differentiation markers, FGFs may act on other functions in osteoblasts. For example, FGF-2 downregulates the expression of connexin-43 in mouse calvarial cells, resulting in a decrease in gap junctional intercellular communication (98). FGF-2 was also found to increase sodium-dependent phosphate transport in mouse calvarial cells, which may contribute to the regulation of intramembranous calcification (99). Thus, FGFs regulate bone cells by acting at early and late stages of the osteoblast phenotype. Additionally, FGF-2 was found to affect apoptosis of osteoblasts (100). In the rat calvarial cell system, osteoblasts undergo apoptosis at the end of the differentiation pathway (101) and apoptosis occurs during normal mouse suture development *in vivo* (102). It is thus possible that FGFs may play a role in the control of cranial vault development by inhibiting apoptosis in cells of the osteoblastic lineage.

FGFs also have important effects on osteoblastic cell differentiation and bone matrix formation in long-term culture, although the effects are dependent on the cell culture system. In rat calvariae, FGF-1 blocks the progression of the osteoblast developmental sequence and reduces bone nodule formation (94). FGF-2 also reduces osteoblast markers in human marrow stromal cells and trabecular bone cells in long-term culture (103). In contrast, in the rat bone marrow stromal system, growth stimulation induced by FGF-2 is followed by increased cell differentiation and matrix mineralization (83,84). FGF-2 also stimulates the growth and expression of the osteogenic phenotype of dexamethasone-treated rat (85) and human (104) bone marrow stromal cells. In the rat model, the osteogenic effect of FGF-2 and BMP-2 appears to be synergistic, suggesting that FGF-2 enhances the marrow stromal cell population that is responsive to BMP-2 and dexamethasone (86). In neonatal human calvarial preosteoblastic cells (105), short treatment with FGF-2 initially increases cell growth and reduces osteoblast differentiation markers, whereas prolonged FGF-2 treatment increases osteocalcin synthesis and matrix mineralization in long-term culture (Fig. 12.4), showing that FGF-2 effects are dependent on

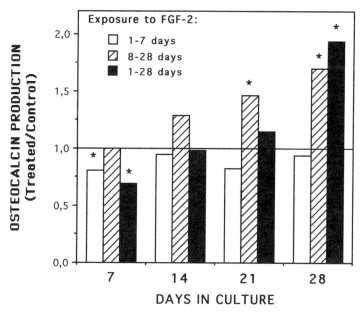

FIG. 12.4. Dual effects of transient (1–7 days), late (8–28 days) and continuous (1–28 days) treatments with FGF-2 (50 ng/ml) on osteocalcin production by human calvarial osteoblastic cells in culture, showing that the effects of FGF-2 on osteoblast differentiation are maturation stage–specific. Data are the mean ± SEM (*: p < 0.05 vs. untreated cells). (Redrawn from Debiais et al., *J Bone Miner Res* 1998;13:645–654, with permission of the American Society for Bone and Mineral Research).

the stage of osteoblast maturation (23). These *in vitro* osteogenic effects of FGF-2 may be relevant to the *in vivo* situation, where FGF-2 acts on osteoblast precursor cells to increase endosteal bone formation, as discussed below.

Some of the effects of FGFs on bone cells may be mediated by local growth factors. For example, FGF-1 and FGF-2 increase the production of TGF-β *in vitro* and *in vivo* (94,106–108) and TGF-β increases FGF-2 expression in osteoblastic cells (24). In addition, TGF-β and FGF-1 and FGF-2 interact to modulate their mitogenic effects in osteoblasts (24). In human calvarial cells, FGF-2 decreases TGF-β2 production in immature cells and has opposite effects in differentiated cells, indicating that FGF-2 modulates the production of TGF-β2 differently depending on the stage of cell maturation (22). In addition to TGF-βs, other local growth factors may mediate the effects of FGFs. For example, FGF-2 decreases the expression of IGF-I, IGF-II, and IGF-I binding proteins 2 through 6 in osteoblastic cells (109). The synthesis of IGF binding protein-5, an important regulatory protein of IGFs in bone cells, is also inhibited by FGF-2 through transcriptional mechanisms (109). Recent data indicates that FGF-2 induces hepatocyte growth factor expression in osteoblasts (110). These factors may thus mediate some of the actions of FGF-2 on osteoblasts.

The signaling mechanisms involved in regulation of the osteoblast phenotype by FGFs remain relatively unknown. In many cell types, binding of FGFs to FGFRs leads to receptor dimerization, activation of intrinsic tyrosine phosphorylation, and initiation of downstream kinase cascades, which culminate in altered gene transcription (26). Activation of FGFRs initiates a sequence of events leading to mitogen-activated protein (MAP) kinase phosphorylation. However, FGFRs also activate phospholipase C, leading to activation of protein kinase C (PKC) and mobilization of intracellular calcium. Additionally, exogenous FGF-2 bound to FGFRs may be internalized by endocytosis and translocated into the nucleus, where it may activate gene transcription (111–113). In osteoblastic cells, FGF-2 was found to activate MAP kinase signal transduction and extracellular signal–reg-

ulated kinase 2 (ERK2) (114,115); however, FGF actions in osteoblastic cells may involve several complex pathways. For example, it was recently found that the FGF-2 transcriptional activation of the matrix metalloproteinase MMP1 in mouse osteoblasts is independent of ERK1/ERK2 MAP kinase activity (115). In the clonal rat osteoblastic cell line Py1a, inhibition of the PKC pathway inhibits c-fos and the mitogenic response to FGF-2 but not the FGF-2 effects on MAP kinase phosphorylation (116). In addition, the FGF-2-induced increase in interleukin-6 synthesis was found to involve p38 mitogen-activated protein kinase in osteoblasts (117). Thus, the respective roles of MAP kinases and other signaling pathways involved in the FGF effects on osteoblastic cell function begins to be clarified.

In Vivo Effects of Fibroblast Growth Factors

There is considerable evidence that FGF–FGFR interactions play important roles in the control of fetal skeletal development *in vivo*. In mice, FGFR-1 disruption results in embryonic lethality in null FGFR-1 mice, and this receptor is required for early embryonic mesodermal development (118). In transgenic mice, FGFR-2 is required for epithelial morphogenesis (119), and homozygous FGFR-2-deficient mice die during embryogenesis (120). On the other hand, excess exogenous FGF-2 results in developmental abnormalities in limb patterning (121). In addition, transgenic mice overexpressing FGF-2 display chondrodysplasia and shortening of long bones (122,123). FGF-2 inhibits growth plate chondrocyte proliferation *in vivo* (124), further indicating that FGFs play a key role in endochondral bone formation (125). FGFR-3 knockout in the mouse causes overgrowth of long bones and vertebrae (45), supporting the inhibitory effect of FGFR-3 signaling on cartilage growth (46). Moreover, excessive FGF signaling associated with mutations of FGFRs 1 through 3 results in several abnormalities in bone morphogenesis in humans (42–44), showing that the FGF–FGFR system is an essential mechanism regulating cartilage and longitudinal bone growth during development *in vivo*.

Evidence that FGFs also influence bone formation *in vivo* in postnatal life comes from experimental studies. In growing rats, exogenous FGF-2 at low dose stimulates endosteal bone formation (106,107,126,127), and intraosseous application of FGF-2 in normal rabbits increases bone formation and bone mineral density at the sites of injection (128). Additionally, FGF-2 administration produces hyperosteosis in long or spongious bone (129). Systemic administration of FGF-1 (130) or local application of FGF-2 stimulates bone formation and restores bone volume in ovariectomized rodents (131), showing that FGFs have anabolic effects on bone formation in both normal and osteopenic animals. The mechanisms that are involved in the stimulatory effects of FGF-2 on endosteal bone formation *in vivo* appear to be multiple. The formation of new bone in treated rats results from the initial effect of exogenous FGF-1 and FGF-2 on the recruitment of osteoblast precursor cells, which differentiate into preosteoblasts and then into osteoblasts (106). This is consistent with the *in vitro* FGF effects on bone marrow stromal cells in long-term cultures (83,84,132,133). In addition, FGF-2 may increase the local expression of TGF-β, as increased immunoreactivity for TGF-β1 was found in osteoblasts and bone matrix after FGF-2 treatment in rats (106,107). Since FGF-2 enhances TGF-β expression in mature osteoblastic cells *in vitro* (23,94,108), part of the anabolic effect of FGF-2 on bone formation *in vivo* may be related to the stimulation of endogenous TGF-β synthesis in osteoblasts.

FIBROBLAST GROWTH FACTOR RECEPTOR MUTATIONS AND INTRAMEMBRANOUS BONE FORMATION

The importance of FGF–FGFR interactions in skeletal development in humans is demonstrated by the recent discoveries that mutations in FGFRs are associated with heritable human skeletal disorders involving craniofacial and limb abnormalities, such as Apert, Crouzon, Pfeiffer, and Jackson-Weiss syndromes (42–44) and achondroplasia (47,48). Craniosynostotic syndromes related to FGFR-1 and FGFR-2 mutations were shown to be associated with mutations in the immunoglobulin (Ig) III domain or in the linker between Ig II and Ig III domains (Fig. 12.5). Most of the FGFR mutations are missense, with a smaller number of splice mutations or small insertions or deletions (134). Experimental studies suggest that some of these mutations may engender gain of function (135–139). FGFR-2 and FGFR-3 mutations induce constitutive activation of the receptor, which may result from complex functional alterations of the mutant receptor (134). For example, in Crouzon syndrome, transfection of NIH3T3 cells with C342Y-mutated FGFR-2 results in ligand-independent activation of FGFR-2 signaling, associated with decreased binding of FGF-2 to the mutated receptor (140). In Apert syndrome, FGFR-2 mutations were found to enhance receptor occupancy by FGF ligands and/or to induce prolongation of the duration of receptor signaling rather than increased tyrosine kinase phosphorylation (141–143). It has been postulated that FGFR-2 mutations in the linker region may be involved both in stabilizing the structure of Ig II and Ig III and in ligand binding. The disulfide bond may stabilize the whole structure by increasing hydrophobic interactions between amino acid residues inside the Ig fold, leading to major conformational changes of the secondary structure. In addition, the S–S bridge formation or dissociation may result in the creation of free cysteine residues and abnormal disulfide bonding with other mutant FGFR molecules or FGF ligands (142). Interestingly, use of the dominant-negative FGFR-2 loss-of-function approach in mice showed that the secreted soluble dominant-negative FGFR-2 causes skull and limb malformations reminiscent of human skeletal disorders associated with FGFR mutations (144). Thus, it appears that too much or too little FGFR signaling can induce similar skeletal abnormalities, at least in mice. However, the signaling mechanisms linking the genotypic and phenotypic alterations induced by FGFR mutations in human bone cells remain to be established.

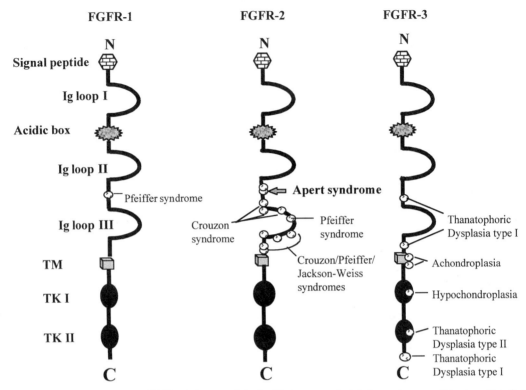

FIG. 12.5. Mutations in FGFRs 1-3 associated with human skeletal syndromes. The location for each syndrome on FGFRs is shown on the structure of the receptors. TM, transmembrane domain; TK I and TK II, tyrosine kinase domain.

Developmentally, the problem of syndromic craniosynostosis may be posed as follows: What causes the suture to fail in the execution of its proliferative and antidifferentiative programs? To answer this question, different mutations in FGFR-2 have been generated in several organisms to examine the function of these receptors during development. The phenotypic consequences of these mutations are diverse and seem to differ from those known in humans because of species-specific differences in FGFR functions (134). Using *ex utero* surgical techniques on fetal mice, it was recently shown that implantation of FGF-2-soaked beads over the coronal suture accelerates suture closure (51,52), possibly by inducing the proliferation and differentiation of immature osteoblasts, leading to increased production of matrix (52). In this murine model, FGFR-2 expression is high in areas of rapid cell proliferation but not in domains of osteogenic

differentiation, suggesting downregulation of the receptor (51). Application of exogenous FGF-4 also accelerates osteoblast differentiation in the mouse cranial suture (52). This suggests that excessive FGF-2 signaling results in osteogenic differentiation and is associated with downregulation of FGFR-2 expression. Using a newly developed human calvarial cell model (105), we recently investigated the phenotypic consequences of FGFR-2 mutations in humans at the tissue and cellular levels (55,145,146). *In vivo*, we found that the fused suture in Apert syndrome is characterized by increased deposition of new bone matrix by preosteoblasts at the subperiosteal level compared to the normal suture (55). While cell growth in proliferating mesenchymal cells or preosteoblasts appears to be normal, type I collagen, osteopontin, and osteocalcin were found to be prematurely expressed in preosteoblasts (Fig. 12.6). Using a human cal-

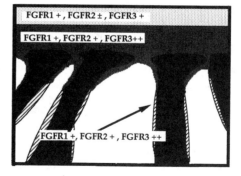

A. NORMAL

FGFR1 + , FGFR2 ± , FGFR3 +

FGFR1 + , FGFR2 ++, FGFR3 ++

FGFR1 +, FGFR2 ++ , FGFR3 ++

B. APERT

FGFR1 + , FGFR2 ± , FGFR3 +

FGFR1 +, FGFR2 + , FGFR3++

FGFR1 +, FGFR2 + , FGFR3 ++

Mesenchymal Cells

Normal Pre-Osteoblasts (Col 1±, OC ±, OP±)   Apert Pre-Osteoblasts (Col 1+, OC+, OP+)

Osteoblasts (Col 1+, OC+, OP+)   Bone Matrix

FIG. 12.6. Schematic representation of the normal human fetal suture **(A)** and Apert fused suture **(B)** showing the alterations of preosteoblast differentiation induced by the Ser252Trp FGFR-2 Apert mutation. The mutation induces premature expression of type 1 collagen (*Col 1*), osteocalcin (*OC*) and osteopontin (*OP*) in preosteoblasts, and downregulation of FGFR-2 in preosteoblasts and osteoblasts, resulting in increased de novo matrix deposition and premature ossification (from Lomri et al., 1998; Marie, 1999).

varial cell line with the Apert FGFR-2 Ser252Trp mutation, we found that the mutant cells display increased expression of osteoblast marker genes and osteogenesis *in vitro* (145), showing that the Apert FGFR-2 mutation constitutively induces a selective increase in the process of the differentiation pathway in preosteoblasts (Fig. 12.6). This is consistent with our finding in human nonsyndromic craniosynostosis, in which premature osteogenesis results from increased bone formation and osteoblast differentiation with normal cell proliferation (147). However, distinct FGFR-2 mutations associated with alterations of the FGFR transduction pathway, may lead to different cellular phenotypes in vitro (148). Interestingly, we also found that the Ser252Trp FGFR-2 mutation induces a selective downregulation of FGFR-2 in preosteoblasts and osteoblasts in the fused suture *in vitro* and *in vivo*, whereas FGFR-1, FGFR-3, and syndecan expression is not reduced (55). This is consistent with the downregulation of FGFR-2 in Crouzon syndrome (149) and in FGF-2 treated mouse suture cells (51). The FGFR-2 downregulation in mutant cells may lead to alteration of FGFR downstream signal-

ing, which may contribute to the observed premature osteoblast differentiation (55,149). Premature ossification induced by FGFR mutations may thus result from dysregulation of the osteoblast proliferation/differentiation program associated with a time- and space-related alteration of specific genes. Recent data from our laboratory also demonstrated that the Ser252Trp FGFR-2 mutation in Apert syndrome selectively increases E- and N-cadherin expression in human fetal calvarial cells *in vitro* and *in vivo*, resulting in increased cell–cell adhesion, increased preosteoblast differentiation, and osteogenesis (150). Thus, FGFR-2 mutations may activate signaling pathways leading to increased expression of specific genes and premature osteoblast phenotype in the cranial suture. The identification of differentially expressed genes between normal and mutated human suture cells may help us to better understand the mechanisms controlling sutural closure.

FIBROBLAST GROWTH FACTORS AND BONE RESORPTION

Besides controlling bone formation, FGF-1 and FGF-2 were shown to activate bone resorption *in vitro* (82,151–153). Several mechanisms may be involved in the FGF-induced increase in bone resorption. In cultured fetal rat long bones, FGF-2 stimulates bone resorption by a prostaglandin-independent mechanism in the presence of heparin (151). In mouse calvaria and fetal rat long bone cultures, however, prostaglandins mediate some of the effects of FGF-1 and FGF-2 on bone resorption (82,153). Recently, FGF-2 was found to increase the formation of multinuclear, tartrate-resistant acid phosphatase–positive, and calcitonin receptor–positive resorbing osteoclast-like cells in mouse bone marrow cultures. In this model, the induction of osteoclast formation by FGF-2 is mediated by an increased prostaglandin E_2 (PGE_2) production in the culture (153). Accordingly, FGF-2 was found to rapidly stimulate PGE_2 production in mouse calvarial cells through transcriptional regulation of prostaglandin G/H synthase-2 (PGHS-2), the major enzyme involved in arachidonic acid conversion to prostaglandins (154). On the other hand, FGF-2 was found to increase interleukin (IL-6) transcripts and protein in mouse calvarial osteoblastic cells (155). This effect is dependent on intracellular calcium mobilization and is autoregulated by PKC activation (156). Since IL-6 is an important activator of bone resorption *in vitro,* the inducing effect of FGF-2 on IL-6 synthesis may partially mediate the effect of FGF-2 on resorbing cells (155). Thus, FGF-2 may have both direct and indirect effects on osteoclast precursor recruitment and bone resorption.

FGF was also found to control the proteolytic enzymes that are involved in bone matrix degradation and resorption. In rat calvarial bone cells, FGFs increase interstitial collagenase mRNA and protein in part by a prostaglandin- and PKC-dependent pathway (94,157). In addition, FGF-2 induces the expression of tissue inhibitors of metalloproteinases (TIMP) 1 and 3 (157), which are important regulators of collagenase activity. In mouse calvarial osteoblastic cells, FGF-2 transcriptionally regulates collagenase gene expression through a prostaglandin-independent and protein tyrosine kinase–dependent pathway (158). Recently, the FGF response elements involved in the FGF-2 activation of the human interstitial collagenase promoter in mouse osteo-blastic cells were identified (115). Although the role of collagenase in osteoblasts remains uncertain, these data suggest that FGF-2 may modulate bone matrix degradation by regulating collagenase expression and activity. In addition, FGF-2 was found to affect stromelysin-3 expression in mouse calvarial cells. FGF-2 acutely decreases stromelysin-3 mRNA stability, whereas prolonged treatment increases gene transcription; this mechanism may contribute to matrix degradation (159). It can then be hypothesized that the FGF-2-induced proteolysis of the matrix may result in the release of HSPGs, which may in turn regulate the activity of FGFs on bone cells.

FIBROBLAST GROWTH FACTORS AND BONE REPAIR

Experimental data indicate that FGFs may play an important role in the control of fracture repair. At the early stage of fracture repair, FGF-1 and FGF-2 are expressed in the granulation tissue at the fracture site (160). At this stage, the local production of FGFs may increase cell migration and angiogenesis (161). During the formation of the callus, FGF-1 expression increases whereas FGF-2 expression is stable, suggesting distinct roles of these factors in fracture repair (162). Evidence for FGF regulation of fracture repair comes from experimental studies testing FGF response in models of fracture repair. The local application of FGF-2 was found to stimulate callus formation and to facilitate fracture repair in normal rats and to restore the impaired repairing process in diabetic rats (163). The healing effect of FGF-2 appears to result from the early increase in recruitment of mesenchymal cells, which are essential for fracture repair as they differentiate into chondroblasts and osteoblasts (163). However, FGF-2 may also act by increasing the local production of TGF-β (108), which has a major regulatory role in fracture repair (162). Although FGF-1 increases the proliferation of chondrocyte precursors in the early stages of chondrogenesis (164) and increases fibrous callus in the fracture site in rats, it does not enhance bone repair (165), possibly because of the different biological activities of the two factors. In addition to having a potential role in enhancement of bone healing, FGF-2 at low dose was reported to stimulate chondrogenesis or bone formation in various models of bone defect (166–171). Collectively, these experimental data suggest that FGFs may have therapeutic effects on bone regeneration (172).

CONCLUSION

Recent studies on the expression and biology of FGFs and FGFRs at the tissue, cellular, and molecular levels point to an important role of FGF–FGFR interactions in the control of endochondral and intramembranous bone formation. This is highlighted in particular by the spatiotemporal expression of FGF, FGFR and HSPG coreceptors, the complex cellular and molecular effects of FGFs in bone cells, and the phenotypic consequences of FGFR mutations in human skeletal syndromes. However, several points need to be addressed for a better understanding of the effects of FGFs on skeletogenesis. While the expression of FGFs and FGFRs during skeletal development has been determined, the precise role of the distinct FGFs and FGFR isoforms in the control of osteoprogenitor cell proliferation and osteoblast differentiation is not known. In addition, the cellular and molecular mechanisms underlying the effects of exogenous FGFs or the FGFR mutations on osteogenesis need to be determined. The identification of the signal-transduction pathways that are activated by FGFR mutations and that lead to the expression of specific genes and abnormal phenotypes in human bone cells may help us to understand the molecular regulatory effects of FGFs during osteoblast differentiation and osteogenesis *in vivo* and perhaps to develop new therapeutic approaches to stimulate bone formation in human bone disorders.

ACKNOWLEDGMENTS

The senior author (P.J. Marie) wish to thank other members of his group, D. Modrowski, A. Molténi, and Ph. Delannoy, for their contribution to the work presented in this review and A.-L. Delezoide for permission to use published material.

REFERENCES

1. Aubin JE, Liu F. The osteoblast lineage. In: Bilezikian J, Raisz LG, Rodan GA, eds. *Principles of bone biology.* San Diego: Academic Press, 1996:51–67.
2. Marie PJ. Osteoblasts and bone formation. In: Zaidi M, ed. *Advances in organ biology.* Stamford: JAI Press, 1998:445–473.
3. Canalis E, McCarthy TL, Centrella M. Growth factors and cytokines in bone cell metabolism. *Annu Rev Med* 1991;42:17–24.
4. Baylink DJ, Finkelman RD, Subburaman M. Growth factors to stimulate bone formation. *J Bone Miner Res* 1993;8:S565–S572.
5. Marie PJ, Hott M, Lomri A. Regulation of endosteal bone formation and osteoblasts in rodent vertebrae. *Cells Mater* 1994;4:143–154.
6. Mundy GR. Local control of bone formation by osteoblasts. *Clin Orthop Rel Res* 1995;313:19–26.
7. Gospodarowicz D. Fibroblast growth factor. *Crit Rev Oncog* 1989;1:1–26.
8. Bikfalvi A, Klein S, Pintucci G, et al. Biological roles of fibroblast growth factor-2. *Endocr Rev* 1997;18,1:26–45.
9. Kimelman D, Kirschner M. Synergistic induction of mesoderm by FGF and TGF-β and the identification of an mRNA coding for FGF in the early *Xenopus* embryo. *Cell* 1987;51:869–877.
10. Amaya E, Stein PA, Musci TJ, et al. FGF signaling in the early specification of mesoderm in *Xenopus. Development* 1993;118:477–487.
11. Yamaguchi TP, Rossant J. Fibroblast growth factors in mammalian development. *Curr Opin Genet Dev* 1995;5:485–491.
12. Niswander L. Growth factor interactions in limb development. *Ann NY Acad Sci* 1996;785:23–26.
13. Johnson RL, Tabin CJ. Molecular models for vertebrate limb development. *Cell* 1997;90:979–990.
14. Naski MC, Ornitz DM. FGF signaling in skeletal development. *Front Biosci* 1998;3:d781–d794.
15. Kettunen P, Thesleff I. Expression and function of FGFs-4, -8, and -9 suggest functional redundancy and repetitive use as epithelial signals during tooth morphogenesis. *Dev Dyn* 1998;211:256–268.
16. Fu YM, Spirito P, Yu ZX, et al. Acidic fibroblast growth factor in the developing rat embryo. *J Cell Biol* 1991;114:1261–1273.
17. Gonzalez AM, Hill DJ, Logan A, et al. Distribution of fibroblast growth factor (FGF)-2 and FGF receptor-1 messenger RNA expression and protein presence in the mid-trimester human fetus. *Pediat Res* 1996;39:375–385.
18. Twal WO, Vasilatos-Younken R, Gay CV, et al. Isolation and localization of basic fibroblast growth factor-immunoreactive substance in the epiphyseal growth plate. *J Bone Miner Res* 1994;9:1737–1744.
19. Tajima Y, Kawasaki M, Kurihara K, et al. Immunohistochemical profile of basic fibroblast growth factor and heparan sulphate in adult rat mandibular condylar cartilage. *Arch Oral Biol* 1998;43:873–877.
20. Hauschka PW, Mavrakos AE, Iafrati MD, et al. Growth factors in bone matrix: isolation of multiple types by affinity chromatography on heparin-sepharose. *J Biol Chem* 1986;261:12665–12674.
21. Globus RK, Plouet J, Gospodarowicz D. Cultured bo-

vine bone cells synthesize basic fibroblast growth factor and store it in their extracellular matrix. *Endocrinology* 1989;124:1539–1547.

22. Debiais F, Graulet AM, Marie PJ. Fibroblast growth
factor-2 differently affects human neonatal calvaria osteoblastic cells depending on the stage of cell differentiation. *J Bone Miner Res* 1998;13:645–654.

23. Hurley MM, Abreu C, Gronowicz G, et al. Expression
and regulation of basic fibroblast growth factor mRNA
levels in mouse osteoblastic MC3T3-E1 cells. *J Biol
Chem* 1994;269:9392–9396.

24. Sabbieti MG, Marchetti L, Abreu C, et al. Prostaglandins regulate the expression of fibroblast growth fac-
tor-2 in bone. *Endocrinology* 1999;140:434–444.

25. Hurley MM, Tetradis S, Huang YF, et al. Parathyroid
hormone regulates the expression of fibroblast growth
factor-2 mRNA and fibroblast growth factor receptor
mRNA in osteoblastic cells. *J Bone Miner Res* 1999;
14:776–783.

26. Jaye M, Schlessinger J, Dionne CA. Fibroblast growth
factor receptor kinases: molecular analysis and signal
transduction. *Biochem Biophys Acta* 1992;1135:185–
199.

27. Johnson DE, Lee PL, Lu L, et al. Diverse forms of a
receptor for acidic and basic fibroblast growth factors.
Mol Cell Biol 1990;10:4728–4736.

28. Ornitz DM, Xu J, Colvin JS, et al. Receptor specificity
of the fibroblast growth factor family. *J Biol Chem*
1996;271:15292–15297.

29. Hughes SE. Differential expression of the fibroblast
growth factor receptor (FGFR) multigene family in
normal human adult tissues. *J Histochem Cytochem*
1997;45:1005–1019.

30. Orr-Urtreger A, Givol D, Yayon A, et al. Developmental expression of two murine fibroblast growth factor receptors, flg and bek. *Development* 1991;113:
1419–1434.

31. Wanaka A, Milbrandt EM, Johnson M. Expression of
FGF receptor gene in rat development. *Development*
1991;111:455–468.

32. Peters KG, Werner S, Chen G, et al. Two FGF receptor
genes are differentially expressed in epithelial and
mesenchymal tissues during limb formation and organogenesis in the mouse. *Development* 1992;114:233–
243.

33. Orr-Urtreger A, Bedford MT, Burakova T, et al. Developmental localization of the splicing alternatives of fibroblast growth factor receptor-2. *Dev Biol* 1993;158:
475–486.

34. Patstone G, Pasquale EB, Maher PA. Different members of the fibroblast growth factor receptor family are
specific to distinct cell types in the developing chicken
embryo. *Dev Biol* 1993;155:107–123.

35. Peters K, Ornitz DM, Werner S, et al. Unique expression pattern of the FGF receptor 3 gene during mouse
organogenesis. *Dev Biol* 1993;155:423–430.

36. Partanen J, Vainikka S, Korhonen J, et al. Diverse receptors for fibroblast growth factors. *Prog Growth
Factor Res* 1992;4:69–83.

37. Wilke TA, Gubbels S, Schwartz J, et al. Expression
of fibroblast growth factor receptors (FGFR-1, FGFR-
2, FGFR-3) in the developing head and face. *Dev Dyn*
1997;210:41–52.

38. Delezoide AL, Benoist-Lasselin C, Legeai-Mallet L,
et al. Spatio-temporal expression of FGFR 1, 2 and 3

genes during human embryo-fetal ossification. *Mech
Dev* 1998;77:19–30.

39. Kettunen P, Karavanova I, Thesleff I. Responsiveness
of developing dental tissues to fibroblast growth factors: expression of splicing alternatives of FGFR1,
-2, -3, and of FGFR4; and stimulation of cell proliferation by FGF-2, -4, -8, and -9. *Dev Genet* 1998;22:
374–385.

40. Molténi A, Modrowski D, Hott M, et al. Differential
expression of fibroblast growth factor receptor-1, -2,
and -3 and syndecan-1, -2, and -4 in neonatal rat mandibular condyle and calvaria during osteogenic differentiation *in vitro*. *Bone* 1999;24:337–347.

41. Xu X, Weinstein M, Li C, et al. Fibroblast growth
factor receptor 2 (FGFR2)-mediated reciprocal regulation loop between FGF8 and FGF10 is essential for
limb induction. *Development* 1998;125:753–765.

42. Park WJ, Bellus GA, Jabs EW. Mutations in fibroblast
growth factor receptors: phenotypic consequences during eukaryotic development. *Am J Hum Genet* 1995;
57:748–754.

43. Muenke M, Schelle U. Fibroblast growth-factor receptor mutations in human skeletal disorders. *Trends
Genet* 1995;11:308–313.

44. Wilkie AOM. Craniosynostosis—genes and mechanisms. *Hum Mol Genet* 1997;6:1647–1656.

45. Colvin JS, Bohne BA, Harding GW, et al. Skeletal
overgrowth and deafness in mice lacking fibroblast
growth factor receptor 3. *Nat Genet* 1996;12:390–397.

46. Deng C, Wynshaw-Boris A, Zhou F, et al. Fibroblast
growth factor receptor 3 is a negative regulator of bone
growth. *Cell* 1996;84:911–921.

47. Rousseau F, Bonaventure J, Legeal-Mallet L, et al.
Mutations in the gene encoding fibroblast growth factor receptor-3 in achondroplasia. *Nature* 1994;371:
252–254.

48. Shiang R, Thompson LM, Zhu YZ, et al. Mutations in
the transmembrane domain of FGFR-3 cause the most
common genetic form of dwarfism, achondroplasia.
Cell 1994;78:335–342.

49. Szebenyi G, Savage MP, Olwin BB, et al. Changes
in the expression of fibroblast growth factor receptors
mark distinct stages of chondrogenesis *in vitro* and
during chick limb skeletal patterning. *Dev Dyn* 1995;
204:446–456.

50. Cohen J. Sutural biology and the correlates of craniosynostosis. *Am J Med Genet* 1993;47:581–616.

51. Iseki S, Wilkie AOM, Heath JK, et al. FGFR-2 and
osteopontin domains in the developing skull vault are
mutually exclusive and can be altered by locally applied FGF-2. *Development* 1997;124:3375–3384.

52. Kim H-J, Rice DPC, Kettunen PJ, et al. FGF-, BMP-
and Shh-mediated signaling pathways in the regulation
of cranial suture morphogenesis and calvaria bone development. *Development* 1998;125:1241–1251.

53. Mehrara BJ, Mackool RJ, McCarthy JG, et al. Immunolocalization of basic fibroblast growth factor and fibroblast growth factor receptor-1 and receptor 2 in rat
cranial sutures. *Plast Reconstr Surg* 1998;102:1805–
1820.

54. Most D, Levine JP, Chang J, et al. Studies in cranial
suture biology: up-regulation of transforming growth
factor-β1 and basic fibroblast growth factor mRNA
correlates with posterior frontal cranial suture fusion
in the rat. *Plast Reconstr Surg* 1998;101:1431–1440.

55. Lemonnier J, Hott M, Delannoy P, et al. Selective down-regulation of fibroblast growth factor receptor-2 mRNA and protein in Apert syndromic craniosynostosis. *Calcif Tissue Int* 1999 *(in press)*.

56. Roth DA, Gold LI, Han VK, et al. Immunolocalization of transforming growth factor beta 1, beta 2, and beta 3 and insulin-like growth factor I in premature cranial suture fusion. *Plast Reconstr Surg* 1997;99:300–309.

57. Opperman LA, Nolen AA, Ogle RC. TGF-beta 1, TGF-beta 2, and TGF-beta 3 exhibit distinct patterns of expression during cranial suture formation and obliteration *in vivo* and *in vitro*. *J Bone Miner Res* 1997;12:301–310.

58. Opperman LA, Passarelli RW, Morgan EP, et al. Cranial sutures require tissue interactions with dura mater to resist osseous obliteration *in vitro*. *J Bone Miner Res* 1995;10:1978–1987.

59. Cohen MM. Transforming growth factor betas and fibroblast growth factors and their receptors: role in sutural biology and craniosynostosis. *J Bone Miner Res* 1997;12:322–331.

60. Klagsbrun M, Baird A. A dual receptor system is required for basic fibroblast growth factor activity. *Cell* 1991;67:229–231.

61. Hurley MM, Kream BE, Raisz LG. Structural determinants of the capacity of heparin to inhibit collagen synthesis in 21-day fetal rat calvariae. *J Bone Miner Res* 1990;5:1127–1133.

62. Simmons HA, Thomas KA, Raisz LG. Effects of acidic and basic growth factor and heparin on resorption of cultured fetal rat long bone. *J Bone Miner Res* 1991;6:1301–1305.

63. Hurley MM, Kessler M, Gronowicz G, et al. The interaction of heparin and basic fibroblast growth factor on collagen synthesis in 21-day fetal rat calvariae. *Endocrinology* 1992;130:2675–2682.

64. Yayon A, Klagsbrun M, Esko JD, et al. Cell surface, heparin-like molecules are required for binding of basic fibroblast growth factor to its high affinity receptor. *Cell* 1991;64:841–848.

65. David G. Integral membranes heparan sulfate proteoglycans. *FASEB J* 1993;7:1023–1030.

66. Rapraeger AC. The coordinated regulation of heparan sulfate, syndecans and cell behavior. *Curr Opin Cell Biol* 1993;5:844–853.

67. Bernfield M, Hinkes MT, Gallo RL. Developmental expression of the syndecans: possible function and regulation. *Development* 1993;205–212.

68. Vainio S, Jalkanen M, Vaahtokari A, et al. Expression of syndecan gene is induced early, is transient, and correlates with changes in mesenchymal cell proliferation during tooth organogenesis. *Dev Biol* 1991;147:322–333.

69. Solursh M, Reiter RS, Jensen KL, et al. Transient expression of a cell surface heparan sulfate proteoglycan (syndecan) during limb development. *Dev Biol* 1990;140:83–92.

70. Dhodapkar MV, Abe E, Theus A, et al. Syndecan-1 is a multifunctional regulator of myeloma pathobiology: control of tumor cell survival, growth, and bone cell differentiation. *Blood* 1998;8:2679–2688.

71. Gould SE, Upholt WB, Kosher RA. Syndecan-3: a member of the syndecan family of membrane-intercalated proteoglycans that is expressed in high amounts at the onset of chicken limb cartilage differentiation. *Proc Natl Acad Sci USA* 1992;89:3271–3275.

72. Dealy CN, Sheghatoleslami MR, Ferrari D, et al. FGF-stimulated outgrowth and proliferation of limb mesoderm is dependent on syndecan-3. *Dev Biol* 1997;184:343–350.

73. Shimazu A, Nah HD, Kirsch T, et al. Syndecan-3 and the control of chondrocyte proliferation during endochondral ossification. *Exp Cell Res* 1996;229:126–136.

74. Kim CW, Goldberger OA, Gallo RL, et al. Members of the syndecan family of heparan sulfate proteoglycans are expressed in distinct cell, tissue-, and development specific patterns. *Mol Cell Biol* 1994;5:797–805.

75. Molténi A, Modrowski D, Hott M, et al. Alterations of matrix- and cell-associated proteoglycans inhibit osteogenesis and growth response to FGF-2 in cultured rat mandibular condyle and calvaria. *Cell Tissue Res* 1999;295:523–536.

76. Modrowski D, Lomri A, Marie PJ. Glycosaminoglycans bind granulocyte macrophage colony-stimulating factor and modulate its mitogenic activity and signaling in human osteoblastic cells. *J Cell Physiol* 1998;177:187–195.

77. Modrowski D, Lomri A, Baslé MF, et al. Syndecan-2 binds GM-CSF and controls its mitogenic activity in human osteoblastic cells. *J Bone Miner Res* 1997;12[suppl 1]:230.

78. Cizmeci-Smith G, Langan E, Youkey J, et al. Syndecan-4 is a primary-response gene induced by basic fibroblast growth factor and arterial injury in vascular smooth muscle cells. *Arterioscler Thromb Vasc Biol* 1997;17:172–180.

79. Elenius K, Maatta A, Salmivirta M, et al. Growth factors induce 3T3 cells to express bFGF-binding syndecan. *J Biol Chem* 1992;25:6435–6441.

80. Globus RK, Patterson-Buckendahl P, Gospodarowicz D. Regulation of bovine bone cell proliferation by fibroblast growth factor and transforming growth factor β. *Endocrinology* 1988;123:98–105.

81. McCarthy TL, Centrella M, Canalis E. Effects of fibroblast growth factors on deoxyribonucleic acid and collagen synthesis in rat parietal cells. *Endocrinology* 1989;125:2118–2126.

82. Shen V, Kohler G, Huang J, et al. An acidic fibroblast growth factor stimulates DNA synthesis, inhibits collagen and alkaline phosphatase synthesis and induces resorption in bone. *Bone Miner* 1989;7:205–219.

83. Noff D, Pitaru S, Savion N. Basic fibroblast growth factor enhances the capacity of bone marrow cells to form bone-like nodules *in vitro*. *FEBS Lett* 1989;250:619–621.

84. Pitaru S, Kotev-Emeth S, Noff D, et al. Effect of basic fibroblast growth factor on the growth and differentiation of adult stromal bone marrow cells: enhanced development of mineralized bone-like tissue in culture. *J Bone Miner Res* 1993;8:919–929.

85. Locklin R, Williamson MC, Beresford JN, et al. *In vitro* effects of growth factors and dexamethasone on rat marrow stromal cells. *Clin Orthop* 1995;313:27–35.

86. Hanada K, Dennis JE, Caplan AI. Stimulatory effects of basic fibroblast growth factor and bone morphogenetic protein-2 on osteogenic differentiation of rat bone

marrow-derived mesenchymal stem cells. *J Bone Miner Res* 1997;12:1606–1614.

87. Canalis E, Centrella M, McCarthy T. Effects of basic fibroblast growth factor on bone formation *in vitro*. *J Clin Invest* 1988;81:1572–1577.

88. Kato H, Matsuo R, Komiyama O, et al. Decreased mitogenic and osteogenic responsiveness of calvarial osteoblasts isolated from aged rats to basic fibroblast growth factor. *Gerontology* 1995;41[Suppl 1]:20–27.

89. Hurley MM, Abreu C, Harrison JR, et al. Basic fibroblast growth factor inhibits type I collagen gene expression in osteoblastic MC3T3-E1 cells. *J Biol Chem* 1993;268:5588–5593.

90. Rodan SB, Wesolowski G, Thomas KA, et al. Effects of acidic and basic fibroblast growth factors on osteoblastic cells. *Connect Tissue Res* 1989;20:283–288.

91. Shiba H, Nakamura S, Shirakawa M, et al. Effects of basic fibroblast growth factor on proliferation, the expression of osteonectin (SPARC) and alkaline phosphatase, and calcification in cultures of human pulp cells. *Dev Biol* 1995;170:457–466.

92. Delany AM, Canalis E. Basic fibroblast growth factor destabilizes osteonectin mRNA in osteoblasts. *Am J Physiol* 1998;43:C734.

93. Rodan SB, Wesolowski G, Yoon K, et al. Opposing effects of fibroblast growth factor and pertussis toxin on alkaline phosphatase, osteopontin, osteocalcin, and type I collagen mRNA levels in ROS 17/2.8 cells. *J Biol Chem* 1989;264:19934–19941.

94. Tang KT, Capparelli C, Stein JL, et al. Acidic fibroblast growth factor inhibits osteoblast differentiation *in vitro:* altered expression of collagenase, cell growth-related, and mineralization-associated genes. *J Cell Biochem* 1996;61:152–166.

95. Schedlich LJ, Flanagan JL, Crofts LA, et al. Transcriptional activation of the human osteocalcin gene by basic fibroblast growth factor. *J Bone Miner Res* 1994; 9:143–152.

96. Boudreaux JM, Towler DA. Synergistic induction of osteocalcin gene expression: identification of a bipartite element conferring fibroblast growth factor 2 and cyclic AMP responsiveness in the rat osteocalcin promoter. *J Biol Chem* 1996;271:7508–7515.

97. Newberry EP, Boudreaux JM, Towler DA. The rat osteocalcin fibroblast growth factor (FGF)–responsive element: an okadaic acid-sensitive, FGF-selective transcriptional response motif. *Mol Endocrinol* 1996;10:1029–1040.

98. Shiokawa-Sawada M, Mano H, Hanada K, et al. Down-regulation of gap junctional intercellular communication between osteoblastic MC3T3-E1 cells by basic fibroblast growth factor and a phorbol ester (12-*O*-tetradecanoylphorbol-13-acetate). *J Bone Miner Res* 1997;12:1165–1173.

99. Suzuki A, Palmer G, Bonjour JP, et al. Basic fibroblast growth factor selectively stimulates inorganic phosphate transport in MC3T3-E1 osteoblast-like cells. *Bone* 1998;23:5S.

100. Hill PA, Tumber A, Meikle MC. Multiple extracellular signals promote osteoblast survival and apoptosis. *Endocrinology* 1997;138:3849–3858.

101. Lynch MP, Capparelli C, Stein JL, et al. Apoptosis during bone-like tissue development. *J Cell Biochem* 1998;68:31–49.

102. Bourez RLJH, Mathijssen IMJ, Vaandrager JM, et al. Apoptotic cell death during normal embryogenesis of the coronal suture: early detection of apoptosis in mice using annexin V. *J Craniofac Surg* 1997;8:441–445.

103. Berrada S, Lefebvre F, Harmand MF. The effect of recombinant human basic fibroblast growth factor rhFGF-2 on human osteoblast in growth and phenotype expression. *In Vitro Cell Dev* 1995;31:698–702.

104. Pri-Chen S, Pitaru S, Lokiec F, et al. Basic fibroblast growth factor enhances the growth and expression of the osteogenic phenotype of dexamethasone-treated human bone marrow-derived bone-like cells in culture. *Bone* 1998;23:111–117.

105. De Pollak C, Arnaud E, Renier D, et al. Age-related changes in bone formation, osteoblastic cell proliferation and differentiation during postnatal osteogenesis in human calvaria. *J Cell Biochem* 1997;64:128–139.

106. Nakamura T, Hanada K, Tamura M, et al. Stimulation of endosteal bone formation by systemic injections of recombinant basic fibroblast growth factor in rats. *Endocrinology* 1995;136:1276–1284.

107. Kawaguchi H, Kurokawa T, Hanada K, et al. Stimulation of fracture repair by recombinant human basic fibroblast growth factor in normal and streptozotocin-diabetic rats. *Endocrinology* 1994;135:774–781.

108. Noda M, Vogel R. Fibroblast growth factor enhances type β1 transforming growth factor gene expression in osteoblast-like cells. *J Cell Biol* 1989;109:2529–2535.

109. Hurley MM, Abreu C, Hakeda Y. Basic fibroblast growth factor regulates IGF-I binding proteins in the clonal osteoblastic cell line MC3T3-E1. *J Bone Miner Res* 1995;10:222–230.

110. Blanquaert F, Delany AM, Canalis E. Fibroblast growth factor-2 induces hepatocyte growth factor/scatter factor expression in osteoblasts. *Endocrinology* 1999;140:1069–1074.

111. Baldin V, Roman A-M, Bosc-Bierne I, et al. Translocation of bFGF to the nucleus is G1 phase cell cycle specific in bovine aortic endothelial cells. *EMBO J* 1990;9:1511–1517.

112. Nakanishi Y, Kihara K, Mizuno K, et al. Direct effect of basic fibroblast growth factor on gene transcription in a cell-free system. *Proc Natl Acad Sci USA* 1992; 89:5216–5220.

113. Mason IJ. The ins and outs of fibroblast growth factors. *Cell* 1994;78:547–552.

114. Chaudhary LR, Avioli LV. Activation of extracellular signal-regulated kinases 1 and 2 (ERK1 and ERK2) by FGF-2 and PDGF-BB in normal human osteoblastic and bone marrow stromal cells: differences in mobility and in-gel renaturation of ERK1 in human, rat, and mouse osteoblastic cells. *Biochem Biophys Res Commun* 1997;238:134–139.

115. Newberry EP, Willis D, Latifi T, et al. Fibroblast growth factor receptor signaling activates the human interstitial collagenase promoter via the bipartite Ets-AP1 element. *Mol Endocrinol* 1997;11:1129–1144.

116. Hurley MM, Marcello K, Abreu C, et al. Signal transduction by basic fibroblast growth factor in rat osteoblastic Py1a cells. *J Bone Miner Res* 1996;11:1256–1263.

117. Kozawa O, Tokuda H, Matsuno H, Uematsu T. Involvement of p38 mitogen-activated protein kinase in basic fibroblast growth factor-induced interleukin-6 synthesis in osteoblasts. *J Cell Biochem* 1999;74:479–485.

118. Deng C, Bedford M, Li C, et al. Fibroblast growth

factor receptor-1 (FGFR-1) is essential for normal neural tube and limb development. *Dev Biol* 1997;185:42–54.

119. Yamaguchi TP, Harpal K, Henkemeyer M, et al. Fgfr-1 is required for embryonic growth and mesodermal patterning during mouse gastrulation. *Genes Dev* 1994;8:3032–3044.

120. Olwin BB, Arthur K, Hannon K, et al. Role of FGFs in skeletal muscle and limb development. *Mol Reprod Dev* 1994;39:90–101.

121. Cohn MJ, Izpisua-Belmonte JC, Abud H, et al. Fibroblast growth factors induce additional limb development from the flank of chick embryos. *Cell* 1995;80:1–20.

122. Coffin JD, Florkiewicz RZ, Jneumann J, et al. Abnormal bone growth and selective translational regulation in basic fibroblast growth factor (FGF-2) transgenic mice. *Mol Cell Biol* 1995;6:1861–1873.

123. Lightfoot PS, Swisher R, Coffin JD, et al. Ontogenetic limb bone scaling in basic fibroblast growth factor (FGF-2) transgenic mice. *Growth Dev Aging* 1997;61:127–139.

124. Mancilla EE, de Luca F, Uyeda JA, et al. Effects of fibroblast growth factor-2 on longitudinal bone growth. *Endocrinology* 1998;139:2900–2904.

125. Kato Y, Iwamoto M. Fibroblast growth factor is an inhibitor of chondrocyte terminal differentiation. *J Biol Chem* 1990;265:5903–5909.

126. Mayahara H, Ito T, Nagal H, et al. *In vivo* stimulation of endosteal bone formation by basic fibroblast growth factor in rats. *Growth Factors* 1993;9:73–80.

127. Nagai H, Tsukuda R, Mayahara H. Effects of basic fibroblast growth factor (bFGF) on bone formation in growing rats. *Bone* 1995;16:367–373.

128. Nakamura K, Kurokawa T, Kato T, et al. Local application of basic fibroblast growth factor into the bone increases bone mass at the applied site in rabbits. *Arch Orthop Trauma Surg* 1996;115:344–346.

129. Mazue G, Bertolero F, Garofano L, et al. Experience with the preclinical assessment of fibroblast growth factor. *Toxicol Lett* 1992;65:329–338.

130. Dunstan CR, Boyce R, Boyce BF, et al. Systemic administration of acidic fibroblast growth factor (FGF-1) prevents bone loss and increases new bone formation in ovariectomized rats. *J Bone Miner Res* 1999;14:953–959.

131. Nakamura K, Kawaguchi H, Aoyama I, et al. Stimulation of bone formation by intraosseous application of recombinant basic fibroblast growth factor in normal and ovariectomized rabbits. *J Orthop Res* 1997;15:307–313.

132. Martin I, Muraglia A, Campanile G, et al. Fibroblast growth factor-2 supports *ex vivo* expansion and maintenance of osteogenic precursors from human bone marrow. *Endocrinology* 1997;138:4456–4462.

133. Scutt A, Bertram P. Basic fibroblast growth factor in the presence of dexamethasone stimulates colony formation, expansion, and osteoblastic differentiation by rat bone marrow stromal cells. *Calcif Tissue Int* 1999;64:69.

134. Webster MK, Donoghue DJ. FGFR activation in skeletal disorders: too much of a good thing. *Trends Genet* 1997;13:178–182.

135. Neilson KM, Friesel RE. Constitutive activation of fibroblast growth factor receptor-2 by a point mutation associated with Crouzon syndrome. *J Biol Chem* 1995;270:26037–26040.

136. Galvin BD, Hart KC, Meyer AN, et al. Constitutive receptor activation by Crouzon syndrome mutations in fibroblast growth factor receptor (FGFR)2 and FGFR2/Neu chimeras. *Proc Natl Acad Sci USA* 1996;93:7894–7899.

137. Neilson KM, Friesel R. Ligand-independent activation of fibroblast growth factor receptors by point mutations in the extracellular, transmembrane, and kinase domains. *J Biol Chem* 1996;271:25049–25057.

138. Naski MC, Wang Q, Xu J, et al. Graded activation of fibroblast growth factor receptor 3 by mutations causing achondroplasia and thanatophoric dysplasia. *Nat Genet* 1996;13:233–237.

139. Webster MK, Donoghue DJ. Constitutive activation of fibroblast growth factor receptor 3 by the transmembrane domain point mutation found in achondroplasia. *EMBO J* 1996;15:520–527.

140. Mangasarian K, Li Y, Mansukhani A, et al. Mutation associated with Crouzon syndrome causes ligand-independent dimerization and activation of FGF receptor-2. *J Cell Physiol* 1997;172:117–125.

141. Park WJ, Theda C, Maestri NE, et al. Analysis of phenotypic features and FGFR-2 mutations in Apert syndrome. *Am J Hum Genet* 1995;57:321–328.

142. Anderson J, Burns HD, Enriquez-Harris P, et al. Apert syndrome mutations in fibroblast growth factor receptor 2 exhibit increased affinity for FGF ligand. *Hum Mol Genet* 1998;7:1475–1483.

143. Burke D, Wilkes D, Blundell TL, et al. Fibroblast growth factor receptors: lessons from the genes. *Trends Biochem Sci* 1998;23:59–62.

144. Celli G, LaRochelle WJ, Mackem S, et al. Soluble dominant-negative receptor uncovers essential roles for fibroblast growth factors in multi-organ induction and patterning. *EMBO J* 1998;17:1642–1655.

145. Lomri A, Lemonnier J, Hott M, et al. Increased calvaria cell differentiation and bone matrix formation induced by fibroblast growth factor receptor-2 mutations in Apert syndrome. *J Clin Invest* 1998;101:1310–1317.

146. Marie PJ. Cellular and molecular alterations of osteoblasts in human disorders of bone formation. *Histo Pathol* 1999;14:525–538.

147. De Pollak C, Renier D, Hott M, et al. Increased bone formation and osteoblastic cell phenotype in premature cranial suture ossification (craniosynostosis). *J Bone Miner Res* 1996;11:401–407.

148. Fragale A, Tartaglia M, Bernardini S, et al. Decreased proliferation and altered differentiation in osteoblasts from genetically and clinically distinct craniosynostotic disorders. *Am J Pathol* 1999;154:1465–1477.

149. Bresnick S, Schendel S. Crouzon's disease correlates with low fibroblast growth factor receptor activity in stenosed cranial sutures. *J Craniofac Surg* 1995;6:245–250.

150. Lemonnier J, Modrowski D, Hott M, et al. The Ser252Trp FGFR-2 mutation in Apert syndrome selectively increases E-cadherin and N-cadherin expression in human calvaria osteoblasts *in vitro* and *in vivo*. *J Bone Miner Res* 1998;23:S188.

151. Simmons HA, Raisz LG. Effects of acid and basic fibroblast growth factor and heparin on resorption of cultured fetal rat long bones. *J Bone Miner Res* 1991;6:1301–1305.

152. Kawaguchi H, Kurogawa T, Tanaka S, et al. Basic fibroblast growth factor stimulates bone resorption through mitogenic effects on immature osteoblastic cells as well as cyclooxygenase-2 induction. *J Bone Miner Res* 1997;12:S209.

153. Hurley MM, Lee SK, Raisz LG, et al. Basic fibroblast growth factor induces osteoclast formation in murine bone marrow cultures. *Bone* 1998;22:309–316.

154. Kawaguchi H, Pilbeam CC, Gronowicz G, et al. Transcriptional induction of prostaglandin G/H synthase-2 by basic fibroblast growth factor. *J Clin Invest* 1995; 96:923–930.

155. Hurley MM, Abreu C, Marcello K, et al. Regulation of NFIL-6 and IL-6 expression by basic fibroblast growth factor in osteoblasts. *J Bone Miner Res* 1996;11:760–767.

156. Kozawa O, Suzuki A, Uematsu T. Basic fibroblast growth factor induces interleukin-6 synthesis in osteoblasts: autoregulation by protein kinase C. *Cell Signal* 1997;9:463–468.

157. Varghese S, Ramsby ML, Jeffrey JJ, et al. Basic fibroblast growth factor stimulates expression of interstitial collagenase and inhibitors of metalloproteinases in rat bone cells. *Endocrinology* 1995;136:2156–2162.

158. Hurley MM, Marcello K, Abreu C, et al. Transcriptional regulation of the collagenase gene by basic fibroblast growth factor in osteoblastic MC3T3-E1 cells. *Biochem Biophys Res Commun* 1995;214:331–339.

159. Delany AM, Canalis E. Dual regulation of stromelysin-3 by fibroblast growth factor-2 in murine osteoblasts. *J Biol Chem* 1998;273:16595–16600.

160. Scully SP, Joyce ME, Abidi N, et al. The use of polymerase chain reaction generated sequences as probes for hybridization. *Mol Cell Probes* 1990;4:485–495.

161. Thomas KA, Rios-Candelore M, Gimenez-Gallego G, et al. Pure brain-derived acidic fibroblast growth factor is a potent angiogenic vascular endothelial cell mitogen with sequence homology to interleukin 1. *Proc Natl Acad Sci USA* 1985;82:6409–6413.

162. Joyce ME, Jingushi S, Scully SP. Role of growth factors in fracture healing. In: Barbule A, Caldwell MD, Eaglstein WH, eds. *Clinical and experimental approaches to dermal and epidermal repair: normal and chronic wounds.* New York: Wiley-Liss, 1991: 391–416.

163. Hiroshi K, Takahide K, Keigo H, et al. Stimulation of fracture repair by recombinant human basic fibroblast growth factor in normal and streptozotocin-diabetic rats. *Endocrinology* 1994;135:774–781.

164. Cuevas P, Burgos J, Baird A. Basic fibroblast growth factor (FGF) promotes cartilage repair *in vivo. Biochem Biophys Res Commun* 1988;156:611–618.

165. Jingushi S, Heydeman S, Kana L, et al. Acidic fibroblast growth factor (aFGF) injection stimulates cartilage enlargement and inhibits cartilage gene expression in rat fracture healing. *J Orthop Res* 1990;8:364–371.

166. Wang JS. Basic fibroblast growth factor for stimulation of bone formation in osteoinductive or conductive implants. *Acta Orthop Scand* 1996;269[Suppl]:1–33.

167. Aspenberg P, Thorngren K, Lohmander LS. Dose-dependent stimulation of bone induction by basic growth factor in rats. *Acta Orthop Scand* 1991;62:481–484.

168. Andreshak JL, Rabin SI, Patwardhan AG, et al. Tibial segmental defect repair: chondrogenesis and biomedical strength modulated by basic fibroblast growth factor. *Anat Rec* 1997;248:198–204.

169. Yamada K, Tabata Y, Yamamoto K, et al. Potential efficacy of basic fibroblast growth factor incorporated in biodegradable hydrogels for skull bone regeneration. *J Neurosurg* 1997;86:871–875.

170. Inui K, Maeda H, Sano A, et al. Local application of basic fibroblast growth factor minipellet induces the healing of segmental bony defects in rabbits. *Biol Trace Elem Res* 1998;63:490.

171. Kimoto T, Hosokawa R, Kubo T, et al. Continuous administration of basic fibroblast growth factor (FGF-2) accelerates bone induction on rat calvaria—an application of a new drug delivery system. *J Dent Res* 1998;77:1965–1969.

172. Radomsky ML, Thompson AY, Spiro RC, et al. Potential role of fibroblast growth factor in enhancement of fracture healing. *Clin Orthop* 1998;355[Suppl]:S283–S293.

Skeletal Growth Factors,
edited by Ernesto Canalis.
Lippincott Williams & Wilkins, Philadelphia, © 2000.

13

Fibroblast Growth Factors, Chondrogenesis, and Related Clinical Disorders

David M. Ornitz

Department of Molecular Biology and Pharmacology, Washington University Medical School, St. Louis, Missouri 63110

Fibroblast growth factor (FGF) was discovered in the 1970s as an activity that stimulated the proliferation of 3T3 fibroblasts (1) and chondrocytes (2). The discovery that chondrocytes provide a rich source of FGF suggested that FGF was an essential factor regulating chondrocyte growth and development. Indeed, over the past 25 years, a variety of studies have demonstrated roles for FGF signaling in the earliest stages of bone development, mesenchymal condensation, and regulation of both intramembranous and endochondral bone growth.

Recent genetic evidence has identified mutations in FGF receptors (FGFRs) that result in skeletal diseases in humans. Gene targeting studies in mice have also identified specific roles for FGFR signaling in chondrogenesis. In this chapter, the FGF and FGFR families are discussed in terms of their roles in regulating early cartilage development and in diseases that affect chondrogenesis.

THE FIBROBLAST GROWTH FACTOR FAMILY

Nineteen members of the FGF family have been identified in mammals. Thus far, all but six of the FGF ligands have been shown to activate one of the four high-affinity cell surface FGFRs (Ornitz, unpublished data; 3,4–10). Each FGF and FGFR has specific spatial and temporal patterns of expression throughout development. Additionally, some of the FGFs and FGFRs overlap in their expression pattern. This suggests that FGF signaling is at least in part determined by the specificity of FGF ligands for their receptors. Additionally, the affinity and specificity of the FGFRs is modulated by alternative splicing, and the interaction of FGF with the FGFR is dependent on heparin sulfate. Heparin sulfate side chains of cell surface and extracellular matrix–associated proteoglycans facilitate ligand binding and limit ligand diffusion (reviewed in 5,11,12). Furthermore, tissue-specific chemical modifications of heparin sulfate may further affect the activity of FGFs (12–14).

FIBROBLAST GROWTH FACTOR EXPRESSION IN MESENCHYMAL CONDENSATIONS, DEVELOPING CARTILAGE, AND BONE

Mesenchymal condensation is the first morphologic event leading to bone formation (15,16). Although at present there is little direct genetic evidence that FGFs regulate skeletal development at the level of mesenchymal condensation, expression of both FGFs and FGFRs have been observed in condensing mesenchyme. These observations suggest a role for FGF signaling at this stage of development.

FGFR2 is one of the first markers of prechondrogenic condensation in humans and mice. In day 33 human embryos or day 10.5 mouse embryos, FGFR2 RNA is intensely expressed in mesenchymal condensation and in epidermis but

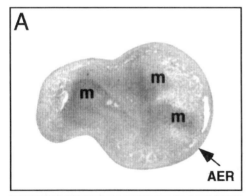

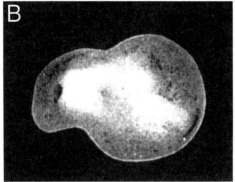

FIG. 13.1. Expression of fibroblast growth factor receptor 2 (*Fgfr2*) in the mesenchymal condensation (*m*) and apical ectodermal ridge (*AER*) of a Carnegie stage 16 human embryo. **A:** Hemotoxylin and eosin–stained longitudinal section of the distal upper extremity. **B:** Dark-field image of the same section hybridized with a probe for FGFR2. (From ref. 18, with permission.)

associated long bone abnormalities. This may result from abnormal activity of FGFR1 or FGFR2 at the condensation stage of development or in the periosteum later in development.

The ligands that activate FGFRs in the mesenchymal condensation as well as in the growth plate (see below) have been difficult to identify. At the mesenchymal condensation stage, FGF9 expression has been observed in limb mesenchymal condensations (Ornitz et al., unpublished observation). However, mice lacking FGF9 show no apparent defects in skeletal development (Colvin and Ornitz, unpublished observation). Similarly, FGF5 and FGF6 are expressed in limb mesenchyme outside the condensation (20,21). However, gene knockout experiments indicate no involvement of these ligands in skeletal development (22,23). At present, the data suggest that if these or other FGF ligands are mediators of the mesenchymal condensation they do not act alone. Future experiments in which multiple FGF ligands are knocked out will be required to address these issues of possible redundancy.

EXPRESSION IN THE GROWTH PLATE

Unique expression patterns of FGFRs have been identified in the growth plate. FGFR3 is expressed in the epiphyseal growth plate and is most highly expressed in a histomorphologic domain that encompasses proliferating and prehypertrophic chondrocytes (Fig. 13.2). This expression pattern suggests a direct role for FGFR3 in regulating chondrocyte proliferation and possibly differentiation (18,24,25). In contrast, FGFR1 is prominently expressed in hypertrophic chondrocytes (Fig. 13.2) (18,26), suggesting a role for FGFR1 in maintaining the hypertrophic phenotype of these cells (cell survival), in regulating the production of unique extracellular matrix products of hypertrophic chondrocytes, or in signaling their eventual apoptotic death.

Studies of FGFR3 null mice show that prolonged expression of markers for cell proliferation (27) and overexpression of activated FGFR3 (achondroplasia mutation) in a chondrocytic cell line or in the growth plate of transgenic

is not expressed in the surrounding loose connective tissue (17,18) (Fig. 13.1). In contrast, FGFR1 is expressed diffusely in the loose and condensed precartilaginous mesenchyme (18). Later in development, both FGFR1 and FGFR2 are expressed in primary bone collar (perichondrium and periosteum) (18). Similarly, in chick limb development, FGFR2 is expressed in regions where mesenchymal condensations take place but prior to morphologic differentiation. By stage 27, FGFR2 expression is prominent within the condensation. As in mammals, FGFR1 is expressed in loose mesenchyme surrounding the condensations (19).

Patients with mutations in FGFR1 and FGFR2 develop craniosynostosis but in addition have

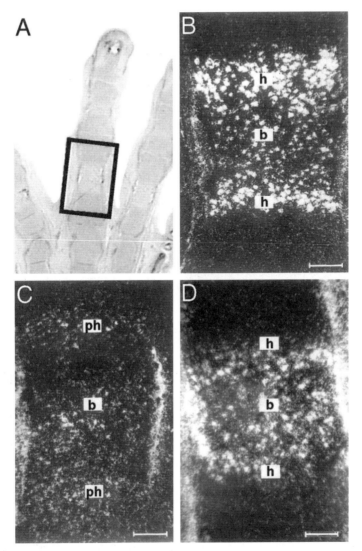

FIG. 13.2. Fibroblast growth factor receptor 1 (FGFR1) FGFR3, and *ColX* gene expression during human endochondral bone formation. Serial sections of a developing hand from a 12-week-old human fetus. **A:** Hematoxylin–eosin staining of the developing carpal bones and phalanges. **B–D:** Higher magnification of the inset in **(A)** showing ColX **(B)**, FGFR3 **(C)**, and FGFR1 **(D)** expression in the hypertrophic chondrocytes of the P1 phalange growth plate. *ph,* prehypertrophic chondrocytes; *h,* hypertrophic chondrocytes; *b,* bone. (From ref. 106, with permission.)

mice results in diminished cell proliferation (Ornitz, et al., unpublished data) (25). In addition to affecting chondrocyte proliferation, evidence suggests that FGFR3 may regulate chondrocyte differentiation. The addition of FGF to cultured chondrocytes has been shown to inhibit chondrocyte differentiation (28). Histologic studies

of biopsies from individuals with achondroplasia show either extensive or focal disorganization of the growth plate (29–31). Furthermore, FGFR3 $-/-$ mice have an expanded zone of hypertrophy in the epiphyseal growth plate (27,32) and mice overexpressing activated FGFR3 in the growth plate show decreased numbers of cells in the prehypertrophic and hypertrophic zones (25). These observations suggest that FGFR3 signaling regulates chondrocyte differentiation *in vivo*.

The physiologic FGF ligand(s) for FGFR3 in the epiphyseal growth plate has not been unambiguously identified. FGF2 is abundantly expressed in growth plate chondrocytes (2,33,34) and for many years was thought to be a candidate physiologic ligand in the growth plate. Furthermore, FGF2 is a potent mitogen for growth plate (35) or articular (36) chondrocytes in culture, FGF2 can accelerate the regeneration of cartilage tissue in *in vivo* subcutaneous cartilage implants (37), and FGF2 is a ligand for the mesenchymal splice forms of FGFRs 1, 2, and 3 (38). The addition of FGF2 to chondrocytes cultured in soft agar, as well as monolayer culture, resulted in a dramatic increase in cell proliferation (39–41). When compared to other known mitogens for chondrocytes, FGF2 was a more potent mitogen than insulin-like growth factor-I, transforming growth factor-β (TGF-β), and epidermal growth factor (39,42). Surprisingly, however, mice lacking FGF2 have no overt skeletal defects (43–45). This suggests that FGF2 is not the physiologic ligand for FGFR3 in the growth plate. Alternatively, FGF2 may cooperate with other members of the family to regulate chondrogenesis. Because FGF2 lacks a signal peptide, it has been proposed that it may be released from stressed or damaged cells to allow a rapid physiologic response to injury (46,47). Thus, FGF2 may have a more subtle function in shaping bones in response to stress rather than regulating bone elongation. Detailed analysis of FGF2 null mice may address these issues.

The expression of two ligands for FGFR3, FGF8 and FGF17 has recently been observed in developing bone in the mouse between embryonic day 14.5 (E14.5) and E16.5. Both ligands were expressed in dorsal costal cartilage and in costal perichondrium. FGF8 expression was observed in the osteoblast compartment of calvarial bone, the mandible, cortical bone, and growth plate of long bones. FGF17 expression was not detected in long bones but was detected in some intramembranous bone, such as the maxilla and the scapula (48). After E16.5, expression of these ligands decreased in the growth plate, and it is not yet known whether they are reexpressed in the growth plate of long bones after birth. Besides these ligands, other FGFs can function as ligands for FGFR3 *in vitro* yet have not been rigorously examined for expression in the growth plate of developing bones. Because the ligand for FGFR3 appears to be limiting, the regulation of such a ligand, in terms of its expression or bioavailability, will be an important component of the complex regulatory cascades controlling longitudinal bone growth.

EXPRESSION IN CRANIAL SUTURES

Mutations in FGFR1 and FGFR2 give rise to many of the craniosynostosis syndromes (see chapter 12 and below), demonstrating that FGF signaling is clearly also involved in the development of intramembranous bones. Several studies have identified FGFR1 and FGFR2 expression in intramembranous bone (49). FGFR2 is expressed at the growing margins of the flat bones of the skull in areas of rapid proliferation but is excluded from areas of osteogenic differentiation (50,51).

FGF9, a ligand for the mesenchymal splice form of FGFR2, is highly expressed in the dura and calvarial mesenchyme beneath cranial sutures (51). FGF2, also a ligand for FGFR3, was identified in dural cells during late embryogenesis and postnatally, in osteoblasts on the endocranial surface of the suture, and in sutural connective tissue (49). These expression patterns suggest that FGF9 may signal from underlying tissue to its receptor to induce growth and differentiation of the osteogenic front and that it may modulate the expression of FGF2 during suture fusion. This hypothesis is supported by experiments in which FGF4 beads (also a ligand for FGFR2), placed on the osteogenic front, induce proliferation and partial fusion of the cranial suture (51).

MUTATIONS IN FIBROBLAST GROWTH FACTOR RECEPTORS CAUSE SKELETAL DISEASES

Genetic evidence that FGF signaling is required for normal bone development has recently emerged from the linkage of several human skeletal dysplasias to the genes encoding FGFRs *1, 2,* and *3.* These disorders can be broadly classified into two groups: the dwarfing chondrodysplasia syndromes and the craniosynostosis syndromes. The chondrodysplasia syndromes generally involve mutations in FGFR3 (Fig. 13.3) and include the diseases hypochon-

droplasia (HCH) (52), achondroplasia (ACH) (53–56), and thanatophoric dysplasia (TD) (57–60). Craniosynostosis syndromes frequently involve mutations in *FGFR1* or *FGFR2* (Fig. 13.3) and include Crouzon syndrome (CS) (61–71), Pfeiffer syndrome (PS) (62,64,68,72,73), Jackson-Weiss syndrome (JWS) (63,64,67), Beare-Stevenson cutis gyrata (BS) (74), Apert syn-

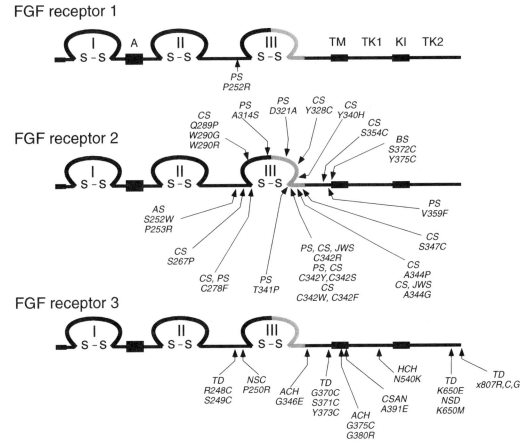

FIG. 13.3. Mutations in fibroblast growth factor (*FGF*) receptors 1-3 in human skeletal diseases. **Top:** FGFR1 showing a single-point mutation causing Pfeiffer syndrome (*PS*). The *shaded region* within immunoglobulin (Ig)-like domain III represents the sequence subject to alternative splicing in FGFRs 1–3. *SP,* signal peptide; *A,* acidic region; *I, II, III,* Ig-like domains; *TM,* transmembrane domain; *KI,* kinase insert; *S-S,* disulfide bond. **Middle:** FGFR2 showing the position of mutations responsible for Crouzon syndrome (*CS*), Jackson-Weiss syndrome (*JWS*), PS, Apert syndrome (*AS*), and Beare-Stevenson cutis gyrata (*BS*). **Bottom:** FGFR3 showing the mutations responsible for achondroplasia (*ACH*), thanatophoric dysplasia (*TD*), hypochondroplasia (*HCH*), CS associated with acanthosis nigricans (*CSAN*), and a nonsyndromic craniosynostosis (*NSC*). The *stippled line* attached to the end of FGFR3 represents an extension of the protein resulting from mutations in the stop codon of the receptor. The *numbers* represent the position of the amino acid in the coding sequence for the human receptor. Amino acids are abbreviated using standard single-letter abbreviations. (From ref. 25, with permission.)

drome (AS) (75), and a nonsyndromic cranio-synostosis (76).

CRANIOSYNOSTOSIS SYNDROMES

The craniosynostosis syndromes PS, CS, JWS, BS, and AS have in common craniosynostosis (premature closure of the cranial sutures), resulting in clinically abnormal skull shape. The coronal suture is most commonly affected in AS, BS, CS, JWS, and PS (71,74). In addition to the involvement of the cranial sutures, many of these patients have distinct facial features and develop a variety of phenotypes that affect the appendicular skeleton. The types of abnormality seen in the distal extremities include syndactyly of the hands and feet or broadening of the thumbs and big toes. A more detailed discussion of the clinical features of the craniosynostosis syndromes can be found in chapter 12.

In general, the mutations affecting craniofacial development result from mutations in FGFR 1 or 2. Recently, however, mutations in FGFR3 have also been shown to cause a syndrome resembling CS and a nonsyndromic craniosynostosis (70,76; for review of FGFR mutations and the corresponding clinical abnormalities, see 77,78). The developmental origin of these phenotypes in relationship to the expression patterns of FGFR3 is not known. The contrast between phenotypes affecting suture closure and those affecting endochondral ossification suggests distinct biochemical activities of the respective mutations. Alternatively, nonlinked secondary genetic mutations or epigenetic events may alter the consequences of similarly acting mutations, resulting in these very distinct syndromes.

CHONDRODYSPLASIAS

The dwarfing chondrodysplasias include HCH (52), ACH (53,54), and TD (57,60). Several recent reviews cover both molecular and clinical features of the FGFR3-associated chondrodysplasia syndromes (5,77,79). ACH, HCH, and TD are briefly described here. All of these diseases result from dominant mutations in the *FGFR3* gene. HCH is a mild and relatively common skeletal disorder with clinical features similar to those of ACH. ACH is the most common

form of genetic dwarfism. ACH is characterized by shortening of the proximal and, to a lesser extent, distal long bones. The cranium of ACH patients is characterized by frontal bossing, and the face is characterized by a depressed nasal bridge. Rare homozygous cases of ACH usually result in neonatal lethality (80). These individuals have features similar to those of TD. TD results from several dominant mutations in the *FGFR3* gene. TD is the most common lethal neonatal skeletal disorder and is clinically similar to homozygous ACH (80).

In contrast to dwarfing chondrodysplasia syndromes resulting from activating mutations in FGFR3, mice homozygous for null alleles of *FGFR3* exhibit skeletal overgrowth (27,32). The opposite phenotypes between the *FGFR3* null mice and ACH suggest that the mutations causing dwarfism are gain-of-function alleles. These data show that *FGFR3* negatively regulates bone growth and leads to the paradoxical question of how signaling through a growth factor receptor can inhibit growth.

Several biochemical studies have shown that mutations causing ACH and TD are gain-of-function mutations, resulting in increased receptor tyrosine kinase activity (81–84). The G380R mutation in the transmembrane domain of FGFR3 (responsible for most cases of ACH) partially activates receptor signaling (81). The basal mitogenic activity of this receptor (assayed as a chimeric receptor containing the tyrosine kinase domain from FGFR1) could be augmented by the addition of ligand, and the dose-response curve suggested that this receptor has a similar ligand-binding affinity to that of the wild-type receptor. Studies of receptor tyrosine phosphorylation showed ligand-independent receptor autophosphorylation. The K650E and R248C mutations of TD are also activating mutations. These mutations result in ligand-independent receptor activation, as evidenced by ligand-independent cell proliferation and receptor tyrosine phosphorylation. Significantly, the mutations causing TD were more strongly activating than the mutation causing ACH. This suggested a correlation between the degree of receptor activation and the severity of the dwarfing chondrodysplasia. In this study, it was also demonstrated that the FGFR3 R248C mutation constitutively activates the receptor by forming a disulfide-linked receptor homodimer in which an unpaired cysteine residue in the extracellular domain of the receptor forms an intermolecular disulfide linkage (81). The FGFR3 K650E mutation occurs in a highly conserved lysine residue in the activation loop of the receptor (85,86). This mutation results in a constitutively active tyrosine kinase, presumably by altering the structure of the activation loop. Unlike the R248C mutation, which shows constitutive activation matching that of maximally stimulated wild-type receptor, the K650E mutant receptor can be activated by ligand to a level greater than that of the wild-type receptor. These observations are consistent with the observed covalent homodimerization consequence of the R248C mutation and the deregulation of the kinase domain by the K650E mutation.

Transgenic mice in which an FGFR3 cDNA containing the G380R mutation (ACH) is over-expressed in the growth plate develop a phenotype resembling ACH. Mice in which the K650E (TD type II) mutation is introduced into the FGFR3 genomic locus by homologous recombination showed a similar phenotype (87). These studies demonstrate that activated FGFR3 signaling inhibits chondrocyte proliferation and slows chondrocyte differentiation *in vivo* (25,87). Studies in which tissue from TD type I patients was examined showed that the constitutive activation of FGFR3 (R248C) does not prevent chondrocyte proliferation but rather alters their differentiation by triggering premature apoptosis through activation of the STAT1 signaling pathway (88). Similarly, FGFR3 containing the K650E mutation has constitutive tyrosine kinase activity which can specifically activate the transcription factor STAT1, leading to growth arrest *in vitro* (89) and *in vivo* (87).

MIXED CASES OF CHONDRODYSPLASIA AND CRANIOSYNOSTOSIS

A few rare cases have been described in which both chondrodysplasia and craniosynostosis phenotypes occur within a single patient. In one case, a patient with an FGFR3 N540K mutation presented with HCH and a cloverleaf skull (90).

Additionally, in patients with an FGFR3 R248C mutation (TD type I), the cloverleaf skull deformity is observed in about half of the cases and is likely due to variable expressivity of the mutation. In patients with an FGFR3 K650E mutation (TD type II), the cloverleaf skull deformity occurs often (57).

MUTATIONS IN FIBROBLAST GROWTH FACTOR RECEPTORS INCREASE RECEPTOR ACTIVITY OR RESPONSE TO LIGAND

All of the mutations identified in FGFRs are autosomal dominant and frequently arise sporadically. The great majority of these disorders result from point mutations in the coding sequence of an FGFR that result in a single amino acid substitution; however, a few mutations alter the stop codon and thus extend the length of the reading frame (Fig. 13.3).

Functional studies of the FGFRs have localized ligand-binding domains to the second and third immunoglobulin (Ig) domains (91–93). Interestingly, many of the mutations that affect FGFR activity are localized to three highly conserved amino acid residues (RSP) within the linker sequence between Ig domains II and III (Fig. 13.4) and to sequences around the conserved cysteine residues within Ig domain III (Fig. 13.3). The conserved RSP motif is itself embedded within a highly conserved sequence that is thought to function as a receptor dimerization domain (94). The conserved cysteine residues within the Ig domains, as well as other nearby residues, are required for the proper folding of the Ig domain (95). It is hypothesized, and in some cases demonstrated, that some of these mutations disrupt the tertiary structure of the Ig domain and lead to constitutive or activated receptor signaling (96).

THE PARADOX OF FIBROBLAST GROWTH FACTOR SIGNALING PATHWAYS IN THE GROWTH PLATE

Classically, FGFs are considered powerful mitogens for many cell types, including primary chondrocytes (2,33,97). It is therefore surprising and provocative that FGFR3 signaling inhibits

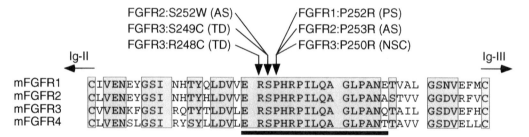

FIG. 13.4. Conserved sequence in the linker region between immunoglobulin (Ig)-like domains II and III of fibroblast growth factor receptors (FGFRs) 1–3. The relative position of mutations occurring in FGFRs 1–3 clustered within three conserved amino acid residues are indicated. The conserved region thought to serve as a receptor dimerization domain is *underlined* (94). *AS*, Apert syndrome; *TD*, thanatophoric dysplasia; *PS*, Pfeiffer syndrome; *NSC*, nonsyndromic craniosynostosis.

chondrocyte proliferation *in vivo* in the growth plate. This paradoxical activity may be a unique property of FGFR3 or may result from a unique response of the growth plate chondrocyte to an FGFR-derived signal. Interestingly, *in vitro*, FGFR3 activation by ligand or by activating mutations results in a poor mitogenic response compared to FGFR1 activation (81,98,99). Recent *in vitro* studies, in which a constitutively active FGFR3 (containing the K650E mutation) was overexpressed in a nonchondrocytic cell line, showed decreased cell proliferation and a coincident increase in STATI activity, suggesting that activated FGFR3 may stimulate growth-inhibitory pathways (89).

The effects of activating mutations in FGFR3 on the proliferation and differentiation of epiphyseal chondrocytes are now well described. It is clear that activating mutations in FGFR3 dramatically inhibit both chondrocyte proliferation (either directly or by slowing the entry of resting chondrocytes into the proliferating zone) and differentiation. The consequence of these mutations on chondrogenesis is a histologically shortened growth plate and a gross phenotype resembling the human skeletal disorders ACH and TD (25,53,54,79,100). The signaling pathways linking FGFR3 to stat1 that negatively regulate chondrocyte proliferation are not known. Furthermore, it is not known whether these pathways are specific to FGFR3 (versus FGFR1) or whether this response is unique to the chondrocyte.

WHAT IS THE RATE-LIMITING STEP IN ENDOCHONDRAL OSSIFICATION?

The physiologic FGF ligand that regulates endochondral ossification is not known. However, gain-of-function and loss-of-function mutations in FGFR3 and comparison to transgenic mice that overexpress an FGF in the growth plate suggest that an FGF ligand is the rate-limiting step in the FGF pathway regulating endochondral ossification. Transgenic mice that overexpress wild-type FGFR3 in the growth plate do not show signs of abnormal chondrocyte proliferation or abnormal growth plate morphology (25). However, postnatal transgenic mice overexpressing activated FGFR3 or ectopic FGF2 in proliferating chondrocytes develop a dwarfing condition similar to ACH (25,101). These observations suggest that in the postnatal growth plate the concentration of an as-yet-unidentified FGF ligand is limiting relative to that of FGFR3.

In contrast, during embryonic development, the activated FGFR3 transgene has no effect on the proliferation of chondrocytes, and loss of FGFR3 results in a broadened growth plate. This suggests that during embryonic development chondrocyte proliferation is insensitive to FGFR signaling, either because the concentration of FGF is in excess, saturating FGFR signaling pathways, or other mitogens function dominantly during embryonic life and mask the growth-inhibitory effects of FGFR3.

HOW FIBROBLAST GROWTH FACTOR SIGNALING PATHWAYS INTERACT WITH OTHER SIGNALING PATHWAYS TO COORDINATE BONE GROWTH AND CHONDROGENESIS

Along with FGFs, endochondral bone growth is regulated by many signaling molecules, including growth hormone, insulin-like growth factor-1, parathyroid hormone–related protein (PTHrP), Indian hedgehog (Ihh), and bone mor-phogenetic proteins (BMPs) (102,103). The expression pattern of FGFRs as well as some of these other molecules is summarized in Fig. 13.5. A feedback loop has been identified in which Ihh and PTHrP interact to coordinate chondrocyte differentiation (104,105). The relationship between the Ihh/PTHrP and FGF signaling pathways has been investigated by examining the expression of *Ihh* and its receptor, *patched*, and of *PTHrP* in the growth plate of mice that either lack FGFR3 or overexpress

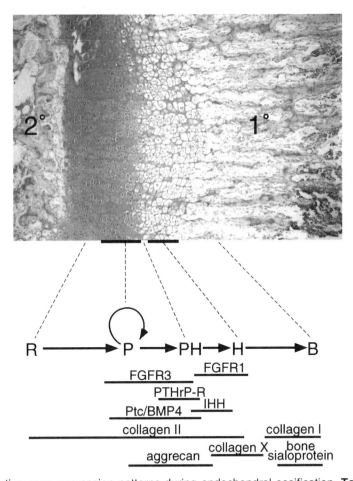

FIG. 13.5. Relative gene expression patterns during endochondral ossification. **Top:** Hematoxylin and eosin–stained section of the epiphyseal growth plate from the proximal tibia of a 2-week-old mouse. *1°*, primary ossification center; *2°*, secondary ossification center. **Bottom:** A linear model of differentiation in which chondrocytes sequentially transit through resting (*R*), proliferating (*P*), prehypertrophic (*PH*), and hypertrophic (*H*) stages of differentiation. The hypertrophic chondrocytes are ultimately replaced by trabecular bone (*B*) and bone marrow. *Lines* indicate the relative spatial patterns of gene expression. *BMP4*, bone morphogenetic protein 4; *FGFR*, fibroblast growth factor receptor; *IHH*, Indian hedgehog; *Ptc*, Patched; *PTHrP-R*, parathyroid hormone–related peptide receptor.

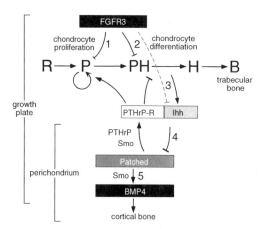

FIG. 13.6. Model for the effects of fibroblast growth factor receptor 3 (*FGFR3*) on the growth plate showing feedback signaling pathways which act to coordinate the steps of skeletal growth and differentiation (From ref. 25, with permission.) The *rectangles* indicate the relative expression domains in the growth plate as described in Fig. 13.5 [Patched and bone morphogenetic protein 4 (*BMP4*) are also expressed in the perichondrium]. FGFR3 inhibits skeletal growth by inhibiting chondrocyte proliferation or the entry of cells into the proliferative zone (*step 1*) and differentiation (*step 2.*) The inhibition of differentiation may occur near the prehypertrophic region. This may be the result of a direct action of FGFR3 *(solid line)* or indirectly as a result of inhibiting Indian hedgehog *(Ihh)* expression *(gray dashed line, step 3)*. Ihh is normally upregulated during chondrocyte hypertrophy and can bind to and inactivate its receptor, Patched, within the growth plate and perichondrium *(step 4)*. The interaction of Ihh with Patched releases the inhibitory actions of Patched on Smoothened *(Smo)*, thereby activating downstream signaling events, which result in the stimulation of parathyroid hormone–related protein *(PTHrP)* and *patched* expression. The PTHrP receptor in turn stimulates chondrocyte proliferation and slows differentiation. In the proposed signaling pathway, FGFR3 inhibits *Ihh* expression in the growth plate, which in turn inhibits *patched* and *Bmp4* expression (107,108) in both the growth plate and perichondrium *(step 5)*. In this manner, FGFR3 can globally coordinate skeletal growth by controlling the growth of both bone and cartilage. *R,* resting chondrocytes; *P,* proliferating chondrocytes; *PH,* prehypertrophic chondrocytes; *H,* hypertrophic chondrocytes; *B,* trabecular bone and bone marrow. (From ref. 25, with permission.)

FGFR3 containing the activating mutation, G380R. In mice that overexpress FGFR3 G380R, *Ihh* expression and signaling, as assessed by examining *patched* expression, are inhibited. Furthermore, expression of *Bmp4,* a molecule thought to be downstream of *Ihh,* is also suppressed in both growth plate cartilage and in the surrounding perichondrium (Fig. 13.6) (25). In contrast, in mice lacking FGFR3, the expression of these molecules is increased relative to wild-type mice (25). These data suggest that FGFR3 signaling is genetically upstream of the Ihh, BMP, and PTHrP signaling pathways and that FGFR3 signaling may serve to globally coordinate endochondral bone growth.

ACKNOWLEDGMENTS

This work was supported by grants HD35692 and CA60673 from the National Institutes of Health.

REFERENCES

1. Gospodarowicz D, Moran JS. Mitogenic effect of fibroblast growth factor on early passage cultures of human and murine fibroblasts. *J Cell Biol* 1975;66: 451–457.
2. Klagsbrun M, Langner R, Levenson R, et al. The stimulation of DNA synthesis and cell division in chondrocytes and 3T3 cells by a growth factor isolated from cartilage. *Exp Cell Res* 1977;105:99–108.
3. Smallwood PM, Munozsanjuan I, Tong P, et al. Fibroblast growth factor (FGF) homologous factors—new members of the FGF family implicated in nervous system development. *Proc Natl Acad Sci USA* 1996;93: 9850–9857.
4. Coulier F, Pontarotti P, Roubin R, et al. Of worms and men: an evolutionary perspective on the fibroblast growth factor (FGF) and FGF receptor families. *J Mol Evol* 1997;44:43–56.
5. Naski MC, Ornitz DM. FGF signaling in skeletal development. *Front Biosci* 1998;3:D781–D794.
6. McWhirter JR, Goulding M, Weiner JA, et al. A novel fibroblast growth factor gene expressed in the developing nervous system is a downstream target of the chimeric homeodomain oncoprotein E2A-Pbx1. *Development* 1997;124:3221–3232.
7. Miyake A, Konishi M, Martin FH, et al. Structure and expression of a novel member, FGF-16, of the fibroblast growth factor family. *Biochem Biophys Res Commun* 1998;243:148–152.
8. Hoshikawa M, Ohbayashi N, Yonamine A, et al. Structure and expression of a novel fibroblast growth factor, *Fgf17,* preferentially expressed in the embryonic brain. *Biochem Biophys Res Commun* 1998;244:187–191.

9. Greene JM Li LY, Yourey PA, et al. Identification and characterization of a novel member of the fibroblast growth factor family. *Eur J Neurosci* 1998;10:1911–1925.

10. Nishimura T, Utsunomiya Y, Hoshikawa M, et al. Structure and expression of a novel human FGF, FGF-19, expressed in the fetal brain. *Biochem Biophys Acta* 1999;1444:148–151.

11. Ornitz DM, Waksman G. Fibroblast growth factor receptors. In: *Growth factors and wound healing: basic science and potential clinical applications.* New York: Springer-Verlag, 1997;151–174.

12. McKeehan WL, Wang F, Kan M. The heparan sulfate-fibroblast growth factor family: diversity of structure and function. *Prog Nucleic Acid Res Mol Biol* 1998; 59:135–176.

13. Dietrich CP, Nader HB, Strauss AH. Structural differences of heparan sulfates according to the tissue and species of origin. *Biochem Biophys Res Commun* 1983; 111:865–871.

14. Vlodavsky I, Miao HQ, Medalion B, et al. Involvement of heparan sulfate and related molecules in sequestration and growth promoting activity of fibroblast growth factor. *Cancer Metastasis Rev* 1996;15:177–186.

15. Hall BK. Earliest evidence of cartilage and bone development in embryonic life. *Clin Orthop* 1987;255: 255–272.

16. Hall BK, Miyake T. The membranous skeleton: the role of cell condensations in vertebrate skeletogenesis. *Anat Embryol (Berl)* 1992;186:107–124.

17. Orr-Urtreger A, Givol D, Yayon A, et al. Developmental expression of two murine fibroblast growth factor receptors, *flg* and *bek. Development* 1991;113: 1419–1434.

18. Delezoide AL, Benoist-Lasselin C, Legeaimallet L, et al. Spatio-temporal expression of Fgfr 1, 2 and 3 genes during human embryo-fetal ossification. *Mech Dev* 1998;77:19–30.

19. Noji S, Koyama E, Myokai F, et al. Differential expression of three chick FGF receptor genes, FGFR1, FGFR2 and FGFR3, in limb and feather development. *Prog Clin Biol Res* 1993;383B:645–654.

20. Haub O, Goldfarb M. Expression of the fibroblast growth factor-5 gene in the mouse embryo. *Development* 1991;112:397–406.

21. deLapeyriere O, Ollendorff V, Planche J, et al. Expression of the Fgf6 gene is restricted to developing skeletal muscle in the mouse embryo. *Development* 1993;118: 601–611.

22. Hebert JM, Rosenquist T, Gotz J, et al. FGF5 as a regulator of the hair growth cycle: evidence from targeted and spontaneous mutations. *Cell* 1994;78: 1017–1025.

23. Fiore F, Planche J, Gibier P, et al. Apparent normal phenotype of Fgf6−/− mice. *Int J Dev Biol* 1997;41: 639–642.

24. Peters K, Ornitz DM, Werner S, et al. Unique expression pattern of the FGF receptor 3 gene during mouse organogenesis. *Dev Biol* 1993;155:423–430.

25. Naski MC, Colvin JS, Coffin JD, et al. Repression of hedgehog signaling and BMP4 expression by fibroblast growth factor receptor 3 in growth plate cartilage of transgenic mice. *Development* 1998;125:4977–4988.

26. Peters KG, Werner S, Chen G, et al. Two FGF receptor genes are differentially expressed in epithelial and mesenchymal tissues during limb formation and organogenesis in the mouse. *Development* 1992;114:233–243.

27. Deng C, Wynshaw-Boris A, Zhou F, et al. Fibroblast growth factor receptor 3 is a negative regulator of bone growth. *Cell* 1996;84:911–921.

28. Kato Y, Iwamoto M. Fibroblast growth factor is an inhibitor of chondrocyte terminal differentiation. *J Biol Chem* 1990;265:5903–5909.

29. Briner J, Giedion A, Spycher MA. Variation of quantitative and qualitative changes of endochondral ossification in heterozygous achondroplasia. *Pathol Res Pract* 1991;187:271–278.

30. Rimoin DL, Hughes GN, Kaufman RL, et al. Endochondral ossification in achondroplastic dwarfism. *N Engl J Med* 1970;283:728–735.

31. Ponseti IV. Skeletal growth in achondroplasia. *J Bone Joint Surg Am* 1970;52-A:701–716.

32. Colvin JS, Bohne BA, Harding GW, et al. Skeletal overgrowth and deafness in mice lacking fibroblast growth factor receptor 3. *Nat Genet* 1996;12:390–397.

33. Gospodarowicz D, Mescher AL. A comparison of the responses of cultured myoblasts and chondrocytes to fibroblast and epidermal growth factors. *J Cell Physiol* 1977;93:117–127.

34. Twal WO, Vasilatos-Younken R, Gay CV, et al. Isolation and localization of basic fibroblast growth factor-immunoreactive substance in the epiphyseal growth plate. *J Bone Miner Res* 1994;9:1737–1744.

35. Quarto R, Campanile G, Cancedda R, et al. Modulation of commitment, proliferation, and differentiation of chondrogenic cells in defined culture medium. *Endocrinology* 1997;138:4966–4976.

36. Jones KL, Addison J. Pituitary fibroblast growth factor as a stimulator of growth in cultured rabbit articular chondrocytes. *Endocrinology* 1975;97:359–365.

37. Fujisato T, Sajiki T, Liu Q, et al. Effect of basic fibroblast growth factor on cartilage regeneration in chondrocyte-seeded collagen sponge scaffold. *Biomaterials* 1996;17:155–162.

38. Ornitz DM, Xu J, Colvin JS, et al. Receptor specificity of the fibroblast growth factor family. *J Biol Chem* 1996;271:15292–15297.

39. Kato Y, Iwamoto M, Koike T. Fibroblast growth factor stimulates colony formation of differentiated chondrocytes in soft agar. *J Cell Physiol* 1987;133:491–498.

40. Wroblewski J, Edwall-Arvidsson C. Inhibitory effects of basic fibroblast growth factor on chondrocyte differentiation. *J Bone Miner Res* 1995;10:735–742.

41. Trippel SB, Wroblewsk J, Makower A-M, et al. Regulation of growth-plate chondrocytes by insulin-like growth factor I and basic fibroblast growth factor. *J Bone Joint Surg* 1993;75:177–189.

42. Koike T, Iwamoto M, Shimazu A, et al. Potent mitogenic effects of parathyroid hormone (PTH) on embryonic chick and rabbit chondrocytes. *J Clin Invest* 1990; 85:626–631.

43. Zhou M, Sutliff RL, Paul RJ, et al. Fibroblast growth factor 2 control of vascular tone. *Nat Med* 1998;4: 201–207.

44. Tobe T, Ortega S, Luna JD, et al. Targeted disruption of the FGF2 gene does not prevent choroidal neovascularization in a murine model. *Am J Pathol* 1998;153: 1641–1646.

45. Dono R, Texido G, Dussel R, et al. Impaired cerebral cortex development and blood pressure regulation in Fgf-2-deficient mice. *EMBO J* 1998;17:4213–4225.
46. Lindner V, Reidy MA. Proliferation of smooth muscle cells after vascular injury is inhibited by an antibody against basic fibroblast growth factor. *Proc Natl Acad Sci USA* 1991;88:3739–3743.
47. Cheng GC, Briggs WH, Gerson DS, et al. Mechanical strain tightly controls fibroblast growth factor-2 release from cultured human vascular smooth muscle cells. *Circ Res* 1997;80:28–36.
48. Xu J, Lawshe A, MacArthur CA, et al. Genomic structure, mapping, activity and expression of fibroblast growth factor 17. *Mech Dev* 1999;83:165–178.
49. Mehrara BJ, Mackool RJ, McCarthy JG, et al. Immunolocalization of basic fibroblast growth factor and fibroblast growth factor receptor-1 and receptor-2 in rat cranial sutures. *Plast Reconstr Surg* 1998;102:1805–1820.
50. Iseki S, Wilkie AOM, Heath JK, et al. Fgfr2 and osteopontin domains in the developing skull vault are mutually exclusive and can be altered by locally applied FGF2. *Development* 1997;124:3375–3384.
51. Kim HJ, Rice DP, Kettunen PJ, et al. FGF-, BMP- and Shh-mediated signalling pathways in the regulation of cranial suture morphogenesis and calvarial bone development. *Development* 1998;125:1241–1251.
52. Bellus GA, McIntosh I, Smith EA, et al. A recurrent mutation in the tyrosine kinase domain of fibroblast growth factor receptor 3 causes hypochondroplasia. *Nat Genet* 1995;10:357–359.
53. Rousseau F, Bonaventure J, Legeal-Mallet L, et al. Mutations in the gene encoding fibroblast growth factor receptor-3 in achondroplasia. *Nature* 1994;371:252–254.
54. Shiang R, Thompson LM, Zhu Y-Z, et al. Mutations in the transmembrane domain of FGFR3 cause the most common genetic form of dwarfism, achondroplasia. *Cell* 1994;78:335–342.
55. Superti-Furga A, Eich G, Bucher HU, et al. A glycine 375-to-cysteine substitution in the transmembrane domain of the fibroblast growth factor receptor-3 in a newborn with achondroplasia. *Eur J Pediatr* 1995;154:215–219.
56. Ikegawa S, Fukushima Y, Isomura M, et al. Mutations of the fibroblast growth factor receptor-3 gene in one familial and six sporadic cases of achondroplasia in Japanese patients. *Hum Genet* 1995;96:309–311.
57. Tavormina PL, Shiang R, Thompson LM, et al. Thanatophoric dysplasia (types I and II) caused by distinct mutations in fibroblast growth factor receptor 3. *Nat Genet* 1995;9:321–328.
58. Rousseau F, el Ghouzzi V, Delezoide AL, et al. Missense FGFR3 mutations create cysteine residues in thanatophoric dwarfism type I (TD1). *Hum Mol Genet* 1996;5:509–512.
59. Rousseau F, Saugier P, Le Merrer M, et al. Stop codon *FGFR3* mutations in thanatophoric dwarfism type 1. *Nat Genet* 1995;10:11–12.
60. Tavormina PL, Rimoin DL, Cohn DH, et al. Another mutation that results in the substitution of an unpaired cysteine residue in the extracellular domain of FGFR3 in thanatophoric dysplasia type I. *Hum Mol Genet* 1995;4:2175–2177.
61. Reardon W, Winter RM, Rutland P, et al. Mutations

in the fibroblast growth factor receptor 2 gene cause Crouzon syndrome. *Nat Genet* 1994;8:98–103.
62. Rutland P, Pulleyn LJ, Reardon W, et al. Identical mutations in the FGFR2 gene cause both Pfeiffer and Crouzon syndrome phenotypes. *Nat Genet* 1995;9:173–176.
63. Jabs EW, Li X, Scott AF, et al. Jackson-Weiss and Crouzon syndromes are allelic with mutations in fibroblast growth factor receptor 2. *Nat Genet* 1994;8:275–279.
64. Meyers GA, Day D, Goldberg R, et al. FGFR2 exon IIIa and IIIc mutations in Crouzon, Jackson-Weiss, and Pfeiffer syndromes: evidence for missense changes, insertions, and a deletion due to alternative RNA splicing. *Am J Hum Genet* 1996;58:491–498.
65. Oldridge M, Wilkie AOM, Slaney SF, et al. Mutations in the third immunoglobulin domain of the fibroblast growth factor receptor-2 gene in Crouzon syndrome. *Hum Mol Genet* 1995;4:1077–1082.
66. Gorry MC, Preston RA, White GJ, et al. Crouzon syndrome: mutations in two spliceoforms of FGFR2 and a common point mutation shared with Jackson-Weiss syndrome. *Hum Mol Genet* 1995;4:1387–1390.
67. Park WJ, Meyers GA, Li X, et al. Novel FGFR2 mutations in Crouzon and Jackson-Weiss syndromes show allelic heterogeneity and phenotypic variability. *Hum Mol Genet* 1995;4:1229–1233.
68. Schell U, Hehr A, Feldman GJ, et al. Mutations in FGFR1 and FGFR2 cause familial and sporadic Pfeiffer syndrome. *Hum Mol Genet* 1995;4:323–328.
69. Steinberger D, Mulliken JB, Muller U. Predisposition for cysteine substitutions in the immunoglobulin-like chain of FGFR2 in Crouzon syndrome. *Hum Genet* 1995;96:113–115.
70. Meyers GA, Orlow SJ, Munrow IR, et al. Fibroblast growth factor receptor 3 transmembrane mutation in Crouzon syndrome with acanthosis nigricans. *Nat Genet* 1995;11:462–464.
71. Wilkie AOM, Morriss-Kay GM, Jones EY, et al. Functions of fibroblast growth factors and their receptors. *Curr Biol* 1995;5:500–507.
72. Muenke M, Schell U, Hehr A, et al. A common mutation in the fibroblast growth factor receptor 1 gene in Pfeiffer syndrome. *Nat Genet* 1994;8:269–274.
73. Lajeunie E, Ma HW, Bonaventure J, et al. FGFR2 mutations in Pfeiffer syndrome. *Nat Genet* 1995;9:108.
74. Przylepa KA, Paznekas W, Zhang M, et al. Fibroblast growth factor receptor 2 mutations in Beare-Stevenson cutis gyrata syndrome. *Nat Genet* 1996;13:492–494.
75. Wilkie AOM, Slaney SF, Oldridge M, et al. Apert syndrome results from localized mutations of FGFR2 and is allelic with Crouzon syndrome. *Nat Genet* 1995;9:165–172.
76. Bellus GA, Gaudenz K, Zackai EH, et al. Identical mutations in three different fibroblast growth factor receptor genes in autosomal dominant craniosynostosis syndromes. *Nat Genet* 1996;14:174–176.
77. Webster MK, Donoghue DJ. FGFR activation in skeletal disorders: too much of a good thing. *Trends Genet* 1997;13:178–182.
78. Wilkie AOM. Craniosynostosis—genes and mechanisms. *Hum Mol Genet* 1997;6:1647–1656.
79. Horton WA. Fibroblast growth factor receptor 3 and the human chondrodysplasias. *Curr Opin Pediatr* 1997;9:437–442.

80. Stanescu R, Stanescu V, Maroteaux P. Homozygous achondroplasia: morphologic and biochemical study of cartilage. *Am J Med Genet* 1990;37:412–421.

81. Naski MC, Wang Q, Xu J, et al. Graded activation of fibroblast growth factor receptor 3 by mutations causing achondroplasia and thanatophoric dysplasia. *Nat Genet* 1996;13:233–237.

82. Webster MK, Donoghue DJ. Constitutive activation of fibroblast growth factor receptor 3 by the transmembrane domain point mutation found in achondroplasia. *EMBO J* 1996;15:520–527.

83. Webster MK, D'Avis PY, Robertson SC, et al. Profound ligand-independent kinase activation of fibroblast growth factor receptor 3 by the activation loop mutation responsible for a lethal skeletal dysplasia, thanatophoric dysplasia type II. *Mol Cell Biol* 1996;16:4081–4087.

84. Li Y, Mangasarian K, Mansukhani A, et al. Activation of FGF receptors by mutations in the transmembrane domain. *Oncogene* 1997;14:1397–1406.

85. Hanks SK, Quinn AM, Hunter T. The protein kinase family: conserved features and deduced phylogeny of the catalytic domains. *Science* 1988;241:42–52.

86. Mohammadi M, Schlessinger J, Hubbard SR. Structure of the FGF receptor tyrosine kinase domain reveals a novel autoinhibitory mechanism. *Cell* 1996;86:577–587.

87. Li CL, Chen L, Iwata T, et al. A Lys644Glu substitution in fibroblast growth factor receptor 3 (FGFR3) causes dwarfism in mice by activation of STATs and ink4 cell cycle inhibitors. *Hum Mol Genet* 1999;8:35–44.

88. Legeai-Mallet L, Benoist-Lasselin C, Delezoide AL, et al. Fibroblast growth factor receptor 3 mutations promote apoptosis but do not alter chondrocyte proliferation in thanatophoric dysplasia. *J Biol Chem* 1998;273:13007–13014.

89. Su WCS, Kitagawa M, Xue NR, et al. Activation of Stat1 by mutant fibroblast growth-factor receptor in thanatophoric dysplasia type II dwarfism. *Nature* 1997;386:288–292.

90. Angle B, Hersh JH, Christensen KM. Molecularly proven hypochondroplasia with cloverleaf skull deformity—a novel association. *Clin Genet* 1998;54:417–420.

91. Chellaiah A, Yuan W, Chellaiah M, et al. Mapping ligand binding domains in chimeric FGF receptor molecules: multiple domains determine ligand binding specificity. *J Biol Chem* 1999;274:34785–34794.

92. Johnson DE, Lee PL, Lu J, et al. Diverse forms of a receptor for acidic and basic fibroblast growth factors. *Mol Cell Biol* 1990;10:4728–4736.

93. Wang F, Kan M, Yan G, et al. Alternately spliced NH_2-terminal immunoglobulin-like loop I in the ectodomain of the fibroblast growth factor (FGF) receptor 1 lowers affinity for both heparin and FGF-1. *J Biol Chem* 1995;270:10231–10235.

94. Wang F, Kan M, McKeehan K, et al. A homeo-interaction sequence in the ectodomain of the fibroblast growth factor receptor. *J Biol Chem* 1997;272:23887–23895.

95. Glockshuber R, Schmidt T, Pluckthun A. The disulfide bonds in antibody variable domains: effects on stability, folding *in vitro*, and functional expression in *Escherichia coli. Biochemistry* 1992;31:1270–1279.

96. Galvin BD, Hart KC, Meyer AN, et al. Constitutive receptor activation by Crouzon syndrome mutations in fibroblast growth factor receptor (FGFR)2 and FGFR2/Neu chimeras. *Proc Natl Acad Sci USA* 1996;93:7894–7899.

97. Basilico C, Moscatelli D. The FGF family of growth factors and oncogenes. *Adv Cancer Res* 1992;59:115–165.

98. Lin HY, Xu JS, Ornitz DM, et al. The fibroblast growth factor receptor-1 is necessary for the induction of neurite outgrowth in PC12 cells by aFGF. *J Neurosci* 1996;16:4579–4587.

99. Lin H-Y, Xu J, Ischenko I, et al. Identification of the cytoplasmic regions of fibroblast growth factor (FGF) receptor 1 which play important roles in the induction of neurite outgrowth in PC12 cells by FGF-1. *Mol Cell Biol* 1998;18:3762–3770.

100. Horton WA. Molecular genetic basis of the human chondrodysplasias. *Endocrinol Metab Clin North Am* 1996;25:683–697.

101. Coffin JD, Florkiewicz RZ, Neumann J, et al. Abnormal bone growth and selective translational regulation in basic fibroblast growth factor (FGF-2) transgenic mice. *Mol Cell Biol* 1995;6:1861–1873.

102. Erlebacher A, Filvaroff EH, Gitelman SE, et al. Toward a molecular understanding of skeletal development. *Cell* 1995;80:371–378.

103. Reddi AH. Bone and cartilage differentiation. *Curr Opin Genet Dev* 1994;4:737–744.

104. Vortkamp A, Lee K, Lanske B, et al. Regulation of rate of cartilage differentiation by Indian hedgehog and PTH-related protein. *Science* 1996;273:613–622.

105. Lanske B, Karaplis AC, Lee K, et al. PTH/PTHrP receptor in early development and Indian hedgehog-regulated bone growth. *Science* 1996;273:663–666.

106. Delezoide AL, Benoist-Lasselin C, Legeai-Mallet L, et al. Abnormal FGFR 3 expression in cartilage of thanatophoric dysplasia fetuses. *Hum Mol Genet* 1997;6:1899–1906.

107. Zou H, Wieser R, Massague J, et al. Distinct roles of type I bone morphogenetic protein receptors in the formation and differentiation of cartilage. *Genes Dev* 1997;11:2191–2203.

108. Zou H, Choe KM, Lu Y, et al. BMP signaling and vertebrate limb development. *Cold Spring Harb Symp Quant Biol* 1997;62:269–272.

Skeletal Growth Factors,
edited by Ernesto Canalis.
Lippincott Williams & Wilkins, Philadelphia, © 2000.

14

Hepatocyte Growth Factor

Alberta Zallone, Maria Grano, and *Paolo M. Comoglio

Institute of Human Anatomy, University of Bari, Bari, Italy
°Department of Biomedical Sciences, Instituto di Ricerea e Cura del Canero,
University of Torino, Torino, Italy

HEPATOCYTE GROWTH FACTOR AND ITS RECEPTOR, C-MET

Hepatocyte growth factor (HGF) was discovered independently as a strong growth-promoting agent in liver cells and as a fibroblast-derived effector of dissociation and motility events such as scattering activity in polarized epithelial cells (1–6). After biochemical purification and cDNA cloning (7,8), the two proteins were shown to be the same molecule (9). In epithelia, HGF is a potent survival and regeneration factor after severe tissue damage. Its ability to accelerate organ regeneration resides in both enhancement of cell growth and modulation of events that contribute to the reestablishment of normal tissue patterning. A vast number of studies following its identification demonstrated that HGF has functions in virtually every tissue of the body. Hematopoiesis (10,11), bone formation and resorption (12), chondrogenesis (13), angiogenesis (14,15), and axonal chemoattraction (16,17) are all critically controlled by HGF. HGF appears to be a powerful mitogenic and morphogenic molecule and plays a role in liver and tissue repair. During embryogenesis, the HGF receptor is expressed in the epithelial component of various organs, whereas HGF is expressed in the adjacent mesenchyme (18). HGF-dependent epithelial morphogenesis is based on a finely tuned interplay between related phenomena including cell proliferation, motility, extracellular matrix degradation, and survival (2,3,6). In transformed epithelia, this interplay is responsible for invasive growth.

The HGF receptor is encoded by the MET protooncogene (19,20) The protein product of this oncogene (21,22) is a single-pass, disulfide-linked $\alpha\beta$ heterodimer arising by proteolytic processing of a common precursor in the post-Golgi compartment (23–25). The α chain is an extracellular glycoprotein, whereas the β chain is a transmembrane subunit responsible for the tyrosine kinase activity (Fig. 14.1). The intracellular domain of this receptor includes well-conserved tyrosine kinase catalytic sites flanked by distinctive juxtamembrane and carboxy-terminal sequences. Phosphorylation of tyrosine residues in positions 1234 and 1235 has a positive regulatory effect on the enzyme activity (26–28), whereas phosphorylation of a serine residue in the juxtamembrane domain negatively regulates the kinase (29,30). The carboxy-terminal domain of the receptor includes two critical tyrosine residues that, when phosphorylated, together form a specific docking site for multiple signal transducers and adaptors (31–41).

From a structural viewpoint, the overall domain organization of HGF is remarkably similar to that of the blood protease plasminogen. During evolution, HGF has lost protease activity but has retained the proteolytic mechanism of activation of the proteases (42,43). Therefore, the activity of this growth factor also relies on proteolytic events that occur in the extracellular milieu, the same ones that initiate blood clotting and fibrinolysis. This indicates that one possible way to inhibit HGF activity is to interfere with its acti-

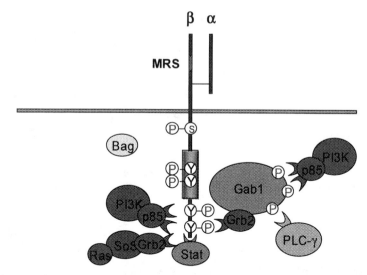

FIG. 14.1 Schematic representation of the structure of the Met receptor. The receptor is a disulfide-linked heterodimer. The α chain is an extracellular glycoprotein; the β chain is a transmembrane subunit responsible for the tyrosine kinase activity. The intracellular domain of the receptor includes a tyrosine kinase catalytic site. Two phosphorylated tyrosine residues contained within the kinase domain have a positive regulatory effect on the enzyme activity, whereas a serine residue in the juxtamembrane domain negatively regulates the kinase. The carboxy-terminal portion includes two tyrosine residues that, when phosphorylated, together form a specific docking site for multiple signal transducers and adaptors.

vation mechanism either at the site of production or at the level of target cells.

HGF belongs to a family of proteins defined by the presence of at least one peculiar domain known as kringle (an 80–amino acid, double-looped structure formed by three internal disulfide bridges), a serine protease domain, and an activation segment located between the kringle and the protease domains. HGF does not possess intrinsic enzymatic activity and is a ligand for a transmembrane tyrosine kinase, the MET receptor. HGF is secreted as a single-chain, biologically inert glycoprotein precursor (pro-HGF). Under appropriate conditions, pro-HGF is converted into its bioactive form by proteolytic digestion within two positively charged amino acids (the so-called dibasic site Arg[494]-Val[495]). Mature HGF is a heterodimer consisting of a 62-kDa α chain and a 32- to 34-kDa β chain held together by a disulfide bond (Fig. 14.2). The nucleotide sequences of human, rat, and mouse HGF cDNA predict that both chains are encoded by a single open reading frame, resulting in a

728–amino acid polypeptide. Starting from the amino terminus, the α chain of HGF contains a hairpin loop of about 27 amino acids, followed by four kringles, whereas the β chain contains the serine protease-like structure (8).

To characterize the receptor-binding domain of HGF, individual deletions of each kringle

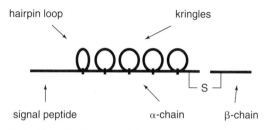

FIG. 14.2 A diagram of the structure of hepatocyte growth factor (HGF). The protein is a heterodimer consisting of a heavy α chain and a light β chain held together by a disulfide bond. Starting from the amino-terminal signal peptide, the α chain contains a hairpin loop followed by four kringles.

have been carried out (44). Only deletion of the first kringle is accompanied by a substantial reduction in receptor-binding capacity, suggesting that the primary receptor-binding site is located within this region. The functional domain responsible for motogenic response resides within the amino terminus and the first two kringle domains. The α chain contributes to receptor activation, and cleavage of HGF into the two subunits is required for proper induction of the biological response (45).

Proteoglycans, which are abundant and ubiquitous tissue components, are likely to capture and immobilize those growth factors and cytokines that have affinity for glycosaminoglycans; in this way, they provide a molecular reservoir aimed at accumulating growth factors on the cell surface, protecting them from degradation, or transferring them to the high-affinity receptors that initiate the cellular response. Other possible functional consequences of growth factors binding to proteoglycans include ligand stabilization, induced fit for receptor binding, and oligomerization. Indeed, analysis of the binding properties of HGF indicates the existence of two classes of site with affinities one order of magnitude apart. The high-affinity binding site (K_d in the 10^{-10} M range) has been identified as the receptor encoded by the MET protooncogene; the lower-affinity, large-capacity site, with a K_d in the range of 10^{-9} M, corresponds to matrix or cell surface–associated heparin sulfate proteoglycans. This is indicated by the presence of a heparin-binding domain on the HGF α chain (6). The presentation of multivalent HGF molecules, induced by the binding of HGF to sulfated epitopes on heparin sulfate proteoglycan chains, may facilitate subsequent receptor dimerization and triggering of biological response. The finding that heparin is crucial for inducing HGF dimerization and that cellular responses to HGF depend on the glycosaminoglycan composition of the cell membrane further support the hypothesis that receptor activation requires cooperative participation by multiple surface and soluble components. According to the aforementioned data, one could speculate that HGF, weakly adsorbed onto matrix or cell surface proteoglycans and then assembled into oligomeric moieties, displays multivalent interactions with preclus-

tered receptors; proper growth factor activation at target cell sites would be accomplished by noncovalent interactions with urokinase plasminogen activator (uPA) and uPA receptor.

HEPATOCYTE GROWTH FACTOR AND BONE CELLS

A Fully Functional Hepatocyte Growth Factor Receptor Is Expressed by Primary Osteoclasts and by Osteoclast Cell Lines

HGF is produced by stromal cells (11) and can stimulate hemopoiesis. This finding induced us and others (12,46) to investigate a possible role of HGF in bone biology. We first investigated whether c-MET, the HGF receptor, was expressed by osteoclasts, utilizing both freshly dissected human osteoclasts obtained from surgical samples and osteoclast-like cell lines (giant cell tumor [GCT] 23 and giant cell tumor 51) obtained from giant cell tumor of bone and stabilized *in vitro*. The presence of the HGF receptor in normal, freshly prepared human osteoclasts and in GCT cells was investigated by indirect immunofluorescence, using antibodies specific for the extracellular domain of the receptor. Human osteoclasts and GCT cells were strongly positive at their surface and partially stained in intracellular compartments (Fig. 14.3). Since it is extremely difficult to obtain large numbers of fresh human osteoclasts, the biochemical features of the HGF receptor were investigated in the osteoclast-like lines GCT-23, -24, -31, -32, and -51 (47). Cell lysates were extracted and probed in Western blots with antibodies directed against the N-terminal portion of the HGF receptor. In the presence of β-mercaptoethanol, a single band of 145 kDa, corresponding to the β chain, and an additional band of 170 kDa, corresponding to the precursor, could be shown. The expected 190-kDa protein corresponding to the $\alpha\beta$ dimer could be demonstrated under nonreducing conditions (12). To investigate whether the HGF receptor molecule was functional in GCT cells, we tested its tyrosine phosphorylation upon ligand binding. Cells were stimulated for 10 minutes at 37°C with nanomolar concentrations of human recombinant HGF. Cell lysates were immunoprecipitated with anti-HGF

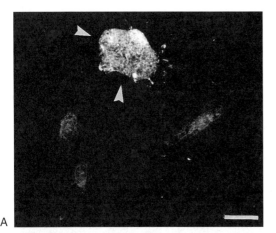

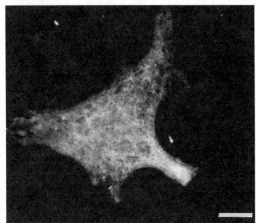

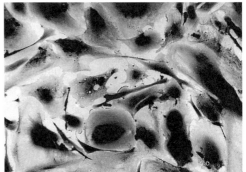

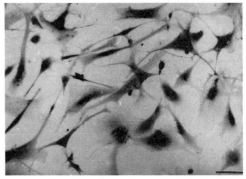

FIG. 14.4 Morphological changes of osteoclast-like GCT cells in response to hepatocyte growth factor (HGF). Cells plated onto coverslips were treated with 5 ng/ml HGF for 24 hours, then fixed with glutaraldehyde and stained with crystal violet. The spread morphology of untreated cells **(a)** switches to a spindle motile phenotype after stimulation **(b)**. Bar: 50 μm.

FIG. 14.3 Detection of hepatocyte growth factor (HGF) receptor at the cell surface of primary human osteoclasts explanted in vitro. The HGF receptor is visualized by immunofluorescence, using monoclonal antibodies directed against the extracellular domain of the β chain. The receptor is expressed on a small osteoclast precursor (panel **a**, *arrow*) and in a large mature multinucleated osteoclast **(b)**. Fibroblastic cells present in the same field **(a)** are negative. Bars: **a**, 20 μm; **b**, 30 μm.

receptor antibodies and probed in Western blots with antiphosphotyrosine antibodies. Specific tyrosine autophosphorylation of the receptor β chain in response to HGF was found.

Hepatocyte Growth Factor Induces Morphological Changes and Motility in GCT Cells

Osteoclast morphology changes according to the functional state of the cell, varying from a flat to a spindle-refractile cell shape. GCT cells were plated on coverslips and treated with nanomolar concentrations of recombinant HGF; observation of the cells under the phase contrast microscope showed that the treatment induced a dramatic switch from a flat morphology to a spindle-refractile appearance. The changes became evident after 2 hours and were maximal after 24 hours of treatment (Fig. 14.4). The effect of HGF on osteoclast motility was investigated in a Boyden chamber assay, using either GCT cells or freshly prepared osteoclasts. Without stimulation, cells were virtually unable to cross the filter between the upper and the lower sides of the chamber. HGF induced chemotactically oriented migration, both in the presence and in the absence of serum; the effect was dose-dependent (12).

Hepatocyte Growth Factor Stimulation Induces Activation of pp60[c-Src] in GCT Cells

It is known that, upon ligand binding, the HGF receptor triggers intracellular signals by activation of several downstream transducers, including proteins of the *Src* family (48,34). It is well established that activation of c-*Src* is a characteristic feature of osteoclasts (49,50). Lysates from cells stimulated with nanomolar concentrations of HGF were extracted and immunoprecipitated with specific anti-pp60[c-Src] antibodies. The kinase activity of immunoprecipitates was then measured on the exogenous substrate [Val[5]]-angiotensin II. A significant increase in pp60[c-Src] kinase activity was measured. This degree of stimulation was comparable to the extent of Src kinase stimulation observed in epithelial cells stimulated by HGF (34) and in fibroblasts or macrophages stimulated by platelet-derived growth factor (PDGF) or colony-stimulating factor-I (CSF-I), respectively (51, 52).

Hepatocyte Growth Factor Triggers a Rise in Intracellular Calcium Concentration in Primary Osteoclasts and in GCT Cells

As shown previously, activation of the HGF receptor by the ligand generates a complex cascade of intracellular signals involving phospholipase C (PLC)-γ (34). PLC-γ in turn induces elevation of the intracellular calcium concentration $[Ca^{2+}]_i$. The effect of HGF stimulation on

$[Ca^{2+}]_i$ was measured by single-cell fluorimetry, after loading with the Ca^{2+}-sensitive probe Fura-2. Fresh human osteoclasts or multinucleated GCT cells containing at least three nuclei were analyzed. In both cases, HGF induced an increase of $[Ca^{2+}]_i$ in a dose-dependent manner (Table 14.1). The maximum response was reached at 2.5 ng/ml HGF: the $[Ca^{2+}]_i$ in basal conditions was 122 ± 10 nM; upon addition of HGF, we measured an increase of $[Ca^{2+}]_i$ peaking at 310 ± 38 nM within 240 ± 0.4 seconds, followed by a sustained phase at peak values and a slow decrease reaching a plateau within 240 ± 0.7 seconds at 214 ± 23 nM. These values were similar to those observed in several other cell types, including osteoclasts of different species, upon stimulation by different ligands (53).

To investigate whether the HGF-induced $[Ca^{2+}]_i$ increase depends on release of Ca^{2+} from intracellular stores or from influx from the extracellular environment, the intracellular stores were depleted by treatment with the Ca^{2+}-ATPase inhibitor thapsigargin. As expected, the treatment produced a transient increase of $[Ca^{2+}]_i$ (419 ± 36 nM), slowly returning toward baseline (272 ± 33 nM); addition of HGF failed to generate a further increase of $[Ca^{2+}]_i$. To investigate the role of extracellular calcium, experiments were repeated in a nominally calcium-free buffer. Under these conditions, HGF still induced the $[Ca^{2+}]_i$ increase (102 ± 62 to 295 ± 49 nM), but the peak was followed by an immediate return toward baseline (136 ± 35 nM) and the plateau was abolished.

TABLE 14.1. *Response of human osteoclasts to HGF*

			$[CA^{2+}]i$ nM			
Treatment	n	Concentration ng/ml	Basal	Peak	Plateau	Δ Peak
HGF	4	0.5	196 ± 58	209 ± 53	—	33 ± 0
"	4	1.25	71 ± 23	**221 ± 27	115 ± 33	149 ± 27
"	6	2.5	115 ± 16	*310 ± 38	**214 ± 23	195 ± 29
"	5	5	111 ± 11	*294 ± 43	**210 ± 28	182 ± 83
"	6	7.5	127 ± 16	*243 ± 13	164 ± 22	116 ± 9
"	5	12.5	120 ± 4	*227 ± 5	162 ± 6	106 ± 7
TG2μM + HGF	4	2.5	272 ± 33	226 ± 24	—	—
EGTA3mM + HGF	4	2.5	102 ± 62	*295 ± 49	136 ± 35	192 ± 68

* p < 0.001 (vs Basal)
** p < 0.01 (vs Basal)

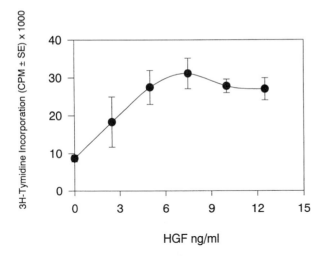

FIG. 14.5 Hepatocyte growth factor (HGF) stimulates thymidine incorporation by osteoclast-like GCT cells. Growth-arrested cells were pulsed with 1 μCi/ml of [^{3}H]-thymidine for 24 hours in serum-free medium in the presence or absence of the indicated concentrations of recombinant HGF. Values on the ordinate indicate cycles per minute $\times$ 10^3 incorporated in trichloroacetic acid precipitates harvested from quadruplicate wells. Bars show the standard error.

Hepatocyte Growth Factor Stimulates [^{3}H]-Thymidine Incorporation in GCT Cells

The activity of HGF in promoting thymidine incorporation was also evaluated. GCT cells, growth-arrested by 24-hour incubation in serum-free medium, were pulsed with 1 μCi/ml of [^{3}H]-thymidine for 24 hours, in the presence of increasing concentrations of HGF. Untreated cells were used as a control. At a concentration of 7.5 ng/ml, HGF induced a fourfold increase in DNA synthesis. The stimulatory activity was dose-dependent, and the maximal effect occurred between 5 and 7.5 ng/ml (Fig. 14.5).

Hepatocyte Growth Factor Inhibits Bone Resorption

The ability to resorb the bone matrix is a distinctive feature of the osteoclastic phenotype. In GCT cells, bone resorption activity has been previously demonstrated and shown to be modulated by different factors, including the hormone calcitonin and the extracellular Ca^{2+} concentration (48,54). To investigate the possible role of HGF in the modulation of bone-resorption activity, GCT cells were incubated with radiolabeled bone fragments in the presence of different concentrations of recombinant HGF. At intervals between 2 and 6 days, bone resorption was quantified by measuring the ^{3}H-proline released in the spent medium. HGF treatment reduced bone resorption in a dose-dependent manner. The inhibitory effect was observed at concentrations between 12.5 and 62.5 ng/ml; lower concentrations were ineffective. Bone resorption was reduced in a dose-dependent manner to a maximum of about 50%. The effect of HGF was reversible since removal of the factor from the culture medium after 48 hours completely restored the capability of resorbing bone (Grano et al., personal communication, 1998).

Hepatocyte Growth Factor Is Produced by Osteoclasts

It has been shown that HGF is found in fragments obtained from giant cell tumors of bone (55). In order to investigate whether the factor was endogenously produced, we tested the culture medium conditioned by osteoclastic cells and found a secretion as high as 3.5 ng/ml of biologically active growth factor.

Hepatocyte Growth Factor and Integrin Activation

Integrins mediate cell adhesion and can induce different cellular responses, including changes in intracellular pH, changes and oscillation in intracellular free calcium, and protein phosphorylation on tyrosine. During bone resorption, the integrin $\alpha_v\beta_3$ regulates adhesion of osteoclasts to bone extracellular matrix proteins, such as osteopontin. Adhesion via $\alpha_v\beta_3$ is followed by osteoclast polarization onto the bone surface and by the onset of bone resorption. Several studies indicate that $\alpha_v\beta_3$ is involved both in migration and in the organization of the sealing zones, such that the same integrin may mediate different functions. It has been recently demonstrated that $\alpha_v\beta_3$ exists in two different conformational states, basal and activated, analogous to the conformational states of the platelet integrin $\alpha_{IIb}\beta_3$ (56). That study was performed with a murine monoclonal activating antibody, AP5, that binds a linear epitope corresponding to the amino terminus of the β_3 subunit, classified as a ligand-inducible binding site. The different conformational states may regulate ligand-binding properties and modulate different cellular behaviors induced by ligands. The states of the integrin can be considered two functionally distinct receptors (57). This property of $\alpha_v\beta_3$ offers a potential explanation for the different osteoclast behavior in response to its ligands. Antibody-activated integrin endowed the osteoclasts with increased affinity for ligand and increased motility. With the aim of understanding how $\alpha_v\beta_3$ integrin can be activated in physiological conditions, we pretreated osteoclasts with HGF or CSF before performing motility or adhesion experiments. We discovered that both growth factors were able to switch most of the integrin in the activated status, increasing motility. $\alpha_v\beta_3$,

searched by immunostaining with the appropriate antibodies, was localized in undulating membrane and in ruffles, and podosomes were almost absent. This last finding can explain the inhibitory role of high doses of HGF in bone resorption. The cells are mainly motile, and for bone resorption, a stable adhesive ring, where all of the proteins of podosomes are found in a proper organization, is necessary.

Hepatocyte Growth Factor and Osteoblasts

Whereas unstimulated osteoblasts express immunoreactive c-met and c-met transcripts, they do not express detectable HGF protein under basal conditions (12). However, recent studies have demonstrated that fibroblast growth factor-2 (FGF-2) and PDGF-BB induce HFG transcripts and protein concentrations in primary cultures of rodent osteoblasts and osteoblast cell lines (58). FGF-2 and PDGF-BB appear to play a role in tissue and fracture repair, and their ability to induce HGF synthesis in osteoblasts is consistent with a possible role of HGF in fracture healing. This possibility is substantiated by the demonstration that HGF increases [³H]-thymidine incorporation in osteoblasts, a marker of DNA synthesis. The increase was dose-dependent and HGF was effective at 2 ng/ml (Fig. 14.6). Conversely, osteocalcin secretion and alkaline phosphatase activity were decreased, in-

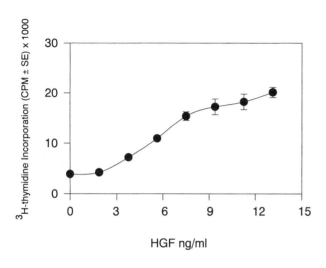

FIG. 14.6 Hepatocyte growth factor (HGF) stimulates thymidine incorporation by human osteoblast cells. Growth-arrested cells were pulsed with 1 μCi/ml of [³H]-thymidine for 24 hours in serum-free medium in the presence or absence of the indicated concentrations of recombinant HGF. Values on the ordinate indicate cycles per minute $\times$ 10³ incorporated in trichloroacetic acid precipitates harvested from quadruplicate wells. Bars show the standard error.

dicating a switch toward proliferation and not toward osteoblast differentiation.

Role of Hepatocyte Growth Factor in Bone Remodeling

The aforementioned findings indicate that HGF has a role in bone remodeling, inducing biological responses in both osteoclasts and os- teoblasts. In osteoclasts, HGF stimulates chemo- tactically oriented migration. Cell migration is important in early steps of bone resorption, when osteoclast precursors are attracted toward the bone matrix. In these cells, HGF stimulates DNA synthesis, therefore controlling both mi- gration and proliferation. In osteoblasts, HGF stimulates DNA synthesis but fails to induce cell migration. The finding that HGF triggers prolif- eration of both osteoclasts and osteoblasts is only apparently a paradox. In fact, bone resorp- tion and formation are tightly coupled. HGF in- creases the number of resorbing cells by chemo- tactic attraction of osteoclasts and by stimulation of their proliferation. At the same time, the fac- tor balances the number of osteogenic cells re- quired for bone remodeling. These cells arrive *in situ* together with endothelial sprout (whose migration and proliferation is also stimulated by HGF) and actively proliferate in the presence of HGF, secreted by osteoclasts and stromal cells, and transforming growth factor, released from the bone matrix by resorbing osteoclasts. In con- clusion, HGF can produce an autocrine–para- crine loop effective in the control of bone remod- eling.

ACKNOWLEDGMENTS

This work was supported by funds of the Ital- ian Association for Cancer Research (AIRC) granted to A.Z. and to P.M.C.

REFERENCES

1. Nakamura T, Teramoro H, Ichihara A. Purification and characterization of a growth factor from rat platelets for mature parenchymal hepatocytes in primary cultures. *Proc Natl Acad Sci USA* 1986;83:6489–6493.
2. Stoker M, Gherardi E, Perryman M, et al. Scatter factor is a fibroblast-derived modulator of epithelial cell motil- ity. *Nature* 1987;327:239–242.
3. Gherardi E, Gray J, Stoker M, et al. Purification of scat- ter factor, a fibroblast derived basic protein that modu- lates epithelial interjunctions and movement. *Proc Natl Acad Sci USA* 1989;86:5844–5848.
4. Godha E, Yamasaki T, Tsubouchi H, et al. Biological and immunological properties of human hepatocyte growth factor from plasma of patients with fulminant hepatic failure. *Biochim Biophys Acta* 1990;1053: 21–26.
5. Zarnegar R, Michalopoulos G. Purification and biologi- cal characterization of human hepatopoietin A, a poly- peptide growth factor for hepatocytes. *Cancer Res* 1989; 49:3314–3320.
6. Weidner KM, Behrens J, Vanderkerckove J, et al. Scat- ter factor: molecular characteristics and effect on the invasiveness of epithelial cells. *J Cell Biol* 1990;111: 2097–2198.
7. Miyazawa K, Tsubouchi H, Naka D, et al. Molecular cloning and sequence analysis of cDNA for human he- patocyte growth factor. *Biochem Biophys Res Commun* 1989;163:967–973.
8. Nakamura T, Nishizawa T, Hagiya M, et al. Molecular cloning and expression of human hepatocyte growth fac- tor. *Nature* 1989;342:440–443.
9. Naldini L, Weidmer KM, Vigna E, et al. Scatter factor and hepatocyte growth factor are indistinguishable lig- ands for the Met receptor. *EMBO J* 1991;10:2867–2878.
10. Galimi F, Bagnara GP, Bonsi L, et al. Hepatocyte growth factor induces proliferation and differentiation of multipotent and erythroid hemopoietic progenitors. *J Cell Biol* 1994;127:1743–1754.
11. Takai K, Hara J, Matsumoto K, et al. Hepatocyte growth factor is constitutively produced by human bone marrow stromal cells and indirectly promotes hemopoiesis. *Blood* 1997;89:1560–1565.
12. Grano M, Galimi F, Zambonin G, et al. Hepatocyte growth factor is a coupling factor for osteoclasts and osteoblasts *in vitro*. *Proc Natl Acad Sci USA* 1996;93: 7644–7648.
13. Takebayashi T, Iwamoto M, Jikko A, et al. Hepatocyte growth factor/scatter factor modulates cell motility, pro- liferation and proteoglycan synthesis of chondrocytes. *J Cell Biol* 1995;129:1411–1419.
14. Bussolino F, Di Renzo MF, Ziche M, et al. Hepatocyte growth factor is a potent angiogenic factor which stimu- lates endothelial cell motility and growth. *J Cell Biol* 1992;119:629–640.
15. Grant DS, Kleinman HK, Goldberg JD, et al. Scatter factor induces blood vessel formation *in vivo*. *Proc Natl Acad Sci USA* 1993;90:1937–1941.
16. Honda S, Kagoshima M, Wanaka A, et al. Localization and functional coupling of HGF and cMET/HGF recep- tor in rat brain: implication as neurotrophic factor. *Brain Res Mol Brain Res* 1995;32:197–210.
17. Ebens A, Brose K, Leonardo ED, et al. Hepatocyte growth factor/scatter factor is an axonal chemoattractant and a neurotrophic factor for spinal motor neurons. *Neu- ron* 1996;17:1157–1172.
18. Sonnenberg E, Meyer D, Weidner KM, et al. Scatter factor/hepatocyte growth factor and its receptor, the c- met tyrosine kinase, can mediate a signal exchange be- tween mesenchyme and epithelia during development. *J Cell Biol* 1993;123:223–235.

19. Bottaro DP, Rubin JS, Faletto DL, et al. Identification of the hepatocyte growth factor receptor as the c-met proto-oncogene product. *Science* 1991;251:802–804.

20. Naldini L, Vigna E, Narsimhan RP, et al. Hepatocyte growth factor (HGF) stimulates the tyrosine kinase activity of the receptor encoded by the proto-oncogene c-MET. *Oncogene* 1991;6:501–504.

21. Cooper CS, Park M, Blair DG, et al. Molecular cloning of a new transforming gene from a chemically transformed human cell line. *Nature* 1984;311:29–33.

22. Park M, Dean M, Kaul K, et al. Sequence of MET protooncogene cDNA has features characteristic of the tyrosine kinase family of growth factor receptors. *Proc Natl Acad Sci USA* 1987;84:6379–6383.

23. Giordano S, Ponzetto C, Di Renzo MF, et al. Tyrosine kinase receptor indistinguishable from the c-met protein. *Nature* 1989;990:155–156.

24. Giordano S, Di Renzo MF, Narsimhan RP, et al. Biosynthesis of protein encoded by the c-met proto-oncogene. *Oncogene* 1989;4:1383–1388.

25. Crepaldi T, Prat M, Giordano S, et al. Generation of a truncated hepatocyte growth factor receptor in the endoplasmic reticulum. *J Biol Chem* 1994;269:1750–1755.

26. Ferracini R, Longati P, Naldini L, et al. Identification of the major autophosphorylation site of the Met/hepatocyte growth factor receptor tyrosine kinase. *J Biol Chem* 1991;266:19558–19564.

27. Naldini L, Vigna E, Ferracini R, et al. The tyrosine kinase encoded by the MET proto-oncogene is activated by autophosphorylation. *Mol Cell Biol* 1991;11:1793–1805.

28. Longati P, Bardelli A, Ponzetto C, et al. Tyrosines 1234–1235 are critical for activation of the tyrosine kinase encoded by the MET proto-oncogene (HGF receptor). *Oncogene* 1994;9:49–57.

29. Gandino L, Di Renzo MF, Giordano S, et al. Protein kinase C activation inhibits tyrosine phosphorylation of the c-met protein. *Oncogene* 1990;5:721–725.

30. Gandino L, Longati P, Medico E, et al. Phosphorylation of serine 985 negatively regulates the hepatocyte growth factor receptor kinase. *J Biol Chem* 1994;269:1815–1820.

31. Graziani A, Gramaglia D, Cantley LC, et al. The tyrosine phosphorylate hepatocyte growth factor/scatter factor receptor associates with phosphatidylinositol 3-kinase. *J Biol Chem* 1991;266:22087–22090.

32. Graziani A, Gramaglia D, Della Zonca P, et al. Hepatocyte growth factor/scatter factor stimulates the Ras–guanine nucleotide exchanger. *J Biol Chem* 1993;268:9165–9168.

33. Ponzetto C, Bardelli A, Maina F, et al. A novel recognition motif for phosphatidylinositol 3-kinase binding mediates its association with the hepatocyte growth factor/scatter factor receptor. *Mol Cell Biol* 1993;13:4600–4606.

34. Ponzetto C, Bardelli A, Zhen Z, et al. A multifunctional docking site mediates signaling and transformation by the hepatocyte growth factor/scatter factor receptor family. *Cell* 1994;77:261–271.

35. Villa-Moruzzi E, Lapi S, Prat M, et al. A protein tyrosine phosphatase activity associated with the hepatocyte growth factor/scatter factor receptor. *J Biol Chem* 1993;268:18176–18180.

36. Lee CC, Yamada KM. Alternatively spliced juxtamembrane domain of a tyrosine kinase receptor is a multi-

functional regulatory site. Deletion alters cellular tyrosine phosphorylation pattern and facilitates binding of phosphatidylinositol-3′-kinase to the hepatocyte growth factor receptor. *J Biol Chem* 1995;270:507–510.

37. Pellicci G, Giordano S, Zhen Z, et al. The motogenic and mitogenic responses to HGF are amplified by the Shc adaptor protein. *Oncogene* 1995;10:1631–1638.

38. Iwama A, Yamaguchi N, Suda T. STK/RON receptor tyrosine kinase mediates both apoptotic and growth signals via the multifunctional docking site conserved among the HGF receptor family. *EMBO J* 1996;15:5866–5875.

39. Weidner K, Di Cesare S, Sachs M, et al. Interaction between Gab 1 and the c-met receptor tyrosine kinase is responsible for epithelial morphogenesis. *Nature* 1996;384:173–176.

40. Nguyen L, Holgado Madruga M, Maroun C, et al. Association of the multisubstrate docking protein Gab1 with the hepatocyte growth factor receptor requires a functional Grb2 binding site involving tyrosine 1356. *J Biol Chem* 1997;272:20811–20819.

41. Bardelli A, Longati P, Gramaglia D, et al. Gab1 coupling to the HGF/Met receptor multifunctional docking site requires binding of Grb2 and correlates with the transforming potential. *Oncogene* 1997;15:3103–3111.

42. Naldini L, Tamagnone L, Vigna E, et al. Extracellular proteolytic cleavage by urokinase is required for activation of hepatocyte growth factor/scatter factor. *EMBO J* 1992;11:4825–4883.

43. Mars WM, Zarnegar R, Michalopoulos GK. Activation of hepatocyte growth factor by the plasminogen activators uPA and tPA. *Am J Pathol* 1993;145:949–956.

44. Lokker NA, Mark MR, Luis EA, et al. Structure–function analysis of hepatocyte growth factor: identification of variants that lack mitogenic activity yet retain high affinity receptor binding. *EMBO J* 1992;11:2503–2510.

45. Trusolino L, Pugliese L, Comoglio PM. Interactions between scatter factors and their receptors: hints for therapeutic applications. *FASEB J* 1998;12:1267–1280.

46. Fuller K, Owens J, Chambers TJ. The effect of hepatocyte growth factor on the behavior of osteoclasts. *Biochem Biophys Res Commun* 1995;212:334–340.

47. Grano M, Colucci S, De Bellis M, et al. A new model for bone resorption study *in vitro:* human osteoclast-like cells from giant cell tumors of bone. *J Bone Miner Res* 1994;9:1013–1020.

48. Bardelli AF, Maina I, Gout MJ, et al. Autophosphorylation promotes complex formation of recombinant hepatocyte growth factor receptor with cytoplasmic effector containing SH2 domain. *Oncogene* 1992;7:1973–1978.

49. Horne WC, Neff L, Chatterjee D, et al. Osteoclasts express high levels of pp60c-src in association with intracellular membranes. *J Cell Biol* 1992;119:1003–1013.

50. Soriano PC, Montgomery C, Geske R, et al. Targeted disruption of the c-src proto-oncogene leads to osteopetrosis in mice. *Cell* 1991;64:693–702.

51. Courtneidge SA, Dhand R, Pilat D, et al. Activation of the Src family kinases by colony stimulating factor-1, and their association with its receptor. *EMBO J* 1993;12:943–950.

52. Kypta RM, Goldberg Y, Ulug ET, et al. Association between the PDGF receptor and members of the src family of tyrosine kinases. *Cell* 1990;62:481–492.

53. Malgaroli A, Meldolesi J, Zambonin Zallone A, et al.

Control of cytosolic free calcium in rat and chicken osteoclasts. The role of extracellular calcium and calcitonin. *J Biol Chem* 1989;264:14342–14347.

54. Miyauchi A, Hruska KA, Greenfield EM, et al. Osteoclast cytosolic calcium, regulated by voltage-gated calcium channel and extracellular calcium, controls podosomes assembly and bone resorption. *J Cell Biol* 1990; 111:2543–2552.

55. Ferracini R, Di Renzo MF, Scotlandi K, et al. The Met/HGF receptor is overexpressed in human osteosarcoma and is activated by either a paracrine or an autocrine circuit. *Oncogene* 1995;10:739–749.

56. Pelletier AJ, Kunicki TJ, Quaranta V. Activation of the integrin $\alpha_v\beta_3$ involves a discrete cation-binding site that regulates conformation. *J Biol Chem* 1996;271: 1364–1370.

57. Pelletier AJ, Kunicki TJ, Ruggeri ZM, et al. The activation state of the integrin $\alpha IIb\beta_3$ affects outside-in signals leading to cell spreading and focal adhesion kinase phosphorylation. *J Biol Chem* 1995;270:18133–18140.

58. Blanquaert F, Delany AM, Canalis E. Fibroblast growth factor-2 induces hepatocyte growth factor/scatter factor expression in osteoblasts. *Endocrinology* 1999;140: 1069.

Skeletal Growth Factors,
edited by Ernesto Canalis.
Published by Lippincott Williams & Wilkins, Philadelphia, 2000.

15

Transforming Growth Factor-β

Anita B. Roberts

Laboratory of Cell Regulation and Carcinogenesis, National Cancer Institute, Bethesda, Maryland 20892-5055

The transforming growth factor-βs (TGF-βs) are multifunctional peptides expressed in mammals as three highly homologous isoforms, TGF-βs 1, 2, and 3. While the initial characterization of the TGF-βs in 1983 was based on their ability to transform cells *in vitro* and in the context of their being proximal effectors of transformation, it was immediately apparent that these proteins also were present in large amounts in platelets and in bone and that they must be involved in normal physiology as well as in disease pathogenesis (for review, see 1). Now the TGF-βs serve as the paradigmatic molecules for a superfamily of over 40 different related proteins, presumably derived from a common ancestral gene (2), which includes the bone morphogenetic proteins (Chapters 19–21), activins (Chapters 17 and 18), inhibins, and müllerian inhibitory substance, among others. Distinguished initially for their ability to inhibit the growth of most epithelial and hematopoietic cells and to regulate the production of extracellular matrix by mesenchymal cells, the TGF-βs are now known to act via autocrine, paracrine, and endocrine modes to control a wide variety of developmental processes and to play key roles in the pathogenesis of many diseases, including especially fibrotic diseases, parasitic diseases, autoimmune diseases, and carcinogenesis. Moreover, the unique mitogenic actions of TGF-β on osteoblasts (3), coupled with its abilities to stimulate matrix formation and to induce expression of parathyroid hormone–related protein (4) (Chapter 25), implicate it as a major

physiological regulator of bone formation and fracture repair (Chapter 16). Key to its multifunctional activities are not only complex transcriptional regulatory mechanisms governing the tissue-specific expression of both the ligand and its receptors but also intricate post-transcriptional mechanisms which control the trafficking and activation of the latent forms of TGF-β as well as extensive crosstalk between signal-transduction pathways downstream of TGF-β, of tyrosine kinase receptors, and even of nuclear hormone receptors. Because of the extensive literature on TGF-β, recent reviews of the subject are cited whenever possible in lieu of the primary references.

MOLECULAR BIOLOGY OF THE TRANSFORMING GROWTH FACTOR-βs

The three mammalian isoforms of TGF-β, TGF-βs 1, 2, and 3, are expressed in cell-specific patterns, with the type 1 isoform in most cases being the most abundant or, as in the platelet α-granule, the only isoform present (1). TGF-βs 1, 2, and 3 are localized to three different chromosomes (human chromosomes 19q13, 1q41, and 14q24, respectively) and are transcribed as mRNAs characterized by long 3' and 5'-untranslated regions, implicating posttranscriptional regulation. While such mechanisms are only beginning to be studied (5,6), the transcriptional regulation of the three isoforms has been studied in detail and has provided insight into the unique role of the type 1 isoform in response to injury and in disease.

The promoter for TGF-β1 is distinguished from those of TGF-βs 2 and 3 by its lack of a classic TATAA box and by the presence of multiple regulatory sites which can be activated by immediate-early genes, including c-jun, c-fos, and egr-1 and by a variety of oncogenes, including abl, fos, jun, ras, and src (7). The promoter has several GC boxes proximal to the transcriptional start site which mediate its regulation by both Sp1 and Zf9/CPBP, a core-promoter binding protein in the Kruppel-like zinc-finger transcription factor family which has been implicated in the upregulation of expression of both TGF-β1 and its receptors in response to injury (8). Other transcriptional regulatory sites include activator protein-1 (AP-1) sites, which figure prominently in the autoinduction of TGF-β1 as well as in oncogenic induction by activated jun and fos genes (9), and early growth response-1 (Egr-1) GC-rich sites (10). Importantly, these same sites also mediate the action of a variety of viral transactivator proteins on transcription of TGF-β1, including the Tat transcriptional transactivator produced by human immunodeficiency virus type 1 (HIV-1), which binds to GC/GA sites (11); human T-lymphotropic virus type 1 (HTLV-1) Tax transactivator protein, which activates transcription of TGF-β1 through AP-1 sites (12); and both hepatitis B virus X protein (13) and the human cytomegalovirus IE2 regulatory protein, which activate TGF-β1 through direct interaction with Egr-1 and its binding sites in the promoter (14). The TGF-β1 promoter is also regulated by the products of the retinoblastoma susceptibility gene (15) and the Wilms' tumor gene (16). These unique and distinguishing features of the TGF-β1 promoter provide a mechanistic basis for the selective overexpression of this isoform seen in repair of injury, in response to stress, in the pathogenesis of viral-mediated disease, and in carcinogenesis.

The promoters for TGF-βs 2 and 3 are distinct from that of TGF-β1 and more similar to each other. Each is characterized by the presence of a TATA box marking the transcriptional initiation site and a proximal cyclic adenosine monophosphate (cAMP)–response element (CRE)/activating transcription factor (ATF) site, which strongly influences transcription via binding of ATF-1 (17). A novel mechanism of transcriptional regulation by 17-β-estradiol and a synthetic estrogen-response modifier, raloxifene, through a proximal polypurine sequence called the raloxifene-response element (RRE) has been described for TGF-β3 (18). This activation, which is independent of the DNA-binding domain of the estrogen receptor and presumably mediated by an adaptor protein, is proposed to contribute to the effects of estrogen on maintenance of bone. Members of the steroid hormone receptor family, including retinoids, vitamin D, and the antiestrogen tamoxifen, also upregulate expression of various TGF-β isoforms by posttranscriptional mechanisms that include stabilization of mRNA transcripts (19).

The nonredundant expression of the three isoforms is supported by studies of mice in which the TGF-β1, TGF-β2, or TGF-β3 genes have been deleted by homologous recombination. TGF-β1 null mice die at about 3 weeks of age from multifocal inflammation and autoimmune disease, with profound dysregulation of hematopoietic homeostasis (20). TGF-β2 null mice have multiple developmental defects of the heart, lungs, skeleton, eyes, and ears that result in perinatal mortality and that are nonoverlapping with those of TGF-β1 or TGF-β3 null mice. In contrast, mice lacking TGF-β3 die perinatally from more limited and consistent features, including delayed pulmonary development and defective palatogenesis resulting from impaired adhesion of the medial edge epithelium of the apposing palatal shelves.

LATENT FORMS OF TRANSFORMING GROWTH FACTOR-β AND THEIR ACTIVATION

Although expression of the TGF-βs and their receptors might at first appear ubiquitous, based on in vitro observations of the ability of most cell lines to both produce and respond to TGF-β, there is now known to be a complex array of mechanisms regulating the bioactivity of TGF-β (for review see 21). TGF-βs 1, 2, and 3 are encoded as 390– to 412–amino acid precursors

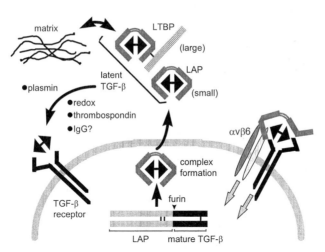

FIG. 15.1. Multiple mechanisms for activation and trafficking of latent forms of transforming growth factor-β *(TGF-β)*. Following intracellular processing, mature TGF-β is secreted from cells in the form of either a small latent complex with its own latency-associated peptide *(LAP)* protein or a large latent complex involving latent TGF-β binding protein *(LTBP)*. The latent forms can associate with matrix and be activated by a variety of mechanisms, ultimately permitting the binding of mature TGF-β to its signaling receptor (21). In the case of activation by binding to the $\alpha_v\beta_6$ integrin receptor, reciprocal activation of integrin signaling has been shown to occur (29).

that are processed proteolytically at conserved tetrabasic sites by furin, a member of the mammalian convertase family of endoproteases. Expression of furin has recently been shown to be upregulated by TGF-β, resulting in increased processing of the TGF-β precursor and possibly representing an important mechanism for dysregulation of the bioavailability of TGF-β in disease pathogenesis (22). TGF-β is unique in the superfamily in that the N-terminal portion of its precursor, called latency-associated peptide (LAP), then associates noncovalently with the processed, biologically active 112–amino acid C-terminal domain (mature TGF-β) to form what is called the small (100 kDa) latent complex, in which the receptor-binding domains of the mature TGF-βs are masked (Fig. 15.1). Mutations in the LAP domain result in intracellular retention of TGF-β, demonstrating a requirement for association of TGF-β with its LAP for secretion from cells (23). Although the LAP proteins for TGF-βs 1, 2, and 3 differ significantly, TGF-β1 LAP confers latency on mature TGF-β2 and TGF-β3 with equal or even enhanced potency when compared to TGF-β1, possibly contributing to cross-regulation of the activity of the different isoforms (24).

Many cells secrete TGF-β in the form of a tertiary large (220 kDa) latent complex in which a large secretory glycoprotein, the latent TGF-β binding protein (LTBP), is covalently bound to LAP (21). Three LTBP genes have been identified thus far and shown to be important both in secretion of TGF-β and in targeting it to extracellular matrix (25). Interestingly, in human platelets, where more than 95% of the total TGF-β1 can be accounted for in the form of the large and small latent complexes, the molecular composition of the latent complex has been shown to determine its fate (26). Upon clotting of blood and degranulation of platelets, the large latent complex is released into the serum, whereas the small latent complex remains associated with the clot and is released slowly upon proteolysis of the clot. The different temporal patterns of bioavailability of these two pools of latent TGF-β in platelets suggest that the particular molecular form of latent TGF-β complexes may be important in control of both its activity and its trafficking. Not only wound and fracture healing but also disease pathogenesis may involve, in part, subtle changes in the composition, and consequently the fate, of such complexes.

Activation of latent TGF-β, studied intensively *in vitro*, is still poorly understood *in vivo*, where mobilization of extracellular matrix stores of TGF-β represents a key epigenetic mechanism for regulating the local concentration of active TGF-β. *In vitro* studies of the mechanisms of activation of the latent complex have been focused on nonenzymatic activation by extremes of pH, heat, or chaotropic agents which disrupt the interaction between LAP and mature TGF-β and on proteolytic mechanisms. The latter have been investigated in detail in activated macrophages cultured *in vitro* and in heterotypic coculture of endothelial cells and smooth muscle cells, where latent TGF-β is activated by a complex process involving binding of the latent form to the mannose-6-phosphate [insulin-like growth factor-II (IGF-II)] receptor and the concerted action of both transglutaminase and the serine protease plasminogen/plasmin (21). Plasmin-dependent activation of latent TGF-β has also been implicated in control of proliferation of vascular smooth muscle cells *in vivo* since activation of TGF-β is inhibited in the aortic wall and serum of mice expressing apolipoprotein(a), a homologue of plasminogen which inhibits its cleavage to plasmin (27). However, in contrast to the purported involvement of plasmin in pathological activation of TGF-β, it would appear to be dispensable in the basal activation of latent TGF-β since there is no detectable dysfunction of TGF-β-dependent processes in mice in which the genes encoding various components of the plasminolytic pathway have been deleted (28). Recently, it has been shown that latent TGF-β can also become activated by binding the $\alpha_v\beta_6$ integrin receptor through an RGD sequence in the TGF-β1 or TGF-β3 LAP protein (29). These data suggest a novel mechanism whereby activation of latent TGF-β could be regulated by controlling cellular expression of this integrin receptor on epithelial cells and further that upregulated expression of $\alpha_v\beta_6$ might contribute to the excessive activation of latent TGF-β in inflammatory disease.

Another mechanism of activation of latent TGF-β involves a putative protease-independent conformational change of the latent complex following its binding to thrombospondin, a component of platelet α-granules and of extracellular matrix. Binding of a unique sequence, RFK, of thrombospondin to the LAP protein is thought to unmask the receptor-binding epitope of latent TGF-β, thereby activating the complex (30). An intrinsic role for this mechanism is supported by the considerable overlap of phenotypes in mice null for TGF-β1 and for thrombospondin-1 (31). Immunoglobulin (Ig) G, implicated in activation of latent TGF-β in autoimmune disease, has also been suggested to act by changing the conformation of the latent complex or, alternatively, by activating TGF-β indirectly following internalization of the IgG/TGF-β complex through Fc receptors (32). TGF-β, bound noncovalently to α-macroglobulin, is also latent, but whether this complex functions as a clearance mechanism or can be activated by certain cells is controversial (33). Ionizing radiation and changes in redox status have also been implicated in activation of latent TGF-β (34,35); the mechanisms involved are not yet known. Nonetheless, the breadth and variety of mechanisms available for masking the activity of TGF-β, for directing secreted TGF-β to matrix stores, and subsequently for activating these latent forms in response to a variety of physiological and pathological stimuli underscore the importance of this posttranscriptional regulation of TGF-β activity.

Recent studies demonstrating the ability of systemic recombinant LAP to neutralize the antiproliferative activity of TGF-β during liver regeneration (24) and of locally secreted decorin to inhibit matrix protein deposition in a model of glomerulonephritis (36) suggest that molecules such as LAP or decorin, which can block the activity of TGF-β, or thrombospondin peptides, which activate TGF-β (30), may ultimately find clinical application in modulation of the bioavailability of TGF-β.

AUTOCRINE, PARACRINE, AND ENDOCRINE MODES OF TRANSFORMING GROWTH FACTOR-β ACTION

TGF-β1 has the ability to stimulate the activity of its own promoter through AP-1 sites, leading to the concept of "autoregulation" and providing the mechanistic basis for prolongation of secretion and autocrine action of TGF-β following an initial stimulus (9). Recent studies in transgenic mice in which TGF-β receptor function has been inactivated in target cells by expression of a dominant negative type II receptor driven by the metallothionein promoter suggest that inactivation of TGF-β signaling pathways, as is characteristic of most malignant cells, may contribute directly to stimulation of paracrine pathways (37). In this transgenic model, increased levels of TGF-β secreted by pancreatic acinar cells expressing the dominant negative receptor and no longer sensitive to TGF-β stimulate responsive stromal tissue elements, resulting in paracrine stimulation of angiogenesis and matrix deposition.

Whereas autocrine and paracrine modes of action are key to processes such as organogenesis and morphogenesis and to repair of injury, it is now appreciated that TGF-β action is not limited to the local environment of the cells that produce it and that endocrine circulation of TGF-β contributes prominently to the pathogenesis of chronic fibrotic and autoimmune diseases and serves as a prognostic marker in several diseases, including carcinogenesis and atherosclerosis. Evidence for a physiological role of circulating TGF-β1 comes from the unexpected observation in TGF-β1 null mice that TGF-β1 protein is transferred both transplacentally and lactationally from heterozygous mothers to their TGF-β1 ($-/-$) progeny (38). The carrier protein(s) involved in this endocrine trafficking of TGF-β1 is not known, although IgG is a likely candidate, as discussed previously.

The presence of physiologically significant levels of TGF-β1 (approximately 5 ng/ml) in plasma of normal human subjects suggests that endocrine trafficking of TGF-β1 may play an important physiological role (39). Since the half-life of active TGF-β is only 2 to 3 minutes, it is likely that plasma TGF-β1 is in the form of the small or large latent complex or possibly bound to a carrier molecule such as thrombospondin, IgG, or α-macroglobulin (40). Although the tissue source of plasma TGF-β1 is unknown, this mode of trafficking is unique to the type 1 isoform; TGF-βs 2 and 3 are restricted to more localized autocrine and paracrine modes of action and are undetectable in plasma.

It is now clear that dysregulation of endocrine trafficking of TGF-β1 may predispose to or be indicative of certain pathologies. Transgenic mice overexpressing TGF-β1 driven by the albumin promoter have elevated plasma levels of TGF-β1 and develop progressive renal dysfunction characterized by fibrosis (41). Similarly, in breast cancer patients, elevated plasma TGF-β1 has been found to be a strong positive predictor for lethal fibrotic sequelae in liver and lung following bone marrow transplantation (42), and in men with prostate disease, it has been shown to be the best marker of invasive prostatic adenocarcinoma (43). In a broader context, the distinct pathologies related to elevated plasma levels of TGF-β suggest that the pool of "excessive" TGF-β1 is likely to be distinct from that of basal levels and that understanding the nature of the different molecular complexes of TGF-β secreted into the circulation, as well as the mechanisms of sequestration and uptake of these complexes by target tissues, will be essential to the design of appropriate therapies.

Deficient levels of plasma TGF-β1 also correlate with disease. Patients having previously been diagnosed with significant stenoses of all three major coronary vessels uniformly showed severe deficiencies in plasma TGF-β1 levels, contrasting with the normal range of plasma TGF-β1 levels in healthy patients free of atherosclerotic lesions (44). Moreover, a polymorphism in the signal peptide of TGF-β1 has been shown to correlate with serum concentrations of TGF-β1 and with susceptibility to osteoporosis, suggesting that it may be one of the genetic determinants in this disease (45).

CELL BIOLOGY OF TRANSFORMING GROWTH FACTOR-β

TGF-β has unique effects on cells, inhibiting the growth of most epithelial, endothelial, and hematopoietic cell lineages and often antagonizing the effects of more classic "growth" factors such as epidermal growth factor (EGF) or platelet-derived growth factor (1). While the molecular basis of this distinctive mode of action is now understood in terms of the unique receptors and signal-transduction pathways (see below), one must be cautious in adopting a reductionist approach and attempting to link a particular end point with a particular extracellular signal. Rather, the multifunctional and pleiotropic activities of TGF-β are best modeled by the concept of switches that can be wired to different cellular functions depending on the cellular context (46).

Since most cells are capable of expressing TGF-β receptors and secreting TGF-β, its cellular activities are extremely diverse. The major cellular end points of TGF-β action could be defined broadly to include effects on chemotaxis and cell growth, differentiation, and function (1,47). TGF-β stimulates the chemotaxis of several cell types, including fibroblasts, macrophages, lymphocytes, and neutrophils. These effects underlie the action of TGF-β in tissue repair as well as in inflammation and fibrosis (48,49). Inhibition of growth by TGF-β is mediated, in part, by direct effects on molecules regulating the cell cycle, including especially retinoblastoma protein (pRb) and the cyclin–cyclin-dependent kinase (cdk) inhibitors p15^{Ink4b}, p21$^{WAF1/Cip1}$, p27^{Kip1}, and p57^{Kip2} (50). The critical role of TGF-β1 in control of homeostasis of epithelia and of bone marrow–derived cell lineages has been underscored by study of TGF-β1 null mice (51). Moreover, the discovery that epithelial and lymphoid cells, which together form the basis of most human cancers, escape from regulation by TGF-β during malignant progression has led to elucidation of the tumor-suppressive activity of TGF-β and to identification of a variety of mechanisms by which tumor cells escape from regulation by TGF-β (52). TGF-β also plays a key role in regulating immune cell function, as illustrated both in escape from immune surveillance by cancer cells secreting excessive levels of TGF-β and in autoimmune disease, where it mediates tolerance and suppresses immune responses to local autoreactivity (51). Recently, it has been shown that TGF-β induces apoptosis of certain cells and that this mechanism may mediate, in part, its regulation of the balance of lineages of bone marrow–derived cells (53), its control of hepatic regeneration (54), and its effects on tissue

regression following hormone ablation in hormone-dependent tissues such as mammary gland and prostate (55).

The most prominent effects of TGF-β on mesenchymal cells involve regulation of target gene activity rather than of growth per se. Key to many of the effects of TGF-β on tissue repair and fibrosis are its multiple actions on regulation of extracellular matrix production by stromal cells (48,56). These involve (a) enhancement of the expression of many matrix proteins, including fibronectin, several collagen isotypes, and the proteoglycans biglycan and decorin; (b) suppression of expression and activity of serine, thiol, and metalloproteinases, including plasminogen activator, collagenase, elastase, and stromelysin; (c) stimulation of expression of inhibitors of metalloproteinases such as plasminogen activator inhibitor-1 (PAI-1) and tissue inhibitor of metalloproteinases (TIMP-1); and (d) regulation of integrin expression and thereby the ability of cells to interact with specific matrix proteins. Combined, these effects contribute to a prominent role of endocrine, paracrine, or autocrine TGF-β in fibrogenesis in many tissues, including liver, lung, and kidney, as demonstrated by the beneficial outcome in terms of accumulation of matrix protein deposition by specific treatments targeted at blocking the activity of TGF-β (57).

TRANSFORMING GROWTH FACTOR-β RECEPTORS

Transmembrane receptors for TGF-β family ligands are distinguished from those of other growth factors and cytokines by their specificity for phosphorylation on serine or threonine rather than on tyrosine residues (for reviews see 58,59). Receptor complexes are heterotetrameric, consisting of two types of receptor, which are distinguished both structurally and functionally. The assembly of the heteromeric complex is initiated by ligand binding to the type II receptor (75 to 85 kDa) and stabilized by interactions between the cytoplasmic domains of the type II and type I (50 to 60 kDa), or signal-transducing, receptor. This model for receptor activation involves activation of the kinase activity of the type I receptor by phosphorylation of several serine and threonine residues in a glycine-serine–rich juxtamembrane domain (GS domain) by the type II receptor kinase. Mutation of a single threonine residue to glutamine (T204D) at the interface between the GS domain and the kinase domain of the TGF-β type I receptor results in its constitutive activation, demonstrating that the activated type I kinase alone is sufficient to transduce downstream signals. Mutationally activated type I receptors are often used in studies of signal transduction by members of the TGF-β family since they eliminate the need for ligand and the type II receptor. Signals from all three isoforms of TGF-β appear to be mediated by a single type II receptor called TβR-II and one type I receptor referred to as either TβR-I or ALK-5 (activin receptor-like kinase). Another type I receptor, ALK-1, expressed on endothelial cells and mutated in the autosomal-dominant disorder hereditary hemorrhagic telangiectasia (HHT), can also complex with ligand-bound TβR-II; but its role in signaling is presently not understood (60).

Two other cell surface binding proteins also participate in TGF-β receptor binding in certain cells (reviewed in 58,59). Betaglycan, formerly called the type III receptor, binds all isoforms of TGF-β but may play a selective role in facilitating interaction of TGF-β2 with TβR-II since this isoform binds to the type II receptor with significantly lower affinity than that of TGF-β1 and TGF-β3. Sharing some homology with Betaglycan is endoglin, which is expressed at its highest levels on endothelial cells and is inactivated in forms of HHT. Unlike Betaglycan, endoglin binds TGF-β1 and TGF-β3 selectively. The specific roles of these two proteins are not fully understood, though it has been suggested that they may constrain the conformation of the TGF-βs in such a way as to enhance binding to TβR-II.

THE SMAD SIGNAL-TRANSDUCTION PATHWAY

Recent studies, based in large part on genetic analyses in *Drosophila* and *Caenorhabditis elegans,* have identified a family of cytoplasmic mediators, termed Smad proteins, which share highly conserved N- and C-terminal domains [called Mad homology 1 and 2 (MH1 and MH2) based on homology to the *Drosophila* Mad protein] connected by highly divergent proline-rich linker regions (for reviews see 58,59,61). These proteins contain no recognizable protein–protein interaction motifs or enzymatic activities. To date, eight different mammalian *Smad* genes have been described, which fall into three distinct functional sets: receptor-activated Smads, which includes Smads 1, 2, 3, 5, and 8; a single common mediator Smad, Smad 4/DPC4; and inhibitory Smads, Smads 6 and 7 (see also Chapter 19).

The present model for downstream signaling via the Smad pathway is that (a) receptor-activated Smads bind to and are phosphorylated on two C-terminal serine residues in their MH2 domain by the type I receptor kinase; (b) the phosphorylated, pathway-specific Smads then heterooligomerize in the cytoplasm with the common mediator, Smad4; and (c) the heteromeric Smad4-containing complex is then translocated to the nucleus, where it mediates transcriptional activation of the target gene. Data suggest that this funneling of multiple signals through a single node can serve to modulate crosstalk between different receptors of the TGF-β family in that the relative strength of each signal can be controlled by competition for a limited pool of Smad4 (62). Inhibitory Smads, induced by TGF-β family ligands, function in a negative feedback loop to terminate or reduce the strength of the signal.

Of the five receptor-activated Smads identified thus far, Smads 2 and 3 have been shown to mediate signals from TGF-β and activin receptors, whereas Smads 1, 5, and 8 mediate signals from bone morphogenetic protein (BMP) receptors (58,59). There are indications, however, that this delineation may not be so strictly defined. Smad1 is phosphorylated by TGF-β treatment of human breast cancer cells with either BMP-2 or TGF-β (63) and the *Smad5* gene has been implicated in inhibition by TGF-β of proliferation of primitive human hematopoietic progenitor cells (64). All of the receptor-activated Smad proteins share a common C-terminal motif, SSXS-COOH, in which the two carboxyl-terminal serine residues are phosphorylated by the activated type I receptor kinase. Mutations in this phosphorylation motif (3S>A) result in dominant negative function, presumably by their stable association with the type I receptor and their subsequent failure to associate with Smad4.

Key roles of these proteins in signaling are clear from the observations that targeted deletion of Smad2 (65,66) or Smad4 (67) results in early embryonic lethality. In contrast, deletion of Smad3 results in a variety of adult phenotypes, including colon carcinogenesis (68) and defects in humoral immunity (69). Smads 2 and 4 have been found to be mutated in certain cancers, and Smad3 can be inactivated by complexing with an oncogene, Evi-1, expressed in certain myeloid malignancies (70,71).

An important development in our understanding of the mechanism of signal transduction by Smad proteins has been the identification of inhibitory Smads or anti-Smads. These proteins, which have as their counterparts the SOCS/SSI proteins of the Jak/Stat signaling pathways (72), are rapidly induced by treatment of cells with TGF-β, suggesting that anti-Smads might function to terminate a ligand-induced signal (73). They are also important targets of signaling crosstalk, as discussed below.

TRANSCRIPTIONAL ACTIVATION OF NUCLEAR TARGET GENES BY SMADS

The nuclear translocation of phosphorylated, receptor-activated Smads is consistent with their proposed direct role in transcriptional activation of target genes. However, unlike the specific cis elements which led to the identification of the Stat transducers of signals from receptor tyrosine kinases (74), the diversity of response elements identified in target genes activated by TGF-β and other superfamily members has proved challenging in terms of understanding the mechanisms of transcriptional activation by Smads. Present models suggest that while Smad proteins can bind DNA directly, they likely also require the cooperation of multiple, diverse, sequence-specific DNA-binding proteins as well

as coactivator molecules such as CRE binding protein (CBP)/p300 to mediate their transcriptional effects (for review, see 61). An excellent example of this is the collagen VII promoter, where an AP-1 binding site is central to a bipartite Smad binding element, resulting in a unique 52-bp minimal TGF-β response element (75). The complexity of such a multifactorial response element adds both to the specificity of the response patterns in particular cell types and to the degree of crosstalk between different pathways which may modulate the levels of activity of the transcription factors or the coactivators themselves.

The MH1 domain of Smad proteins can bind DNA directly. The only exception to this rule is Smad2, in which an inserted 30–amino acid sequence precludes DNA binding. A naturally occurring splice variant has been described in which this region is deleted, restoring DNA-binding activity comparable to that of Smad3 (76). Two DNA-binding sequences have been identified, one a consensus GC-rich binding sequence, GCCCnCGc, found in several Dpp response elements in Drosophila genes (reviewed in 61), and the other a palindromic Smad binding element, GTCTAGAC, defined by a screen with random oligonucleotides (77) and found in the promoters of many TGF-β-responsive genes, including PAI-1, type VII collagen, and JunB.

Ligand-activated Smad1, Smad2, and Smad3, as well as Smad4 have been shown to be capable of binding to the coactivator CBP or its closely related functional homologue p300 (78). The essential nature of this interaction is demonstrated by the fact that disruption of the Smad–CBP/p300 interaction by the adenoviral transforming protein E1A, which binds the coactivators, blocks nearly all Smad-stimulated transcriptional responses in cells (79). MSG1, another nuclear protein that strongly activates transcription without binding to DNA, has been shown to interact with the SAD domain in the middle linker region of Smad4 and to be required for activation of Smad4-dependent transcription in certain cells (80). This protein is also downregulated by both ras and E1A, again suggesting crosstalk between different pathways to modulate the activity of TGF-β signaling.

In summary, it can be said that the inability to define specific consensus TGF-β-responsive elements in target genes results from the diversity of transcription factors that cooperate with Smad signaling protein complexes and the added complexity of the need for an adjacent cooperating Smad DNA-binding site (61).

OTHER SIGNALING PATHWAYS

Activation by TGF-β of classic mitogen-activated protein kinase (MAPK/ERK) pathways (81), stress-activated protein kinase (SAPK/JNK) pathways (82), and TGF-β-activated kinase (TAK-1) pathways (83) has been described in several cell types; and one common target of TGF-β, the fibronectin gene, has recently been shown to be activated by a Smad-independent SAPK/JNK pathway (84). However, the demonstration of a direct interaction between Smad 3/Smad4 and c-Jun and c-Fos, targets of MAPK/SAPK pathways, suggests that the interplay between these pathways in mediating signals from TGF-β receptors will be complex (85).

RECEPTOR CROSSTALK MEDIATED BY SMAD PROTEINS

Not only do Smad proteins transduce direct signals from TGF-β receptors, but they also mediate signaling crosstalk between the receptor serine-threonine kinases of the TGF-β family, receptor tyrosine kinases, and even nuclear hormone receptors (Fig. 15.2). Both inhibitory phosphorylation of the middle linker region of Smad1 at consensus sites for MAPK/ERK kinase (MEK) pathways stimulated by EGF (86) and activating phosphorylation of Smad2 by hepatocyte growth factor–stimulated kinases downstream of MEK-1 (87) and by the SAPK/JNK pathway have been described (88). Inhibitory Smads are also now emerging as major targets of inputs from other pathways. Induction of Smads 6 and 7 by EGF and phorbol myristate acetate (73) or of Smad7 by interferon-γ(89) has been proposed to underlie antagonistic effects of these ligands on TGF-β signaling. In the case of interferon-γ, the transcriptional activation of

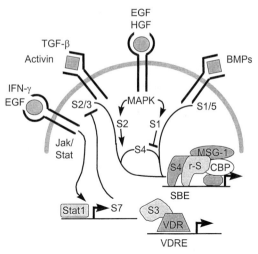

FIG. 15.2. Signaling crosstalk via Smad proteins contributes to the multifunctionality and complexity of transforming growth factor-β *(TGF-β)* responses. Smad *(S)* proteins not only mediate direct signals from receptors of the TGF-β superfamily to gene targets (*SBE,* Smad binding element) but also have been recently shown to integrate inputs from other signaling pathways. These include competition for common coactivators (CBP/p300) possibly regulated by availability of the superactivator MSG-1 (78,80); the inhibitory *(S1)* or stimulatory *(S2)* phosphorylation of Smads by mitogen-activated protein kinase *(MAPK)* pathways downstream of epidermal growth factor *(EGF)* and hepatocyte growth factor *(HGF)* receptors (86–88); enhanced expression of inhibitory Smads (S7) by interferon-γ *(IFN-γ)* via Jak/Stat-dependent pathways (73, 89); and enhancement by Smad3 *(S3)* of vitamin D receptor–dependent transcription (90). *r-S,* receptor-activated Smad.

Smad7 is mediated by the Jak1/Stat1 pathway. Activation of vitamin D–dependent reporter genes by direct 1,25-dihydroxyvitamin D$_3$–dependent interaction of the MH1 domain of Smad3 with the vitamin D receptor has also been reported, but it is unclear at present whether this requires C-terminal phosphorylation of Smad3 (90). These exciting findings suggest that Smad proteins are sensors of signaling inputs from a variety of pathways and that activation of selected gene targets by Smads likely reflects an integrated signal from diverse pathways.

SUMMARY

The general features of the molecular and cellular biology of TGF-β are now fairly well understood, and information concerning specific signaling pathways and mechanisms involved in mediating the effects of TGF-β on target cells is accumulating rapidly. The new frontier will now be to use this information to formulate novel therapeutic strategies for many diseases in which either upregulation or suppression of TGF-β activity might be of advantage.

REFERENCES

1. Roberts AB, Sporn MB. The transforming growth factors-β. In: Sporn MB, Roberts AB, eds. *Handbook of experimental pharmacology, Peptide growth factors and their receptors.* New York: Springer-Verlag, 1990: 419–472.
2. Kingsley DM. The TGF-beta superfamily: new members, new receptors, and new genetic tests of function in different organisms. *Genes Dev* 1994;8:133–146.
3. Robey PG, Young MF, Flanders KC, et al. Osteoblasts synthesize and respond to transforming growth factor-type beta (TGF-beta) *in vitro. J Cell Biol* 1987;105: 457–463.
4. Yin JJ, Selander K, Chirgwin JM, et al. TGF-beta signaling blockade inhibits PTHrP secretion by breast cancer cells and bone metastases development. *J Clin Invest* 1999;103:197–206.
5. Romeo DS, Park K, Roberts AB, et al. An element of the transforming growth factor-beta 1 5'-untranslated region represses translation and specifically binds a cystolic factor. *Mol Endocrinol* 1993;7:759–766.
6. Arrick BA, Lee AL, Grendell RL, et al. Inhibition of translation of transforming growth factor-beta 3 mRNA by its 5' untranslated region. *Mol Cell Biol* 1991;11: 4306–4313.
7. Roberts AB, Sporn MB. Differential expression of the TGF-beta isoforms in embryogenesis suggests specific roles in developing and adult tissues. *Mol Reprod Dev* 1992;32:91–98.
8. Kim Y, Ratziu V, Choi SG, et al. Transcriptional activation of transforming growth factor beta1 and its receptors by the kruppel-like factor Zf9/Core promoter-binding protein and sp1. Potential mechanisms for autocrine fibrogenesis in response to injury. *J Biol Chem* 1998; 273:33750–33758.
9. Kim SJ, Angel P, Lafyatis R, et al. Autoinduction of transforming growth factor beta 1 is mediated by the AP-1 complex. *Mol Cell Biol* 1990;10:1492–1497.
10. Kim SJ, Park K, Rudkin BB, et al. Nerve growth factor induces transcription of transforming growth factor-beta 1 through a specific promoter element in PC12 cells. *J Biol Chem* 1994;269:3739–3744.
11. Thatikunta P, Sawaya BE, Denisova L, et al. Identification of a cellular protein that binds to Tat-responsive element of TGF beta-1 promoter in glial cells. *J Cell Biochem* 1997;67:466–477.

12. Kim SJ, Kehrl JH, Burton J, et al. Transactivation of the transforming growth factor beta 1 (TGF-beta 1) gene by human T lymphotropic virus type 1 tax: a potential mechanism for the increased production of TGF-beta 1 in adult T cell leukemia. *J Exp Med* 1990;172:121–129.
13. Yoo YD, Ueda H, Park K, et al. Regulation of transforming growth factor-beta 1 expression by the hepatitis B virus (HBV) X transactivator. Role in HBV pathogenesis. *J Clin Invest* 1996;97:388–395.
14. Yoo YD, Chiou CJ, Choi KS, et al. The IE2 regulatory protein of human cytomegalovirus induces expression of the human transforming growth factor beta1 gene through an Egr-1 binding site. *J Virol* 1996;70: 7062–7070.
15. Kim SJ, Wagner S, Liu F, et al. Retinoblastoma gene product activates expression of the human TGF-beta 2 gene through transcription factor ATF-2. *Nature* 1992; 358:331–334.
16. Dey BR, Sukhatme VP, Roberts AB, et al. Repression of the transforming growth factor-beta 1 gene by the Wilms' tumor suppressor WT1 gene product. *Mol Endocrinol* 1994;8:595–602.
17. Kingsley-Kallesen M, Johnson L, Scholtz B, et al. Transcriptional regulation of the TGF-beta 2 gene in choriocarcinoma cells and breast carcinoma cells: differential utilization of Cis-regulatory elements. *In Vitro Cell Dev Biol Anim* 1997;33:294–301.
18. Yang NN, Venugopalan M, Hardikar S, et al. Identification of an estrogen response element activated by metabolites of 17beta-estradiol and raloxifene. *Science* 1996; 273:1222–1225.
19. Roberts AB, Sporn MB. Mechanistic interrelationships between two superfamilies: the steroid/retinoid receptors and transforming growth factor-β. *Cancer Surv* 1992;14:205–219.
20. Letterio JJ, Bottinger EP. TGF-beta knockout and dominant-negative receptor transgenic mice. *Miner Electrolyte Metab* 1998;24:161–167.
21. Munger JS, Harpel JG, Gleizes PE, et al. Latent transforming growth factor-beta: structural features and mechanisms of activation. *Kidney Int* 1997;51: 1376–1382.
22. Blanchette F, Day R, Dong W, et al. TGF-beta1 regulates gene expression of its own converting enzyme furin. *J Clin Invest* 1997;99:1974–1983.
23. Lopez AR, Cook J, Deininger PL, et al. Dominant negative mutants of transforming growth factor-beta 1 inhibit the secretion of different transforming growth factor-beta isoforms. *Mol Cell Biol* 1992;12:1674–1679.
24. Bottinger EP, Factor VM, Tsang ML, et al. The recombinant proregion of transforming growth factor beta1 (latency-associated peptide) inhibits active transforming growth factor beta1 in transgenic mice. *Proc Natl Acad Sci USA* 1996;93:5877–5882.
25. Taipale J, Miyazono K, Heldin CH, et al. Latent transforming growth factor-beta 1 associates to fibroblast extracellular matrix via latent TGF-beta binding protein. *J Cell Biol* 1994;124:171–181.
26. Grainger DJ, Mosedale DE, Metcalfe JC, et al. Active and acid-activatable TGF-beta in human sera, platelets and plasma. *Clin Chim Acta* 1995;235:11–31.
27. Grainger DJ, Kemp PR, Liu AC, et al. Activation of transforming growth factor-beta is inhibited in transgenic apolipoprotein(a) mice. *Nature* 1994;370: 460–462.

28. Carmeliet P, Bouche A, De Clercq C, et al. Biological effects of disruption of the tissue-type plasminogen activator, urokinase-type plasminogen activator, and plasminogen activator inhibitor-1 genes in mice. *Ann NY Acad Sci* 1995;748:367–381.

29. Munger JS, Huang X, Kawakatsu H, et al. The integrin alpha v beta 6 binds and activates latent TGF beta 1: a mechanism for regulating pulmonary inflammation and fibrosis. *Cell* 1999;96:319–328.

30. Schultz-Cherry S, Chen H, Mosher DF, et al. Regulation of transforming growth factor-beta activation by discrete sequences of thrombospondin 1. *J Biol Chem* 1995; 270:7304–7310.

31. Crawford SE, Stellmach V, Murphy-Ullrich JE, et al. Thrombospondin-1 is a major activator of TGF-beta1 *in vivo. Cell* 1998;93:1159–1170.

32. Caver TE, O'Sullivan FX, Gold LI, et al. Intracellular demonstration of active TGFbeta1 in B cells and plasma cells of autoimmune mice. IgG-bound TGFbeta1 suppresses neutrophil function and host defense against *Staphylococcus aureus* infection. *J Clin Invest* 1996;98: 2496–2506.

33. Webb DJ, Crookston KP, Figler NL, et al. Differences in the binding of transforming growth factor beta 1 to the acute-phase reactant and constitutively synthesized alpha-macroglobulins of rat. *Biochem J* 1995;312: 579–586.

34. Barcellos-Hoff MH, Derynck R, Tsang ML, et al. Transforming growth factor-beta activation in irradiated murine mammary gland. *J Clin Invest* 1994;93:892–899.

35. Barcellos-Hoff MH, Dix TA. Redox-mediated activation of latent transforming growth factor-beta 1. *Mol Endocrinol* 1996;10:1077–1083.

36. Isaka Y, Brees DK, Ikegaya K, et al. Gene therapy by skeletal muscle expression of decorin prevents fibrotic disease in rat kidney. *Nat Med* 1996;2:418–423.

37. Bottinger EP, Jakubczak JL, Roberts IS, et al. Expression of a dominant-negative mutant TGF-beta type II receptor in transgenic mice reveals essential roles for TGF-beta in regulation of growth and differentiation in the exocrine pancreas. *EMBO J* 1997;16:2621–2633.

38. Letterio JJ, Geiser AG, Kulkarni AB, et al. Maternal rescue of transforming growth factor-beta 1 null mice. *Science* 1994;264:1936–1938.

39. Wakefield LM, Letterio JJ, Chen T, et al. Transforming growth factor-beta1 circulates in normal human plasma and is unchanged in advanced metastatic breast cancer. *Clin Cancer Res* 1995;1:129–136.

40. Wakefield LM, Winokur TS, Hollands RS, et al. Recombinant latent transforming growth factor beta 1 has a longer plasma half-life in rats than active transforming growth factor beta 1, and a different tissue distribution. *J Clin Invest* 1990;86:1976–1984.

41. Kopp JB, Factor VM, Mozes M, et al. Transgenic mice with increased plasma levels of TGF-beta 1 develop progressive renal disease. *Lab Invest* 1996;74: 991–1003.

42. Anscher MS, Peters WP, Reisenbichler H, et al. Transforming growth factor beta as a predictor of liver and lung fibrosis after autologous bone marrow transplantation for advanced breast cancer. *N Engl J Med* 1993; 328:1592–1598.

43. Ivanovic V, Melman A, Davis-Joseph B, et al. Elevated plasma levels of TGF-beta 1 in patients with invasive prostate cancer. *Nat Med* 1995;1:282–284.

44. Grainger DJ, Kemp PR, Metcalfe JC, et al. The serum concentration of active transforming growth factor-beta is severely depressed in advanced atherosclerosis. *Nat Med* 1995;1:74–79.

45. Yamada Y, Miyauchi A, Goto J, et al. Association of a polymorphism of the transforming growth factor-beta1 gene with genetic susceptibility to osteoporosis in postmenopausal Japanese women. *J Bone Miner Res* 1998; 13:1569–1576.

46. Nathan C, Sporn M. Cytokines in context. *J Cell Biol* 1991;113:981–986.

47. Fynan TM, Reiss M. Resistance to inhibition of cell growth by transforming growth factor-beta and its role in oncogenesis. *Crit Rev Oncog* 1993;4:493–540.

48. Roberts AB. Transforming growth factor-*β*: activity and efficacy in animal models of wound healing. *Wound Rep Reg* 1995;3:408–418.

49. McCartney-Francis NL, Wahl SM. Transforming growth factor beta: a matter of life and death. *J Leukoc Biol* 1994;55:401–409.

50. Massagué J, Polyak K. Mammalian antiproliferative signals and their targets. *Curr Opin Genet Dev* 1995;5: 91–96.

51. Letterio JJ, Roberts AB. Regulation of immune responses by TGF-beta. *Annu Rev Immunol* 1998;16: 137–161.

52. Markowitz SD, Roberts AB. Tumor suppressor activity of the TGF-beta pathway in human cancers. *Cytokine Growth Factor Rev* 1996;7:93–102.

53. Buske C, Becker D, Feuring-Buske M, et al. TGF-beta inhibits growth and induces apoptosis in leukemic B cell precursors. *Leukemia* 1997;11:386–392.

54. Takiya S, Tagaya T, Takahashi K, et al. Role of transforming growth factor beta 1 on hepatic regeneration and apoptosis in liver diseases. *J Clin Pathol* 1995;48: 1093–1097.

55. Hsing AY, Kadomatsu K, Bonham MJ, et al. Regulation of apoptosis induced by transforming growth factor-beta1 in nontumorigenic rat prostatic epithelial cell lines. *Cancer Res* 1996;56:5146–5149.

56. Border WA, Noble NA. Transforming growth factor beta in tissue fibrosis. *N Engl J Med* 1994;331: 1286–1292.

57. Border WA, Noble NA. TGF-beta in kidney fibrosis: a target for gene therapy. *Kidney Int* 1997;51:1388–1396.

58. Massagué J. TGF-*β* signal transduction. *Annu Rev Biochem* 1998;67:753–791.

59. Derynck R, Feng XH. TGF-beta receptor signaling. *Biochim Biophys Acta* 1997;1333:F105–F150.

60. Lux A, Attisano L, Marchuk D. Assignment of TGF-*β*1, *β*3, and a third new ligand to the type I receptor ALK-1. *J Biol Chem* 1999;274:9984–9992.

61. Derynck R, Zhang Y, Feng XH. Smads: transcriptional activators of TGF-beta responses. *Cell* 1998;95: 737–740.

62. Candia AF, Watabe T, Hawley SH, et al. Cellular interpretation of multiple TGF-beta signals: intracellular antagonism between activin/BVg1 and BMP-2/4 signaling mediated by Smads. *Development* 1997;124:4467–4480.

63. Liu X, Yue J, Frey RS, et al. Transforming growth factor beta signaling through Smad1 in human breast cancer cells. *Cancer Res* 1998;58:4752–4757.

64. Bruno E, Horrigan SK, Van Den Berg D, et al. The Smad5 gene is involved in the intracellular signaling

pathways that mediate the inhibitory effects of transforming growth factor-beta on human hematopoiesis. *Blood* 1998;91:1917–1923.

65. Waldrip WR, Bikoff EK, Hoodless PA, et al. Smad2 signaling in extraembryonic tissues determines anterior–posterior polarity of the early mouse embryo. *Cell* 1998;92:797–808.

66. Nomura M, Li E. Smad2 role in mesoderm formation, left–right patterning and craniofacial development. *Nature* 1998;393:786–790.

67. Sirard C, de la Pompa JL, Elia A, et al. The tumor suppressor gene Smad4/Dpc4 is required for gastrulation and later for anterior development of the mouse embryo. *Genes Dev* 1998;12:107–119.

68. Zhu Y, Richardson JA, Parada LF, et al. Smad3 mutant mice develop metastatic colorectal cancer. *Cell* 1998; 94:703–714.

69. Yang X, Letterio JJ, Lechleider RJ, et al. Targeted disruption of SMAD3 results in impaired mucosal immunity and diminished T cell responsiveness to TGF-beta. *EMBO J* 1999;18:1280–1291.

70. Kurokawa M, Mitani K, Imai Y, et al. The t(3;21) fusion product, AML1/Evi-1, interacts with smad3 and blocks transforming growth factor-beta-mediated growth inhibition of myeloid cells. *Blood* 1998;92:4003–4012.

71. Kurokawa M, Mitani K, Irie K, et al. The oncoprotein Evi-1 represses TGF-beta signalling by inhibiting Smad3. *Nature* 1998;394:92–96.

72. Hilton DJ, Richardson RT, Alexander WS, et al. Twenty proteins containing a C-terminal SOCS box form five structural classes. *Proc Natl Acad Sci USA* 1998;95: 114–119.

73. Afrakhte M, Moren A, Jossan S, et al. Induction of inhibitory Smad6 and Smad7 mRNA by TGF-beta family members. *Biochem Biophys Res Commun* 1998;249: 505–511.

74. Darnell JE Jr. STATs and gene regulation. *Science* 1997; 277:1630–1635.

75. Vindevoghel L, Lechleider RJ, Kon A, et al. SMAD3/4-dependent transcriptional activation of the human type VII collagen gene (COL7A1) promoter by transforming growth factor beta. *Proc Natl Acad Sci USA* 1998;95: 14769–14774.

76. Yagi K, Goto D, Hamamoto T, et al. Alternatively spliced variant of smad2 lacking exon 3. Comparison with wild-type smad2 and smad3. *J Biol Chem* 1999; 274:703–709.

77. Zawel L, Dai JL, Buckhaults P, et al. Human Smad3 and Smad4 are sequence-specific transcription activators. *Mol Cell* 1998;1:611–617.

78. Feng XH, Zhang Y, Wu RY, et al. The tumor suppressor Smad4/DPC4 and transcriptional adaptor CBP/p300 are coactivators for smad3 in TGF-beta-induced transcriptional activation. *Genes Dev* 1998;12:2153–2163.

79. Topper JN, DiChiara MR, Brown JD, et al. CREB binding protein is a required coactivator for Smad-dependent, transforming growth factor beta transcriptional responses in endothelial cells. *Proc Natl Acad Sci USA* 1998;95:9506–9511.

80. Shioda T, Lechleider RJ, Dunwoodie SL, et al. Transcriptional activating activity of Smad4: roles of SMAD hetero-oligomerization and enhancement by an associating transactivator. *Proc Natl Acad Sci USA* 1998;95: 9785–9790.

81. Hartsough MT, Mulder KM. Transforming growth factor-beta signaling in epithelial cells. *Pharmacol Ther* 1997;75:21–41.

82. Atfi A, Buisine M, Mazars A, et al. Induction of apoptosis by DPC4, a transcriptional factor regulated by transforming growth factor-beta through stress-activated protein kinase/c-Jun N-terminal kinase (SAPK/JNK) signaling pathway. *J Biol Chem* 1997;272: 24731–24734.

83. Yamaguchi K, Shirakabe K, Shibuya H, et al. Identification of a member of the MAPKKK family as a potential mediator of TGF-beta signal transduction. *Science* 1995; 270:2008–2011.

84. Hocevar BA, Brown TL, Howe PH. TGF-beta induces fibronectin synthesis through a c-Jun N-terminal kinase-dependent, Smad4-independent pathway. *EMBO J* 1999;18:1345–1356.

85. Zhang Y, Feng XH, Derynck R. Smad3 and Smad4 co-operate with c-Jun/c-Fos to mediate TGF-beta-induced transcription. *Nature* 1998;394:909–913.

86. Kretzschmar M, Doody J, Massagué J. Opposing BMP and EGF signalling pathways converge on the TGF-beta family mediator Smad1. *Nature* 1997;389:618–622.

87. de Caestecker MP, Parks WT, Frank CJ, et al. Smad2 transduces common signals from receptor serine-threonine and tyrosine kinases. *Genes Dev* 1998;12: 1587–1592.

88. Brown JD, DiChiara MR, Anderson KR, et al. MEKK-1, a component of the stress (stress-activated protein kinase/c-Jun N-terminal kinase) pathway, can selectively activate Smad2-mediated transcriptional activation in endothelial cells. *J Biol Chem* 1999;274: 8797–8805.

89. Ulloa L, Doody J, Massagué J. Inhibition of transforming growth factor-beta/SMAD signalling by the interferon-gamma/STAT pathway. *Nature* 1999;397:710–713.

90. Yanagisawa J, Yanagi Y, Masuhiro Y, et al. Convergence of transforming growth factor-beta and vitamin D signaling pathways on SMAD transcriptional coactivators. *Science* 1999;283:1317–1321.

Skeletal Growth Factors,
edited by Ernesto Canalis.
Lippincott Williams & Wilkins, Philadelphia, © 2000.

16

Transforming Growth Factor-β in Skeletal Development and Maintenance

Tamara N. Alliston and Rik Derynck

Departments of Growth and Development and of Anatomy, Programs in Cell Biology and Developmental Biology, University of California at San Francisco, San Francisco, California 94143

Skeletal development is precisely regulated by a variety of hormones and growth and differentiation factors, including several members of the transforming growth factor-β (TGF-β) superfamily. This group of structurally related, secreted, dimeric polypeptides includes members from species as diverse as *Drosophila* and *Caenorhabditis elegans* to vertebrates. TGF-β-related growth and differentiation factors regulate a large number of developmental processes ranging from pattern formation to tissue differentiation and organ morphogenesis. Studies on skeletal development have been particularly focused on the TGF-β-related bone morphogenetic proteins (BMPs) because of their ability to induce ectopic cartilage and bone formation. In fact, this activity led to their initial identification. TGF-β, the best-characterized member and prototype of the TGF-β superfamily, has also received considerable attention for its role in cartilage and bone development for several reasons. TGF-β was the first identified member of this growth factor family and is readily available. In addition, bone is the major source of TGF-β in vertebrates, and TGF-β has been identified as a cartilage-inducing factor. Furthermore, chondrocytes and osteoblasts both secrete TGF-β and respond to TGF-β with alterations in their differentiation and function. Also, the bone-resorbing activity of osteoclasts is regulated by TGF-β, further emphasizing its possible role in skeletal development and metabolism. In this chapter,

we focus on the role of TGF-β in skeletal development and physiology, both *in vitro* and *in vivo*, without discussing the activities and roles of the other TGF-β-related factors.

TRANSFORMING GROWTH FACTOR-β RELEASE AND ACTIVATION

Among the more than 50 TGF-β superfamily members, three are named TGF-β, TGF-β1, 2 and 3 (1). TGF-β1 was the first member of the superfamily to be identified and characterized. TGF-βs 2 and 3 were subsequently identified as closely related polypeptides, each encoded by a unique gene. Although the three TGF-β species are closely related, their temporal and spatial expression patterns during development are highly distinct. All three TGF-βs are encoded as precursors, which undergo a proteolytic cleavage between the propolypeptide and the mature polypeptide sequences. Fully active TGF-β consists of two disulfide-linked, mature TGF-β polypeptides. This mature form is most often a homodimer, although heterodimers of TGF-β have been detected as well. TGF-β is, however, not secreted in its mature, fully active form but rather as a latent complex with two noncovalently bound propolypeptides and, often, an associated latent TGF-β binding protein (LTBP) (2,3). The LTBP itself can be one of three closely related polypeptides encoded by unique genes. Following secretion, these complexes are often deposited in extracellular matrices, including the bone matrix, through their ability to interact with a select set of proteins. Thus, although high levels of TGF-β are present in bone matrix, it is present in one of two types of latent complex, i.e., with or without LTBP, from which it must be released and activated to exert its functions on osteoblasts and osteoclasts (4,5). The existence of different latent complexes for TGF-βs 1, 2, and 3, possibly with different affinities for each of the three LTBPs, strongly suggests a complex regulation of both deposition and activation of the latent TGF-β. In many cases, the activation of TGF-β complexes may result from proteolysis of the propolypeptides, presumably by proteases such as plasmin (2). On the other hand, latent TGF-β is also efficiently activated in the acidic microenvironment created by osteoclasts (6). Thus, TGF-β, released and activated during the process of bone resorption, can exert its activity on both osteoblasts and osteoclasts.

TRANSFORMING GROWTH FACTOR-β RECEPTOR SIGNALING

Following activation of the latent TGF-β complexes, the mature and active TGF-β dimer interacts with the cell surface TGF-β receptors and induces multiple cell type–dependent responses, such as changes in cell proliferation and differentiation, and gene expression. The functional TGF-β receptor complex is heterotetrameric, consisting of two type II and two type I receptors (7–9). The type II and type I receptors are structurally related transmembrane serine/threonine kinases, which exist as homodimers prior to ligand binding. The heteromeric interactions between the type I and type II receptor dimers are stabilized by the binding of TGF-β, thereby creating a functional heterotetrameric complex. This ligand-induced stabilization then allows the type II receptors to phosphorylate, and consequently activate, the type I receptors, which in turn phosphorylate other specific downstream effectors. Whereas only one type II receptor for TGF-β, i.e., TβRII, has been identified, several type I receptors may have the ability to mediate TGF-β responses. The best-charac-

terized type I receptor, TβRI [or activin receptor-like kinase (ALK-5)], has been shown to induce several TGF-β-specific responses and is generally considered "the" TGF-β type I receptor. However, other type I receptors, TSR-1/ALK-1 and Tsk7L/ActRI/ALK-2, also bind TGF-β under physiological conditions and are likely to mediate specific TGF-β effects, albeit possibly in defined cell types and for defined responses (1).

Although additional mechanisms of TGF-β signal transduction may exist, the only well characterized effectors of TGF-β signaling are the Smads, a family of structurally related intracellular proteins known to activate transcription (7–10). The most conserved regions of the structurally related Smads are the N-terminal segment [the N-, or Mad homology 1 (MH1), domain] and the C-terminal segment (the C-, or MH2, domain). These two domains are separated by the middle third of the protein, the much-less-conserved "linker" segment. Based on structural and functional features, the Smads can be divided into three classes: receptor-activated Smads, common Smads, and inhibitory Smads. Among the nine vertebrate Smads known so far, five are able to transiently interact with type I receptors and are phosphorylated at their C termini. Following their phosphorylation, these receptor-activated Smads dissociate from the receptor to form a heterotrimeric complex with Smad4. Smads 1, 5, and 8 are phosphorylated by BMP type I receptors and mediate BMP signaling, whereas Smads 2 and 3 are phosphorylated by TGF-β and activin receptors and mediate their signaling. Smad3 is most likely the major effector of TGF-β-induced gene expression, although for some genes cooperation with Smad2 may be required. Smad2 is most likely the major effector of activin signaling. Thus, in response to TGF-β, a heterotrimeric complex of Smad3 (and/or Smad2) and Smad4 is formed, while BMP receptor activation results in the activation and heteromerization of Smad1, -5, or -8 with Smad4. The receptor-activated Smad/Smad4 complex then translocates into the nucleus, where it mediates the ligand-induced changes in transcription (7–10).

The mechanism of Smad-induced transcription is conceptually well understood (11). Heteromeric Smad complexes interact with promoter sequences but exert their activities through physical interaction and functional cooperativity with other transcription factors bound to defined promoter sequences. For example, in response to activin, the Smad2/4 complex can induce expression of the goosecoid and Mix.2 genes through physical interaction with the FAST-1 or FAST-2 winged helix transcription factors, which themselves are bound to activin-responsive promoter elements. In a conceptually similar way, the Smad3/4 complex interacts with c-Jun/c-Fos at the activator protein-1 (AP-1) binding site of the collagenase I promoter and cooperatively activates TGF-β-inducible transcription. The Smad2/4 and Smad3/4 complexes are now known to interact and cooperate with a variety of transcription factors. The multiplicity of these interactions may explain the complex cellular responses to the ligands of the TGF-β superfamily (11). Most relevant to osteoblast function is the interaction between Smad3 and the vitamin D_3 receptor, a transcription factor which is activated by vitamin D_3 binding (12). The functional interaction of the vitamin D_3 receptor with the Smad3/4 complex results in cooperative activation of some genes, although this interaction may also explain the inhibitory effect of TGF-β on vitamin D_3–induced expression of other genes or in other cell contexts.

EXPRESSION OF TRANSFORMING GROWTH FACTOR-β AND ITS RECEPTORS DURING SKELETAL DEVELOPMENT

One approach to evaluate the way in which TGF-β and its receptors regulate skeletal development is to assess their expression patterns during development. As a first step in endochondral bone formation, mesenchymal cells form condensations at the sites of future long bone formation and differentiate into chondroblasts. As chondroblasts differentiate into chondrocytes, they deposit the cartilage matrix, thereby forming the cartilaginous anlagen, which provide the pattern for bone formation. The cartilage is surrounded by layers of perichondrial cells, which

compose the perichondrium that is responsible for appositional growth of the structures. The longitudinal growth of long bones occurs through a complicated series of differentiation and proliferation events, which involve chondrocytes, osteoblasts, osteoclasts, and endothelial cells. Following initial replacement of the central portion of the cartilage mold with bone matrix and bone marrow cavity, an epiphyseal growth plate forms, which marks the zone at which the cartilage matrix is degraded and replaced by bone. Osteoblasts deposit the bone matrix, which subsequently becomes mineralized, and as the osteoblasts become surrounded by mineralized matrix, they terminally differentiate into osteocytes. During and following the replacement of the cartilage primordia by bone, the perichondrium is converted into a periosteum, in which the mesenchymal cells differentiate into osteoblasts. In the case of intramembranous bone formation, the mesenchymal cells organize themselves into bone primordia and differentiate into bone matrix–secreting osteoblasts. Thus, in contrast to endochondral bone formation, intramembranous bones are formed without a cartilage precursor.

Several studies have evaluated the expression of the three TGF-β species during skeletal development, primarily focusing on prenatal mouse development. All three TGF-β isoforms are expressed during skeletal development, often in overlapping temporal and spatial patterns, although some discrepancies are apparent between the *in situ* localization of the mRNAs and the immunohistochemical localization of the protein. Whereas all three TGF-β species are expressed at low levels in the mesenchyme, the expression of each is increased during mesenchymal condensation, which gives rise to the perichondrium and periosteum. TGF-β1 mRNA is found at high levels in perichondrial cells and at much lower levels in the center of the cartilage anlagen (13). Although TGF-β2 mRNA is localized in the perichondrium and in chondroblasts, the highest levels are detected in the periosteum and at sites of intramembranous bone formation (14). TGF-β2 mRNA is not detected in proliferating or mature chondrocytes. Finally, TGF-β3 mRNA is highly expressed in the condensing mesenchyme surrounding developing bone structures. Thus, the perichondrium expresses mRNAs for all three TGF-β isoforms, albeit with different intensities and somewhat different patterns (15). Although the TGF-β mRNAs are present at low levels in the central cartilaginous tissue, all three TGF-β proteins have been localized to this region using immunohistochemistry, and high TGF-β3 levels were found in the chondrocytes of the developing ribs and vertebrae (16).

TGF-β has been localized in the growth plate, although again with somewhat different patterns for the different TGF-β species (17–19), as assessed by both immunohistochemistry (17,19, 20) and in situ hybridization (18,19). Whereas TGF-β2 was detected in all zones of the growth plate, TGF-β1 and TGF-β3 levels were highest in the proliferative and hypertrophic zone chondrocytes (19). Furthermore, the coexpression of TGF-β2 and TGF-β3 with collagen type II mRNA in transitional chondrocytes (20) is consistent with the ability of TGF-β to regulate chondrocyte differentiation.

In bone, TGF-βs 1, 2, and 3 are easily detected in bone cells and tissues, including the osteoblasts, the perichondrium, and sites of intramembranous bone formation. Despite discrepancies between relative levels and localization of RNA and protein for each isoform, these data collectively support an important regulatory role for TGF-β in osteoblast function and skeletal development. Specifically, while TGF-β1 and TGF-β3 mRNAs are detected in the periosteum and at sites of intramembranous bone formation (13–15,18), high levels of TGF-β2 mRNA are particularly striking at these locations (14). On the other hand, TGF-β1 protein levels in the periosteum are much higher than TGF-β2 and TGF-β3 levels (16). Nevertheless, these data strongly suggest that osteoblasts and the surrounding bone tissue contain all three TGF-β isoforms in vivo (14,17,18). Finally, osteoclasts also express TGF-β, possibly primarily, TGF-β1 (17,21), suggesting that TGF-β may influence osteoclast activity.

The colocalization of the TGF-β receptors with the TGF-β ligand throughout skeletal development suggests that TGF-β exerts its effects by autocrine or paracrine signaling. Whereas the expression of the type I TGF-β receptor mRNA in the mouse fetus is ubiquitous (22), high levels of the type II TGF-β receptor mRNA are apparent in mesenchyme that gives rise to skeletal elements and in mesenchyme that surrounds the cartilage anlagen (22,23). A role for TGF-β in maturing cartilage is supported by coexpression of the type I and type II receptor mRNAs with the ligands in articular cartilage (24) and in the epiphyseal growth plate (19,25). In articular cartilage, the receptors were coexpressed with the ligands in the proliferative and least mature zones (24), whereas in the growth plate, the receptors were predominantly expressed in the maturing and hypertrophic zones (19,25). TGF-β receptors are also expressed at sites of bone formation. Thus, both TGF-β and the receptors are expressed at sites of intramembranous bone formation and in the periosteum and endosteum of developing endochondral bones, strongly suggesting an autocrine role of TGF-β in preosteoblasts and osteoblasts (19,25). Finally, recent studies have evaluated the expression of different Smads during endochondral ossification of the epiphyseal growth plate. Whereas Smad4 was broadly expressed in all zones of the growth plate, Smad2 was strongly expressed in proliferating chondrocytes and Smad3 was primarily expressed in maturing chondrocytes. Smads 6 and 7, which can inhibit signaling by the TGF-β receptor–activated Smads 2 and 3, were most highly expressed in mature chondrocytes. Thus, the TGF-β-activated Smads and the inhibitory Smads are generally colocalized with TGF-β and TGF-β receptor expression (26).

Little is known about possible alterations in expression of TGF-β and its receptors during chondrocyte or osteoblast maturation in vivo. Some relevant data have been obtained in cell culture experiments, although the changes in expression of TGF-β1 and the type II TGF-β receptor may depend on the cell culture conditions. Nevertheless, changes in patterns of ligand and receptor expression may occur during osteoblastic maturation. For example, retinoic acid–induced differentiation of osteoblasts stimulates expression of TGF-β2 and, to a lesser extent, TGF-β1 (27). In addition, with progressive osteoblastic differentiation, the type II receptor levels decrease, an effect that also can be induced by treatment with BMP-2 (28). Concomitantly, expression of the TGF-β type I receptor increases (28), possibly because of the ability of CBFA1, a key osteogenic differentiation factor, to enhance its expression (29). Accordingly, the relative ratio of type I to type II receptors may increase with progressive osteoblastic differentiation (28). Consistent with this observation, glucocorticoid suppression of osteoblastic differentiation is accompanied by a decrease in type I TGF-β receptor expression (30). In addition, retinoic acid–induced osteoblastic differentiation results in an overall decrease in TGF-β receptors at the cell surface (27).

TRANSFORMING GROWTH FACTOR-β REGULATES CHONDROCYTE DIFFERENTIATION AND CARTILAGE FORMATION

Consistent with its localization in the perichondrium and in differentiating chondrocytes, TGF-β is a potent regulator of chondrocyte differentiation *in vitro* and of cartilage formation *in vivo. In vitro,* mesenchymal cells derived from several sources can be induced by TGF-β to differentiate into chondrocytes. However, some seemingly contradictory results may reflect the complexity of the differentiation process and the interactions of TGF-β with other growth factors.

The ability of TGF-β to induce cartilage formation was first demonstrated by the isolation of TGF-β2 as cartilage-inducing factor (CIF) from demineralized bone extract. CIF was purified based on its ability to induce chondrogenic differentiation of rat muscle cells seeded in agarose gel culture (31). Chondrocyte differentiation was assessed based on morphological changes into rounded cells, resembling cartilage cells, and the synthesis of proteoglycan and the chondrocyte marker collagen II. Sequence analysis showed CIF to be identical to TGF-β2, and purified TGF-β1 was similarly able to induce chondrocyte differentiation (31,32). The chondrogenic effect of TGF-β has also been demonstrated using embryonic chick limb mesenchymal cells. When grown in high-density

micromass cultures, TGF-β induced cartilage matrix and glycosaminoglycan synthesis and collagen II expression. In addition, TGF-β promoted chondrocyte differentiation of these cells in subconfluent cultures, which do not allow spontaneous differentiation (33). Finally, TGF-β can also induce chondrocyte characteristics in established mesenchymal cell lines. For example, the multipotential fibroblast-like cell line C3H10T1/2, when grown in micromass culture, responds to TGF-β with increased production of sulfated proteoglycans and expression of collagen II and cartilage link protein, markers of chondrocyte differentiation. However, these cells do not acquire the characteristic morphology of chondrocytes, suggesting incomplete differentiation (34).

As is the case with many other responses to TGF-β, its ability to induce chondrocyte differentiation depends on the experimental conditions and the presence of other growth factors. For example, chondrocyte differentiation of embryonic chick limb mesenchymal cells depends on the duration and time of TGF-β administration, suggesting that other factors may cooperate with TGF-β and be required for the differentiation response (35). Accordingly, TGF-β and basic fibroblast growth factor (FGF) cooperate in the stimulation of cartilage differentiation of chick limb bud cells. While TGF-β by itself was able to induce chondrocyte differentiation, addition of FGF enhanced this differentiation and induced the formation of cartilaginous nodules (36). Extracellular matrix may also stimulate cartilage formation in response to TGF-β. This is illustrated by the differentiation of cartilage cells grown on Matrigel, which can be inhibited by antibodies to TGF-β1 and stimulated by addition of TGF-β, thus indicating a cooperativity between TGF-β and an extracellular matrix component(s). When these cells were grown on plastic or collagen I, they reverted to a nonchondrocytic phenotype (37). Finally, the importance of culture conditions and differentiation stage is also illustrated by the ability of TGF-β to induce dedifferentiation of chondrocytes into a fibroblastic phenotype, when the cells are grown at low density or in serum-free conditions (38–40).

Although TGF-β stimulates early chondrocytic differentiation, it inhibits the later stages, such as the formation of hypertrophic cartilage in culture. This has been documented in several types of experiments. For example, rabbit growth plate chondrocytes, grown as a pelleted mass, undergo mineralization similarly to hypertrophic chondrocytes, and this process can be inhibited by TGF-β (41). TGF-β also prevents terminal differentiation of rat epiphyseal chondrocytes, grown as three-dimensional pellets, into hypertrophic cartilage cells, yet stabilizes the prehypertrophic chondrocyte phenotype. However, as mentioned, when the cells are subconfluent, the chondrocytic phenotype is stabilized, and the chondrocytes consequently dedifferentiate into fibroblast-like cells (40). The inhibitory effect of TGF-β1 on cartilage maturation is also apparent in defined organ cultures of long bone rudiments. In this system, TGF-β apparently inhibits chondrocyte proliferation, hypertrophic differentiation, and matrix mineralization (42,43). Since TGF-β1 stimulates parathyroid hormone (PTH)–related protein (PTHrP) expression and PTHrP inhibits hypertrophic differentiation and matrix differentiation, TGF-β likely exerts some of its activities on cartilage through induction of PTHrP (43).

The potent ability of TGF-β to regulate chondrogenic differentiation is also apparent *in vivo*. Injection of TGF-β1 or TGF-β2 under the periosteum of the rat femur induces a high level of chondrocyte differentiation and the formation of a cartilaginous mass, presumably as a result of recruitment and mitogenic stimulation of periosteal mesenchymal cells and their subsequent differentiation. Following cessation of the TGF-β injections, cartilage is replaced by bone, thus reiterating the process of endochondral bone formation (44). Although *in vitro* TGF-β1 and TGF-β2 are largely equipotent at inducing chondrocytic differentiation (45), TGF-β2 was considerably more potent than TGF-β1 in these *in vivo* experiments. TGF-β also induces the formation of endochondral bone when applied adjacent to the cartilage in rabbit ear wounds (46) or at the site of a tibial fracture in the rabbit (47) and has even been shown to induce endochondral bone formation at extraskeletal sites in the baboon (48). Consistent with the ability of TGF-

β to induce cartilage formation, antisense oligonucleotides specific for TGF-β3 inhibited the growth of Meckel's cartilage in mandibular explant cultures (49). Taken together, the ability of TGF-β to regulate chondrogenesis *in vitro* and *in vivo* and the localization of TGF-β at sites of cartilage formation strongly suggest a normal physiological role for TGF-β in chondrocyte differentiation and cartilage formation during development.

Finally, TGF-β may also play a role in the pathogenesis of osteoarthritis, a degenerative joint disease characterized by destruction of articular cartilage. Transgenic mice, which express a cytoplasmically truncated type II TGF-β receptor in articular chondrocytes and, consequently, have impaired TGF-β responsiveness in these cells, show pathological characteristics of osteoarthritic joints (50). The articular cartilage of these joints has a reduced proteoglycan content, which is consistent with the ability of TGF-β to induce proteoglycan synthesis. These mice also showed areas of hypertrophic and disorganized cartilage, confirming the ability of TGF-β to inhibit terminal hypertrophic cartilage differentiation and mineralization (50). Consistent with the decreased proteoglycan content of these joints, injection of TGF-β into arthritic mouse joints has been reported to stimulate proteoglycan synthesis and cartilage repair (51). On the other hand, unlike the phenotype of these transgenic mice, osteoarthritic chondrocytes show increased sensitivity to TGF-β when compared to normal joint chondrocytes (52). It thus appears that TGF-β plays a role in the maintenance of normal articular cartilage and that impairment of this signaling pathway results in decreased proteoglycan synthesis and premature hypertrophic cartilage differentiation and mineralization, both characteristics of osteoarthritis.

TRANSFORMING GROWTH FACTOR-β REGULATES OSTEOBLAST DIFFERENTIATION AND FUNCTION

In addition to its role in chondrocyte differentiation and cartilage formation, TGF-β regulates osteoblast differentiation. Both TGF-β1 and TGF-β2 are deposited by osteoblasts into the bone matrix, although TGF-β1 is approximately eightfold more abundant than TGF-β2. Once released from bone matrix and activated, TGF-β has the ability to regulate the differentiation and function of osteoblasts and their progenitors. As with chondrocyte differentiation, the many studies in cell culture again illustrate how the effect of TGF-β depends on the culture conditions and the differentiation stage of the cells.

Little is known about the regulation of TGF-β expression by osteoblasts *in vivo*. The presence of TGF-β1 and TGF-β2 in bone matrix suggests a high-level expression of both isoforms by the matrix-depositing osteoblasts, although osteoclasts could also contribute to the TGF-β1 deposition. Whether or not TGF-β expression is altered with progressive osteoblast differentiation is unknown, although vitamin D$_3$, which stimulates osteoblastic differentiation, enhances TGF-β2 expression by osteoblasts in culture (53). In addition, PTH, which also promotes osteoblast differentiation, and estrogen stimulate TGF-β production (54,55). The regulation of TGF-β1 in cell culture may, however, not be predictive for the *in vivo* context since expression of TGF-β1 may primarily be a response to cell culture on plastic, as is known for other cell types (56).

Consistent with its mitogenic effect on fibroblasts and undifferentiated mesenchymal cells, TGF-β stimulates the proliferation of osteoprogenitors and osteoblast-enriched cell cultures. On the other hand, TGF-β has also been reported to inhibit proliferation of certain bone cell cultures or osteosarcoma cell lines, suggesting that the proliferative response may depend on the differentiation stage of the cells (57). The proliferative effect suggests that a major role of TGF-β *in vivo* may be to expand the osteoprogenitor cell population, thereby increasing the pool of committed osteoblasts. This is supported by *in vivo* data from transgenic mice, which overexpress "activated" TGF-β2 in preosteoblasts and show a strongly increased number of preosteoblasts and an increased density of osteoblasts and osteocytes (58).

TGF-β is also a chemoattractant for osteoblasts and their progenitors and, thus, may recruit these cells to the site of TGF-β activation (59,60). Together with the proliferative effect of TGF-β on osteoprogenitor cells, the chemotactic effect may explain the high number of osteoprogenitor cells at sites of TGF-β injection or at sites of bone repair, where TGF-β is expressed and activated.

The effect of TGF-β on differentiation of preosteoblasts and osteoblasts varies with the culture conditions and differentiation state of the cells. Bone marrow, which forms colonies in culture, responds to TGF-β with increases in alkaline phosphatase, osteonectin, and osteocalcin, indicative of a stimulatory effect of TGF-β on osteoblastic differentiation (61). On the other hand, many reports illustrate an inhibitory effect of TGF-β on osteoblast differentiation. In these studies, treatment of osteoblasts or osteoblast-like cell lines with TGF-β often decreases alkaline phosphatase and osteocalcin expression and cyclic adenosine monophosphate (cAMP) production in response to PTH (39,62–65). In addition, TGF-β alters the cellular response to vitamin D$_3$: for example, it inhibits vitamin D$_3$–induced osteocalcin production, while synergizing with vitamin D$_3$ to increase alkaline phosphatase activity (66). Finally, whereas TGF-β also inhibits nodule formation and mineralization (67), it stimulates the expression of collagen I, osteopontin, and osteonectin, which are major extracellular matrix proteins that compose the bone matrix (39,62,65,68–70).

Collectively, and in spite of some apparent contradictions, the numerous reports on the effects of TGF-β on osteoblasts *in vitro* suggest that one of its major roles in bone is to expand the pool of osteoprogenitors, largely through its ability to induce proliferation and chemotaxis. Importantly, the available data also suggest that TGF-β blocks later stages of differentiation, even though it acts as a potent inducer of extracellular matrix synthesis and bone matrix deposition. Thus, the effect of TGF-β on osteoblast differentiation may be conceptually similar to its effects on chondrocyte differentiation: TGF-β stimulates cell proliferation and early differentiation stages, thus expanding the pool of progenitor cells, yet inhibits the later stages of chondrocyte or osteoblast differentiation.

Several studies have evaluated the effects of

TGF-β on osteoblasts *in vivo*. As mentioned, local injection or application of TGF-β usually induces endochondral bone formation, whereby its primary effect may be to stimulate mesenchymal cell proliferation and chondrocyte differentiation. Consequently, the increased bone formation in these studies may be a consequence of the endochondral bone formation process rather than a direct effect of TGF-β on osteoblasts. A transgenic mouse model in which TGF-β was specifically expressed in preosteoblasts and osteoblasts may provide a more informative system to assess the effect of TGF-β on osteoblasts *in vivo*. Mice expressing "activated" TGF-β2 from the osteocalcin promoter display increased bone deposition and increased bone resorption (58), reflecting the combined effects of TGF-β on both osteoblasts and osteoclasts. They also have dramatically increased numbers of preosteoblasts in both the periosteum and endosteum, indicative of a strong proliferative effect of TGF-β on the progenitor cell population. In addition, and presumably in part as a consequence of the increased progenitor cell pool, the osteoblast and osteocyte numbers and densities are also increased, thus suggesting that TGF-β also enhances the differentiation rate (58,71). Consistent with this observation, overexpression of a dominant negative TGF-β type II receptor results in a decreased number of osteocytes, further supporting the notion that autocrine signaling by TGF-β is a determinant of preosteoblast proliferation and differentiation (72). Mice overexpressing activated TGF-β2 in their osteoblasts also have increased bone matrix deposition. Although this observation is consistent with the ability of TGF-β to induce matrix deposition, this effect also depends, at least in part, on the increased osteoclast activity in this transgenic model. Finally, the bones of these transgenic mice often show an irregular and incomplete calcification of the bone matrix, which may be related to the ability of TGF-β to regulate expression of bone matrix proteins (58). Taken together, both the *in vitro* and *in vivo* observations support the notion that TGF-β is an important regulator of osteoblast differentiation, with a predominant role in the early stages of the osteogenitor pool expansion and differentiation process.

OSTEOCLAST DIFFERENTIATION AND FUNCTION IS REGULATED BY TRANSFORMING GROWTH FACTOR-β

Besides its ability to regulate osteoblast differentiation and function, TGF-β also regulates osteoclast function and, consequently, bone resorption (57). Unlike the mesenchymally derived chondrocytes and osteoblasts, osteoclasts descend from the monocyte phagocyte lineage (73,74). These terminally differentiated, multinucleated giant cells are exquisitely structured to perform the unique function of bone resorption (75). The cell's ruffled border secretes lysosomal enzymes and produces the acidic microenvironment required for bone resorption. As a consequence, the latent TGF-β, which is stored in the bone matrix, is released and exposed to the acidic conditions and proteolytic enzymes secreted by the osteoclast, thus resulting in its activation (6,76). The activated TGF-β can then also communicate with the bone-forming osteoblast, thereby regulating its function and bone matrix deposition. Exposure of osteoblasts to TGF-β stimulates them to produce an array of factors which in turn can regulate osteoclast function. In this manner, TGF-β provides a mechanism to coordinate the bone-forming activities of the osteoblasts with the bone-resorbing activities of the osteoclasts (74,75,77). In part because of the dependence of osteoclast differentiation and function on osteoblasts, the effects of TGF-β on osteoclast differentiation and function are not well understood. Nevertheless, several *in vitro* and *in vivo* findings emphasize the potent ability of TGF-β to regulate osteoclast differentiation, activation, function, and apoptosis.

While some studies reveal a stimulatory effect of TGF-β on osteoclast differentiation and bone resorption, others document inhibitory effects. For example, TGF-β was first reported to stimulate bone resorption of mouse calvaria in culture (78) but was subsequently shown to inhibit resorption of fetal rat long bones in culture at higher concentrations than those used to stimulate calvarial bone resorption (79). In addition, TGF-β treatment of bone marrow cultures has been shown to inhibit proliferation and differentiation of hematopoietic progenitors (80), including those that give rise to osteoclasts (81). These seemingly contradictory reports may be due to a concentration dependence of the TGF-β effect on osteoclast differentiation and bone resorption. Accordingly, vitamin D_3–induced osteoclast differentiation of bone marrow cells shows a biphasic response to TGF-β such that low doses of TGF-β (10 to 100 pg/ml) stimulate osteoclast differentiation and function and high doses (1 to 4 ng/ml) strongly inhibit osteoclast formation (82). Correlated with the ability of low levels of TGF-β to stimulate osteoclast differentiation is the observation that low-dose TGF-β stimulates prostaglandin production in these cultures, presumably by the mesenchymal cells. Thus, prostaglandins induce osteoclast differentiation, and this stimulation was inhibited by a TGF-β antibody in this system. In addition, indomethacin, an inhibitor of prostaglandin production, blocked the osteoclast differentiation–inducing activity of TGF-β (82). Thus, the stimulatory effect of TGF-β at low doses may be due to the induction of prostaglandins by stromal cells, without inhibiting the proliferation and differentiation of hematopoietic precursors (78,82–84). At higher doses, TGF-β may directly inhibit the proliferation and differentiation of the osteoclast progenitors. The presence of osteoblasts or stromal cells and their response to TGF-β is thus also an important determinant for the effect of TGF-β on osteoclast differentiation. In the presence of osteoblasts (but not in the presence of nonosteoblastic cells), TGF-β exposure stimulated osteoclastic resorption, whereas without the cocultured osteoblasts TGF-β did not detectably affect the resorbing activity of osteoclasts (85).

The stimulatory effect of TGF-β on osteoclastic bone resorption may also be due to the ability of TGF-β to induce expression and secretion of macrophage colony-stimulating factor (CSF-I) by stromal mesenchymal cells and osteoblasts (86). CSF-I is essential for osteoclast differentiation (73), as was shown in *op/op* mice, which lack functional osteoclasts and consequently

have an osteopetrotic phenotype (87). These mice have an inactivated CSF-I gene, and their stromal cells and osteoblasts no longer produce CSF-I (86), which would normally activate its cognate receptor on osteoclast precursors and stimulate their differentiation (73). Accordingly, osteoclast differentiation can be rescued by providing exogenous CSF-I or wild-type osteoblasts (88,89). Also in this way TGF-β may exert an indirect stimulatory effect on osteoclast differentiation. Consistent with a stimulatory role of osteoblasts on osteoclast function, transgenic mice in which the osteoblasts have an impaired responsiveness to TGF-β also exhibit an osteopetrotic phenotype (72).

The recent identification of a novel transmembrane cytokine and its receptor, as well as a secreted decoy receptor, has provided further insight into the mechanism of cellular crosstalk between osteoblasts and osteoclasts and its regulation by TGF-β (90,91). This cytokine, which has been named osteoprotegerin ligand (OPGL), receptor activation of NFκB ligand (RANKL), and osteoclast differentiation factor (ODF), is a member of the tumor necrosis factor (TNF) family of transmembrane ligands and induces osteoclast differentiation and activity (92,93). Expressed by osteoblasts and mesenchymal cells, OPGL binds to and activates the OPGL receptor, named RANK, which is expressed on osteoclast progenitors and osteoclasts (91). Thus, activation of the OPGL receptor by OPGL through cell–cell contact may explain the differentiation-inducing effect of this coculture. The activity of OPGL on osteoclast progenitors is further regulated by osteoprotegerin (OPG) or osteoclast-inhibitory factor (OCIF) (92,94). OPG is a soluble receptor, related to the TNF receptor, which also binds OPGL and in this way acts as a decoy receptor and prevents the interaction of OPGL with its signaling receptor on osteoclast progenitors. Like OPGL, OPG is produced by stromal cells and osteoblasts, thereby providing this cell type with an additional means to profoundly regulate osteoclast differentiation. Thus, stromal cells express OPGL as a stimulator of osteoclast differentiation on their cell surface and secrete OPG as an inhibitor of OPGL-induced osteoclast differentiation.

Recent studies have revealed a connection between the OPGL signaling system and the ability of TGF-β to inhibit osteoclast differentiation. TGF-β was shown to induce the expression and secretion of OPG in osteoblast and bone marrow stromal cell lines (95,96), whereas other agents that stimulate bone resorption, such as 1,25 (OH)$_2$vitamin D$_3$, prostaglandin E$_2$ (PGE$_2$), interleukin-1α (IL-1α), and PTH, reduced the levels of OPG mRNA (96). Furthermore, OPGL expression was inhibited by TGF-β (95). Therefore, the TGF-β-induced stimulation of OPG production and inhibition of OPGL expression may explain the inhibitory effect of TGF-β on osteoclast differentiation and function. Accordingly, antibodies against OPG decreased the inhibition of bone resorption by TGF-β (95,96). Finally, because OPGL may act as an osteoclast survival factor (91), the TGF-β-regulated decrease of OPGL and the concomitant increase of OPG may result in increased osteoclast apoptosis.

A potential role of TGF-β in osteoclast apoptosis has been most extensively studied within the context of osteoporosis. In postmenopausal osteoporosis, the decreased levels of ovarian steroids lead to bone loss (97). Several studies have implicated TGF-β in this process. First, at the cellular level, estrogen stimulates the expression of TGF-β2 by osteoblasts (54,98,99). In addition, while both TGF-β and estrogen induce osteoclast apoptosis, estrogen-induced apoptosis is blocked by an anti-TGF-β antibody (100). These findings at the cellular level together with in vivo data that are discussed in the next section suggest that TGF-β may play a role in the estrogen-mediated inhibition of bone resorption.

Although the observations summarized above emphasize the important role of TGF-β in osteoclast differentiation and function, additional studies are required to more fully characterize its direct effect on osteoclasts and its indirect effects mediated by bone marrow stromal cells and osteoblasts.

ROLE OF TRANSFORMING GROWTH FACTOR-β IN BONE REPAIR AND MAINTENANCE

The effects of TGF-β on the differentiation and function of chondrocytes, osteoblasts, and osteoclasts suggest that, in vivo, TGF-β functions as an important regulator of bone repair and maintenance. Several types of in vivo study have allowed characterization of the role of TGF-β. Some of these evaluated the consequences of local or systemic administration of TGF-β (44,83,101,102), whereas in other studies mice were genetically manipulated to overexpress TGF-β or to alter TGF-β signaling (50,58,71,72). In addition mice which lack expression of one of the three TGF-β species were generated through targeted gene inactivation, and the consequent changes in bone formation and remodeling were studied (103,104).

The anabolic effects of TGF-β on bone formation in vivo were first demonstrated by injecting TGF-β1 or TGF-β2 under the periosteum of rat calvariae (83,101) or long bones (44). These injections stimulated intramembranous bone formation from the periosteum and increased bone thickness (83,101) or caused the formation of a cartilaginous mass that was replaced by bone through endochondral ossification (44). In addition, short-term systemic administration of TGF-β2 increased the rate of bone formation and mineral apposition (102), further supporting the anabolic role of TGF-β in bone. These and other studies illustrate the stimulatory effect of TGF-β on the events that are normally associated with endochondral or intramembranous bone development (46,48,105). Thus, TGF-β injection near bones made by intramembranous bone formation, such as calvariae, stimulated mesenchymal cell differentiation into osteoblasts, which then deposit bone (83). At these sites, TGF-β presumably promotes bone growth by amplifying the pool of osteoprogenitors, thereby increasing the number of differentiating osteoblasts and bone deposition (106). The increased thickness of long bones, observed as a result of systemic TGF-β administration, also occurs through a direct stimulation of the proliferation and differentiation of periosteal osteoprogenitors and subsequent appositional bone matrix deposition (102). On the other hand, injection of TGF-β into areas that are derived from endochondral bone formation induces the events characteristics of endochondral bone formation. At these sites, injected TGF-β induces chondroprogenitor and osteoprogenitor proliferation, and chondrocytic differentiation and the cartilage matrix is eventually replaced by bone (44). Thus, in the context of endochondral bone formation, the TGF-β-induced bone formation may, in part, be a direct consequence of its primary effect on cartilage formation. Importantly, TGF-β is not a potent inducer of exogenous cartilage or bone formation, as are BMPs 2 and 4 (57). This may be due to the inability of TGF-β to convert myogenic satellite cells into chondrocytes or osteoblasts and the need for a chondrogenic or osteogenic environment.

The observed effects of local TGF-β application also provide insight into the role of endogenous TGF-β in bone repair. At sites of bone fractures, the expression of TGF-β, i.e., primarily TGF-β1, is upregulated, and latent TGF-β is activated (107). The release of TGF-β by platelets at the fracture site provides an additional source of TGF-β (108). During the repair process of long bones, a cartilaginous callus is formed, which, through endochondral ossification, is converted into bone. This bone callus is then remodeled to return the mended bone to its original shape (108). Consistent with the effects of experimental injection of TGF-β into the periosteum (44), TGF-β accelerates and/or enhances bone repair (46,109). Therefore, increased levels of active endogenous TGF-β at the site of bone repair may be important for the bone fracture–healing process. The role of endogenous and exogenous TGF-β in bone repair is also consistent with its role in soft-tissue wound repair (110).

Mice in which one of the three TGF-β genes is inactivated through gene targeting have also provided information about the role of TGF-β in bone formation. Inactivation of the TGF-β1 gene results in a prenatally lethal vasculogenesis defect for approximately half of the offspring and, for the mice that are born alive, a severe multifocal inflammation which results in lethality after 2 to 3 weeks (111,112). The nature of this phenotype severely limits investigation since any observed abnormalities could be due to consequences of the massive inflammatory phenotype. Nevertheless, analyses of young mice and immunosuppression of the inflammatory phenotype with rapamycin in adult mice have allowed characterization of the bone phe-

notype in TGF-β1-deficient mice (103). These mice exhibited defective bone elasticity, reduced bone mineral content, and a smaller growth plate and bone size (103). These observations collectively suggest a role for TGF-β1 in maintaining the mineral and matrix quality of bone and in regulating growth plate and bone size. TGF-β2-deficient mice exhibit a large number of malformations, including defects in palate closure and lung development which result in perinatal death. For this reason, a thorough analysis of the bone phenotype has not been possible. Nonetheless, malformations in the craniofacial, appendicular, and axial skeletons are apparent in the TGF-β2-deficient mice, with the most prominent defects observed in the cranial bones, the mandible, the ribs, and the tuberosities of long bones (104). This phenotype reflects a critical role for TGF-β2 in the developmental patterning of bone. TGF-β3-deficient mice also die perinatally because of defects in palatogenesis and lung development. Histologically, the TGF-β3-deficient mouse phenotype suggests an essential role for TGF-β3 in epithelial–mesenchymal interactions (113,114). These mice display no skeletal abnormalities. Collectively, these phenotypes suggest an important role for TGF-β1 and TGF-β2 in bone formation and maintenance. Because of the severity and lethality of the phenotypes, no evaluation of the phenotype in the absence of both TGF-β1 and TGF-β2 has been possible.

Another way to characterize the function of TGF-β is to overexpress a cytoplasmically truncated TGF-β receptor, which interferes in a dominant negative way with the endogenous signaling by all three TGF-β species. Thus, transgenic mice that overexpress a dominant negative type II TGF-β receptor show impaired TGF-β responsiveness in the cartilage of joints and consequently develop an osteoarthritic phenotype (50). The importance of this finding for the characterization of the effect of TGF-β on cartilage differentiation and maintenance has been discussed above. To specifically evaluate the role of TGF-β signaling in (pre)osteoblasts, transgenic mice were generated which express the same dominant negative version of the type II TGF-β receptor from the osteocalcin promoter, thus resulting in impaired TGF-β responsiveness of the osteoblasts. These mice had increased levels of trabecular bone, despite the fact that they had a reduced osteocyte density in the femoral epiphysis and no change in the mineral apposition rate (72). Although the osteoclast numbers did not differ between the long bones of the wild-type and transgenic mice, a decreased level of osteoclastic activity and decreased osteoclast numbers were apparent in calvarial bones. Analysis of this phenotype suggested that the increased trabeculation in these mice resulted from reduced osteoclast activity and decreased bone resorption. In addition, the decreased osteocyte density is consistent with the stimulatory effect of TGF-β on the proliferation and differentiation of the osteoblastic progenitors. The impaired osteoblastic responsiveness to TGF-β also resulted in altered mechanical qualities of the transgenic bones. The transgenic bones were tougher and the increased trabecular volume resulted in greater bone strength (72).

In complementary experiments, transgenic mice were generated with increased expression of activated TGF-β2 in osteoblasts. These TGF-β2-overexpressing mice exhibited a severe, progressive osteoporotic phenotype, due to an imbalance between increased bone resorption and increased bone deposition (58). They also showed a strongly increased number of osteoprogenitor cells and an increased osteocyte density. Comparative analyses of these mice with those that overexpress the dominant negative TGF-β receptors and of crosses between these two transgenic mouse strains revealed that autocrine production of TGF-β and osteoblast responsiveness to TGF-β are required for direct stimulation of osteoblastic differentiation and osteocyte density (71). In contrast, the increased mineral apposition rate and increase in bone turnover when TGF-β2 is overexpressed by osteoblasts are indirect consequences of the stimulatory effect of TGF-β2 on osteoclastic bone resorption (71). Accordingly, alendronate, a compound which blocks osteoclast activity, decreased the elevated mineral apposition rate in bones of transgenic mice with increased osteoblastic expression of TGF-β2 (71).

These transgenic studies together with the bone phenotype of TGF-β1-deficient mice reveal a key role for TGF-β in bone metabolism. TGF-β secreted by osteoblasts and deposited in bone is a direct regulator not only of osteoblast differentiation and function but also of osteoclast activity. The latter activity is in part dictated by the osteoblastic response to TGF-β, suggesting that TGF-β mediates the functional crosstalk between both cell types and could function as a "coupling factor." Considering the importance of the required balance between bone resorption and bone deposition, TGF-β may play a key role in the control of bone remodeling. Slight changes in the levels of active TGF-β or in the osteoblastic responsiveness to TGF-β may thus upset this balance and result in severe phenotypic consequences that affect the mechanical properties of the bones and can manifest themselves as an osteoporotic or osteopetrotic phenotype (58,72).

The extent to which TGF-β plays a role in metabolic bone disease in humans is as yet unclear. Some informative correlations have been made, although their significance for human disease remains to be demonstrated. First, *in vitro,* TGF-β expression in osteoblasts is induced by estrogen, suggesting that TGF-β may participate in the osteoprotective effect of ovarian steroids (54,98,99). TGF-β has also been implicated as a mediator of the apoptotic effects of estrogen on osteoclasts (100), perhaps by its induction of OPG and inhibition of OPGL expression (95,96). Furthermore, injection of TGF-β into the marrow cavity of long bones decreased ovariectomy-induced osteoclastic resorption (115). Accordingly, several studies report a decrease of TGF-β in the bone matrix of ovariectomized rats or in postmenopausal women (99,116–118). In many of these studies, the loss of TGF-β correlated with decreased bone mass (99,115,117), and administration of estrogen resulted in an increase of both bone mass and TGF-β levels (99). Interestingly, a polymorphism in the TGF-β1 gene in a group of Japanese women has been correlated with increased resistance to osteoporosis (119). This polymorphism correlated with elevated levels of TGF-β in bone and serum and a reduced number of bone fractures (119). It is important to note, however, that another study reported elevated TGF-β1 levels in the iliac crest of postmenopausal women, relative to premenopausal women or postmenopausal women who used hormone-replacement therapy (120). The increased TGF-β1 levels correlated with increased bone remodeling and increased osteoblast and osteoclast densities but not with a change in overall bone mass. While these observations collectively suggest a role for TGF-β in osteoporosis, further research is clearly required to characterize the relationship between TGF-β and osteoporosis.

In summary, TGF-β has clearly been shown to regulate chondrocyte, osteoblast, and osteoclast differentiation and function both *in vitro* and *in vivo*. Some of the findings may appear confusing and contradictory, largely because of the use of different model systems and the difficulties associated with investigation of these cell types *in vitro*. Nevertheless, the available results have characterized some important functions of TGF-β on these cell types. While the importance of TGF-β in cartilage and bone development and maintenance *in vivo* has been convincingly illustrated, extensive further characterization will be required before we will fully comprehend its role *in vivo*. Only then will we begin to understand how deregulation of TGF-β expression, activation, or responsiveness contributes to metabolic bone disease in humans.

ACKNOWLEDGMENTS

The authors thank Ernesto Canalis for his patience and support throughout the writing of this chapter. Work in the laboratory of the authors was supported by a postdoctoral fellowship from the Arthritis Foundation to T.N.A. and by National Institutes of Health grants CA63101, AR41126, and DE-10306 and a grant from the Arthritis Foundation to R.D.

REFERENCES

1. Derynck R, Choy L. *Transforming growth factor-β and its receptors*. In: Thomsen A, ed. The cytokine handbook. 3rd ed, San Diego: Academic Press, 1998: 593–636.
2. Munger JS, Harpel JG, Gleizes PE, et al. Latent transforming growth factor-β: structural features and mechanisms of activation. *Kidney Int* 1997;51:1376–1382.
3. Taipale J, Saharinen J, Keski-Oja J. Extracellular matrix-associated transforming growth factor-β: role in cancer cell growth and invasion. *Adv Cancer Res* 1998; 75:87–134.
4. Bonewald LF, Dallas SL. Role of active and latent transforming growth factor β in bone formation. *J Cell Biochem* 1994;55:350–357.
5. Bonewald LF. Regulation and regulatory activities of transforming growth factor β. *Crit Rev Eukaryot Gene Expr* 1999;9:33–44.
6. Oursler MJ. Osteoclast synthesis and secretion and activation of latent transforming growth factor β. *J Bone Miner Res* 1994;9:443–452.
7. Massagué J. TGF-β signal transduction. *Annu Rev Biochem* 1998;67:753–791.
8. Derynck R, Feng XH. TGF-β receptor signaling. *Biochim Biophys Acta* 1997;1333:F105–F150.
9. Heldin CH, Miyazono K, ten Dijke P. TGF-β signalling from cell membrane to nucleus through SMAD proteins. *Nature* 1997;390:465–471.
10. Whitman M. Smads and early developmental signaling by the TGFβ superfamily. *Genes Dev* 1998;12: 2445–2462.
11. Derynck R, Zhang Y, Feng XH. Smads: transcriptional activators of TGF-β responses. *Cell* 1998;95:737–740.
12. Yanagisawa J, Yanagi Y, Masuhiro Y, et al. Convergence of transforming growth factor-β and vitamin D signaling pathways on SMAD transcriptional coactivators. *Science* 1999;283:1317–1321.
13. Lehnert SA, Akhurst RJ. Embryonic expression pattern of TGF β type-1 RNA suggests both paracrine and autocrine mechanisms of action. *Development* 1988; 104:263–273.
14. Pelton RW, Nomura S, Moses HL, et al. Expression of transforming growth factor β2 RNA during murine embryogenesis. *Development* 1989;106:759–767.
15. Pelton RW, Dickinson ME, Moses HL, et al. *In situ* hybridization analysis of TGF β3 RNA expression during mouse development: comparative studies with TGF β1 and β2. *Development* 1990;110:609–620.
16. Pelton RW, Saxena B, Jones M, et al. Immunohistochemical localization of TGF β1, TGF β2, and TGF β3 in the mouse embryo: expression patterns suggest multiple roles during embryonic development. *J Cell Biol* 1991;115:1091–1105.
17. Sandberg M, Vuorio T, Hirvonen H, et al. Enhanced expression of TGF-β and c-fos mRNAs in the growth plates of developing human long bones. *Development* 1988;102:461–470.
18. Millan FA, Denhez F, Kondaiah P, et al. Embryonic gene expression patterns of TGF β1, β2 and β3 suggest different developmental functions *in vivo*. *Development* 1991;111:131–143.
19. Horner A, Kemp P, Summers C, et al. Expression and distribution of transforming growth factor-β isoforms and their signaling receptors in growing human bone. *Bone* 1998;23:95–102.
20. Thorp BH, Anderson I, Jakowlew SB. Transforming growth factor-β1, -β2 and -β3 in cartilage and bone cells during endochondral ossification in the chick. *Development* 1992;114:907–911.
21. Sandberg M, Autio-Harmainen H, Vuorio E. Localization of the expression of types I, III, and IV collagen,

TGF-β1 and c-fos genes in developing human calvarial bones. *Dev Biol* 1988;130:324–334.

22. Iseki S, Osumi-Yamashita N, Miyazono K, et al. Localization of transforming growth factor-β type I and type II receptors in mouse development. *Exp Cell Res* 1995; 219:339–347.

23. Lawler S, Candia AF, Ebner R, et al. The murine type II TGF-β receptor has a coincident embryonic expression and binding preference for TGF-β1. *Development* 1994;120:165–175.

24. Fukumura K, Matsunaga S, Yamamoto T, et al. Immunolocalization of transforming growth factor-βs and type I and type II receptors in rat articular cartilage. *Anticancer Res* 1998;18:4189–4193.

25. Kabasawa Y, Ejiri S, Matsuki Y, et al. Immunoreactive localization of transforming growth factor-β type II receptor-positive cells in rat tibiae. *Bone* 1998;22: 93–98.

26. Sakou T, Onishi T, Yamamoto T, et al. Localization of Smads, the TGF-β family intracellular signaling components during endochondral ossification. *J Bone Miner Res* 1999;14:1145–1152.

27. Gazit D, Ebner R, Kahn AJ, et al. Modulation of expression and cell surface binding of members of the transforming growth factor-β superfamily during retinoic acid-induced osteoblastic differentiation of multipotential mesenchymal cells. *Mol Endocrinol* 1993;7: 189–198.

28. Centrella M, Casinghino S, Kim J, et al. Independent changes in type I and type II receptors for transforming growth factor β induced by bone morphogenetic protein 2 parallel expression of the osteoblast phenotype. *Mol Cell Biol* 1995;15:3273–3281.

29. Ji C, Casinghino S, Chang DJ, et al. CBFA (AML/PEBP2)-related elements in the TGF-β type I receptor promoter and expression with osteoblast differentiation. *J Cell Biochem* 1998;69:353–363.

30. Chang DJ, Ji C, Kim KK, et al. Reduction in transforming growth factor β receptor I expression and transcription factor CBFA1 on bone cells by glucocorticoid. *J Biol Chem* 1998;273:4892–4896.

31. Seyedin SM, Thomas TC, Thompson AY, et al. Purification and characterization of two cartilage-inducing factors from bovine demineralized bone. *Proc Natl Acad Sci USA* 1985;82:2267–2271.

32. Seyedin SM, Segarini PR, Rosen DM, et al. Cartilage-inducing factor-β is a unique protein structurally and functionally related to transforming growth factor-β. *J Biol Chem* 1987;262:1946–1949.

33. Kulyk WM, Rodgers BJ, Greer K, et al. Promotion of embryonic chick limb cartilage differentiation by transforming growth factor-β. *Dev Biol* 1989;135: 424–430.

34. Denker AE, Nicol SB, Tuan RS. Formation of cartilage-like spheroids by micromass cultures of murine C3H10T1/2 cells upon treatment with transforming growth factor-β1. *Differentiation* 1995;59:25–34.

35. Carrington JL, Reddi AH. Temporal changes in the response of chick limb bud mesodermal cells to transforming growth factor β type 1. *Exp Cell Res* 1990; 186:368–373.

36. Schofield JN, Wolpert L. Effect of TGF-β1, TGF-β2, and bFGF on chick cartilage and muscle cell differentiation. *Exp Cell Res* 1990;191:144–148.

37. Basic N, Basic V, Bulic K, et al. TGF-β and basement

membrane Matrigel stimulate the chondrogenic phenotype in osteoblastic cells derived from fetal rat calvaria. *J Bone Miner Res* 1996;11:384–391.

38. Tschan T, Bohme K, Conscience-Egli M, et al. Autocrine or paracrine transforming growth factor-β modulates the phenotype of chick embryo sternal chondrocytes in serum-free agarose culture. *J Biol Chem* 1993; 268:5156–5161.

39. Rosen DM, Stempien SA, Thompson AY, et al. Transforming growth factor-β modulates the expression of osteoblast and chondroblast phenotypes *in vitro*. *J Cell Physiol* 1988;134:337–346.

40. Ballock RT, Heydemann A, Wakefield LM, et al. TGF-β1 prevents hypertrophy of epiphyseal chondrocytes: regulation of gene expression for cartilage matrix proteins and metalloproteases. *Dev Biol* 1993;158: 414–429.

41. Kato Y, Iwamoto M, Koike T, et al. Terminal differentiation and calcification in rabbit chondrocyte cultures grown in centrifuge tubes: regulation by transforming growth factor β and serum factors. *Proc Natl Acad Sci USA* 1988;85:9552–9556.

42. Dieudonné SC, Semeins CM, Goei SW, et al. Opposite effects of osteogenic protein and transforming growth factor β on chondrogenesis in cultured long bone rudiments. *J Bone Miner Res* 1994;9:771–780.

43. Serra R, Karaplis A, Sohn P. Parathyroid hormone–related peptide (PTHrP)–dependent and–independent effects of transforming growth factor β (TGF-β) on endochondral bone formation. *J Cell Biol* 1999;145: 783–794.

44. Joyce ME, Roberts AB, Sporn MB, et al. Transforming growth factor-β and the initiation of chondrogenesis and osteogenesis in the rat femur. *J Cell Biol* 1990; 110:2195–2207.

45. Chimal-Monroy J, Diaz de Leon L. Differential effects of transforming growth factors β1, β2, β3 and β5 on chondrogenesis in mouse limb bud mesenchymal cells. *Int J Dev Biol* 1997;41:91–102.

46. Beck LS, DeGuzman L, Lee WP, et al. TGF-β1 induces bone closure of skull defects. *J Bone Miner Res* 1991;6:1257–1265.

47. Critchlow MA, Bland YS, Ashurst DE. The effect of exogenous transforming growth factor-β2 on healing fractures in the rabbit. *Bone* 1995;16:521–527.

48. Ripamonti U, Duneas N, Van Den Heeven B, et al. Recombinant transforming growth factor-β1 induces endochondral bone in the baboon and synergizes with recombinant osteogenic protein-1 (bone morphogenetic protein-7) to initiate rapid bone formation. *J Bone Miner Res* 1997;12:1584–1595.

49. Chai Y, Mah A, Crohin C, et al. Specific transforming growth factor-β subtypes regulate embryonic mouse Meckel's cartilage and tooth development. *Dev Biol* 1994;162:85–103.

50. Serra R, Johnson M, Filvaroff EH, et al. Expression of a truncated, kinase-defective TGF-β type II receptor in mouse skeletal tissue promotes terminal chondrocyte differentiation and osteoarthritis. *J Cell Biol* 1997; 139:541–552.

51. Glansbeek HL, van Beuningen HM, Vitters EL, et al. Stimulation of articular cartilage repair in established arthritis by local administration of transforming growth factor-β into murine knee joints. *Lab Invest* 1998;78: 133–142.

52. Lafeber FP, van Roy HL, van der Kraan PM, et al. Transforming growth factor-β predominantly stimulates phenotypically changed chondrocytes in osteoarthritic human cartilage. *J Rheumatol* 1997;24:536–542.

53. Wu Y, Craig TA, Lutz WH, et al. Identification of 1β,25-dihydroxyvitamin D3 response elements in the human transforming growth factor β2 gene. *Biochemistry* 1999;38:2654–2660.

54. Oursler MJ, Cortese C, Keeting P, et al. Modulation of transforming growth factor-β production in normal human osteoblast-like cells by 17β-estradiol and parathyroid hormone. *Endocrinology* 1991;129:3313–3320.

55. Oursler MJ, Riggs BL, Spelsberg TC. Glucocorticoid-induced activation of latent transforming growth factor-β by normal human osteoblast-like cells. *Endocrinology* 1993;133:2187–2196.

56. Streuli CH, Schmidhauser C, Kobrin M, et al. Extracellular matrix regulates expression of the TGF-β1 gene. *J Cell Biol* 1993;120:253–260.

57. Centrella M, Horowitz MC, Wozney JM, et al. Transforming growth factor-β gene family members and bone. *Endocr Rev* 1994;15:27–39.

58. Erlebacher A, Derynck R. Increased expression of TGF-β2 in osteoblasts results in an osteoporosis-like phenotype. *J Cell Biol* 1996;132:195–210.

59. Hughes FJ, Aubin JE, Heersche JN. Differential chemotactic responses of different populations of fetal rat calvaria cells to platelet-derived growth factor and transforming growth factor β. *Bone Miner* 1992;19:63–74.

60. Pfeilschifter J, Wolf O, Naumann A, et al. Chemotactic response of osteoblastlike cells to transforming growth factor β. *J Bone Miner Res* 1990;5:825–830.

61. Long MW, Robinson JA, Ashcraft EA, et al. Regulation of human bone marrow–derived osteoprogenitor cells by osteogenic growth factors [erratum in *J Clin Invest* 1995;96:2541]. *J Clin Invest* 1995;95:881–887.

62. Centrella M, McCarthy TL, Canalis E. Transforming growth factor β is a bifunctional regulator of replication and collagen synthesis in osteoblast-enriched cell cultures from fetal rat bone. *J Biol Chem* 1987;262:2869–2874.

63. Guenther HL, Cecchini MG, Elford PR, et al. Effects of transforming growth factor type β upon bone cell populations grown either in monolayer or semisolid medium. *J Bone Miner Res* 1988;3:269–278.

64. ten Dijke P, Iwata KK, Goddard C, et al. Recombinant transforming growth factor type β3: biological activities and receptor-binding properties in isolated bone cells. *Mol Cell Biol* 1990;10:4473–4479.

65. Centrella M, McCarthy TL, Canalis E. Skeletal tissue and transforming growth factor β. *FASEB J* 1988;2:3066–3073.

66. Bonewald LF, Kester MB, Schwartz Z, et al. Effects of combining transforming growth factor β and 1,25-α dihydroxyvitamin D3 on differentiation of a human osteosarcoma (MG-63). *J Biol Chem* 1992;267:8943–8949.

67. Antosz ME, Bellows CG, Aubin JE. Effects of transforming growth factor β and epidermal growth factor on cell proliferation and the formation of bone nodules in isolated fetal rat calvaria cells. *J Cell Physiol* 1989;140:386–395.

68. Wrana JL, Maeno M, Hawrylyshyn B, et al. Differential effects of transforming growth factor-β on the synthesis of extracellular matrix proteins by normal fetal rat calvarial bone cell populations. *J Cell Biol* 1988;106:915–924.

69. Noda M, Rodan GA. Type β transforming growth factor (TGF β) regulation of alkaline phosphatase expression and other phenotype-related mRNAs in osteoblastic rat osteosarcoma cells. *J Cell Physiol* 1987;133:426–437.

70. Noda M, Yoon K, Prince CW, et al. Transcriptional regulation of osteopontin production in rat osteosarcoma cells by type β transforming growth factor. *J Biol Chem* 1988;263:13916–13921.

71. Erlebacher A, Filvaroff EH, Ye JQ, et al. Osteoblastic responses to TGF-β during bone remodeling. *Mol Biol Cell* 1998;9:1903–1918.

72. Filvaroff E, Erlebacher A, Ye JQ, et al. Inhibition of TGF-β receptor signaling in osteoblasts leads to decreased bone remodeling and increased trabecular bone mass. *Development* 1999;126:4267–4279.

73. Cecchini MG, Hofstetter W, Halasy J, et al. Role of CSF-1 in bone and bone marrow development. *Mol Reprod Dev* 1997;46:75–83.

74. Suda T, Takahashi N, Martin TJ. Modulation of osteoclast differentiation [erratum in *Endocr Rev* 1992;13:191]. *Endocr Rev* 1992;13:66–80.

75. Suda T, Nakamura I, Jimi E, et al. Regulation of osteoclast function. *J Bone Miner Res* 1997;12:869–879.

76. Oreffo RO, Mundy GR, Seyedin SM, et al. Activation of the bone-derived latent TGF β complex by isolated osteoclasts. *Biochem Biophys Res Commun* 1989;158:817–823.

77. Suda T, Takahashi N, Udagawa N, et al. Modulation of osteoclast differentiation and function by the new members of the tumor necrosis factor receptor and ligand families. *Endocr Rev* 1999;20:345–357.

78. Tashjian AH Jr, Voelkel EF, Lazzaro M, et al. Alpha and beta human transforming growth factors stimulate prostaglandin production and bone resorption in cultured mouse calvaria. *Proc Natl Acad Sci USA* 1985;82:4535–4538.

79. Pfeilschifter J, Seyedin SM, Mundy GR. Transforming growth factor β inhibits bone resorption in fetal rat long bone cultures. *J Clin Invest* 1988;82:680–685.

80. Jacobsen FW, Stokke T, Jacobsen SE. Transforming growth factor-β potently inhibits the viability-promoting activity of stem cell factor and other cytokines and induces apoptosis of primitive murine hematopoietic progenitor cells. *Blood* 1995;86:2957–2966.

81. Chénu C, Pfeilschifter J, Mundy GR, et al. Transforming growth factor β inhibits formation of osteoclast-like cells in long-term human marrow cultures. *Proc Natl Acad Sci USA* 1988;85:5683–5687.

82. Shinar DM, Rodan GA. Biphasic effects of transforming growth factor-β on the production of osteoclast-like cells in mouse bone marrow cultures: the role of prostaglandins in the generation of these cells. *Endocrinology* 1990;126:3153–3158.

83. Marcelli C, Yates AJ, Mundy GR. *In vivo* effects of human recombinant transforming growth factor β on bone turnover in normal mice. *J Bone Miner Res* 1990;5:1087–1096.

84. Dieudonné SC, Foo P, van Zoelen EJ, et al. Inhibiting and stimulating effects of TGF-β1 on osteoclastic bone resorption in fetal mouse bone organ cultures. *J Bone Miner Res* 1991;6:479–487.

85. Hattersley G, Chambers TJ. Effects of transforming growth factor β1 on the regulation of osteoclastic development and function. *J Bone Miner Res* 1991;6: 165–172.

86. Takaishi T, Matsui T, Tsukamoto T, et al. TGF-β-induced macrophage colony-stimulating factor gene expression in various mesenchymal cell lines. *Am J Physiol* 1994;267:C25–C31.

87. Yoshida H, Hayashi S, Kunisada T, et al. The murine mutation osteopetrosis is in the coding region of the macrophage colony stimulating factor gene. *Nature* 1990;345:442–444.

88. Takahashi N, Udagawa N, Akatsu T, et al. Deficiency of osteoclasts in osteopetrotic mice is due to a defect in the local microenvironment provided by osteoblastic cells. *Endocrinology* 1991;128:1792–1796.

89. Felix R, Cecchini MG, Fleisch H. Macrophage colony stimulating factor restores *in vivo* bone resorption in the op/op osteopetrotic mouse. *Endocrinology* 1990; 127:2592–2594.

90. Filvaroff E, Derynck R. Bone remodelling: a signalling system for osteoclast regulation. *Curr Biol* 1998;8: R679–R682.

91. Suda T, Takahashi N, Udagawa N, et al. Modulation of osteoclast differentiation and function by the new members of the tumor necrosis factor receptor and ligand families. *Endocr Rev* 1999;20:345–357.

92. Yasuda H, Shima N, Nakagawa N, et al. Osteoclast differentiation factor is a ligand for osteoprotegerin/osteoclastogenesis-inhibitory factor and is identical to TRANCE/RANKL. *Proc Natl Acad Sci USA* 1998;95:3597–3602.

93. Lacey DL, Timms E, Tan HL, et al. Osteoprotegerin ligand is a cytokine that regulates osteoclast differentiation and activation. *Cell* 1998;93:165–176.

94. Simonet WS, Lacey DL, Dunstan CR, et al. Osteoprotegerin: a novel secreted protein involved in the regulation of bone density. *Cell* 1997;89:309–319.

95. Takai H, Kanematsu M, Yano K, et al. Transforming growth factor-β stimulates the production of osteoprotegerin/osteoclastogenesis inhibitory factor by bone marrow stromal cells. *J Biol Chem* 1998;273: 27091–27096.

96. Murakami T, Yamamoto M, Ono K, et al. Transforming growth factor-β1 increases mRNA levels of osteoclastogenesis inhibitory factor in osteoblastic/stromal cells and inhibits the survival of murine osteoclast-like cells. *Biochem Biophys Res Commun* 1998;252: 747–752.

97. Jilka RL. Cytokines, bone remodeling, and estrogen deficiency: a 1998 update. *Bone* 1998;23:75–81.

98. Robinson JA, Riggs BL, Spelsberg TC, et al. Osteoclasts and transforming growth factor-β: estrogen-mediated isoform-specific regulation of production. *Endocrinology* 1996;137:615–621.

99. Yang NN, Bryan HU, Hardikan S, et al. Estrogen and raloxifene stimulate transforming growth factor-β3 gene expression in rat bone: a potential mechanism for estrogen- or raloxifene-mediated bone maintenance. *Endocrinology* 1996;137:2075–2084.

100. Hughes DE, Dai A, Tiffee JC, et al. Estrogen promotes apoptosis of murine osteoclasts mediated by TGF-β. *Nat Med* 1996;2:1132–1136.

101. Noda M, Camilliere JJ. *In vivo* stimulation of bone formation by transforming growth factor-β. *Endocrinology* 1989;124:2991–2994.

102. Rosen D, Miller SC, DeLeon E, et al. Systemic administration of recombinant transforming growth factor β2 (rTGF-β2) stimulates parameters of cancellous bone formation in juvenile and adult rats. *Bone* 1994;15: 355–359.

103. Geiser AG, Zeng QQ, Sato M, et al. Decreased bone mass and bone elasticity in mice lacking the transforming growth factor-β1 gene. *Bone* 1998;23:87–93.

104. Sanford LP, Ormsby I, Gittenberger-de Groot AC, et al. TGF β2 knockout mice have multiple developmental defects that are non-overlapping with other TGF-β knockout phenotypes. *Development* 1997;124: 2659–2670.

105. Taniguchi Y, Tanaka T, Gotoh K, et al. Transforming growth factor β1-induced cellular heterogeneity in the periosteum of rat parietal bones. *Calcif Tissue Int* 1993; 53:122–126.

106. Mundy GR, Boyce B, Hughes D, et al. The effects of cytokines and growth factors on osteoblastic cells. *Bone* 1995;17:71S–75S.

107. Sandberg MM, Aro HT, Vuorio EI. Gene expression during bone repair. *Clin Orthop* 1993;289:292–312.

108. Bolander ME. Regulation of fracture repair by growth factors. *Proc Soc Exp Biol Med* 1992;200:165–170.

109. Nielsen HM, Andreassen TT, Ledet T, et al. Local injection of TGF-β increases the strength of tibial fractures in the rat. *Acta Orthop Scand* 1994;65:37–41.

110. Joyce ME, Jingushi S, Bolander ME. Transforming growth factor-β in the regulation of fracture repair. *Orthop Clin North Am* 1990;21:199–209.

111. Kulkarni AB, Huh CG, Becker D, et al. Transforming growth factor β1 null mutation in mice causes excessive inflammatory response and early death. *Proc Natl Acad Sci USA* 1993;90:770–774.

112. Shull MM, Ormsby I, Kier AB, et al. Targeted disruption of the mouse transforming growth factor-β1 gene results in multifocal inflammatory disease. *Nature* 1992;359:693–699.

113. Kaartinen V, Voncken JW, Shuler C, et al. Abnormal lung development and cleft palate in mice lacking TGF-β3 indicates defects of epithelial–mesenchymal interaction. *Nat Genet* 1995;11:415–421.

114. Proetzel G, Pawlowski SA, Wiles MV, et al. Transforming growth factor-β3 is required for secondary palate fusion. *Nat Genet* 1995;11:409–414.

115. Beaudreuil J, Mbalaviele G, Cohen-Solal M, et al. Short-term local injections of transforming growth factor-β1 decrease ovariectomy-stimulated osteoclastic resorption *in vivo* in rats. *J Bone Miner Res* 1995;10: 971–977.

116. Finkelman RD, Bell NH, Strong DD, et al. Ovariectomy selectively reduces the concentration of transforming growth factor β in rat bone: implications for estrogen deficiency–associated bone loss. *Proc Natl Acad Sci USA* 1992;89:12190–12193.

117. Ikeda T, Shigeno C, Kasai R, et al. Ovariectomy decreases the mRNA levels of transforming growth factor-β1 and increases the mRNA levels of osteocalcin in rat bone *in vivo*. *Biochem Biophys Res Commun* 1993;194:1228–1233.

118. Nicolas V, Prewett A, Bettica P, et al. Age-related decreases in insulin-like growth factor-I and transforming growth factor-β in femoral cortical bone from both men and women: implications for bone loss with aging. *J Clin Endocrinol Metab* 1994;78:1011–1016.

119. Yamada Y, Miyauchi A, Goto J, et al. Association of a polymorphism of the transforming growth factor-β1 gene with genetic susceptibility to osteoporosis in postmenopausal Japanese women. *J Bone Miner Res* 1998; 13:1569–1576.

120. Pfeilschifter J, Diel I, Scheppach B, et al. Concentration of transforming growth factor β in human bone tissue: relationship to age, menopause, bone turnover, and bone volume. *J Bone Miner Res* 1998;13:716–730.

Skeletal Growth Factors,
edited by Ernesto Canalis.
Lippincott Williams & Wilkins, Philadelphia, © 2000.

17

Activin and Follistatin

Hiromu Sugino and Kunihiro Tsuchida

Institute for Enzyme Research, The University of Tokushima, Tokushima, Japan

In the mid-1980s, several hypophysiotropic protein factors that regulate the release of follicle-stimulating hormone (FSH) by pituitary cells were identified from mammalian gonads. These include activins (1,2), which stimulate FSH release, and inhibins (3–6) and follistatins (FS) (7), which inhibit FSH release. These proteins have added a new dimension to the complexity of the hypothalamic–pituitary–gonadal axis system. Activins and inhibins have related dimeric structures, but FS is a glycosylated single-chain protein. Activins and inhibins are members of the transforming growth factor-β (TGF-β) family, the members of which have a wide range of biological actions on cell growth and differentiation. Although the inhibin-specific receptor has not yet been identified, substantial progress has been made recently in the characterization and understanding of activin receptors and their associated signaling mechanisms (reviewed in 8,9). Activins act through two types of transmembrane serine/threonine kinase receptor, types I and II. The cytoplasmic domain of the activated type I receptor interacts with intracellular signaling effectors, Smads, which regulate transcription of selected genes in response to ligand. FS was subsequently found to be an activin-binding protein, forming an inactive complex with activin and neutralizing various activin actions (10,11). As such, the activin–FS system represents a powerful regulatory mechanism that can exert effects on a variety of cellular processes in target organs.

In this chapter, we focus on the biochemical characteristics of activin and follistatin and discuss the emerging role of these proteins as potent tissue regulators.

ACTIVINS

Activins were originally isolated from gonadal fluids based on their ability to stimulate FSH release from cultured primary rat pituitary cells (1,2). *In situ* hybridization and immunohistochemical studies demonstrated that expression of activin subunits is widespread in embryonic and adult tissues other than the gonads, as is that of activin receptors (described below). Subsequent to the identification of the gonadal activins, an erythroid differentiation factor (EDF) was isolated from conditioned medium of the THP-1 human monocytic cell line and found to be identical to activin A (12). In addition, activins have been independently purified on the basis of a number of different biological activities, including nerve cell survival (13), induction of mesoderm in *Xenopus laevis* embryos (14–16), megakaryocyte differentiation (17), promotion of bone growth (18), induction of somatostatin expression (19), and induction of cell cycle arrest and apoptosis (20).

Subunit Structure

Activins and inhibins are functionally antagonistic but structurally related. Inhibins are heterodimeric proteins composed of an α subunit linked by disulfide bonds to one of the related β subunits; activins, on the other hand, are dimers composed of two β subunits. Five β subunits

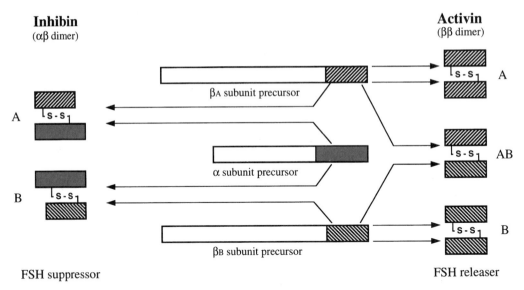

FIG. 17.1. Structures of inhibin and activin. The multiple arrangement of gene products from the α-, β_A-, and β_B-subunit precursors through disulfide bridging yields follicle-stimulating hormone *(FSH)* releasers (activin) and suppressors (inhibin).

have been identified, β_A, β_B, β_C, β_D, and β_E, whereas only a single α subunit has been cloned (21–25). Thus, there is a family of possible dimers. To date, inhibins A ($\alpha\beta_A$) and B ($\alpha\beta_B$) and activins A ($\beta_A\beta_A$), AB ($\beta_A\beta_B$), and B ($\beta_B\beta_B$) have been isolated as dimeric proteins from natural sources (26). DNA sequence analyses showed that all of the subunits are initially synthesized as large precursor proteins, with the mature subunits residing at the COOH-terminal regions of several clusters of multiple basic residues, which can serve as potential proteolytic processing sites (Fig. 17.1). The sizes of the mature forms of the most abundant subunits are 18 kDa for the α subunit and 14 kDa for the β_A and β_B subunits. The proregion in the large precursor is essential for the folding and assembly of activin dimers, indicating that the proregion plays a critical role in biosynthesis (27). The functions of subunits β_C and β_E, cloned from human and mouse liver cDNA libraries (23,25), and β_D, which has been identified only in *Xenopus* (24), are not yet known; and it remains uncertain whether the β_C, β_D, and β_E subunits assemble into homodimers, heterodimers, or both. Thus, depending on the combination of the gene products, protein molecules having

quite different biological activities could be derived from a limited number of genes.

Biological Activities

Inhibin is a functional antagonist of activin in some systems. This antagonism was first observed with regard to FSH secretion by pituitary cells but has also been documented for a number of other responses. There are, however, many activin responses that do not appear to be regulated by inhibin, and no activin-independent effects of inhibin have been described so far. Moreover, the inhibin receptor has not yet been identified and a full understanding of the mechanism of cellular signal transduction and physiological function of inhibin is still far in the future.

In contrast to inhibin, activins have been shown to exert multiple actions on a wide range of tissues and cell types, as might be expected from their structures, which are similar to that of TGF-β. Activins were originally isolated from gonadal fluids by measuring the stimulation of FSH release from cultured primary rat anterior pituitary cells. Indeed, in pituitary cell cultures, activin has been shown to cause dose-dependent and parallel increases in FSH β-subunit mRNA levels and FSH secretion without any effect on luteinizing hormone (LH) β-subunit mRNA levels (28). Furthermore, among activin isoforms, activin B has been reported to act as a local autocrine factor to stimulate FSH production in the pituitary (29). In contrast to their stimulation of FSH release, activins suppress the secretion of growth hormone, prolactin, and corticotrophin from cultured pituitary cells (30–32).

Locally produced activin can modify hormone production in the gonads and regulate folliculogenesis and spermatogenesis. In nondifferentiated ovarian granulosa cells, activin increases FSH-induced progesterone production; conversely, in differentiated granulosa cells, activin inhibits FSH-induced progesterone production. This suggests that activin promotes the initiation of folliculogenesis in small follicles but inhibits the luteinization of large antral follicles (33). In the testis, in addition to stimulating spermatogonial proliferation *in vitro,* activin enhances FSH-induced proliferation of Sertoli cells (34). This synergism between activin and FSH is also observed in immature granulosa cells (35).

Subsequent to the identification of the gonadal activins, EDF was isolated from conditioned medium of the THP-1 human monocytic cell line and found to be identical to activin A (12). A stimulatory effect of activin A on erythropoiesis has also been shown *in vivo* since its administration to mice results in an increase in the number of erythroid progenitors, burst-forming unit, erythroid (BFU-E), and colony-forming unit, erythroid (CFU-E), in the bone marrow and spleen. This stimulatory effect of activin A was abolished by administration of follistatin, which blocked its action by binding to activin (see following), indicating that erythroid progenitors are responsive to, and receive some regulatory signal from, endogenous activin A (36). Maturation of erythroid differentiation requires costimulation by activin A and erythropoietin (EPO): EPO alone scarcely induces differentiation, and cells stimulated by activin A alone undergo apoptotic death (37). Thus, the action of activin appears to commit the cell to death or to differentiation, and the presence of EPO enables differentiation

through suppression of apoptosis. The apoptotic activity of activin derived from macrophages has also been observed in B lineage cells, in which activin induces G_1 arrest by upregulation of $p21^{CIPI/WAFI}$ (38). A stromal protein, designated restrictin-P, that specifically kills plasma-like cells was purified to homogeneity and shown to be identical to activin A (39). The specificity for plasma-like cells stemmed from the ability of activin A to competitively antagonize the proliferation-inducing effects of interleukin-6 (IL-6) and IL-11. The plasmacytoma growth-inhibitory activity of activin A may be mediated in part by inducing apoptotic cell death. Activin was also shown to inhibit capillary endothelial cell growth and may share some of the effects of TGF-β in this system (40).

There is accumulating evidence that activins play important roles in hepatic homeostasis. *In vitro* studies have revealed that activins inhibit DNA synthesis in hepatocytes and induce significant cell loss following subcutaneous administration (41–43). Activin-treated rats developed typical cachexia with severe weight loss. Interestingly, knockout mice lacking the α subunit gene of inhibin also develop hepatic failure resembling that observed in activin-treated rats (44). In the intact liver, activin βA-subunit mRNA is expressed only weakly, but at 20 to 24 hours after 70% hepatectomy, its expression increases markedly and then declines thereafter (45). When FS is infused into the portal vein immediately after hepatectomy, DNA synthesis is accelerated and liver regeneration is significantly augmented. Recently, the activin βC and βE subunits have been isolated from human and mouse cDNA libraries (23,25). The function of these subunits is not yet known, and it remains uncertain if the activin βC and βE subunits assemble into homodimers, heterodimers, or both. It should be noted that both activin βC and βE show striking patterns of liver-restricted expression in adult mice, suggesting that they may play critical roles in normal liver functions (46).

Activin A has also been purified from demineralized bovine bone extract. Activin from bovine bone enhanced ectopic bone formation in rat subcutis when implanted in combination with bone morphogenetic proteins (BMP-2 and

BMP-3) in a collagen/ceramic carrier (18). The role of activin in modulating bone formation is noteworthy, especially in senile osteoporosis (see Chapter 18). Furthermore, recent studies from the dentistry field have shown that activin is identical with mesenchyme-derived diffusible factor, which is required for early tooth bud formation (47).

Although high expression of mRNAs for both activins and activin receptors has been observed in neural tissues, particularly in the hippocampus area, there have been few advances in our understanding of the physiological functions of activins as paracrine factors in the brain. Activins stimulate oxytocin (48) and gonadotropin-releasing hormone (GnRH) (49) production. Activins can induce terminal differentiation of ciliary ganglion neurons, as shown by the production of somatostatin (19). Activins inhibit retinoic acid–induced neural differentiation of P19 teratoma cells and some types of neuroblastoma cell (50). Under some, but not all, conditions, activins also promote the survival of neuronal cells derived from P19 cells and hippocampus (13). Counteracting the activity of activins, FS, an activin-binding protein (see below), suppresses the anchorage-independent growth of P19 cells in soft agar and stimulates neurite outgrowth of IMR-32 neuroblastoma cells (51). Convulsive seizures caused by administration of kainate to rats have been demonstrated to induce the expression of activin β_A mRNA (52). Furthermore, high-frequency stimulation of the perforant pathway, which produces a persistent long-term potentiation (LTP), caused a marked increase in the level of activin β_A mRNA in the dentate gyrus of rat hippocampus. These results suggest a role for activins in the maintenance of neural plasticity in the adult brain.

Activins have profound effects on early embryogenesis, including mesoderm development, axis formation, and the determination of cell fate. In response to members of the TGF-β family, animal caps (ectodermal explant isolated from *Xenopus* blastula-stage embryos) differentiate into mesoderm, instead of their normal epidermal fate. Activin appears to be one of the most intriguing of the family members because it can elicit a broad range of mesodermal cell types and induce mesodermal molecular markers in a concentration-dependent manner (14–16). Ectopic expression of a truncated activin type II receptor (see below) that inhibits activin signaling shows that activin-like molecules are required for mesodermal induction *in vivo* and for patterning of the *Xenopus* embryonic body plan (53). Blocking the activin signal-transduction pathway also reveals autonomous induction of a neural marker (54).

Characterization of Activin Receptors

Affinity labeling and chemical cross-linking of activin-responsive cells using ^{125}I-activin generate two activin–receptor complexes: a type I complex of approximately 65 kDa and a type II complex of approximately 85 kDa (55,56). cDNAs for both types of receptor encode proteins comprising a small extracellular domain, a single transmembrane domain, and a cytoplasmic domain with a protein–serine/threonine kinase motif. Expression cloning identified an activin type II receptor (ActRIIA) as the first vertebrate receptor serine kinase (RSK) (55). Since then, multiple members of this RSK superfamily, including a second subtype of activin type II receptor (ActRIIB) (57,58) and two activin type I receptors [ActRIA and ActRIB, also known as activin receptor-like kinase-2 (ALK-2 and ALK-4, respectively)] (56,59,60), have been identified. The two activin type II receptors (ActRIIA and ActRIIB) bind activin with high affinity ($K_d = 200$ to 700 pM). In contrast, activin type I receptors (ActRIA and ActRIB) do not bind activin directly and need type II receptors to associate with ligand (8). ActRIB appears to be the activin type I receptor responsible for signaling gene transcription and growth inhibition through the activin/TGF-β pathway–specific Smad2 and Smad3 (see below), whereas ActRIA has been found to be responsible for signal transduction of BMP-2 and BMP-7 through activation of the BMP pathway–specific Smad1 (9). Formation of a complex of type I and type II receptors is required to mediate biological responses to activin (60). It is worthy of note that, whereas activins signal mainly through ActRIIs and ActRIB, ActRIIs are also shared by BMP ligands (Fig. 17.2) (9).

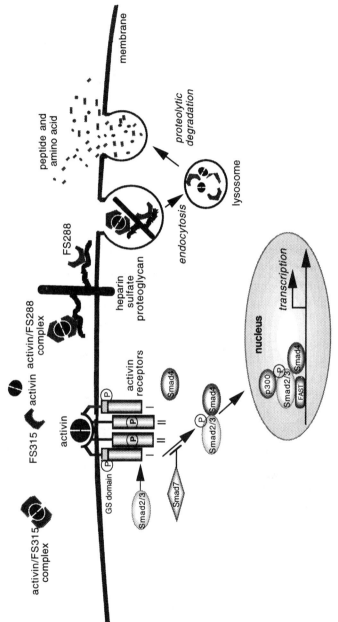

FIG. 17.2. A general model for the initiation of signaling by the activin receptor and regulatory mechanism of activin signal transduction by follistatin *(FS)*. Receptor II is the primary activin receptor and is a constitutively active serine/threonine kinase that recruits receptor I after binding activin. The subsequent phosphorylation of receptor I by receptor II allows the receptor I kinase to propagate the signal to downstream substrates. FS can neutralize activin bioactivity by interfering with the binding of activin to activin type II receptor. Cell surface–bound FS accelerates the endocytotic internalization of activin, leading to its degradation.

Activation of Activin Receptor by Complex Formation and Phosphorylation

A receptor activation model has been proposed for the activin receptor system (61–63) (Fig. 17.2). Type II receptors exhibit a basal level of autophosphorylation that is independent of either type I receptors or ligand binding. Once type I receptors form a complex with type II receptors, they become phosphorylated by the constitutively active type II receptors, mainly in the juxtamembrane GS domain, which is rich in glycine, serine, and threonine. The importance of the kinase activities of both the type II and type I receptors in activin signaling has been shown by using kinase-inactive receptor mutants. Both kinase-defective type II and kinase-defective type I receptors act as dominant negative mutants to block the physiological responses of activin, such as the induction of mesoderm formation in early development and the regulation of gene transcription (61,64). Without the kinase activities of type II receptors, type I receptors do not become phosphorylated. In contrast, even without the kinase activities of type I receptors, both type II and type I receptors become phosphorylated (61). In both cases, downstream signaling is disrupted. Type I receptors specify the signaling of individual TGF-β family members (60,65). This was uncovered by the identification of a constitutively active type I receptor mutant (65). The mutant ActRIB (T206D), in which Thr[206] is replaced by Asp, has been shown to signal antiproliferation and gene transcription even in the absence of activin and ActRIIs. Thr[206] of ActRIB is located in the conserved GS domain of the type I receptor subfamily. These data suggest that type I receptors are the main signal transducers and that, once activated, they are sufficient for downstream signaling.

Intracellular Activin Signal Transduction

Intracellular signaling molecules for activins have only recently been characterized. Clues for possible signaling mediators have come from genetic studies with *Drosophila* and *Caenorhabditis elegans*. The gene called *Mad (Mothers against dpp)* is implicated as a functional molecule interacting with decapentaplegic *(dpp)* during *Drosophila* embryogenesis (66). *Dpp* is a functional homologue of vertebrate BMP-2/4 family members. In *C. elegans,* shortening of body length is caused by mutation of molecules called *Sma*2-4 (67). Recent investigations have identified several mammalian *Sma-* and *Mad*-related proteins (Smads 1–8) involved in signaling by activins and other members of the TGF-β superfamily (9). Among the pathway-restricted Smads, Smads 2 and 3 are phosphorylated by the kinase activity of ActRIB upon ligand binding to activin receptors; phosphorylated Smad2 or Smad3 then forms a complex with Smad4, which is a common mediator Smad for the TGF-β superfamily. Smad2 or Smad3/Smad4 complexes have DNA-binding and transcriptional activities in the nucleus. Coactivators of transcription, including p300/cyclic adenosine monophosphate (cAMP) response element (CRE) binding protein (CREB) and other transcription factors such as activator protein-1 (AP-1), are likely to associate with Smads to exert tissue- and cell-specific transcription. Smads 6 and 7 are inhibitory Smads which associate with type I receptors and inhibit activation of pathway-specific Smads. Smad7 is a potent inhibitor of activin signaling as well as of TGF-β and BMP signaling; the inhibitory effects of Smad6 are not so efficient in terms of activin signaling (Fig. 17.2). Yeast genetic screening has identified several intracellular molecules that can interact with receptor proteins. Among them, immunophilin FK506/rapamycin-binding protein-12 (FKBP-12) may serve as a regulatory protein for signaling of at least some of the TGF-β superfamily members (68,69). Furthermore, a novel mitogen-activated protein (MAP) kinase family member has been identified that specifically transduces TGF-β signaling. The kinase, named TGF-β-activated kinase-1 (TAK-1), is also involved in BMP-4 signaling, although an involvement of the TAK-1 kinase pathway in activin signaling remains to be elucidated (70). Various genes are reported to be induced by activins. For example, in *X. laevis* embryogenesis, induction of *brachyury, goosecoid,* or *myoD* mRNAs is a good marker for assessing the ability of activin to induce mesodermal tissues. Among the immediate-early responsive genes, the mRNA for the protooncogene JunB is dramatically induced by activins in responsive cells (71). Since JunB mRNA is also induced by TGF-β and BMP and overexpression of JunB is capable of mimicking the effects of BMP-2 on the inhibition of myoblast differentiation, this protooncogene is likely to be one of the key molecules mediating the signaling pathway of the TGF-β superfamily, including activins.

FOLLISTATINS

In 1987, a new class of gonadal protein factor, named FSH-suppressing protein (FSP) or FS, was identified in a side fraction derived from the purification of bovine and porcine ovarian inhibins and activins (7,72). FS was characterized initially by its ability to suppress pituitary cellular FSH secretion *in vitro*. The action of FS appears to be similar to that of inhibin, but it is structurally quite different. FS is a single-chain protein that occurs in forms with molecular masses of 31 to 39 kDa, all of which have similar amino acid compositions and identical NH_2-terminal amino acid sequences. In recent studies, an activin-binding protein which was specific for, and had a high affinity for, activin was purified from rat ovary (10) and bovine pituitary (11); it was identical to FS. Interest in the biological significance of FS had diminished because of its weak inhibitory activity compared with that of inhibin. However, the finding that FS is an activin-binding protein sheds new light on its physiological role since it may participate in the regulation of the multiple actions of activin. Indeed, FS mRNA transcripts have been detected in a wide variety of tissues, which may indicate that FS, like activin, has tissue-specific effects or that FS has a universal action on different cell types. The ability of FS to bind to the pleiotropic growth and differentiation factor activin, and thereby to neutralize the actions of activin, makes this glycoprotein a potentially important regulatory factor, capable of modulating autocrine and paracrine functions and the processes of differentiation and development.

Molecular Heterogeneity

FS was originally detected as a mixture containing several bioactive polypeptides in bovine and porcine follicular fluids. Thereafter, processing of the FS gene product was investigated, revealing that alternative splicing generates two types of FS precursor (73,74). One is a pre-FS and the other is its homologue truncated by 27 amino acids at its COOH-terminal end. The corresponding mature FS isoforms comprise 315 (FS-315) and 288 (FS-288) amino acids, respectively.

To date, FS has been purified from rat ovary (10), porcine (26) and human (75) follicular fluids, bovine pituitary (11), and *Xenopus* XTC cell-culture medium (76). Every preparation demonstrated multiple bands in the 32- to 38-kDa molecular mass range when subjected to sodium dodecyl sulfate-polyacrylamide gel electrophoresis under nonreducing conditions. Six molecular forms of FS were isolated, resulting from truncation of the COOH-terminal region and/or the presence of N-linked carbohydrate chains (77). The six FS isoforms can be divided into three groups according to the extent of truncation: full-length core proteins with 315 amino acids (FS-315), FS-315 proteolysis products with 303 amino acids (FS-303), and a COOH-terminally truncated protein with 288 amino acids (FS-288). Characteristically, both FS-315 and FS-303, but not FS-288, contain a highly acidic COOH-terminal extension. The FS-303 molecular form is the major component of FS from mammalian sources. All six isolated FS forms demonstrate almost identical activin-binding activity (K_d = 540 to 680 pM).

Modulation of Activin Action

Immunohistochemical and *in situ* hybridization studies indicate that FS protein and mRNA are ubiquitous in tissues. A similar broad tissue localization has also been demonstrated for activin-subunit mRNA expression. The widespread tissue distributions of activin and FS imply, but do not conclusively demonstrate, that both factors are synthesized locally and that FS regulates the physiological actions of activin in a paracrine or autocrine manner. Several lines of indirect evidence suggest that the biological activities of activin are neutralized by its binding to FS. FS inhibits the functions of activin in pituitary cells (7,10,11,72), granulosa cells (78), erythroid cells (26), embryonal carcinoma cells (51), osteoblasts (79), and embryogenesis (80). An inhibitory effect of FS on erythropoiesis *in vivo* has also been observed. The continuous intraperitoneal administration of FS to normal mice resulted in a decrease of the erythroid progenitors BFU-E and CFU-E in the bone marrow and spleen (36). This supports the hypothesis that endogenous activin participates in murine erythropoiesis, a process in which FS exerts a regulatory function. There is also some evidence that FS does not block all of the bioactivities of activin. Independent of its activin-binding activity, FS itself has stimulatory effects on progesterone production and metabolism by undifferentiated rat granulosa cells (81). Furthermore, in cocultures of rat Sertoli cells and testicular germ cells, FS inhibits activin-stimulated Sertoli cell reaggregation but shows no effect on activin-induced DNA synthesis (82). No explanation for this differential regulation by FS of the actions of activin has so far been elucidated.

The ability of FS to neutralize the activities of activin in various assay systems suggests that there is a stoichiometric relationship between FS and activin. Immunoblotting analysis of partially purified porcine follicular fluid indicated that more than enough FS exists in follicular fluid to generate an activin–FS complex. Interestingly, activins A, AB, and B were found to be present as complexes with FS in the follicular fluid (26). These results indicate that mammalian ovarian cells, probably granulosa cells, synthesize and secrete three activin isoforms as well as FS, which readily form an inert complex in follicular fluid. Gel filtration studies on their stoichiometric interaction indicated that 1 mole of activin binds to 2 moles of FS to form an inactive high-molecular-weight complex and that activin therefore has two binding sites for FS. This relationship between FS and activin closely reflects the antagonistic effect of FS on the actions of activin described previously.

Another activin-binding protein, α_2-macro-globulin (α_2M), is found in human serum and follicular fluid (83,84). α_2M has also been found to bind to FS and inhibin. However, the affinity of activin for α_2M is much lower than that for FS, which could account for the lack of effect of α_2M on the bioactivity of activin. The physiological function of this complex formation is not known, but α_2M may serve a storage or clearance role, as has been shown for other cell growth factors.

Recently, using a surface plasmon resonance biosensor, FS has been demonstrated to interact directly with multiple BMPs, although ligand blotting analyses did not show any detectable binding (85). This interaction may support the idea that FS acts as an organizer factor in early *Xenopus* embryogenesis by inhibiting the activities of BMPs by a different mechanism from that of chordin and noggin, which bind to BMPs and interfere with their ability to bind to their receptors.

Affinity for Heparan Sulfate Proteoglycans

In the course of purification of FS, it was found to possess a strong affinity for sulfated polysaccharides, such as dextran sulfate, heparin, and sulfated cellulose. The interaction between FS and sulfated polysaccharides has been demonstrated to be important in the control of the actions of activin. FS associates with cultured rat granulosa cells, yielding a typical ligand saturation curve with an apparent K_d of 5 nM. Heparin and heparan sulfate, but not chondroitin, keratan, or dermatan sulfates, compete strongly for this binding. Treatment with the glycosaminoglycan-degrading enzymes heparinase and heparitinase results in significant suppression of the binding. These results show that FS has a high affinity for the heparan sulfate side chains of granulosa cell surface proteoglycans (86).

As discussed previously, preparations of FS contain at least six isoforms. Interestingly, the affinity for the heparan sulfate chains was found to differ quite markedly depending on the sequence of the core protein (77). The COOH-terminal truncated form (FS-288) shows a very high affinity for the cells, with a K_d of 2 nM. In contrast, the full-length form (FS-315) shows no affinity, whereas the midsized isoform (FS-303) shows moderate affinity. These results clearly indicate that the COOH-terminal amino acid sequence of FS is important for its binding to the heparan sulfate chains of cell surface proteoglycans.

The biological response first associated with FS was inhibition of activin-induced FSH secretion from cultured rat pituitary cells. FS-288 was more potent than FS-303 and FS-315 in this respect, which is consistent with the differences in the binding affinities of these forms for cell surfaces (77). Moreover, a recent study demonstrated that the *in vivo* FSH-suppressing activity of recombinant FS-288 in ovariectomized rats was greater and longer-lasting than that of inhibin A, which suggests that the COOH-terminal region of FS is important for inhibiting the FSH-releasing activity of activin and probably for exerting other neutralizing effects on the various actions of activin (87).

Inhibitory Mechanism of Activin Actions

Affinity cross-linking analyses using radioiodinated activin and COS cells that transiently expressed the activin type I and/or type II receptors provided more precise information about the effect of FS on the interaction of activin with its receptors. Preincubation of ^{125}I-activin A with FS completely abolished the binding of activin to activin type II receptors and consequently to activin type I receptors. A possibility that cell surface–bound FS-288 presents activin to its receptors, thereby facilitating activin binding, was also tested. FS-288 did bind to the cell surface of transfected COS cells but inhibited the binding of activin to its receptors. These results reveal that FS neutralizes activin bioactivity by interfering with activin binding to activin type II receptors, rather than inhibiting the binding of the type I receptor to the complex of activin and activin type II receptor (88). In addition, unlike basic fibroblast growth factor, cell surface–associated FS cannot present ligand to signaling receptors.

Although the formation of activin–receptor complex was prevented by adding FS, activin is able to associate with the cell surfaces via FS bound to the heparan sulfate side chains of proteoglycans (89). It should be noted that FS isoforms have different roles in the local modulation of activin functions as well as different affinities for cell surfaces. Significant binding of radioiodinated activin to pituitary cell surfaces was observed only in the presence of FS. As expected, FS-288 can markedly promote the cell surface binding of activin and to a greater extent than can FS-315. This implies that when incubated with cells in the presence of FS-288, activin in the medium is trapped by cell-associated FS-288. After being captured on the cell surface, activin, together with FS-288 and proteoglycans, is ingested by endocytotic vesicles, which ultimately fuse with primary lysosomes and are degraded. Most of the vesicle contents were found to be hydrolyzed to small breakdown products and secreted to the exterior. There is little doubt that activin is broken down by such an endocytotic degradation process because various types of inhibitor of each stage of this process significantly blocked degradation of activin. As with radioiodinated activin, proteolytic degradation of ^{125}I-labeled FS-288 in pituitary cells has been observed (89). Taking these findings together, we suggest that the endocytotic degradation of growth factors via cell surface heparan sulfate is necessary to erase the growth factor signals from the surrounding cell surfaces when they accumulate and become redundant. It has been established that the binding of a signaling ligand to its receptor stimulates a biological response and triggers a sequence of events leading to cellular desensitization to the ligand in order to regulate the responsiveness of the target cells to the ligand. In addition to such receptor-mediated endocytosis, there must be a scavenger mechanism for clearing signaling molecules away from their target cell surfaces (Fig. 17.2). These results demonstrated that cell-associated FS-288 (COOH-terminally truncated FS) accelerates the endocytotic internalization of activin into rat pituitary cells, rat granulosa cells, and probably *Xenopus* hemisphere cells, leading to its degradation by lysosomal enzymes. Cell-associated FS therefore plays a role in the system responsible for clearing the activin signal from cell surfaces.

ACKNOWLEDGMENTS

We thank Dr. Y. Eto for providing recombinant human activin A, Dr. S. Shimasaki for the gift of recombinant human follistatins, and Dr. Y. Hasegawa for donating bovine inhibin A. We are grateful to the NIDDK Pituitary Hormone Program for supplying the rat FSH radioimmunoassay kit. This work was supported in part by grants from the Ministry of Education, Science, and Culture of Japan; the Naito Foundation; the Uehara Memorial Foundation; the Mitsubishi Foundation; the Sankyo Foundation of Life Science; and the Kowa Foundation of Life Science.

REFERENCES

1. Vale W, Rivier J, Vaughan J, et al. Purification and characterization of an FSH releasing protein from porcine ovarian follicular fluid. *Nature* 1986;321:776–779.
2. Ling N, Ying SY, Ueno N, et al. Pituitary FSH is released by a heterodimer of the β-subunits from the two forms of inhibin. *Nature* 1986;321:779–782.
3. Robertson DM, Foulds LM, Leversha L, et al. Isolation of inhibin from bovine follicular fluid. *Biochem Biophys Res Commun* 1985;126:220–226.
4. Miyamoto K, Hasegawa Y, Fukuda M, et al. Isolation of porcine follicular fluid inhibin of 32K daltons. *Biochem Biophys Res Commun* 1985;129:396–403.
5. Ling N, Ying SY, Ueno N, et al. Isolation and partial characterization of a M_r 32,000 protein with inhibin activity from porcine follicular fluid. *Proc Natl Acad Sci USA* 1985;82:7217–7221.
6. Rivier J, Spiess J, McClintock R, et al. Purification and partial characterization of inhibin from porcine follicular fluid. *Biochem Biophys Res Commun* 1985;133: 120–127.
7. Ueno N, Ling N, Ying SY, et al. Isolation and partial characterization of follistatin: a single-chain M_r 35,000 monomeric protein that inhibits the release of follicle-stimulating hormone. *Proc Natl Acad Sci USA* 1987;84: 8282–8286.
8. Mathews LS. Activin receptors and cellular signaling by the receptor serine kinase family. *Endocr Rev* 1994; 15:310–325.
9. Heldin CH, Miyazono K, ten Dijke P. TGF-β signaling from cell membrane to nucleus through SMAD proteins. *Nature* 1997;390:465–471.
10. Nakamura T, Takio K, Eto Y, et al. Activin-binding protein from rat ovary is follistatin. *Science* 1990;247: 836–838.
11. Kogawa T, Nakamura T, Sugino K, et al. Activin-binding protein is present in pituitary. *Endocrinology* 1991; 128:1434–1440.
12. Eto Y, Tsuji T, Takezawa M, et al. Purification and characterization of erythroid differentiation factor (EDF) isolated from human leukemia cell line THP-1. *Biochem Biophys Res Commun* 1987;142:1095–1103.
13. Schubert D, Kimura H, LaCorbiere M, et al. Activin is a nerve cell survival molecule. *Nature* 1990;344: 868–870.
14. Asashima M, Nakano H, Shimada K, et al. Mesodermal induction in early amphibian embryos by activin A (erythroid differentiation factor). *Roux Arch Dev Biol* 1990; 198:330–335.
15. Smith JC, Price BMJ, Van Nimmen K, et al. Identification of a potent *Xenopus* mesoderm-inducing factor as a homologue of activin A. *Nature* 1990;345:729–731.
16. van den Eijnden-Van Raaij AJM, van Zoelent EJJ, van Nimmen K, et al. Activin-like factor from a *Xenopus laevis* cell line responsible for mesoderm induction. *Nature* 1990;345:732–734.
17. Fujimoto K, Kawakita M, Kato K, et al. Purification of megakaryocyte differentiation activity from a human fibrous histiocytoma cell line: N-terminal sequence homology with activin A. *Biochem Biophys Res Commun* 1991;174:1163–1168.
18. Ogawa Y, Schmidt DK, Nathan RM, et al. Bovine bone activin enhances bone morphogenetic protein–induced ectopic bone formation. *J Biol Chem* 1992;267: 14233–14237.
19. Coulombe JN, Schwall R, Parent AS, et al. Induction of somatostatin immunoreactivity in cultured ciliary ganglion neurons by activin in choroid cell–conditioned medium. *Neuron* 1993;10:899–906.
20. Nishihara T, Okahashi N, Ueda N. Activin A induces apoptotic cell death. *Biochem Biophys Res Commun* 1993;197:985–991.
21. Mason AJ, Hayflick JS, Ling N, et al. Complementary DNA sequences of ovarian follicular fluid inhibin show precursor structure and homology with transforming growth factor-β. *Nature* 1985;318:659–663.
22. Forage RG, Ring JM, Brown RW, et al. Cloning and sequence analysis of cDNA species coding for the two subunits of inhibin from bovine follicular fluid. *Proc Natl Acad Sci USA* 1986;83:3091–3095.
23. Hötten G, Neidhart H, Shneider C, et al. Cloning of a new member of the TGF-β family: a putative new activin βC chain. *Biochem Biophys Res Commun* 1995; 206:608–613.
24. Oda S, Nishimatsu S, Murakami K, et al. Molecular cloning and functional analysis of a new activin β subunit: a dorsal mesoderm-inducing activity in *Xenopus*. *Biochem Biophys Res Commun* 1995;210:581–588.
25. Fang J, Yin W, Smiley E, et al. Molecular cloning of the mouse activin βE subunit gene. *Biochem Biophys Res Commun* 1996;228:669–674.
26. Nakamura T, Asashima M, Eto Y, et al. Isolation and characterization of native activin B. *J Biol Chem* 1992; 267:16385–16389.
27. Gray AM, Mason AJ. Requirement for activin A and transforming growth factor-β1 pro-regions in homodimer assembly. *Science* 1990;247:1328–1330.
28. Weiss J, Harris PE, Halvorson LM, et al. Dynamic regulation of follicle-stimulating hormone-β messenger ribonucleic acid levels by activin and gonadotropin-releasing hormone in perifused rat pituitary cells. *Endocrinology* 1992;131:1403–1408.
29. Corrigan AZ, Bilezikjian LM, Carroll RS, et al. Evidence for an role of activin B within rat ante-

rior pituitary cultures. *Endocrinology* 1991;128:1682–1684.

30. Kitaoka M, Kojima I, Ogata E. Activin A: a modulator of multiple types of anterior pituitary cells. *Biochem Biophys Res Commun* 1988;157:48–54.

31. Bilezikjian LM, Corrigan AZ, Vale W. Activin-A modulates growth hormone secretion from cultures of rat anterior pituitary cells. *Endocrinology* 1990;126:2369–2376.

32. Bilezikjian LM, Blount AL, Campen CA, et al. Activin A inhibits proopiomelanocortin mRNA accumulation and adrenocorticotropin secretion of AtT20 cells. *Mol Endocrinol* 1991;5:1389–1395.

33. Miro F, Smyth CD, Whitelaw PF, et al. Regulation of 3β-hydroxysteroid dehydrogenase delta 5/delta 4-isomerase and cholesterol side-chain cleavage cytochrome P450 by activin in rat granulosa cells. *Endocrinology* 1995;136:3247–3252.

34. Boitani C, Stefanini M, Fragale A, et al. Activin stimulates Sertoli cell proliferation in a defined period of rat testis development. *Endocrinology* 1995;136:5438–5444.

35. Sugino H, Nakamura T, Hasegawa Y, et al. Erythroid differentiation factor can modulate follicular granulosa cell functions. *Biochem Biophys Res Commun* 1988;153:281–288.

36. Shiozaki M, Sakai R, Tabuchi M, et al. Evidence for the participation of endogenous activin A/erythroid differentiation factor in the regulation of erythropoiesis. *Proc Natl Acad Sci USA* 1992;89:1553–1556.

37. Shiozaki M, Kosaka M, Eto Y. Activin A: a commitment factor in erythroid differentiation. *Biochem Biophys Res Commun* 1998;242:631–635.

38. Yamato K, Koseki T, Ohguchi M, et al. Activin A induction of cell-cycle arrest involves modulation of cyclin D2 and p21$^{\text{CIP1/WAFI}}$ in plasmacytic cells. *Mol Endocrinol* 1997;11:1044–1052.

39. Brosh N, Sternberg D, Honigwachs-Sha'anani J, et al. The plasmacytoma growth inhibitor restrictin-P is an antagonist of interleukin 6 and interleukin 11. Identification as a stroma-derived activin A. *J Biol Chem* 1995;270:29594–29600.

40. McCarthy SA, Bicknell R. Inhibition of vascular endothelial cell growth by activin-A. *J Biol Chem* 1993;268:23066–23071.

41. Schwall RH, Robbins K, Jardieu P, et al. Activin induces cell death in hepatocytes *in vivo* and *in vitro*. *Hepatology* 1993;18:347–356.

42. Yasuda H, Mine T, Shibata H, et al. Activin A: an autocrine inhibitor of initiation of DNA synthesis in rat hepatocytes. *J Clin Invest* 1993;92:1491–1496.

43. Xu J, McKeehan K, Matsuzaki K, et al. Inhibin antagonizes inhibition of liver cell growth by activin by a dominant-negative mechanism. *J Biol Chem* 1995;270:6308–6313.

44. Matzuk MM, Finegold MJ, Su JGJ, et al. α-Inhibin is a tumour-suppressor gene with gonadal specificity in mice. *Nature* 1992;360:313–319.

45. Kogure K, Omata W, Kanzaki M, et al. A single intraportal administration of follistatin accelerates liver regeneration in partially hepatectomized rats. *Gastroenterology* 1995;108:1136–1142.

46. Fang J, Wang SQ, Smiley E, et al. Genes coding for mouse activin beta C and beta E are closely linked and exhibit a liver-specific expression pattern in adult tis-

sues. *Biochem Biophys Res Commun* 1997;231:655–661.

47. Ferguson CA, Tucker AS, Christensen L, et al. Activin is an essential early mesenchymal signal in tooth development that is required for patterning of the murine dentition. *Genes Dev* 1998;12:2636–2649.

48. Sawchenko PE, Plotsky PM, Pfeiffer SW, et al. Inhibin β in central neural pathways involved in the control of oxytocin secretion. *Nature* 1988;334:615–617.

49. Gonzalez-Manchon C, Bilezikjian LM, Corrigan AZ, et al. Activin-A modulates gonadotropin-releasing hormone secretion from a gonadotropin-releasing hormone–secreting neuronal cell line. *Neuroendocrinology* 1991;54:373–377.

50. Hashimoto M, Kondo S, Sakurai T, et al. Activin/EDF as an inhibitor of neural differentiation. *Biochem Biophys Res Commun* 1990;173:193–200.

51. Hashimoto M, Nakamura T, Inoue S, et al. Follistatin is a developmentally regulated cytokine in neural differentiation. *J Biol Chem* 1992;267:7203–7206.

52. Inokuchi K, Kato A, Hiraia K, et al. Increase in activin βA mRNA in rat hippocampus during long-term potentiation. *FEBS Lett* 1996;382:48–52.

53. Hemmati-Brivanlou A, Melton DA. Inhibition of activin receptor signaling promotes neutralization in *Xenopus*. *Cell* 1994;77:273–281.

54. Hemmati-Brivanlou A, Kelly OG, Melton DA. Follistatin, an antagonist of activin, is expressed in the Spemann organizer and displays direct neutralizing activity. *Cell* 1994;77:283–295.

55. Mathews LS, Vale WW. Expression cloning of an activin receptor, a predicted transmembrane serine kinase. *Cell* 1991;65:973–982.

56. Tsuchida K, Mathews LS, Vale WW. Cloning and characterization of a transmembrane serine kinase that acts as an active type I receptor. *Proc Natl Acad Sci USA* 1993;90:11242–11246.

57. Mathews LS, Vale WW, Kintner CR. Cloning of a second type of activin receptor and functional characterization in *Xenopus* embryos. *Science* 1992;255:1702–1705.

58. Attisano L, Wrana JL, Cheifetz S, et al. Novel activin receptors: distinct genes and alternative mRNA splicing generate a repertoire of serine/threonine kinase receptors. *Cell* 1992;68:97–108.

59. Attisano L, Carcamo J, Ventura F, et al. Identification of human activin and TGF beta type I receptors that form heteromeric kinase complexes with type II receptors. *Cell* 1993;75:671–680.

60. Carcamo J, Weis FM, Ventura F, et al. Type I receptors specify growth-inhibitory and transcriptional responses to transforming growth factor β and activin. *Mol Cell Biol* 1994;14:3810–3821.

61. Tsuchida K, Vaughan JM, Wiater E, et al. Inactivation of activin-dependent transcription by kinase-deficient activin receptors. *Endocrinology* 1995;136:5493–5503.

62. Wrana JL, Attisano L, Wieser R, et al. Mechanism of activation of the TGF-beta receptor. *Nature* 1994;370:341–347.

63. Attisano L, Wrana JL, Montalvo E, et al. Activation of signaling by the activin receptor complex. *Mol Cell Biol* 1996;16:1066–1073.

64. Hemmati-Brivanlou A, Melton DA. A truncated activin receptor inhibits mesoderm induction and formation of axial structures in *Xenopus* embryos. *Nature* 1992;359:609–614.

65. Wieser R, Wrana JL, Massagué J. GS domain mutations that constitutively activate TβR-I, the downstream signaling component in the TGF-β receptor complex. *EMBO J* 1995;14:2199–2208.

66. Massagué J. TGFβ signaling: receptors, transducers, and Mad proteins. *Cell* 1996;85:947–950.

67. Savage C, Das P, Finelli AL, et al. *Caenorhabditis elegans* genes sma-2, sma-3, and sma-4 define a conserved family of transforming growth factor beta pathway components. *Proc Natl Acad Sci USA* 1996;93:790–794.

68. Wang T, Li B-Y, Danielson PD, et al. The immunophilin FKBP12 functions as a common inhibitor of the TGFβ family type I receptors. *Cell* 1996;86:435–444.

69. Okadome T, Oeda E, Saitoh M, et al. Characterization of the interaction of FKBP12 with the transforming growth factor-β type I receptor *in vivo*. *J Biol Chem* 1996;271:21687–21690.

70. Yamaguchi K, Shirakabe K, Shibuya H, et al. Identification of a member of the MAPKKK family as a potential mediator of TGFβ signal transduction. *Science* 1995;270:2008–2011.

71. Hashimoto M, Gaddy-Kurten D, Vale W. Protooncogene junB as a target for activin actions. *Endocrinology* 1993;133:1934–1940.

72. Robertson DM, Klein R, de Vos FL, et al. The isolation of polypeptides with FSH suppressing activity from bovine follicular fluid which are structurally different to inhibin. *Biochem Biophys Res Commun* 1987;149:744–749.

73. Shimasaki S, Koga M, Esch F, et al. Porcine follistatin gene structure supports two forms of mature follistatin produced by alternative splicing. *Biochem Biophys Res Commun* 1988;152:717–723.

74. Shimasaki S, Koga M, Esch F, et al. Primary structure of the human follistatin precursor and its genomic organization. *Proc Natl Acad Sci USA* 1988;85:4218–4222.

75. Yokoyama Y, Nakamura T, Nakamura R, et al. Identification of activins and follistatin proteins in human follicular fluid and placenta. *J Clin Endocrinol Metab* 1995;80:915–921.

76. Fukui A, Nakamura T, Sugino K, et al. Isolation and characterization of *Xenopus* follistatin and activins. *Dev Biol* 1993;159:131–139.

77. Sugino K, Kurosawa N, Nakamura T, et al. Molecular heterogeneity of follistatin, an activin-binding protein: higher affinity of the carboxyl-terminal truncated forms for heparan sulfate proteoglycans on the ovarian granulosa cell. *J Biol Chem* 1993;268:15579–15587.

78. Nakamura T, Hasegawa Y, Sugino K, et al. Follistatin inhibits activin-induced differentiation of rat follicular granulosa cells *in vitro*. *Biochem Biophys Acta* 1992;1135:103–109.

79. Hashimoto M, Shoda A, Inouye S, et al. Functional regulation of osteoblastic cells by the interaction of activin A with follistatin. *J Biol Chem* 1992;267:4999–5004.

80. Asashima M, Nakano H, Uchiyama H, et al. Follistatin inhibits the mesoderm-inducing activity of activin A and the vegetalizing factor from chicken embryo. *Roux Arch Dev Biol* 1991;200:4–7.

81. Xiao S, Findlay JK. Interactions between activin and FSH suppressing protein and their mechanisms of action on cultured rat granulosa cells. *Mol Cell Endocrinol* 1991;79:99–107.

82. Mather JP, Roberts PE, Krummen LA. Follistatin modulates activin activity in a cell- and tissue-specific manner. *Endocrinology* 1993;132:2732–2734.

83. Krummen LA, Woodruff TK, DeGuzman G, et al. Identification and characterization of binding proteins for inhibin and activin in human serum and follicular fluids. *Endocrinology* 1993;132:431–443.

84. Vaughan JM, Vale WW. α_2-Macroglobulin is a binding protein of inhibin and activin. *Endocrinology* 1993;132:2038–2050.

85. Iemura S, Yamamoto TS, Takagi C, et al. Direct binding of follistatin to a complex of bone-morphogenetic protein and its receptor inhibits ventral and epidermal cell fates in early *Xenopus* embryo. *Proc Natl Acad Sci USA* 1998;95:9337–9342.

86. Nakamura T, Sugino K, Titani K, et al. Follistatin, an activin-binding protein, associates with heparan sulfate chains of proteoglycans on follicular granulosa cells. *J Biol Chem* 1991;266:19432–19437.

87. Inouye S, Guo Y, DePaolo L, et al. Recombinant expression of human follistatin with 315 and 288 amino acids: chemical and biological comparison with native porcine follistatin. *Endocrinology* 1991;129:815–822.

88. de Winter JP, ten Dijke P, de Vries CJ, et al. Follistatins neutralize activin bioactivity by inhibition of activin binding to its type II receptors. *Mol Cell Endocrinol* 1996;116:105–114.

89. Hashimoto O, Nakamura T, Shoji H, et al. A novel role of follistatin, an activin-binding protein, in the inhibition of activin action in rat pituitary cells: endocytotic degradation of activin and its acceleration by follistatin associated with cell-surface heparan sulfate. *J Biol Chem* 1997;272:13835–13842.

Skeletal Growth Factors,
edited by Ernesto Canalis.
Lippincott Williams & Wilkins, Philadelphia, © 2000.

18

Activin, Follistatin, and Bone

Masayuki Funaba, *Kenji Ogawa, †Takuya Murata, and Matanobu Abe

Department of Nutrition, Azabu University School of Veterinary Medicine, Sagamihara, Japan
°Laboratory Animal Research Center, The Institute of Physical and Chemical Research (RIKEN),
Wako, Japan
†Department of Physiology, Fukui Medical University, Matsuoka, Japan

Activins, dimeric proteins composed of inhibin β subunits, were originally purified from ovarian follicular fluids as stimulators of follicle-stimulating hormone (FSH) secretion from the pituitary. Subsequently, activins have also been purified based on different biological activities, including erythroid differentiation and mesoderm induction in *Xenopus laevis*. In addition, activin β transcripts have been shown to be widely distributed throughout the body. Therefore, at present, activins are believed to be local factors regulating cell proliferation and differentiation, rather than classical hormones (1).

Follistatin, originally purified from follicular fluids as an inhibitor of FSH secretion, neutralizes multiple biological effects of activins by binding with them and preventing activin–receptor interaction. Similar to activins, follistatin is expressed not only in the gonads but also in many other tissues; therefore, follistatin regulates the local action of activins negatively (1).

Activins have been expected to be involved in bone modeling and remodeling since their discovery, based on structural similarity to transforming growth factor-β (TGF-β) and related bone morphogenetic proteins (BMPs). However, because of much weaker activin activity than TGF-β activity on protein synthesis in osteoblasts (2) and because of the limited availability of activins, knowledge of the roles of activins in skeletal tissues is clearly less developed than for TGF-βs and BMPs. Nevertheless, activin β_A transcript is expressed in the skeletal tissue (3),

and activin A, the homodimer of the inhibin β_A subunit, has been purified from bone matrix (4). In addition, type II activin receptor–deficient mice exhibited abnormal cartilage formation (defects in Meckel's cartilage) (5). Furthermore, absence of whiskers and incisors and defects in the formation of the secondary palate were observed in activin β_A-deficient mice (6) and abnormal development of the whiskers was also evident in follistatin-deficient mice (7).

All of these findings suggest a significant role of activins in skeletal tissue. In this chapter, accumulating evidence on the expression of activin, activin receptors, and follistatin is summarized and possible effects of activin on skeletal tissue are described.

EXPRESSION OF ACTIVIN SIGNALING MOLECULES IN BONE

Activin

Roberts et al. (3) first discovered the expression of activins in skeletal tissue by *in situ* hybridization. They showed that during rat embryogenesis activin β_A transcript was detected in the developing skeleton of the snout and the limbs after 14 days post coitum (the time corresponding to chondrogenesis and subsequent osteogenesis), suggesting that activin A is expressed during endochondral bone development. Indeed, activin β_A mRNA was detected in cultured chondrocytes (M. Funaba, K. Ogawa, and

M. Abe, unpublished observation). In addition, immunoreactive activin β_A was localized in proliferating chondrocytes during endochondral bone development ectopically induced by implantation of demineralized bone matrix, suggesting that chondrocytes can produce activin (8).

Activin β_A expression has also been demonstrated in bone as well as in cartilage. Round osteoblasts during the initial stage of osteogenesis in ectopically induced endochondral bone are immunohistochemically activin A-positive (8). In addition, immunoreactive activin A molecules were detected in osteoblasts located in intramembranous ossification during fracture repair (9), and cultured osteoblasts prepared from fetal rat calvaria formed by intramembranous ossification expressed activin β_A mRNA (M. Funaba, K. Ogawa, and M. Abe, unpublished observation). Furthermore, activin protein was detected in culture medium of osteoblast-enriched bone marrow cell culture (10).

Activin A was also detected by antibody staining in tartrate-resistant acid phosphatase (TRAP)-positive multinucleated cells in fetal mouse calvaria culture, suggesting that osteoclasts are also activin A-positive cells (11). However, it is not clear whether osteoclasts produce activin A or whether these molecules reflect products resorbed by osteoclasts.

Activin Receptors and Downstream Signaling Molecules

Similar to the other members of the TGF-β superfamily, activins signal through the sequential activation of two cell surface receptors (type I and type II), both of which are transmembrane serine/threonine protein kinases. Activin binds to type II receptor, resulting in the recruitment of type I receptor into the ligand–receptor complex. Following complex formation, type II receptor phosphorylates type I receptor at a specific glycine/serine-rich site; that phosphorylation is required for intracellular signaling to occur (12,13). At present, two activin type II receptors (ActRII and ActRIIB) and two activin type I receptors (ActRI and ActRIB) are known. However, the type II receptors can bind BMPs

as well as activins and are apparently involved in BMP signaling (14). In addition, ActRI has been shown to function as a BMP type I receptor rather than an activin type I receptor in assays using a synthetic reporter (15), although overexpressed ActRI can form complexes with activin and ActRII (16). Under physiological conditions, precise receptor specificity in activin signaling pathways is not definitive.

Centrella et al. (2) first indicated that activin receptors were expressed in bone cells. They revealed two classes of activin A-binding site (K_d = 0.4 nM and 40 to 50 nM) in cultured osteoblasts from fetal rat parietal bone. In view of the high affinity of activin for ActRII and ActRIIB (K_d = 0.1 to 0.5 nM) (17), the activin binding sites in bone with higher affinity may be type II activin receptors. Activin receptors with higher affinity (K_d = 0.26 nM) were also detected in an osteoblastic cell line, MC3T3-L1 (18). Interestingly, excess TGF-β1 competed with activin A for binding to receptors in osteoblasts (2), although TGF-β had no effect on activin binding to overexpressed activin receptors (17).

Shuto et al. (19) investigated expression of specific activin receptors in skeletal tissue by immunohistochemistry. They showed that ActRII was localized in osteoblasts during both intramembranous and endochondral bone development in the tibia. Activin receptor expression in cartilage during endochondral bone development has not been analyzed, although cultured chondrocytes express ActRI, ActRIB, ActRII, and ActRIIB mRNAs (M. Funaba, K. Ogawa, and M. Abe, unpublished observation) and hypertrophic chondrocytes in pathological ectopic ossified tissue of the paravertebral ligament were ActRI-positive (20). Expression of activin receptors during fracture healing has been reported by Shuto et al. (19) and Nagamine et al. (9): at the mRNA level, expression of ActRI and ActRII increased during rapid intramembranous bone development and initiation of endochondral bone development (19); at the protein level, proliferating and mature chondrocytes and osteoblasts were ActRI-, ActRIB-, ActRII-, and ActRIIB-positive (9).

Type I activin receptors phosphorylated by type II activin receptors transmit the signal downstream. Recent findings indicate that a series of Smad proteins mediates of activin signals; receptor-regulated Smads 2 and 3 are phosphorylated by type I activin receptors, resulting in nuclear translocation and participation in transcriptional activation of activin-induced genes in cooperation with Smad4 (13). Smad2/3 expression in the skeletal tissue is largely unknown, except for a report that Smad2 mRNA was barely detectable in rat osteosarcoma ROS17/2.8 cells (21).

EXPRESSION OF FOLLISTATIN IN BONE

Hashimoto et al. (18) first revealed the expression of follistatin in bone cells. They detected follistatin mRNA in osteoblastic cells and secretion of follistatin protein into the medium. Follistatin expression also changed in a cell stage–specific manner. In undifferentiated osteoblasts, follistatin expression was higher than in differentiated osteoblasts, suggesting that multiple activin functions may be regulated by changing expression of follistatin. This suggestion was consistent with changes in expression of follistatin during endochondral bone development; during the initial stages of chondrogenesis and osteogenesis, immunoreactive follistatin was strongly detected in proliferating chondrocytes and osteoblasts, while hypertrophic chondrocytes and osteoblasts surrounding bone marrow were follistatin-negative (8). Inoue et al. (22) also observed follistatin expression in osteoblasts by *in situ* hybridization and immunohistochemistry. Furthermore, chondrocytes and osteoblasts during endochondral and intramembranous ossification after fracture were also follistatin-positive (9).

Follistatin produced by osteoblasts may also accumulate in the bone matrix. Follistatin content in demineralized bone matrix was higher in younger rats (10 weeks old) than in older rats (6 months old) (23).

FUNCTION OF ACTIVIN AND FOLLISTATIN IN THE CARTILAGE

Activin has been shown to have chondrogenic effects in cultured chondrocytes. In chick limb bud cell cultures, activin A increased amounts of proteoglycan (24). In addition, Luyten et al. (25) observed increased synthesis of sulfated proteoglycans and type II collagen by activin A treatment in articular chondrocyte culture.

Exogenous activin also resulted in increased cartilage formation *in vivo*. When activin A was locally injected near the ectopic implants of demineralized bone matrix during the initial stage of chondrogenesis, the content of C propeptide of type II procollagen was increased and cartilaginous area was enlarged (8). In view of higher expression of follistatin during this period, these findings suggest that activin A has a stimulatory effect on cartilage formation and that chondrogenesis is controlled by changing expression of follistatin. Thus, the net effect of activin is altered by the ratio of local activin to follistatin at the site of chondrogenesis.

FUNCTION OF ACTIVIN AND FOLLISTATIN IN THE BONE

In vitro studies using osteoblast-enriched cultures and osteoblastic cells revealed that activin A increased cellular replication (2,18) and synthesis of collagen as well as noncollagen protein (2). To investigate the role of activin in bone formation *in vivo*, Ogawa et al. (4) used an ectopic bone induction model based on implantation of collagen/ceramic carrier with activin A. These studies revealed that activin A itself had no ability to induce bone development but enhanced bone formation induced by BMPs. Interestingly, implants containing the combination of activin A and BMPs exhibited the presence of well-developed bone with minimal levels of cartilage, whereas an abundance of cartilaginous structures was seen in implants of the combination of TGF-β2 and BMPs. *In vivo* activin effects on bone formation were also examined by Oue et al. (26). They injected activin A onto the periosteum of parietal bone in newborn rats and found increases in bone matrix thickness and alkaline phosphatase–positive osteoblastic cells. All of these findings suggest stimulatory effects of activin for both endochondral and intramembranous ossification. However, activin A was approximately 500-fold less potent than TGF-β1 for *in vitro* bone matrix protein synthesis (2). In addition, stimulation of intramembranous ossification by activin A injection was much weaker than that by TGF-β1 injection (26). Therefore, the physiological significance of activin for bone modeling and remodeling remains to be clarified.

Follistatin binds activin with high affinity (K_d = 0.6 nM), and TGF-β does not compete with activin for binding to follistatin (27). Therefore, to evaluate the physiological role of activin during bone formation, examining the effect of follistatin administration may be effective. In bone marrow cell culture, mineralized osteoblast colony formation was decreased by follistatin addition when activin protein was measured in the medium. These data suggest that activin may be involved in commitment of osteoblast progeni-

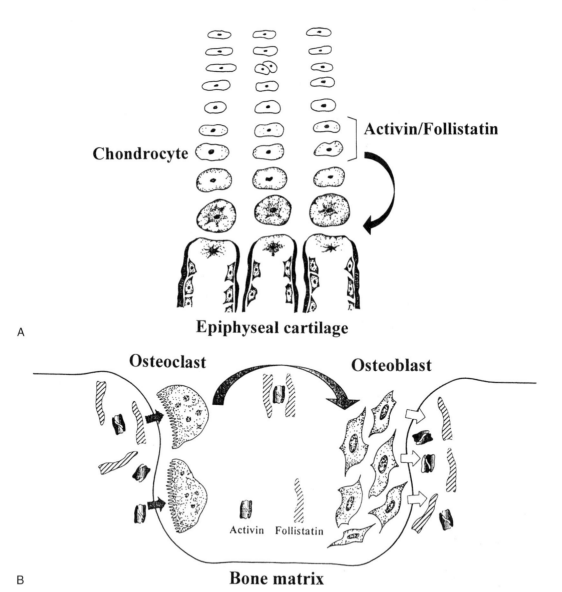

FIG. 18.1. Activin and follistatin in bone modeling and remodeling. Both activin and follistatin are locally produced and involved in the regulation of progression of endochondral bone modeling **(a)** and turnover of bone **(b).**

tors to differentiated osteoblasts (28). Ectopic implantation of demineralized bone matrix with added follistatin resulted in lower bone formation (23). Furthermore, local injections of follistatin near the ectopic implants of demineralized bone matrix during the conversion from cartilage to bone of endochondral ossification, the period of lower follistatin expression, resulted in an abundance of cartilage and lower deposition of calcium, suggesting a role for activin as a positive regulator of conversion of cartilage to bone (8). Recent evidence demonstrates that follistatin can bind to BMP-4 with lower affinity (K_d = 23 nM) than to activin (29). These findings collectively suggest that activins have a stimulatory effect on bone formation, probably in cooperation with the related proteins.

Osteoclasts are believed to be derived from the monocytic lineage (30), and activin is produced by bone marrow cells and has the ability to induce the monocytic differentiation of HL-60 cells (31). Therefore, activin may have some effect on osteoclast formation. Sakai et al. (32) and, more recently, Gaddy-Kurten et al. (33) revealed that activin A enhanced formation of TRAP-positive multinucleated cells in bone marrow cell culture. However, considering that activin A treatment had no effect on bone-resorbing activity *in vitro* (32), the role of activin in bone resorption remains to be clarified.

CONCLUSIONS

Expression of activin, its receptors, and its antagonizing binding protein in skeletal tissue indicates that this signaling system may be involved in bone modeling and remodeling in an autocrine/paracrine manner under the regulation of follistatin (Fig. 18.1). In addition, considering that inhibin can compete with activin for binding to activin receptors (17), circulating inhibins are also likely to be involved in the activin/follistatin regulatory system. Indeed, inhibin treatment of bone marrow cultures has recently been shown to block both osteoblast and osteoclast development (10). To understand the overall function, mechanism, and regulation of activins in skeletal tissues, both *in vivo* and *in*

vitro studies are needed; such approaches should provide greater insight into the significance of the activin/follistatin regulatory system not only in skeletal tissue but also in nonskeletal tissue.

ACKNOWLEDGMENTS

The authors are grateful to D. Gaddy-Kurten, L. S. Mathews, A. Abe, and C. M. Zimmerman for comments on the manuscript.

REFERENCES

1. Vale W, Hsueh A, Rivier C, et al. The inhibin/activin family of hormones and growth factors. In: Sporn MA, Roberts AB, eds. *Peptide growth factors and their receptors.* Berlin: Springer-Verlag, 1990:211–248.
2. Centrella M, McCarthy TL, Canalis E. Activin-A binding and biochemical effects in osteoblast-enriched cultures from fetal-rat parietal bone. *Mol Cell Biol* 1991; 11:250–258.
3. Roberts VJ, Sawchenko PE, Vale W. Expression of inhibin/activin subunit messenger ribonucleic acids during rat embryogenesis. *Endocrinology* 1991;128:3122–3129.
4. Ogawa Y, Schmidt DK, Nathan RM, et al. Bovine bone activin enhances bone morphogenetic protein–induced ectopic bone formation. *J Biol Chem* 1992;267:14233–14237.
5. Matzuk MM, Kumar TR, Bradley A. Different phenotypes for mice deficient in either activins or activin receptor type II. *Nature* 1995;374:356–360.
6. Matzuk MM, Kumar TR, Vassalli A, et al. Functional analysis of activins during mammalian development. *Nature* 1995;374:354–356.
7. Matzuk MM, Lu N, Vogel H, et al. Multiple defects and perinatal death in mice deficient in follistatin. *Nature* 1995;374:360–363.
8. Funaba M, Ogawa K, Murata T, et al. Follistatin and activin in bone: expression and localization during endochondral bone development. *Endocrinology* 1996;137:4250–4259.
9. Nagamine T, Imamura T, Ishidou Y, et al. Immunohistochemical detection of activin A, follistatin, and activin receptors during fracture healing in the rat. *J Orthop Res* 1998;16:314–321.
10. Coker JK, Ballew CB, Jilka RL, et al. Inhibin and activin exert opposing effects on osteoblastogenesis and osteoclastogenesis. In: *Program of the 80th Annual Meeting of The Endocrine Society, New Orleans, LA.* 1998:103.
11. Hosoi T, Inoue S, Hoshino S, et al. Immunohistochemical detection of activin A in osteoclasts. *Gerontology* 1996;42(Suppl):20–24.
12. Gaddy-Kurten D, Tsuchida K, Vale W. Activins and the receptor serine kinase superfamily. *Recent Prog Horm Res* 1995;50:109–129.
13. Massagué J. TGF-β signal transduction. *Annu Rev Biochem* 1998;67:753–791.
14. Yamashita H, ten Dijke P, Huylebroeck D, et al. Osteogenic protein-1 binds to activin type II receptors and induces certain activin-like effects. *J Cell Biol* 1995; 130:217–226.

15. Macías-Silva M, Hoodless PA, Tang SJ, et al. Specific activation of Smad1 signaling pathways by the BMP7 type I receptor, ALK2. *J Biol Chem* 1998;273:25628–25636.

16. Tsuchida K, Mathews LS, Vale WW. Cloning and characterization of a transmembrane serine kinase that acts as an activin type I receptor. *Proc Natl Acad Sci USA* 1993;90:11242–11246.

17. Mathews LS. Activin receptors and cellular signaling by the receptor serine kinase family. *Endocr Rev* 1994;15:310–325.

18. Hashimoto M, Shoda A, Inoue S, et al. Functional regulation of osteoblastic cells by the interaction of activin-A with follistatin. *J Biol Chem* 1992;267:4999–5004.

19. Shuto T, Sarkar G, Bronk JT, et al. Osteoblasts express types I and II activin receptors during early intramembranous and endochondral bone formation. *J Bone Miner Res* 1997;12:403–411.

20. Yonemori K, Imamura T, Ishidou Y, et al. Bone morphogenetic protein receptors and activin receptors are highly expressed in ossification of the posterior longitudinal ligament. *Am J Pathol* 1997;150:1335–1347.

21. Li J, Tsuji K, Komori T, et al. Smad2 overexpression enhances Smad4 gene expression and suppresses CBFA1 gene expression in osteoblastic osteosarcoma ROS17/2.8 cells and primary rat calvaria cells. *J Biol Chem* 1998;273:31009–31015.

22. Inoue S, Nomura S, Hosoi T, et al. Localization of follistatin, an activin-binding protein, in bone tissues. *Calcif Tissue Int* 1994;55:395–397.

23. Funaba M, Murata T, Murata E, et al. Suppressed bone induction by follistatin in spontaneously hypercholesterolemic rat bone. *Life Sci* 1997;61:653–658.

24. Jiang T-X, Yi J-R, Ying S-Y, et al. Activin enhances chondrogenesis of limb bud cells: stimulation of precartilaginous mesenchymal condensations and expression of NCAM. *Dev Biol* 1993;155:545–557.

25. Luyten FP, Chen P, Paralkar V, et al. Recombinant bone morphogenetic protein-4, transforming growth factor-β1, and activin A enhance the cartilage phenotype of articular chondrocytes *in vitro*. *Exp Cell Res* 1994;210:224–229.

26. Oue T, Kanatani H, Kiyoki M, et al. Effect of local injection of activin A on bone formation in newborn rats. *Bone* 1994;15:361–366.

27. Nakamura T, Takio K, Eto Y, et al. Activin-binding protein from rat ovary is follistatin. *Science* 1990;247:836–838.

28. Gaddy-Kurten D, Coker JK, Vaughan JM, et al. Attenuation of osteoblastogenesis in the murine bone marrow by inhibin and follistatin: evidence for distinct effects at different stages of the process. *J Bone Miner Res* 1997;12:S305.

29. Iemura S, Yamamoto TS, Takagi C, et al. Direct binding of follistatin to a complex of bone-morphogenetic protein and its receptor inhibits ventral and epidermal cell fates in early *Xenopus* embryo. *Proc Natl Acad Sci USA* 1998;95:9337–9342.

30. Suda T, Udagawa N, Nakamura I, et al. Modulation of osteoclast differentiation by local factors. *Bone* 1995;17:87S–91S.

31. Yamada R, Suzuki T, Hashimoto M, et al. Induction of differentiation of the human promyelocytic cell line HL-60 by activin/EDF. *Biochem Biophys Res Commun* 1992;187:79–85.

32. Sakai R, Eto Y, Ohtsuka M, et al. Activin enhances osteoclast-like cell formation *in vitro*. *Biochem Biophys Res Commun* 1993;195:39–46.

33. Gaddy-Kurten D, Coker JK, Abe E, et al. Activin substitutes for the BMP2/4 requirement for, and the noggin inhibition of, osteoblastogenesis and osteoclastogenesis in adult murine bone marrow cultures. *J Bone Miner Res* 1998;13:S166.

Skeletal Growth Factors,
edited by Ernesto Canalis.
Lippincott Williams & Wilkins, Philadelphia, © 2000.

19

Bone Morphogenetic Proteins

Masahiro Kawabata and Kohei Miyazono

*Department of Biochemistry, The Cancer Institute, Japanese Foundation for Cancer Research,
Tokyo, Japan*

Bone morphogenetic proteins (BMPs) are secreted polypeptides that exert pleiotropic effects on a variety of lineages of cells. BMPs were originally identified as inducers of bone and cartilage formation in ectopic tissues (1–3), which has given rise to the origin of the name. BMPs regulate growth and differentiation of chondroblasts and osteoblasts. In addition, BMPs are involved in the determination of the fate of other mesenchymal cells, epithelial cells, neuronal cells, and neural crest cells. Various types of cell line, including multipotent progenitor cells, osteoprogenitor cells, osteoblasts, and chondroblasts, have been used to characterize the actions of BMPs (4). BMPs belong to the transforming growth factor-β (TGF-β) superfamily, which includes TGF-βs, activins, and inhibins (5). BMP-related factors account for nearly two-thirds of the whole TGF-β superfamily, which contains over 40 members. BMPs play a pivotal role in the maintenance of homeostasis of organisms, and perturbation of the BMP signaling pathway results in the incipience of various disorders ranging from abnormal morphogenesis of specific organs to embryonal lethality (4,6).

TGF-βs and activins are also pleiotropic growth and differentiation factors (GDFs) that possess activities distinct from those of BMPs. Activins and TGF-βs share similar biological effects, suggesting that these two subfamilies are evolutionarily close. BMPs and activins do not usually compete with each other, although in the development of *Xenopus* embryos they play an opposite role. Activins induce the dorsal meso-derm, whereas BMPs induce the ventral mesoderm of the embryo. The *Xenopus* embryo has, therefore, proved to be a useful system to dissect BMP and activin signals (6). BMPs also inhibit the neural induction of ectodermal cells and convert the cell fate to epidermis in *Xenopus* embryos.

BMPs also have been termed osteogenic protein (OP), cartilage-derived morphogenetic protein (CDMP), and GDF. The terminology of various BMP-related ligands is summarized in Table 19.1. The BMP family comprises BMP-2 to BMP-15. BMP-1 was isolated together with BMP-2, BMP-3, and BMP-4 but does not belong to the TGF-β superfamily since it has different biological activities. BMP-1 is a protease of the astacin family, which cleaves procollagen and induces extracellular matrix deposition (7). BMPs have been identified in various organisms, including invertebrates such as *Drosophila* and *Caenorhabditis elegans*. Decapentaplegic (Dpp) is a BMP-2/4 homologue in *Drosophila*. While BMP-4 rescues defects in the *dpp* gene in *Drosophila* (8), Dpp induces bone formation in mammalian tissues (9), indicating that BMP homologues are functionally interchangeable between vertebrates and invertebrates and that the BMP signaling pathway is conserved between the two distantly related organisms (10,11).

BMPs are secreted as immature precursor proteins and dimerize through a single interchain disulfide bond, followed by subsequent proteolytic cleavage at a characteristic Arg-X-X-Arg consensus site. Seven cysteines are conserved

TABLE 19.1. *Terminology of bone morphogenetic protein (BMP)–related ligands*

BMP	OP	GDF	Others
BMP-1			—[2]
BMP-2			
BMP-3			Osteogenin
BMP-3b		GDF-10	
BMP-4			BMP-2b
BMP-5			
BMP-6			Vgr-1
BMP-7	OP-1		
BMP-8a	OP-2		
BMP-8b	OP-3		
BMP-9			
BMP-10			
BMP-11			
BMP-12		GDF-7	
BMP-13		GDF-6	CDMP-2[c]
BMP-15		GDF-9b	
		GDF-1	
		GDF-3	Vgr-2
		GDF-5	CDMP-1
		GDF-8	Myostatin
		GDF-9	
			Nodal

[a] OP, osteogenic protein
[2] procollagen C-proteinase
[b] CDMP, cartilage-derived morphogenetic protein
GDF, growth and differentiation factors.

among most BMPs, and the overall structure of the mature protein is determined by the invariable spacing of these cysteines. One of these cysteines is involved in the formation of the interchain disulfide bond, as revealed by the crystal structures of TGF-β2 and BMP-7 (12–14). The core of the monomeric structure is a cysteine knot. BMPs bind to a complex of two distinct types of transmembrane receptor with serine-threonine kinase activity. Upon ligand binding, the activated receptors phosphorylate Smad proteins, which serve as intracellular signal mediators. Smads translocate into the nucleus and regulate the expression of target genes in concert with other transcription factors and coactivators (15–17). In this chapter, the nature of each member of the BMP family is first described, with emphasis on the roles *in vivo,* followed by a description of the BMP signaling pathway.

BONE MORPHOGENETIC PROTEINS

Almost 30 members of the BMP family have been identified, and they are further classified into several subgroups based on their structural similarity (Fig. 19.1). Many of the members of the BMP family exert a specific function *in vivo,* and the specificity may be caused by the temporal and spatial expression pattern of the factor in addition to the signaling property of its cognate receptor.

Bone Morphogenetic Proteins 2 and 4

The expression pattern of BMP-2 was examined in mouse by *in situ* hybridization (18–20). In early mouse embryogenesis (days 7.5 to 9.5 of gestation), BMP-2 is expressed in the extra-embryonic mesoderm and promyocardium. At later stages, BMP-2 is expressed in mesenchymal cells in the developing skeletal system, developing limb buds, myocardium, whisker follicles, tooth buds, craniofacial mesenchyme, and other sites. In accordance with the expression pattern, mice deficient in BMP-2 die between day 7.0 and 10.5 from defects in the amnion/chorion and in cardiac development (20). Thus, BMP-2 plays a pivotal role in early development. BMP-2 induces alkaline phosphatase (ALP) activity, one of the markers of osteoblastic differentiation, and collagen synthesis in the MC3T3-E1 osteoblastic cell line (21). BMP-2 also induces early-phase differentiation of ATDC5 chondrogenic cells and inhibits the terminal differentiation of C2C12 myoblasts, converting these into cells of the osteoblast lineage (22,23). Although the molecular target of BMP-2 in the induction of osteoblastic differentiation is not yet known, it inhibits myoblastic differentiation in C2C12 cells by suppressing the transcriptional activity of myogenic factors, such as MyoD and myogenin (24).

BMP-2 and BMP-4, formerly BMP-2b, are 92% identical in the amino acid sequence at the carboxy-terminal region. The earliest expression by day 7.5 of BMP-4 in mice is detected around the time of gastrulation (day 6.5), and BMP-4 is localized in the allantois, amnion, and posterior primitive streak (25,26). Expression is maintained in these regions until day 9 and is also seen in the mesoderm around the hindgut and foregut and in the ventral lateral mesoderm of the posterior body wall and gut. As development

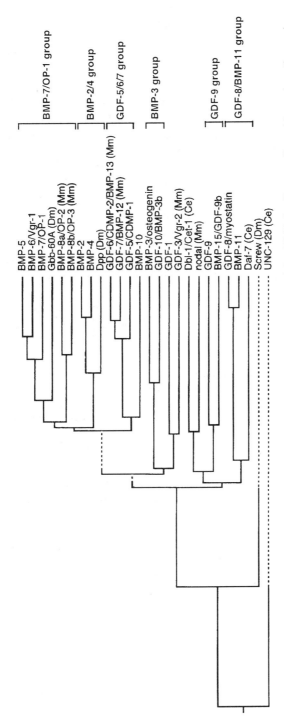

FIG. 19.1. Members of the bone morphogenetic protein (BMP) family. Members of the BMP family are aligned based on the amino acid sequence of the mature region using the Clustal method of DNASTAR. Human, mouse (*Mm*), *Drosophila* (*Dm*), and *Caenorhabditis elegans* (*Ce*) BMPs are presented.

proceeds, expression becomes localized to more specific regions, such as the myocardium, brachial arches, optic vesicle, and diencephalon. In later embryos, BMP-4 is expressed where epithelial–mesenchymal interaction occurs, such as whisker follicles and tooth buds. In addition, BMP-4 is detected in the mesoderm and apical ectodermal ridge of the limb bud. Homozygous BMP-4 null embryos die between days 6.5 and 9.5, with a variable phenotype (26). Most mutant embryos fail to undergo gastrulation and mesoderm formation. Some homozygous mutants have developed to the early somite state or beyond. However, they are developmentally delayed and have truncated or disorganized posterior structures and a reduction in extraembryonic mesoderm. The phenotype of BMP-4 deficiency depends on the genetic background of mice. *Gli3* and *Alx4* were identified as genes that enhance the penetrance and expressivity of polydactyly in BMP-4 heterozygotes (27). BMP-4 is also required for lens induction (28).

Although BMP-2 and BMP-4 are structurally similar and their function *in vitro* is nearly identical, the results of gene disruptive experiments demonstrated that their roles *in vivo* are nonredundant. The roles of BMP-2 and BMP-4 in osteogenesis *in vivo* have not been clarified by gene knockout due to the early death of these animals. In a bone fracture model using mice, BMP-4 was shown to be transiently expressed in less-differentiated osteoprogenitor cells but not in differentiated osteoblasts in the early phase of fracture healing (29); however, osteoblasts from rat calvariae express BMP-2 and BMP-4 *in vitro* (30).

Bone Morphogenetic Protein-7/OP-1 and Related Proteins

BMP-7, or osteogenic protein-1 (OP-1), has been identified as a potent osteogenic factor (31,32). *In situ* hybridization shows that BMP-7/OP-1 is detected earliest in gastrulating embryos and expressed throughout development at diverse sites, including kidneys and eyes, where inductive interactions of different tissues determine the patterning (33). BMP-7/OP-1 is coex-

pressed with BMP-2 in a number of tissues, raising the possibility that BMP-2/7 heterodimers may be the actual ligand at these sites. BMP-7/OP-1-deficient mice die shortly after birth because of poor kidney development. The mice also exhibit eye defects and skeletal patterning defects restricted to the rib cage, the skull, and the hindlimbs (34–36). This phenotype is remarkably different from that of BMP-2 and BMP-4 knockout mice. BMP-7/OP-1 and BMPs 2 and 4 share many biochemical functions, although they have different affinities to specific combinations of receptors. This may explain the different phenotypes of deficient mice but at the molecular level awaits further investigation. Intercrosses of different BMP knockout mice were made to address the possible functional redundancy of BMPs (37). Heterozygous compound mutants of BMP-4 and BMP-7/OP-1 developed minor bone defects in the rib cage and the distal part of the limbs, whereas BMP-2/7 and BMP-5/7 double heterozygous mutants did not present any abnormalities.

In limb development, BMPs play a crucial role. For example, they induce apoptosis in the interdigital mesoderm and remove these areas (38). In chick development, exogenously administered BMP-2 alters the joint shape, whereas exogenous BMP-7/OP-1 inhibits joint formation, although the reason for this difference is unclear (39). BMP-7/OP-1 was shown to induce both chondroblastic and osteoblastic differentiation of newborn rat calvaria-derived cells (40). A low dose of BMP-7/OP-1 induces adipocytic differentiation of C3H10T1/2 cells derived from mouse embryo connective tissue, whereas administration of high-dose BMP-7/OP-1 directed chondrocytic differentiation of the same cells (41).

Other members of the BMP-7/OP-1 subfamily include BMP-5, BMP-6/Vgr-1, BMP-8a/OP-2, and BMP-8b/OP-3. The naturally occurring mutant BMP-5 mouse (the *short ear* mouse) develops abnormalities in the skull and axial parts of the skeleton, such as ears, sternum, ribs, and vertebrate processes (42). BMP-5 is expressed at fibroblast condensations preceding normal skeletal development (day 13.5) and at the periphery of the developing skeletal elements, but the expression in ribs disappears by day 16.5 (43). In addition, BMP-5 is expressed in the soft tissues that are affected in the *short ear* mice. Most BMP-5 expression is in the mesenchymal cells surrounding or underlying an epithelial sheet. The different expression patterns of BMP-2, BMP-5, BMP-6/Vgr-1, and GDF-5 are discussed by King et al. (43). BMP-6/Vgr-1 is expressed in the nervous system and a variety of epithelial tissues including developing skin (18,25,44). BMP-6/Vgr-1 was suggested to regulate early osteoblast differentiation *in vitro* (45–47). Transgenic mice overexpressing BMP-6/Vgr-1 in the epidermis develop varying skin lesions depending on the expression level (48). Gene targeting of BMP-6/Vgr-1 results in no overt defects except for a delay in ossification of the sternum and suggests that BMP-2 may compensate for the loss of BMP-6/Vgr-1 (49). BMP-8a/OP-2 and BMP-8b/OP-3 are expressed in the testis, placenta, and hair follicles and BMP-8b/OP-3 is highly expressed in the decidual cells of the uterus (50). Targeted disruption of the BMP-8b/OP-3 gene results in male infertility due to defects in spermatogenesis (50). Similar to BMP-8b/OP-3, BMP-8a/OP-2 deficiency resulted in defects in the maintenance of spermatogenesis accompanied by germ cell degeneration (51). However, it remains unknown how these closely related factors play nonredundant roles.

Growth and Differentiation Factors 5, 6, and 7

Growth and differentiation factor 5 (GDF-5, also called CDMP-1) is structurally similar to GDF-6 (also called CDMP-2 and BMP-13) and GDF-7 (also called BMP-12), and these members constitute a distinct BMP subfamily. Mice with the mutation *brachypodism* exhibit short limbs and reduced numbers of bones in the digits, and GDF-5 was identified as the gene responsible for the mutation (52). GDF-5 was also isolated from cartilage as CDMP-1, which induces cartilage and bone formation when implanted subcutaneously in rats (53). CDMP-2 was isolated using a similar approach (53). GDF-5/CDMP-1 is expressed in a specific pattern of stripes in the developing limbs of mice

(54). The stripes correspond to the sites where joints will later form. Null mutations in GDF-5/CDMP-1 disrupt normal joint formation, leading to fusions between skeletal elements. The role of GDF-5/CDMP-1 in chick limb development was studied (55). Overexpression of GDF-5/CDMP-1 induced an increase of the skeletal mass. The actions of GDF-5/CDMP-1 were observed at both early and later stages of skeletal development. At an early stage, GDF-5/CDMP-1 increased mesenchymal condensation, probably due to enhancement of cell adhesion. At a later stage, GDF-5/CDMP-1 increased skeletal mass by promoting chondrocyte proliferation. Double knockout of GDF-5/CDMP-1 and BMP-5 caused additional abnormalities, not observed in either of the single mutants, indicating that BMPs have synergistic functions in the regulation of skeletal development (54).

In situ hybridization and immunostaining in human embryos showed that GDF-5/CDMP-1 is predominantly expressed at the sites of mesenchymal condensation of the developing long bones, whereas GDF-6/CDMP-2 expression is restricted to hypertrophic chondrocytes of ossifying long bones (53). Neither gene was detectable in axial skeleton. In accordance with the expression pattern, mutations in GDF-5/CDMP-1 in humans cause autosomal recessive chondrodysplasia, Hunter-Thompson type (CHTT) (56) and Grebe type (CGT) (57). CHTT patients exhibit phenotypes similar to those of the *brachypodism* mutant mice, that is, long-bone shortening, whereas their distal phalanges are relatively normal. CGT resembles CHTT; however, skeletal abnormalities in CGT are much more severe. CHTT is caused by a frameshift mutation, whereas CGT is caused by a missense mutation of the first of the seven highly conserved cysteines to a tyrosine. The CGT mutation creates dominant-negative GDF-5, which interferes with the secretion of other BMPs through the formation of nonfunctional heterodimers. More recently, it was shown that mutations in GDF-5/CDMP-1 cause brachydactyly type C that is autosomal dominant, suggesting the existence of haploinsufficiency of the GDF-5/CDMP-1 gene (58).

Transgenic mice overexpressing GDF-5/

CDMP-1 exhibit chondrodysplasia with an increase of the hypertrophic zone and a reduction of the proliferating chondrocyte zone (59). The results suggest that GDF-5/CDMP-1 promotes the recruitment of mesenchymal cells into the chondrogenic lineage and then accelerates differentiation of chondrocytes to hypertrophy. Using C2C12 cells, GDF-6/CDMP-2/BMP-13 and GDF-7/BMP-12 were shown to inhibit terminal differentiation of myoblasts, but in contrast to BMP-2, they did not induce osteoblastic differentiation (60). Ectopic expression of GDF-5/CDMP-1, GDF-6/CDMP-2/BMP-13, and GDF-7/BMP-12 was shown to induce tendon and ligament formation (61). GDF-7/BMP-12 is the only BMP family member expressed in the roof plate of the neural tube, and recent generation of GDF-7/BMP-12 null mice suggested its involvement in neuronal patterning in the spinal cord (62).

Other Related Proteins

GDF-3/Vgr-2 and GDF-9 were identified through polymerase chain reaction (PCR) homology screening of TGF-β-related polypeptides (63,64). Interestingly, both lacked the conserved cysteine that is involved in the interchain disulfide linkage. GDF-9 is expressed in oocytes and in the testis and hypothalamus in mice (65,66). Development of GDF-9 knockout mice and further characterization revealed that GDF-9 regulates ovarian folliculogenesis through bidirectional somatic cell–germ cell interactions (67,68). BMP-15 is closely related to GDF-9 and is also expressed in oocytes (69).

GDF-8/myostatin was isolated through PCR homology screening as well. GDF-8/myostatin is specifically expressed in skeletal muscles, and disruption of the GDF-8/myostatin gene results in increased muscle volume, suggesting that GDF-8/myostatin negatively regulates the growth of skeletal muscles (70). Furthermore, naturally occurring "double muscled" cattle were shown to have mutation in the GDF-8/myostatin gene (71–73).

BMP-3/osteogenin and BMP-3b/GDF-10 define a distinct BMP subgroup. In situ hybridization of mouse and human embryos showed that BMP-3/osteogenin is expressed in the neural ectoderm, bone matrix, perichondrium, periosteum, osteoblasts, lung bronchial epithelium, and kidney collecting tubules (74,75). BMP-3b/GDF-10 is expressed in bone, brain, and other tissues (76–78). BMP-9, which is similar to BMP-10, was shown to be expressed in developing mouse liver and to stimulate liver cell growth (79). GDF-1 is distantly related to Xenopus Vg-1, but its function in mammals remains to be determined (80). Nodal is required for the formation of the primitive streak during mouse gastrulation and has been implicated in the establishment of the left–right axis (81,82).

BONE MORPHOGENETIC PROTEIN IN INVERTEBRATES

In Drosophila, Dpp, Gbb-60A, and Screw (Scw) have been identified as BMP-related molecules (6). Of the BMP-like ligands in Drosophila, Dpp is best characterized, and genetic analyses of dpp phenotypes have greatly contributed to the elucidation of the mechanism of signaling by the TGF-β superfamily (83). Dpp was isolated as the first member of the BMP family (84). Dpp governs various important steps in Drosophila development. Dpp establishes the dorsal–ventral polarity of the Drosophila embryo, and, at later stages, it is required for gut formation and outgrowth and patterning of imaginal disks (11,83). Dpp belongs to the BMP-2/4 subfamily, whereas Gbb-60A is a Drosophila member of the BMP-7/OP-1 subfamily (Fig. 19.1). Both Dpp and Gbb-60A are required for the patterning of the Drosophila wing, and these two ligands may share common receptors (85). The greater divergence in the sequence of Scw from members of the BMP family suggests that the orthologue of Scw has not been identified in vertebrates. From genetic evidence, it was proposed that Drosophila Dpp and Scw might function as heterodimers (86).

The completion of the genome project of C. elegans has revealed that the worm has four ligands and three receptors in its TGF-β-related signaling pathway (87). Among the ligands, Daf-7 is distantly related to the GDF-8/myostatin and BMP-11 subfamily. The vertebrate homologue of UNC-129 has not been identified. Another as yet anonymous ligand is related to BMP-7/OP-1. Dbl-1/Cet-1 is involved in the Sma/Mab pathway (88), whereas Daf-7 mediates the dauer pathway (89). UNC-129 regulates axon guidance (90).

BONE MORPHOGENETIC PROTEIN HETERODIMERS

As mentioned previously, Scw may form heterodimers with Dpp (86). Coexpression and co-purification of different vertebrate BMPs also suggested that they may form heterodimers (33,91). Recombinant BMP-4/7, BMP-2/7, and BMP-2/6 heterodimers have stronger inductive and osteogenic activities than homodimers of either ligand (91–94). Recently, the possible formation of *Drosophila* Dpp/Gbb-60A heterodimers was proposed (95), whereas Gbb-60A was indicated to act as a homodimer in another report (85). Thus, BMP heterodimers may be physiological ligands under certain conditions.

EXTRACELLULAR REGULATORS OF BONE MORPHOGENETIC PROTEINS

Bone Morphogenetic Protein Activators

BMPs need to be cleaved at the Arg-X-X-Arg sequence to become active proteins (Fig. 19.2). Subtilisin-like proprotein convertases (SPCs) have been implicated in proteolysis (96,97). BMP-4, for example, is cleaved by several SPCs, including SPC1/furin. A recent study showed that the downstream sequence adjacent to the cleavage site determines the cleavage efficiency (97). The same study also showed that the pro domain N-terminal to the cleavage site determines the stability of the processed mature proteins.

Although BMP-1 does not belong to the TGF-β superfamily, it has important functions that may activate BMPs. The gene encodes a procollagen C-proteinase that cleaves procollagens and promotes extracellular matrix deposition (7). The *Drosophila* homologue is tolloid (98), and the *Xenopus* counterpart is xolloid (99). Tolloid was shown to cleave and inactivate the product

of the *short gastrulation (sog)* gene, a Dpp antagonist (Fig. 19.2) (100). Xolloid cleaves chordin, the *Xenopus* homologue of SOG, thereby releasing active BMPs from inactive complexes (101). A similar result was obtained in zebrafish (102). BMP-1 thus may cleave a mammalian BMP antagonist. Interestingly, however, homozygous BMP-1 null mutant mice developed no skeletal abnormalities, with the exception of the reduced ossification of certain skull bones (103). The mice exhibited abnormal extracellular matrix deposition in the amnion and gut herniation.

Bone Morphogenetic Protein Inhibitors

The Spemann organizer dorsalizes the mesoderm and induces the neuralization of the ectoderm in gastrulating *Xenopus* embryos. Noggin was identified as a novel dorsalizing factor localized in the Spemann organizer (104). Noggin binds BMPs 2 and 4 with a higher affinity than it does BMP-7/OP-1 and inhibits BMP binding to cell surface receptors (Fig. 19.2) (105). In mice, noggin is expressed in the node that is a structure similar to the *Xenopus* Spemann organizer, notochord, and dorsal somite through days 7.5 to 10.5 (106) and in condensing cartilage and immature chondrocytes at later stages (107). Noggin knockout mice reveal that noggin is required for patterning of the neural tube and somite at later stages but not for the early induction of neural tissue (106). Noggin-deficient mice also exhibited multiple morphological defects attributed to excessive BMP activity. These included broad and club-shaped limbs, loss of caudal vertebrae, a shortened body axis, and retention of a small vestigial tail. In the mutant mice, cartilage condensation occurred normally but cartilage hyperplasia was observed and the initiation of joint formation failed (107). BMPs induce the expression of noggin in cultured osteoblasts, suggesting that noggin constitutes an autocrine negative-feedback loop in BMP signaling (108).

Other BMP antagonists such as chordin and follistatin may play a redundant role in the early stage of mouse development. Chordin antagonizes BMP signaling by directly binding BMPs, thereby preventing receptor activation (Fig.

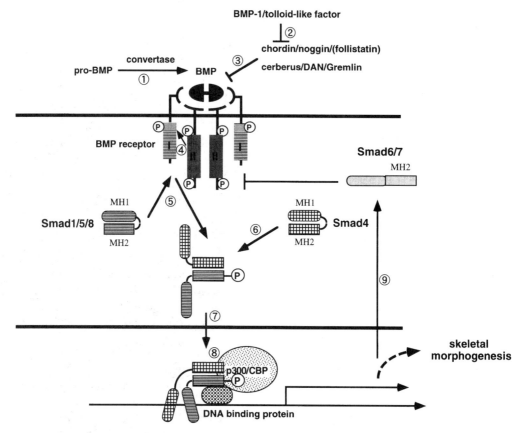

FIG. 19.2. Bone morphogenetic protein (BMP) signaling pathway. BMP signaling from the activation of the pro-BMP protein by cleavage to the transcriptional regulation by Smads is summarized. Each of the signaling steps with the indicated numbers is described in the text. The heterooligomer of Smad1/5/8 and Smad4 may be a trimer (222).

19.2) (109). Although the affinity of chordin to BMP-4 (K_D = 20 nM) is lower than that of noggin (K_D = 30 pM), chordin is more potent than noggin at neural induction in *Xenopus,* suggesting a difference in their *in vivo* functions. Mouse chordin has been identified (110), but its precise physiological role is not known.

Follistatin was originally identified as an activin-binding protein (111) but was later shown to bind with a much lower affinity and antagonize BMP-7/OP-1 and BMP-4 (112,113). Follistatin forms a ternary complex with BMPs and their receptors (114) and binds BMP-4/7 heterodimers with higher affinity than it does homodimers. In mice, follistatin is expressed in the deciduum at an early stage and later in hindbrain, somites, vibrissae, teeth, epidermis, and muscle

(115). Follistatin-deficient mice exhibited multiple defects in ribs, hard palate, skin, diaphragma, and intercostal muscles. These defects are more widespread than those of activin-deficient mice, suggesting that follistatin may regulate the activities of not only activins but also other members of the TGF-β superfamily.

Cerberus, DAN, drm, and Gremlin form another group of BMP antagonists. Cerberus was identified as a head-inducing factor expressed in the Spemann organizer in the *Xenopus* embryo (116). Cerberus-like/cer-1/mCer-1/Cerr1 is the mouse relative of *Xenopus* Cerberus (117–119). DAN was identified as a protein downregulated in v-src-transformed cells (120) and later shown to be a candidate tumor suppressor (121). drm was isolated as a molecule downregulated in mos-transformed rat cells (122). Gremlin is the *Xenopus* homologue of drm, which was identified through screening for factors inducing a secondary axis in the *Xenopus* embryo (123). These factors are secreted proteins that bind BMPs and prevent them from interacting with their receptors (Fig. 19.2), although they are not structurally related to noggin, chordin, or follistatin (123).

BONE MORPHOGENETIC PROTEIN RECEPTORS

Mechanism of Action

The mechanism whereby BMPs bind and activate their cognate receptors is essentially identical to that of TGF-βs, as discussed in Chapter 15. BMPs bind to two types of transmembrane serine-threonine kinase receptor, termed type I and type II (Fig. 19.2) (6,124). The type II kinase is constitutively active. Upon ligand binding, the type I and type II receptors form a heteromeric complex. The type II receptor then transphosphorylates the type I receptor at the juxtamembrane region and activates the type I kinase. In the TGF-β and activin receptor systems, ligands bind directly to the type II receptors, whereas the type I receptors can bind ligands only in the presence of the type II receptors. In contrast, type II receptors for BMPs bind ligands only weakly in the absence of type I receptors, and type I receptors bind ligands by themselves, although the binding affinity is relatively low. Optimal ligand binding is achieved by the presence of both type II and type I receptors. Type I receptors are the effector subunits of the receptor complexes. An amino acid change in the juxta-

membrane region of type I receptors results in constitutive activation of the kinases (5,125). These mutated type I receptors elicit ligand-specific responses in the absence of ligands or type II receptors, indicating that type I receptors phosphorylate downstream signaling components.

Bone Morphogenetic Protein Type II Receptors

Three BMP type II receptors have been identified: (a) the BMP II receptor, (b) the activin type II (ActR-II), and (c) the activin type IIB (ActR-IIB). The terminology of various type I and type II receptors is summarized in Table 19.2. Activin receptors also bind BMPs (126). Thus, the nomenclature of the receptors does not reflect their natural functions. BMP type II receptor (BMPR-II), which ligates exclusively BMPs, was identified through two independent approaches: PCR-based homology screening (127,128) and yeast two-hybrid screening using the cytoplasmic region of TGF-β type II receptor (TβR-II) as bait (129,130).

Two different lengths of BMPR-II have been reported, which are probably derived from alternative splicing (131). The longer receptor contains a long C-terminal tail following the proper kinase domain. The long and short forms are indistinguishable in biochemical assays (130,132), but they may have different functions *in vivo*. BMPR-II is ubiquitously expressed in adult tissues (127,129) and cell lines, such as ROB-C26 osteoprogenitor cells (133).

A minor population of ActR-II-deficient mice exhibit skeletal and facial abnormalities, whereas most lack these defects (134). The mu-

TABLE 19.2. *Terminology of type I and type II receptors*

	Type I receptors	Type II receptors
ALK-1	—	TGF-β type II receptor (TβR-II)
ALK-2	Activin type IA receptor (ActR-IA)	Activin type II receptor (ActR-II)
ALK-3	BMP type IA receptor (BMPR-IA)	Activin type IIB receptor (ActR-IIB)
ALK-4	Activin type IB receptor (ActR-IB)	BMP type II receptor (BMPR-II)
ALK-5	TGF-β type I receptor (TβR-I)	
ALK-6	BMP type IB receptor (BMPR-IB)	
ALK-7	—	

ALK, activin receptor-like kinase; BMP, bone morphogenetic protein; [a] TGF-β, transforming growth factor β.

tant mice had defects in pituitary follicle-stimulating hormone (FSH) secretion, which is normally regulated by activins. In contrast, ActR-IIB-deficient mice exhibit abnormal patterning of the vertebrae and complicated cardiac defects associated with pulmonary and splenic abnormalities, suggesting a role of ActR-IIB in the establishment of the anteroposterior and left–right axes (135). The phenotypes of ActR-II and ActR-IIB null mutations differ from the phenotypes of activin A and B null mutations, indicating that activin receptors mediate signals of other ligands in addition to activins (136).

Bone Morphogenetic Protein Type I Receptors

Two BMP type I receptors with cytoplasmic regions of high structural similarity have been identified (Fig. 19.3). BMP type IA receptor (BMPR-IA) and BMPR-IB are termed activin receptor-like kinase-3 (ALK-3) and ALK-6, respectively. ALK-2 binds activins in the presence of ActR-II or ActR-IIB and has been termed ActR-IA (137,138), although it also binds BMP-7/OP-1 in the presence of ActR-II and mediates BMP signaling (Fig. 19.4) (112,139). In the *Xenopus* embryo, ActR-IB/ALK-4 completely mimics the activities of activins, whereas ALK-2

does not (140). It was recently shown that ALK-2 mediates BMP signaling under physiological conditions (141).

Although BMPR-IA/ALK-3 and BMPR-IB/ALK-6 have similar ligand-binding specificity and target the same Smad species (Fig. 19.4), they may have different activities under certain conditions. C2C12 cells express BMPR-IA/ALK-3, whereas BMPR-IB/ALK-6 is not detected, at least by Northern blotting. The BMP responsiveness of C2C12 cells expressing dominant-negative BMPR-IA/ALK-3 receptor was rescued by overexpressed BMPR-IA/ALK-3 but not by BMPR-IB/ALK-6 (142). In chick limb development, BMPR-IA/ALK-3 and BMPR-IB/ALK-6 are expressed at different stages and places. Dominant-negative BMPR-IB/ALK-6 inhibited the interdigital apoptosis required for normal limb development (143). Misexpression of constitutively active forms of these two receptors resulted in different outcomes. These results indicate that BMPR-IB/ALK-6 is essential for the initial step of cartilage formation as well as apoptosis, whereas BMPR-IA/ALK-3 regulates chondrocyte differentiation (143) and suggest that the two type I receptors have common and distinct downstream signaling pathways. Others have reported that dominant-negative BMPR-IA/ALK-3 inhibits apoptosis (144). The discrep-

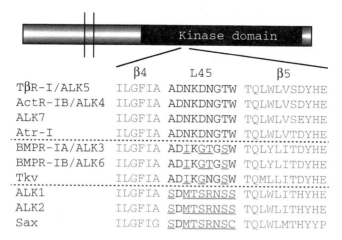

FIG. 19.3. The L45 loop of type I receptors. The L45 loop between β helices 4 and 5 in the kinase domain determines the signaling specificity of type I receptors. Three groups are identified based on the sequence of the L45 loop. Amino acids in the loop different from those of the transforming growth factor-β/activin receptors are underlined.

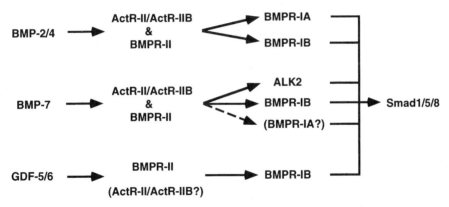

FIG. 19.4. Signaling cascades of various bone morphogenetic proteins (BMPs). The signaling cascades of various BMPs, including ligands, type II receptors, type I receptors, and Smads, are illustrated.

ancy may reflect the difference in experimental conditions. A difference between BMPR-IA/ALK-3 and BMPR-IB/ALK-6 was also observed in 2T3 cells derived from mouse calvariae (145). Dominant-negative BMPR-IA/ALK-3 inhibited adipocyte differentiation of the cells, but not osteoblast differentiation, whereas dominant-negative BMPR-IB/ALK-6 exhibited the opposite effect. The molecular mechanism for these functional differences remains to be explored.

GDF-5 binds to different combinations of type I and type II receptors, but BMPR-IB/ALK-6 has the highest affinity among type I receptors (Fig. 19.4) (133). GDF-5 also binds BMPR-IA/ALK-3 weakly (133,146). GDF-5/CDMP-1 and GDF-6/CDMP-2/BMP-13 bind to BMPR-IB/ALK-6 and BMPR-II and weakly to BMPR-IA/ALK-3 (146).

Of the three type I receptors for BMPs, the gene targeting of BMPR-IA/ALK-3 has been reported (147). BMPR-IA/ALK-3 is expressed ubiquitously during early embryogenesis and in most adult tissues. The mutant mice die by day 9.5 due to defects in mesoderm induction during gastrulation. Thus, the role of BMPR-IA/ALK-3 in skeletal development has not been clarified by gene targeting.

Drosophila **and** *C. elegans* **Receptors**

In *Drosophila*, Punt is the type II receptor for Dpp and Thick veins (Tkv) and Saxophone (Sax) are the type I Dpp receptors (11). Another type I receptor in *Drosophila*, Atr-I/Baboon, binds activin in the presence of Punt (148). Tkv and Sax have at least partial functional overlap *in vivo*, but null mutations of the genes result in distinct phenotypes (149). Null *tkv* homozygotes die during late embryonic stages and fail to undergo dorsal closure (dorsal open). In contrast, *sax* null homozygotes die during late larval stages and produce few or no imaginal disks. Recently, Sax was shown to transmit signals of another *Drosophila* ligand, Scw. Activation of Sax alone has no phenotypic effects, whereas Sax and Tkv synergistically induce dorsal development. Thus, the Dpp/Tkv pathway is indispensable to dorsal patterning, whereas the Scw/Sax pathway is necessary but not sufficient (150, 151). Gbb-60A is proposed to act through Sax, which enhances signaling by Dpp/Tkv in wing disk patterning (152). The difference between the kinase domains of the Tkv and Sax suggests that they may target different substrates. Recently, a short region with nine amino acids between kinase subdomains IV and V of type I receptors, termed the L45 loop, was shown to determine the signaling specificity of type I receptors (153). This region of Tkv is similar to that of BMPR-IA/ALK-3 and BMPR-IB/ALK-6, whereas Sax is related to ALK-1 and ALK-2. Notably, the L45 loop of Atr-I/Baboon is similar to that of TβR-I and ActR-IB/ALK-4 (Fig. 19.3) (126).

C. elegans has one type II receptor, Daf-4, and two type I receptors, Daf-1 and Sma-6 (154,155). Daf-1 was the first identified serine-threonine kinase receptor. Daf-1 and Sma-6 are type I receptors for Daf-7 and Dbl-1/Cet-1, respectively (88,155,156).

SIGNAL TRANSDUCTION

Mechanism of Action

The signaling pathway of the TGF-β superfamily is conserved through invertebrates to vertebrates. Genetic studies using *Drosophila* and *C. elegans* have resulted in the identification of the downstream components of the receptors for BMP-like ligands (15,16). *Mothers against dpp (Mad)* in *Drosophila* and *sma-2, -3,* and *-4* in *C. elegans* share considerable similarity in the amino acid sequence, suggesting that Mad-related proteins mediate intracellular signaling of the serine-threonine kinase receptors. An increased number of vertebrate members belonging to the novel protein family have subsequently been identified and are now denoted Smads. Smads are grouped into three classes based on structure and function (see also Chapter 15). Pathway-specific or receptor-regulated Smads (R-Smads) are directly phosphorylated by type I receptors. Smad2 and Smad3 are substrates of the TGF-β and activin receptors, whereas Smad1, Smad5, and Smad8 propagate BMP-specific signals (Figs. 19.2, 19.4). In contrast, Smad4, which belongs to the second class, is a common mediator (Co-Smad) required by all pathways. Phosphorylated, pathway-specific Smads form heteromeric complexes with Co-Smad, translocate into the nucleus, and activate a certain set of genes. Smads in the third class (Anti-Smads) inhibit signaling by R-Smads and Co-Smads. Smad6 and Smad7 have been shown to inhibit TGF-β/activin and/or BMP signaling.

Smads share two conserved regions, Mad-homology 1 (MH1) domain in the N-terminal part and MH2 in the C-terminal part. R-Smads have, in addition, the SSXS (Ser-Ser-X-Ser) motif at the C-terminal end. The last two serines of the SSXS motif are the sites of direct phosphorylation by the type I receptors. Co-Smads contain the MH1 and MH2 domains but not the SSXS motif. Anti-Smads, however, share only the MH2 domain, and their N-terminal half diverges from the conserved MH1 domain. MH1 and MH2 of R-Smads repress the activation of each other through intramolecular interaction. Phosphorylation of the SSXS motif relieves this mutual repression. MH1 directly binds to DNA, whereas MH2 has an intrinsic transactivation activity. MH2 also mediates various intermolecular interactions, including those of receptor–Smad, Smad–Smad, and Smad–transcription factor.

Three classes of Smads have been identified in *Drosophila* (11). Mad, the founding member of the Smad family, is an R-Smad that is closely related to Smads 1, 5, and 8, consistent with its specificity to the signaling pathway for Dpp, a BMP-like ligand. dSmad2 is closely related to Smads 2 and 3 and is likely to mediate TGF-β/activin-like signals in *Drosophila* (148). Medea is a Co-Smad, whereas Dad is an Anti-Smad.

Receptor-Smads and Common Mediator-Smads in the Bone Morphogenetic Protein Signaling Pathway

Three BMP-specific R-Smads have been identified. Smad1 is the first Smad that was shown to be directly regulated by serine-threonine kinase receptors (157). Smad1 is phosphorylated by BMPR-IA/ALK-3 or BMPR-IB/ALK-6 and then translocates into the nucleus. *Xenopus* Smad1 was shown to induce ventral mesoderm, whereas Smad2 induces dorsal mesoderm (158). Varying doses of Smad1 mimic the activity of BMP-4 as a morphogen, causing concentration-dependent induction of various tissues in the *Xenopus* embryo (159). Smad1 was demonstrated to be a transcriptional activator regulated by BMP-4 (160). Smad1 and Smad5 are directly phosphorylated by BMPR-Is at the C-terminal SSVS motif, form complexes with Smad4, and translocate into the nucleus (161,162). Mutants of both Smads inhibited BMP signaling.

Smad5 induces ventral mesoderm and epidermis from the ectoderm, which otherwise differentiates to neural tissues (163). Smad5 thus phenocopies BMPs as Smad1 does, and these activities of Smad5 depend on the presence of Smad4. Smads 1 and 5 induce ALP activity in C2C12 cells, and dominant-negative Smads 1 and 5 inhibit BMP-induced ALP activity (162,164). BMP-7/OP-1 phosphorylates endogenous Smad5 in ROB-C26 osteoprogenitor cells and Smad1 and Smad5 in P19 embryonic carcinoma cells (141,165). Smads 1, 5, and 8 are also phosphorylated by ALK-2 and heteromerize with Smad4 (Fig. 19.4) (141,166). Smad8 induces the expression of brachyury, a pan-mesodermal marker, but not goosecoid, a dorsal marker, in the *Xenopus* embryo (166). Smad8 has splice variants, but whether they have functional difference is not known (167).

Nuclear Functions of Smads

Nuclear functions of Smads have been extensively characterized in the TGF-β/activin pathway (see Chapter 15). Smads interact with a variety of nuclear proteins, such as sequence-specific DNA-binding proteins and transcriptional coactivators. It has been suggested that the DNA-binding affinities of Smads are relatively low, and that Smads require sequence-specific DNA-binding co-factors for transactivation (17,168). Smad2 interacts with FAST-1, a novel winged-helix/forkhead transcription factor, and activates the expression the *Mix.2* gene upon stimulation by activin in *Xenopus* (169). Smad3 was shown to interact with c-Jun and c-Fos in the transactivation of the *collagenase I* gene (170). However, DNA-binding partners for BMP-specific Smads have not been identified.

Vestigial, labial, and *ultrabithorax* are Dpp-responsive genes in *Drosophila.* Mad was shown to bind directly to the promoter regions of these genes (171). The consensus binding sequence is GCCGnCGC. The MH1 domain binds to DNA and the MH2 domain inhibits the binding. *tinman* is another Dpp-inducible homeobox gene that plays a pivotal role in mesoderm induction. The consensus sequence of the binding sites for Medea and Mad in the Dpp-responsive enhancer in *tinman* is CGCCGC(G/C)G(C/A)C (172), which is almost identical to the previously reported GC-rich Mad binding motif. The bind-

ing site for Smad1/5/8 *in vivo* has not been identified. Screening of Smad3 and Smad4 binding sites using gel-shift PCR selection of oligonucleotides identified a palindromic sequence, GTCTAGAC, to be a consensus binding sequence (SBE, for Smad binding element) (173). *Plasminogen activator inhibitor-1 (PAI-1)* and *junB* are TGF-β-responsive genes. Sequence examination of both promoters resulted in the identification of the CAGACA motif as a common binding site for Smad3 and Smad4 (174,175). SBE and the CAGACA motif have a significant overlap of GTCT or its complementary AGAC sequence. Three-dimensional structural analysis of the MH1 domain of Smad3 revealed the conformation of the Smad–DNA interaction (176). Smad1 was shown to directly bind to SBE (176), but Smad1 did not bind to the CAGACA motif (174,175). The reason for the discrepancy between the results is not clear at present.

A growing number of transcription factors interact with coactivators such as p300 and cyclic adenosine monophosphate (cAMP) response element (CRE) binding protein (CBP) to induce gene expression. Smads were recently shown by several groups to interact directly with p300/CBP (177–182). Smad2 and Smad3 interact with p300/CBP through the MH2 domain, which is consistent with its inherent transactivation activity. In one report, Smad1 was shown to interact with CBP (179). p300/CBP associates with various DNA-binding proteins and may thus act as a stabilizing factor bridging Smads and other transcription factors.

A number of BMP-responsive genes have been reported (6). *Tlx-2* is a BMP-inducible homeobox gene expressed in the primitive streak in the mouse embryo. Smad1 was shown to enhance the BMP responsiveness of *Tlx-2* (183). *Vent.2* is a BMP-responsive gene in *Xenopus.* Indirect evidence was presented that Smad1 mediates the expression of *Vent.2* (184). Smad binding sites and DNA-binding cofactors in these genes have not been identified.

Anti-Smads

Anti-Smads inhibit signaling by R-Smads and Co-Smads (Fig. 19.2). The mechanisms whereby Anti-Smads exert their inhibitory effects have been investigated in the mammalian system. Smad6 and Smad7 associate stably with type I receptors, thereby inhibiting the phosphorylation of R-Smads (185–187). In BMP signaling, Smad6 may also compete with Smad4 in association with Smad1 (188). *Daughters against dpp (Dad)* was identified as a gene whose expression is induced by Dpp (189). Dad is structurally similar to the vertebrate Anti-Smads and antagonizes Dpp signaling. Expression of Dad, Smad6, and Smad7 is induced by ligands, and the autoregulatory feedback loop via Anti-Smads seems to be conserved between invertebrates and vertebrates (Fig. 19.2) (187, 189–191). Smad7 is more efficient at inhibiting TGF-β signals than is Smad6 (192), whereas both Smads equally antagonize BMP signaling (186,193–197; our unpublished observations).

Drosophila Smads

In *Drosophila*, four Smads have been identified. Mad is an R-Smad that transduces signals of Dpp. Medea is a Co-Smad, whereas Dad is an Anti-Smad. Using these three types of Smad, it has been shown that the Smad signaling pathway is conserved between invertebrates and vertebrates at the molecular level (198). Recently, dSmad2 was reported to be an R-Smad that responds to Atr-I/Baboon (148,199). *schnurri (shn)* was isolated as a gene required for the expression of various Dpp-responsive genes (200–202). Several lines of genetic evidence suggest that Shn functions downstream of Dpp. Shn is a large protein with seven C2-H2-type zinc fingers and one C2-HC-type zinc finger, which is homologous to vertebrate transcription factors such as MBP1/HIV-EP1/PRDII-BFI/AT-BP2/αA-CRYBP1 and MBP2/HIV-EP2/AT-BP1/AGIE-BP1. Shn thus may act as a transcriptional cofactor for Mad (203).

Other Signaling Pathways

TGF-β-activated kinase (TAK-1) was isolated as a member of the mitogen-activated protein kinase kinase kinase (MAPKKK) family that is activated by TGF-β and BMP-4 (204).

TAB-1 is a TAK-1-interacting protein that enhances TGF-β signaling (205). In *Xenopus,* TAK-1 induces ventral mesoderm and TAK-1 binding protein (TAB-1) enhances this effect (206). Dominant-negative TAK-1 suppressed the expression of ventral mesoderm markers induced by Smad1 or Smad5. XIAP was isolated as a TAB-1-binding protein (207). XIAP also interacts with BMPR-IA/ALK-3. Thus, the BMPR-IA/ALK-3/XIAP/TAB-1/TAK-1 pathway is likely to mediate BMP signaling. Functional interaction between the Smad pathway and the TAK-1 pathway remains to be determined. BRAM-1 was isolated as a BMPR-IA/ALK-3 binding protein (208). BRAM-1 also interacts with TAB-1 and might be involved in the BMP/TAK-1 pathway.

The Ras/Raf pathway has been implicated in BMP signaling (209). Epidermal growth factor (EGF) induces the phosphorylation of the linker region of Smad1 through activation of the extracellular signal–regulated kinase (ERK) and inhibits its translocation from the cytoplasm to the nucleus. EGF may thus antagonize BMP signaling through Smad1 (210). In another report, however, EGF and hepatocyte growth factor (HGF) were shown to positively regulate Smad signaling (211). HGF induces the phosphorylation of Smad2, probably through MAPKK (MEK-1) and stimulates the activation of transcription by TGF-β. The phosphorylation site has not been determined, and the molecular basis of the positive regulation remains to be shown. Both synergistic and antagonistic regulations between the TGF-β superfamily and the MAPK cascade are known (11), and Smads may be the site of the intersection.

The regulatory mechanism of BMP expression is not fully revealed. In *Drosophila,* hedgehog (Hh) regulates the expression of Dpp in imaginal disks (6). Three mammalian homologues of Hh have been identified: Sonic hedgehog- (Shh), Desert hedgehog (Dhh), and Indian hedgehog (Ihh). Gene disruption of Shh resulted in the absence of distal limb structures, spinal column, and most of the ribs in addition to other abnormalities such as cyclopia (212). Dhh is expressed in the testis, and Dhh-null male mice exhibited complete absence of sperm, whereas female mice showed no obvious phenotype (213). Ihh is expressed in prehypertrophic chondrocytes and has been implicated in chondrocyte differentiation (see Chapter 25) (214). A model in which Ihh positively regulates the expression of BMPs has been proposed (143,215).

CONCLUSION AND PERSPECTIVES

BMPs play pivotal roles in a wide scope of biological phenomena ranging from skeletal morphogenesis to regulation of neural function (6,78,216). Recent identification of signaling molecules of the BMP pathway has greatly contributed to the elucidation of the molecular mechanism of BMP signaling. However, many important questions remain open, particularly regarding the role of BMPs *in vivo*. Results of gene targeting of some BMP members have shed important light on this issue; however, embryonal lethality has impeded the full elucidation of the physiological function of BMPs in the skeletal system. Thus, conditional targetings of BMPs will be the next goal of this approach. The ongoing progress of the human genome project will reveal the relationship of some diseases to BMPs in the near future.

One of the most significant recent achievements in the study of TGF-β superfamily signaling is the identification of proteins of the Smad family. However, the nuclear functions of BMP-specific Smads are largely unknown. The binding DNA sequences and transcriptional cofactors of BMP-specific Smads need to be elucidated. The molecular mechanism whereby BMPs regulate skeletal morphogenesis also remains obscure. Gene targeting of *Cbfa1*/*PEBP2αA*/*AML3* disclosed that the gene is required for osteogenesis (217–220). It was recently reported that BMPs upregulate the expression of *Cbfα1*/*PEBP2αA*/*AML3* (221), but whether *Cbfα1*/*PEBP2αA*/*AML3* is the direct target of BMPs in bone formation awaits further investigation. In *Drosophila,* Dpp regulates the expression of various homeobox genes, such as *labial* (171). Expression of *HoxD13* was altered in mice deficient in BMP-7/OP-1, and the mice developed polydactyly (35). Homeobox genes such as *Tlx-2* might thus be major targets of BMPs also in mammals.

BMPs play crucial roles in the inductive process of various tissues or organs. Other signaling pathways, such as Wnt, Hh, and growth factors including fibroblast growth factors, regulate cell–cell communication as well. Integration of these divergent signaling pathways determines the fate of individual cells and the resulting morphogenesis. It would be a strenuous but fruitful task to disentangle the exquisitely woven threads both *in vitro* and *in vivo*.

ACKNOWLEDGMENTS

We are grateful to Miss A. Nishitoh for her assistance in the preparation of this manuscript.

REFERENCES

1. Urist MR. Bone: formation by autoinduction. *Science* 1965;150:893–899.
2. Wozney JM, Rosen V, Celeste AJ, et al. Novel regulators of bone formation: molecular clones and activities. *Science* 1988;242:1528–1534.
3. Reddi AH. Bone morphogenetic proteins: an unconventional approach to isolation of first mammalian morphogens. *Cytokine Growth Factor Rev* 1997;8: 11–20.
4. Sakou T. Bone morphogenetic proteins: from basic studies to clinical approaches. *Bone* 1998;22:591–603.
5. Derynck R, Feng XH. TGF-β receptor signaling. *Biochim Biophys Acta* 1997;1333:F105–F150.
6. Hogan BL. Bone morphogenetic proteins: multifunctional regulators of vertebrate development. *Genes Dev* 1996;10:1580–1594.
7. Kessler E, Takahara K, Biniaminov L, et al. Bone morphogenetic protein-1: the type I procollagen C-proteinase. *Science* 1996;271:360–362.
8. Padgett RW, Wozney JM, Gelbart WM. Human BMP sequences can confer normal dorsal–ventral patterning in the *Drosophila* embryo. *Proc Natl Acad Sci USA* 1993;90:2905–2909.
9. Sampath TK, Rashka KE, Doctor JS, et al. *Drosophila* transforming growth factor β superfamily proteins induce endochondral bone formation in mammals. *Proc Natl Acad Sci USA* 1993;90:6004–6008.
10. Padgett RW, Das P, Krishna S. TGF-β signaling, Smads, and tumor suppressors. *Bioessays* 1998;20: 382–390.
11. Whitman M. Smads and early developmental signaling by the TGFβ superfamily. *Genes Dev* 1998;12: 2445–2462.
12. Schlunegger MP, Grutter MG. An unusual feature revealed by the crystal structure at 2.2 Å resolution of human transforming growth factor-β2. *Nature* 1992; 358:430–434.
13. Daopin S, Piez KA, Ogawa Y, et al. Crystal structure

of transforming growth factor-β2: an unusual fold for the superfamily. *Science* 1992;257:369–373.

14. Griffith DL, Keck PC, Sampath TK, et al. Three-dimensional structure of recombinant human osteogenic protein 1: structural paradigm for the transforming growth factor β superfamily. *Proc Natl Acad Sci USA* 1996;93:878–883.

15. Heldin CH, Miyazono K, ten Dijke P. TGF-β signalling from cell membrane to nucleus through SMAD proteins. *Nature* 1997;390:465–471.

16. Massagué J. TGF-β signal transduction. *Annu Rev Biochem* 1998;67:753–791.

17. Derynck R, Zhang Y, Feng XH. Smads: transcriptional activators of TGF-β responses. *Cell* 1998;95:737–740.

18. Lyons KM, Pelton RW, Hogan BL. Patterns of expression of murine Vgr-1 and BMP-2a RNA suggest that transforming growth factor-β-like genes coordinately regulate aspects of embryonic development. *Genes Dev* 1989;3:1657–1668.

19. Lyons KM, Pelton RW, Hogan BL. Organogenesis and pattern formation in the mouse: RNA distribution patterns suggest a role for bone morphogenetic protein-2A (BMP-2A). *Development* 1990;109:833–844.

20. Zhang H, Bradley A. Mice deficient for BMP2 are nonviable and have defects in amnion/chorion and cardiac development. *Development* 1996;122:2977–2986.

21. Takuwa Y, Ohse C, Wang EA, et al. Bone morphogenetic protein-2 stimulates alkaline phosphatase activity and collagen synthesis in cultured osteoblastic cells, MC3T3-E1. *Biochem Biophys Res Commun* 1991;174:96–101.

22. Shukunami C, Ohta Y, Sakuda M, et al. Sequential progression of the differentiation program by bone morphogenetic protein-2 in chondrogenic cell line ATDC5. *Exp Cell Res* 1998;241:1–11.

23. Katagiri T, Yamaguchi A, Komaki M, et al. Bone morphogenetic protein-2 converts the differentiation pathway of C2C12 myoblasts into the osteoblast lineage. *J Cell Biol* 1994;127:1755–1766.

24. Katagiri T, Akiyama S, Namiki M, et al. Bone morphogenetic protein-2 inhibits terminal differentiation of myogenic cells by suppressing the transcriptional activity of MyoD and myogenin. *Exp Cell Res* 1997;230:342–351.

25. Jones CM, Lyons KM, Hogan BL. Involvement of bone morphogenetic protein-4 (BMP-4) and Vgr-1 in morphogenesis and neurogenesis in the mouse. *Development* 1991;111:531–542.

26. Winnier G, Blessing M, Labosky PA, et al. Bone morphogenetic protein-4 is required for mesoderm formation and patterning in the mouse. *Genes Dev* 1995;9:2105–2116.

27. Dunn NR, Winnier GE, Hargett LK, et al. Haploinsufficient phenotypes in Bmp4 heterozygous null mice and modification by mutations in Gli3 and Alx4. *Dev Biol* 1997;188:235–247.

28. Furuta Y, Hogan BLM. BMP4 is essential for lens induction in the mouse embryo. *Genes Dev* 1998;12:3764–3775.

29. Nakase T, Nomura S, Yoshikawa H, et al. Transient and localized expression of bone morphogenetic protein 4 messenger RNA during fracture healing. *J Bone Miner Res* 1994;9:651–659.

30. Wada Y, Kataoka H, Yokose S, et al. Changes in osteo-

blast phenotype during differentiation of enzymatically isolated rat calvaria cells. *Bone* 1998;22:479–485.

31. Celeste AJ, Iannazzi JA, Taylor RC, et al. Identification of transforming growth factor β family members present in bone-inductive protein purified from bovine bone. *Proct Natl Acad Sci USA* 1990;87:9843–9847.

32. Ozkaynak E, Rueger DC, Drier EA, et al. OP-1 cDNA encodes an osteogenic protein in the TGF-β family. *EMBO J* 1990;9:2085–2093.

33. Lyons KM, Hogan BL, Robertson EJ. Colocalization of BMP 7 and BMP 2 RNAs suggests that these factors cooperatively mediate tissue interactions during murine development. *Mech Dev* 1995;50:71–83.

34. Dudley AT, Lyons KM, Robertson EJ. A requirement for bone morphogenetic protein-7 during development of the mammalian kidney and eye. *Genes Dev* 1995;9:2795–2807.

35. Luo G, Hofmann C, Bronckers AL, et al. BMP-7 is an inducer of nephrogenesis, and is also required for eye development and skeletal patterning. *Genes Dev* 1995;9:2808–2820.

36. Hofmann C, Luo G, Balling R, et al. Analysis of limb patterning in BMP-7-deficient mice. *Dev Genet* 1996;19:43–50.

37. Katagiri T, Boorla S, Frendo JL, et al. Skeletal abnormalities in doubly heterozygous Bmp4 and Bmp7 mice. *Dev Genet* 1998;22:340–348.

38. Zou H, Niswander L. Requirement for BMP signaling in interdigital apoptosis and scale formation. *Science* 1996;272:738–741.

39. Macias D, Ganan Y, Sampath TK, et al. Role of BMP-2 and OP-1 (BMP-7) in programmed cell death and skeletogenesis during chick limb development. *Development* 1997;124:1109–1117.

40. Asahina I, Sampath TK, Nishimura I, et al. Human osteogenic protein-1 induces both chondroblastic and osteoblastic differentiation of osteoprogenitor cells derived from newborn rat calvaria. *J Cell Biol* 1993;123:921–933.

41. Asahina I, Sampath TK, Hauschka PV. Human osteogenic protein-1 induces chondroblastic, osteoblastic, and/or adipocytic differentiation of clonal murine target cells. *Exp Cell Res* 1996;222:38–47.

42. Kingsley DM, Bland AE, Grubber JM, et al. The mouse short ear skeletal morphogenesis locus is associated with defects in a bone morphogenetic member of the TGF β superfamily. *Cell* 1992;71:399–410.

43. King JA, Marker PC, Seung KJ, et al. BMP5 and the molecular, skeletal, and soft-tissue alterations in short ear mice. *Dev Biol* 1994;166:112–122.

44. Wall NA, Blessing M, Wright CV, et al. Biosynthesis and *in vivo* localization of the decapentaplegic-Vg-related protein, DVR-6 (bone morphogenetic protein-6). *J Cell Biol* 1993;120:493–502.

45. Gitelman SE, Kirk M, Ye JQ, et al. Vgr-1/BMP-6 induces osteoblastic differentiation of pluripotential mesenchymal cells. *Cell Growth Differ* 1995;6:827–836.

46. Boden SD, McCuaig K, Hair G, et al. Differential effects and glucocorticoid potentiation of bone morphogenetic protein action during rat osteoblast differentiation *in vitro*. *Endocrinology* 1996;137:3401–3407.

47. Boden SD, Hair G, Titus L, et al. Glucocorticoid-induced differentiation of fetal rat calvarial osteoblasts

is mediated by bone morphogenetic protein-6. *Endocrinology* 1997;138:2820–2828.

48. Blessing M, Schirmacher P, Kaiser S. Overexpression of bone morphogenetic protein-6 (BMP-6) in the epidermis of transgenic mice: inhibition or stimulation of proliferation depending on the pattern of transgene expression and formation of psoriatic lesions. *J Cell Biol* 1996;135:227–239.

49. Solloway MJ, Dudley AT, Bikoff EK, et al. Mice lacking Bmp6 function. *Dev Genet* 1998;22:321–339.

50. Zhao GQ, Deng K, Labosky PA, et al. The gene encoding bone morphogenetic protein 8B is required for the initiation and maintenance of spermatogenesis in the mouse. *Genes Dev* 1996;10:1657–1669.

51. Zhao GQ, Liaw L, Hogan BL. Bone morphogenetic protein 8A plays a role in the maintenance of spermatogenesis and the integrity of the epididymis. *Development* 1998;125:1103–1112.

52. Storm EE, Huynh TV, Copeland NG, et al. Limb alterations in brachypodism mice due to mutations in a new member of the TGF-β superfamily. *Nature* 1994;368:639–643.

53. Chang SC, Hoang B, Thomas JT, et al. Cartilage-derived morphogenetic proteins. New members of the transforming growth factor-β superfamily predominantly expressed in long bones during human embryonic development. *J Biol Chem* 1994;269:28227–28234.

54. Storm EE, Kingsley DM. Joint patterning defects caused by single and double mutations in members of the bone morphogenetic protein (BMP) family. *Development* 1996;122:3969–3979.

55. Francis-West PH, Abdelfattah A, Chen P, et al. Mechanisms of GDF-5 action during skeletal development. *Development* 1999;126:1305–1315.

56. Thomas JT, Lin K, Nandedkar M, et al. A human chondrodysplasia due to a mutation in a TGF-β superfamily member. *Nat Genet* 1996;12:315–317.

57. Thomas JT, Kilpatrick MW, Lin K, et al. Disruption of human limb morphogenesis by a dominant negative mutation in CDMP1. *Nat Genet* 1997;17:58–64.

58. Polinkovsky A, Robin NH, Thomas JT, et al. Mutations in CDMP1 cause autosomal dominant brachydactyly type C. *Nat Genet* 1997;17:18–19.

59. Tsumaki N, Tanaka K, Arikawa-Hirasawa E, et al. Role of CDMP-1 in skeletal morphogenesis: promotion of mesenchymal cell recruitment and chondrocyte differentiation. *J Cell Biol* 1999;144:161–173.

60. Inada M, Katagiri T, Akiyama S, et al. Bone morphogenetic protein-12 and -13 inhibit terminal differentiation of myoblasts, but do not induce their differentiation into osteoblasts. *Biochem Biophys Res Commun* 1996;222:317–322.

61. Wolfman NM, Hattersley G, Cox K, et al. Ectopic induction of tendon and ligament in rats by growth and differentiation factors 5, 6, and 7, members of the TGF-β gene family. *J Clin Invest* 1997;100:321–330.

62. Lee KJ, Mendelsohn M, Jessel TM. Neuronal patterning by BMPs: a requirement for GDF7 in the generation of a discrete class of commissural interneurons in the mouse spinal cord. *Genes Dev* 1998;12:3394–3407.

63. Jones CM, Simon-Chazottes D, Guenet JL, et al. Isolation of Vgr-2, a novel member of the transforming growth factor-β-related gene family. *Mol Endocrinol* 1992;6:1961–1968.

64. McPherron AC, Lee SJ. GDF-3 and GDF-9: two new members of the transforming growth factor-β superfamily containing a novel pattern of cysteines. *J Biol Chem* 1993;268:3444–3449.

65. McGrath SA, Esquela AF, Lee SJ. Oocyte-specific expression of growth/differentiation factor-9. *Mol Endocrinol* 1995;9:131–136.

66. Fitzpatrick SL, Sindoni DM, Shughrue PJ, et al. Expression of growth differentiation factor-9 messenger ribonucleic acid in ovarian and nonovarian rodent and human tissues. *Endocrinology* 1998;139:2571–2578.

67. Dong J, Albertini DF, Nishimori K, et al. Growth differentiation factor-9 is required during early ovarian folliculogenesis. *Nature* 1996;383:531–535.

68. Carabatsos MJ, Elvin J, Matzuk MM, et al. Characterization of oocyte and follicle development in growth differentiation factor-9-deficient mice. *Dev Biol* 1998;204:373–384.

69. Dube JL, Wang P, Elvin J, et al. The bone morphogenetic protein 15 gene is X-linked and expressed in oocytes. *Mol Endocrinol* 1998;12:1809–1817.

70. McPherron AC, Lawler AM, Lee SJ. Regulation of skeletal muscle mass in mice by a new TGF-β superfamily member. *Nature* 1997;387:83–90.

71. Grobet L, Martin LJ, Poncelet D, et al. A deletion in the bovine myostatin gene causes the double-muscled phenotype in cattle. *Nat Genet* 1997;17:71–74.

72. Kambadur R, Sharma M, Smith TP, et al. Mutations in myostatin (GDF8) in double-muscled Belgian blue and Piedmontese cattle. *Genome Res* 1997;7:910–916.

73. McPherron AC, Lee SJ. Double muscling in cattle due to mutations in the myostatin gene. *Proc Natl Acad Sci USA* 1997;94:12457–12461.

74. Rosen V, Wozney JM, Wang EA, et al. Purification and molecular cloning of a novel group of BMPs and localization of BMP mRNA in developing bone. *Connect Tissue Res* 1989;20:313–319.

75. Vukicevic S, Helder MN, Luyten FP. Developing human lung and kidney are major sites for synthesis of bone morphogenetic protein-3 (osteogenin). *J Histochem Cytochem* 1994;42:869–875.

76. Cunningham NS, Jenkins NA, Gilbert DJ, et al. Growth/differentiation factor-10: a new member of the transforming growth factor-β superfamily related to bone morphogenetic protein-3. *Growth Factors* 1995;12:99–109.

77. Takao M, Hino J, Takeshita N, et al. Identification of rat bone morphogenetic protein-3b (BMP-3b), a new member of BMP-3. *Biochem Biophys Res Commun* 1996;219:656–662.

78. Ebendal T, Bengtsson H, Soderstrom S. Bone morphogenetic proteins and their receptors: potential functions in the brain. *J Neurosci Res* 1998;51:139–146.

79. Song JJ, Celeste AJ, Kong FM, et al. Bone morphogenetic protein-9 binds to liver cells and stimulates proliferation. *Endocrinology* 1995;136:4293–4297.

80. Lee SJ. Identification of a novel member (GDF-1) of the transforming growth factor-β superfamily. *Mol Endocrinol* 1990;4:1034–1040.

81. Collignon J, Varlet I, Robertson EJ. Relationship between asymmetric nodal expression and the direction of embryonic turning. *Nature* 1996;381:155–158.

82. Lowe LA, Supp DM, Sampath K, et al. Conserved left–right asymmetry of nodal expression and alterations in murine situs inversus. *Nature* 1996;381: 158–161.

83. Padgett RW, Savage C, Das P. Genetic and biochemical analysis of TGF β signal transduction. *Cytokine Growth Factor Rev* 1997;8:1–9.

84. Padgett RW, St Johnston RD, Gelbart WM. A transcript from a *Drosophila* pattern gene predicts a protein homologous to the transforming growth factor-β family. *Nature* 1987;325:81–84.

85. Khalsa O, Yoon JW, Torres-Schumann S, et al. TGF-β/BMP superfamily members, Gbb-60A and Dpp, cooperate to provide pattern information and establish cell identity in the *Drosophila* wing. *Development* 1998;125:2723–2734.

86. Arora K, Levine MS, O'Connor MB. The screw gene encodes a ubiquitously expressed member of the TGF-β family required for specification of dorsal cell fates in the *Drosophila* embryo. *Genes Dev* 1994;8: 2588–2601.

87. Ruvkun G, Hobert O. The taxonomy of developmental control in *Caenorhabditis elegans*. *Science* 1998;282: 2033–2041.

88. Suzuki Y, Yandell MD, Roy PJ, et al. A BMP homolog acts as a dose-dependent regulator of body size and male tail patterning in *Caenorhabditis elegans*. *Development* 1999;126:241–250.

89. Estevez M, Attisano L, Wrana JL, et al. The daf-4 gene encodes a bone morphogenetic protein receptor controlling *C. elegans* dauer larva development. *Nature* 1993;365:644–649.

90. Colavita A, Krishna S, Zheng H, et al. Pioneer axon guidance by UNC-129, a *C. elegans* TGF-β. *Science* 1998;281:706–709.

91. Israel DI, Nove J, Kerns KM, et al. Heterodimeric bone morphogenetic proteins show enhanced activity *in vitro* and *in vivo*. *Growth Factors* 1996;13:291–300.

92. Hazama M, Aono A, Ueno N, et al. Efficient expression of a heterodimer of bone morphogenetic protein subunits using a baculovirus expression system. *Biochem Biophys Res Commun* 1995;209:859–866.

93. Aono A, Hazama M, Notoya K, et al. Potent ectopic bone-inducing activity of bone morphogenetic protein-4/7 heterodimer. *Biochem Biophys Res Commun* 1995; 210:670–677.

94. Suzuki A, Kaneko E, Maeda J, et al. Mesoderm induction by BMP-4 and -7 heterodimers. *Biochem Biophys Res Commun* 1997;232:153–156.

95. Chen Y, Riese MJ, Killinger MA, et al. A genetic screen for modifiers of *Drosophila* decapentaplegic signaling identifies mutations in punt, Mothers against dpp and the BMP-7 homologue, 60A. *Development* 1998;125:1759–1768.

96. Cui Y, Jean F, Thomas G, et al. BMP-4 is proteolytically activated by furin and/or PC6 during vertebrate embryonic development. *EMBO J* 1998;17:4735–4743.

97. Constam DB, Robertson EJ. Regulation of bone morphogenetic protein activity by pro domains and proprotein convertases. *J Cell Biol* 1999;144:139–149.

98. Shimell MJ, Ferguson EL, Childs SR, et al. The *Drosophila* dorsal–ventral patterning gene tolloid is related to human bone morphogenetic protein 1. *Cell* 1991; 67:469–481.

99. Goodman SA, Albano R, Wardle FC, et al. BMP1-related metalloproteinases promote the development of ventral mesoderm in early *Xenopus* embryos. *Dev Biol* 1998;195:144–157.

100. Marques G, Musacchio M, Shimell MJ, et al. Production of a DPP activity gradient in the early *Drosophila* embryo through the opposing actions of the SOG and TLD proteins. *Cell* 1997;91:417–426.

101. Piccolo S, Agius E, Lu B, et al. Cleavage of Chordin by Xolloid metalloprotease suggests a role for proteolytic processing in the regulation of Spemann organizer activity. *Cell* 1997;91:407–416.

102. Blader P, Rastegar S, Fischer N, et al. Cleavage of the BMP-4 antagonist chordin by zebrafish tolloid. *Science* 1997;278:1937–1940.

103. Suzuki N, Labosky PA, Furuta Y, et al. Failure of ventral body wall closure in mouse embryos lacking a procollagen C-proteinase encoded by Bmp1, a mammalian gene related to *Drosophila* tolloid. *Development* 1996;122:3587–3595.

104. Smith WC, Harland RM. Expression cloning of noggin, a new dorsalizing factor localized to the Spemann organizer in *Xenopus* embryos. *Cell* 1992;70:829–840.

105. Zimmerman LB, De Jesus-Escobar JM, Harland RM. The Spemann organizer signal noggin binds and inactivates bone morphogenetic protein 4. *Cell* 1996;86: 599–606.

106. McMahon JA, Takada S, Zimmerman LB, et al. Noggin-mediated antagonism of BMP signaling is required for growth and patterning of the neural tube and somite. *Genes Dev* 1998;12:1438–1452.

107. Brunet LJ, McMahon JA, McMahon AP, et al. Noggin, cartilage morphogenesis, and joint formation in the mammalian skeleton. *Science* 1998;280:1455–1457.

108. Gazzerro E, Gangji V, Canalis E. Bone morphogenetic proteins induce the expression of noggin, which limits their activity in cultured rat osteoblasts. *J Clin Invest* 1998;102:2106–2114.

109. Piccolo S, Sasai Y, Lu B, et al. Dorsoventral patterning in *Xenopus:* inhibition of ventral signals by direct binding of chordin to BMP-4. *Cell* 1996;86:589–598.

110. Pappano WN, Scott IC, Clark TG, et al. Coding sequence and expression patterns of mouse chordin and mapping of the cognate mouse chrd and human CHRD genes. *Genomics* 1998;52:236–239.

111. Nakamura T, Takio K, Eto Y, et al. Activin-binding protein from rat ovary is follistatin. *Science* 1990;247: 836–838.

112. Yamashita H, ten Dijke P, Huylebroeck D, et al. Osteogenic protein-1 binds to activin type II receptors and induces certain activin-like effects. *J Cell Biol* 1995;130:217–226.

113. Fainsod A, Deissler K, Yelin R, et al. The dorsalizing and neural inducing gene follistatin is an antagonist of BMP-4. *Mech Dev* 1997;63:39–50.

114. Iemura S, Yamamoto TS, Takagi C, et al. Direct binding of follistatin to a complex of bone-morphogenetic protein and its receptor inhibits ventral and epidermal cell fates in early *Xenopus* embryo. *Proc Natl Acad Sci USA* 1998;95:9337–9342.

115. Matzuk MM, Lu N, Vogel H, et al. Multiple defects and perinatal death in mice deficient in follistatin. *Nature* 1995;374:360–363.

116. Bouwmeester T, Kim S, Sasai Y, et al. Cerberus is a head-inducing secreted factor expressed in the anterior

endoderm of Spemann's organizer. *Nature* 1996;382: 595–601.

117. Belo JA, Bouwmeester T, Leyns L, et al. Cerberus-like is a secreted factor with neutralizing activity expressed in the anterior primitive endoderm of the mouse gastrula. *Mech Dev* 1997;68:45–57.

118. Biben C, Stanley E, Fabri L, et al. Murine cerberus homologue mCer-1: a candidate anterior patterning molecule. *Dev Biol* 1998;194:135–151.

119. Shawlot W, Deng JM, Behringer RR. Expression of the mouse cerberus-related gene, Cerrl, suggests a role in anterior neural induction and somitogenesis. *Proc Natl Acad Sci USA* 1998;95:6198–6203.

120. Ozaki T, Sakiyama S. Molecular cloning and characterization of a cDNA showing negative regulation in v-src-transformed 3Y1 rat fibroblasts. *Proc Natl Acad Sci USA* 1993;90:2593–2597.

121. Enomoto H, Ozaki T, Takahashi E, et al. Identification of human DAN gene, mapping to the putative neuroblastoma tumor suppressor locus. *Oncogene* 1994;9: 2785–2791.

122. Topol LZ, Marx M, Laugier D, et al. Identification of drm, a novel gene whose expression is suppressed in transformed cells and which can inhibit growth of normal but not transformed cells in culture. *Mol Cell Biol* 1997;17:4801–4810.

123. Hsu DR, Economides AN, Wang X, et al. The *Xenopus* dorsalizing factor Gremlin identifies a novel family of secreted proteins that antagonize BMP activities. *Mol Cell* 1998;1:673–683.

124. Kingsley DM. The TGF-β superfamily: new members, new receptors, and new genetic tests of function in different organisms. *Genes Dev* 1994;8:133–146.

125. Wieser R, Wrana JL, Massagué J. GS domain mutations that constitutively activate TβR-I, the downstream signaling component in the TGF-β receptor complex. *EMBO J* 1995;14:2199–2208.

126. Kawabata M, Imamura T, Miyazono K. Signal transduction by bone morphogenetic proteins. *Cytokine Growth Factor Rev* 1998;9:49–61.

127. Rosenzweig BL, Imamura T, Okadome T, et al. Cloning and characterization of a human type II receptor for bone morphogenetic proteins. *Proc Natl Acad Sci USA* 1995;92:7632–7636.

128. Nohno T, Ishikawa T, Saito T, et al. Identification of a human type II receptor for bone morphogenetic protein-4 that forms differential heteromeric complexes with bone morphogenetic protein type I receptors. *J Biol Chem* 1995;270:22522–22526.

129. Kawabata M, Chytil A, Moses HL. Cloning of a novel type II serine/threonine kinase receptor through interaction with the type I transforming growth factor-β receptor. *J Biol Chem* 1995;270:5625–5630.

130. Liu F, Ventura F, Doody J, et al. Human type II receptor for bone morphogenic proteins (BMPs): extension of the two-kinase receptor model to the BMPs. *Mol Cell Biol* 1995;15:3479–3486.

131. Beppu H, Minowa O, Miyazono K, et al. cDNA cloning and genomic organization of the mouse BMP type II receptor. *Biochem Biophys Res Commun* 1997;235: 499–504.

132. Ishikawa T, Yoshioka H, Ohuchi H, et al. Truncated type II receptor for BMP-4 induces secondary axial structures in *Xenopus* embryos. *Biochem Biophys Res Commun* 1995;216:26–33.

133. Nishitoh H, Ichijo H, Kimura M, et al. Identification of type I and type II serine/threonine kinase receptors for growth/differentiation factor-5. *J Biol Chem* 1996; 271:21345–21352.

134. Matzuk MM, Kumar TR, Bradley A. Different phenotypes for mice deficient in either activins or activin receptor type II. *Nature* 1995;374:356–360.

135. Oh SP, Li E. The signaling pathway mediated by the type IIB activin receptor controls axial patterning and lateral asymmetry in the mouse. *Genes Dev* 1997;11: 1812–1826.

136. Matzuk MM, Kumar TR, Vassalli A, et al. Functional analysis of activins during mammalian development. *Nature* 1995;374:354–356.

137. Attisano L, Carcamo J, Ventura F, et al. Identification of human activin and TGF β type I receptors that form heteromeric kinase complexes with type II receptors. *Cell* 1993;75:671–680.

138. Tsuchida K, Mathews LS, Vale WW. Cloning and characterization of a transmembrane serine kinase that acts as an activin type I receptor. *Proc Natl Acad Sci USA* 1993;90:11242–11246.

139. ten Dijke P, Yamashita H, Sampath TK, et al. Identification of type I receptors for osteogenic protein-1 and bone morphogenetic protein-4. *J Biol Chem* 1994;269: 16985–16988.

140. Armes NA, Smith JC. The ALK-2 and ALK-4 activin receptors transduce distinct mesoderm-inducing signals during early *Xenopus* development but do not cooperate to establish thresholds. *Development* 1997; 124:3797–3804.

141. Macías-Silva M, Hoodless PA, Tang SJ, et al. Specific activation of Smad1 signaling pathways by the BMP7 type I receptor, ALK2. *J Biol Chem* 1998;273: 25628–25636.

142. Namiki M, Akiyama S, Katagiri T, et al. A kinase domain–truncated type I receptor blocks bone morphogenetic protein-2-induced signal transduction in C2C12 myoblasts. *J Biol Chem* 1997;272:22046–22052.

143. Zou H, Wieser R, Massagué J, et al. Distinct roles of type I bone morphogenetic protein receptors in the formation and differentiation of cartilage. *Genes Dev* 1997;11:2191–2203.

144. Yokouchi Y, Sakiyama J, Kameda T, et al. BMP-2/-4 mediate programmed cell death in chicken limb buds. *Development* 1996;122:3725–3734.

145. Chen D, Ji X, Harris MA, et al. Differential roles for bone morphogenetic protein (BMP) receptor type IB and IA in differentiation and specification of mesenchymal precursor cells to osteoblast and adipocyte lineages. *J Cell Biol* 1998;142:295–305.

146. Erlacher L, McCartney J, Piek E, et al. Cartilage-derived morphogenetic proteins and osteogenic protein-1 differentially regulate osteogenesis. *J Bone Miner Res* 1998;13:383–392.

147. Mishina Y, Suzuki A, Ueno N, et al. Bmpr encodes a type I bone morphogenetic protein receptor that is essential for gastrulation during mouse embryogenesis. *Genes Dev* 1995;9:3027–3037.

148. Brummel T, Abdollah S, Haerry TE, et al. The *Drosophila* activin receptor baboon signals through dSmad2 and controls cell proliferation but not patterning during larval development. *Genes Dev* 1999;13:98–111.

149. Brummel TJ, Twombly V, Marques G, et al. Character-

ization and relationship of Dpp receptors encoded by the saxophone and thick veins genes in *Drosophila. Cell* 1994;78:251–261.

150. Neul JL, Ferguson EL. Spatially restricted activation of the SAX receptor by SCW modulates DPP/TKV signaling in *Drosophila* dorsal–ventral patterning. *Cell* 1998;95:483–494.

151. Nguyen M, Park S, Marques G, et al. Interpretation of a BMP activity gradient in *Drosophila* embryos depends on synergistic signaling by two type I receptors, SAX and TKV. *Cell* 1998;95:495–506.

152. Haerry TE, Khalsa O, O'Connor MB, et al. Synergistic signaling by two BMP ligands through the SAX and TKV receptors controls wing growth and patterning in *Drosophila. Development* 1998;125:3977–3987.

153. Feng XH, Derynck R. A kinase subdomain of transforming growth factor-β (TGF-β) type I receptor determines the TGF-β intracellular signaling specificity. *EMBO J* 1997;16:3912–3923.

154. Georgi LL, Albert PS, Riddle DL. daf-1, a *C. elegans* gene controlling dauer larva development, encodes a novel receptor protein kinase. *Cell* 1990;61:635–645.

155. Krishna S, Maduzia LL, Padgett RW. Specificity of TGFβ signaling is conferred by distinct type I receptors and their associated SMAD proteins in *Caenorhabditis elegans. Development* 1999;126:251–260.

156. Ren P, Lim CS, Johnsen R, et al. Control of *C. elegans* larval development by neuronal expression of a TGF-β homolog. *Science* 1996;274:1389–1391.

157. Hoodless PA, Haerry T, Abdollah S, et al. MADR1, a MAD-related protein that functions in BMP2 signaling pathways. *Cell* 1996;85:489–500.

158. Graff JM, Bansal A, Melton DA. *Xenopus* Mad proteins transduce distinct subsets of signals for the TGF β superfamily. *Cell* 1996;85:479–487.

159. Wilson PA, Lagna G, Suzuki A, et al. Concentration-dependent patterning of the *Xenopus* ectoderm by BMP4 and its signal transducer Smad1. *Development* 1997;124:3177–3184.

160. Liu F, Hata A, Baker JC, et al. A human Mad protein acting as a BMP-regulated transcriptional activator. *Nature* 1996;381:620–623.

161. Kretzschmar M, Liu F, Hata A, et al. The TGF-β family mediator Smad1 is phosphorylated directly and activated functionally by the BMP receptor kinase. *Genes Dev* 1997;11:984–995.

162. Nishimura R, Kato Y, Chen D, et al. Smad5 and DPC4 are key molecules in mediating BMP-2-induced osteoblastic differentiation of the pluripotent mesenchymal precursor cell line C2C12. *J Biol Chem* 1998;273: 1872–1879.

163. Suzuki A, Chang C, Yingling JM, et al. Smad5 induces ventral fates in *Xenopus* embryo. *Dev Biol* 1997;184: 402–405.

164. Yamamoto N, Akiyama S, Katagiri T, et al. Smad1 and Smad5 act downstream of intracellular signaling of BMP-2 that inhibits myogenic differentiation and induces osteoblast differentiation in C2C12 myoblasts. *Biochem Biophys Res Commun* 1997;238:574–580.

165. Tamaki K, Souchelnytskyi S, Itoh S, et al. Intracellular signaling of osteogenic protein-1 through Smad5 activation. *J Cell Physiol* 1998;177:355–363.

166. Chen Y, Bhushan A, Vale W. Smad8 mediates the signaling of the ALK-2 receptor serine kinase. *Proc Natl Acad Sci USA* 1997;94:12938–12943.

167. Watanabe TK, Suzuki M, Omori Y, et al. Cloning and characterization of a novel member of the human Mad gene family (MADH6). *Genomics* 1997;42:446–451.

168. Kawabata M, Miyazono K. Signal transduction of the TGF-β superfamily by Smad proteins. *J Biochem (Tokyo)* 1999;125:9–16.

169. Chen X, Rubock MJ, Whitman M. A transcriptional partner for MAD proteins in TGF-β signalling. *Nature* 1996;383:691–696.

170. Zhang Y, Feng XH, Derynck R. Smad3 and Smad4 cooperate with c-Jun/c-Fos to mediate TGF-β-induced transcription. *Nature* 1998;394:909–913.

171. Kim J, Johnson K, Chen HJ, et al. *Drosophila* Mad binds to DNA and directly mediates activation of vestigial by Decapentaplegic. *Nature* 1997;388:304–308.

172. Xu X, Yin Z, Hudson JB, et al. Smad proteins act in combination with synergistic and antagonistic regulators to target Dpp responses to the *Drosophila* mesoderm. *Genes Dev* 1998;12:2354–2370.

173. Zawel L, Dai JL, Buckhaults P, et al. Human Smad3 and Smad4 are sequence-specific transcription activators. *Mol Cell* 1998;1:611–617.

174. Dennler S, Itoh S, Vivien D, et al. Direct binding of Smad3 and Smad4 to critical TGF β-inducible elements in the promoter of human plasminogen activator inhibitor-type 1 gene. *EMBO J* 1998;17:3091–3100.

175. Jonk LJ, Itoh S, Heldin CH, et al. Identification and functional characterization of a Smad binding element (SBE) in the JunB promoter that acts as a transforming growth factor-β, activin, and bone morphogenetic protein-inducible enhancer. *J Biol Chem* 1998;273: 21145–21152.

176. Shi Y, Wang YF, Jayaraman L, et al. Crystal structure of a Smad MH1 domain bound to DNA: insights on DNA binding in TGF-β signaling. *Cell* 1998;94: 585–594.

177. Janknecht R, Wells NJ, Hunter T. TGF-β-stimulated cooperation of Smad proteins with the coactivators CBP/p300. *Genes Dev* 1998;12:2114–2119.

178. Feng XH, Zhang Y, Wu RY, et al. The tumor suppressor Smad4/DPC4 and transcriptional adaptor CBP/p 300 are coactivators for smad3 in TGF-β-induced transcriptional activation. *Genes Dev* 1998;12:2153–2163.

179. Topper JN, DiChiara MR, Brown JD, et al. CREB binding protein is a required coactivator for Smad-dependent, transforming growth factor β transcriptional responses in endothelial cells. *Proc Natl Acad Sci USA* 1998;95:9506–9511.

180. Pouponnot C, Jayaraman L, Massagué J. Physical and functional interaction of SMADs and p300/CBP. *J Biol Chem* 1998;273:22865–22868.

181. Nishihara A, Hanai JI, Okamoto N, et al. Role of p300, a transcriptional coactivator, in signalling of TGF-β. *Genes Cells* 1998;3:613–623.

182. Shen X, Hu PP, Liberati NT, et al. TGF-β-induced phosphorylation of Smad3 regulates its interaction with coactivator p300/CREB-binding protein. *Mol Biol Cell* 1998;9:3309–3319.

183. Tang SJ, Hoodless PA, Lu Z, et al. The Tlx-2 homeobox gene is a downstream target of BMP signalling and is required for mouse mesoderm development. *Development* 1998;125:1877–1887.

184. Chen YG, Hata A, Lo RS, et al. Determinants of specificity in TGF-β signal transduction. *Genes Dev* 1998; 12:2144–2152.

185. Hayashi H, Abdollah S, Qiu Y, et al. The MAD-related protein Smad7 associates with the TGFβ receptor and functions as an antagonist of TGFβ signaling. *Cell* 1997;89:1165–1173.

186. Imamura T, Takase M, Nishihara A, et al. Smad6 inhibits signalling by the TGF-β superfamily. *Nature* 1997; 389:622–626.

187. Nakao A, Afrakhte M, Moren A, et al. Identification of Smad7, a TGFβ-inducible antagonist of TGF-β signalling. *Nature* 1997;389:631–635.

188. Hata A, Lagna G, Massagué J, et al. Smad6 inhibits BMP/Smad1 signaling by specifically competing with the Smad4 tumor suppressor. *Genes Dev* 1998;12: 186–197.

189. Tsuneizumi K, Nakayama T, Kamoshida Y, et al. Daughters against dpp modulates dpp organizing activity in *Drosophila* wing development. *Nature* 1997;389: 627–631.

190. Takase M, Imamura T, Sampath TK, et al. Induction of Smad6 mRNA by bone morphogenetic proteins. *Biochem Biophys Res Commun* 1998;244:26–29.

191. Afrakhte M, Moren A, Jossan S, et al. Induction of inhibitory Smad6 and Smad7 mRNA by TGF-β family members. *Biochem Biophys Res Commun* 1998;249: 505–511.

192. Itoh S, Landstrom M, Hermansson A, et al. Transforming growth factor β1 induces nuclear export of inhibitory Smad7. *J Biol Chem* 1998;273:29195–29201.

193. Souchelnytskyi S, Nakayama T, Nakao A, et al. Physical and functional interaction of murine and *Xenopus* Smad7 with bone morphogenetic protein receptors and transforming growth factor-β receptors. *J Biol Chem* 1998;273:25364–25370.

194. Nakayama T, Gardner H, Berg LK, et al. Smad6 functions as an intracellular antagonist of some TGF-β family members during *Xenopus* embryogenesis. *Genes Cells* 1998;3:387–394.

195. Nakayama T, Snyder MA, Grewal SS, et al. *Xenopus* Smad8 acts downstream of BMP-4 to modulate its activity during vertebrate embryonic patterning. *Development* 1998;125:857–867.

196. Casellas R, Brivanlou AH. *Xenopus* Smad7 inhibits both the activin and BMP pathways and acts as a neural inducer. *Dev Biol* 1998;198:1–12.

197. Bhushan A, Chen Y, Vale W. Smad7 inhibits mesoderm formation and promotes neural cell fate in *Xenopus* embryos. *Dev Biol* 1998;200:260–268.

198. Inoue H, Imamura T, Ishidou Y, et al. Interplay of signal mediators of decapentaplegic (Dpp): molecular characterization of mothers against dpp, Medea, and daughters against dpp. *Mol Biol Cell* 1998;9: 2145–2156.

199. Das P, Inoue H, Baker JC, et al. *Drosophila* dSmad2 and Atr-1 transmit activin/TGF-β signals. *Genes Cells* 1999;4:123–134.

200. Grieder NC, Nellen D, Burke R, et al. Schnurri is required for *Drosophila* Dpp signaling and encodes a zinc finger protein similar to the mammalian transcription factor PRDII-BF1. *Cell* 1995;81:781–790.

201. Arora K, Dai H, Kazuko SG, et al. The *Drosophila* schnurri gene acts in the Dpp/TGF β signaling pathway and encodes a transcription factor homologous to the human MBP family. *Cell* 1995;81:781–790.

202. Staehling-Hampton K, Laughon AS, Hoffmann FM. A *Drosophila* protein related to the human zinc finger transcription factor PRDII/MBPI/HIV-EP1 is required for dpp signaling. *Development* 1995;121:3393–3403.

203. Katya D, Henderson KD, Isaac DD, et al. Cell fate specification in the *Drosophila* salivary gland: the integration of homeotic gene function with the DPP signaling cascade. *Dev Biol* 1999;205:10–21.

204. Yamaguchi K, Shirakabe K, Shibuya H, et al. Identification of a member of the MAPKKK family as a potential mediator of TGF-β signal transduction. *Science* 1995;270:2008–2011.

205. Shibuya H, Yamaguchi K, Shirakabe K, et al. TAB1: an activator of the TAK1 MAPKKK in TGF-β signal transduction. *Science* 1996;272:1179–1182.

206. Shibuya H, Iwata H, Masuyama N, et al. Role of TAK1 and TAB1 in BMP signaling in early *Xenopus* development. *EMBO J* 1998;17:1019–1028.

207. Yamaguchi K, Nagai S, Ninomiya-Tsuji J, et al. XIAP, a cellular member of the inhibitor of apoptosis protein family, links the receptors to TAB1-TAK1 in the BMP signaling pathway. *EMBO J* 1999;18:179–187.

208. Kurozumi K, Nishita M, Yamaguchi K, et al. BRAM1, a BMP receptor-associated molecule involved in BMP signalling. *Genes Cells* 1998;3:257–264.

209. Xu RH, Dong Z, Maeno M, et al. Involvement of Ras/Raf/AP-1 in BMP-4 signaling during *Xenopus* embryonic development. *Proc Natl Acad Sci USA* 1996; 93:834–838.

210. Kretzschmar M, Doody J, Massagué J. Opposing BMP and EGF signalling pathways converge on the TGF-β family mediator Smad1. *Nature* 1997;389:618–622.

211. de Caestecker MP, Parks WT, Frank CJ, et al. Smad2 transduces common signals from receptor serine-threonine and tyrosine kinases. *Genes Dev* 1998;12: 1587–1592.

212. Chiang C, Litingtung Y, Lee E, et al. Cyclopia and defective axial patterning in mice lacking Sonic hedgehog gene function. *Nature* 1996;383:407–413.

213. Bitgood MJ, Shen L, McMahon AP. Sertoli cell signaling by Desert hedgehog regulates the male germline. *Curr Biol* 1996;6:298–304.

214. Vortkamp A, Lee K, Lanske B, et al. Regulation of rate of cartilage differentiation by Indian hedgehog and PTH-related protein. *Science* 1996;273:613–622.

215. Naski MC, Colvin JS, Coffin JD, et al. Repression of hedgehog signaling and BMP4 expression in growth plate cartilage by fibroblast growth factor receptor 3. *Development* 1998;125:4977–4988.

216. Mehler MF, Mabie PC, Zhang D, et al. Bone morphogenetic proteins in the nervous system. *Trends Neurosci* 1997;20:309–317.

217. Ducy P, Zhang R, Geoffroy V, et al. Osf2/Cbfa1: a transcriptional activator of osteoblast differentiation. *Cell* 1997;89:747–754.

218. Komori T, Yagi H, Nomura S, et al. Targeted disruption of Cbfa1 results in a complete lack of bone formation owing to maturational arrest of osteoblasts. *Cell* 1997;89:755–764.

219. Otto F, Thornell AP, Crompton T, et al. Cbfa1, a candidate gene for cleidocranial dysplasia syndrome, is essential for osteoblast differentiation and bone development. *Cell* 1997;89:765–771.

220. Mundlos S, Otto F, Mundlos C, et al. Mutations involving the transcription factor CBFA1 cause cleidocranial dysplasia. *Cell* 1997;89:773–779.

221. Tsuji K, Ito Y, Noda M. Expression of the PEBP2alphaA/AML3/CBFA1 gene is regulated by BMP4/7 heterodimer and its overexpression suppresses type I collagen and osteocalcin gene expression in osteoblastic and nonosteoblastic mesenchymal cells. *Bone* 1998;22:87–92.

222. Kawabata M, Inoue H, Hanyu A, et al. Smad proteins exist as monomers *in vivo* and undergo homo- and hetero-oligomerization upon activation by serine/threonine kinase receptors. *EMBO J* 1998;17:4056–4065.

Skeletal Growth Factors,
edited by Ernesto Canalis.
Lippincott Williams & Wilkins, Philadelphia, © 2000.

20

Bone Morphogenetic Proteins and Skeletal and Nonskeletal Development

Gerard Karsenty

*Department of Molecular and Human Genetics, Baylor College of Medicine,
Houston, Texas 77003*

The generic name "bone morphogenetic protein" (BMP) represents an ever-growing subgroup of the transforming growth factor-β (TGF-β) superfamily of growth factors (1–3). With more than 40 members already described, this subgroup represents almost one-third of the TGF-β superfamily. Individually, the members of this subfamily of secreted molecules are termed either BMPs, osteogenic proteins (OPs), cartilage-derived morphogenetic proteins (CDMPs), or growth and differentiation factors (GDFs). As extensive studies of their functions are performed *in vivo,* it becomes increasingly evident that this latter name is more appropriate to describe this subfamily than the term "BMPs." This latter name was proposed by Urist and collaborators (4–6) in their pioneering work demonstrating that demineralized bone extracts could induce *de novo* bone formation when implanted in ectopic sites in rats. This process, which recapitulates all of the events occurring during embryonic skeletal development (7–9), from the beginning generated a great deal of interest among bone biologists and developmental biologists. Indeed, in a sequence that is now very well known, the implant is first colonized by undifferentiated mesenchymal cells, which differentiate into chondrocytes. Later, vascular invasion occurs, followed by osteoblast and osteoclast differentiation and then *de novo* bone formation. These experiments, performed in the 1960s, were followed by the cloning of the first BMPs more than 20 years later and the demonstration that, as isolated or recombinant molecules, these factors could reproduce the bone-forming activity of the bone extracts (1, 10–15).

The availability of cDNA clones for various BMPs and their identification as TGF-β relatives enhanced the interest in these molecules and allowed expression and functional studies to be performed. Unexpectedly maybe, given the nature of the original assay that led to the identification of these proteins, it became rapidly evident that their pattern of expression as well as their physiological functions are not restricted to skeletal development when they affect it. These functions include cell proliferation and differentiation, apoptosis, morphogenesis, patterning of various organs and the skeleton, and organogenesis (16–22). Moreover, recent experiments have shown that several BMP family members cannot induce *de novo* bone formation in the classical subcutaneous implantation assay (23), highlighting the functional heterogeneity of this subfamily. Taking this important fact in account, this review focuses on the few BMP family members whose ability to ectopically form bone in this assay has been demonstrated (12,24–28). This chapter also considers what has been learned about the physiological function of several BMPs *in vivo,* using mostly findings of mouse and human genetics, to delineate the extent to which their physiological role relates to their pharmacological ability.

PATTERN OF EXPRESSION OF BONE MORPHOGENETIC PROTEINS

If the expression pattern of a gene or a family of genes is a reflection of its potential function, one would have predicted, given their spectacular function *in vitro,* that the genes encoding the various BMPs would be expressed preferentially, if not exclusively, in mesenchymal condensations prefiguring the future skeleton, in developing bones, and in differentiated chondrocytes and/or osteoblasts. As it turns out, this is not the case for any of the BMPs for which the pattern of expression has been described. Multiple studies documenting the pattern of expression of *Bmps 2, 4, 5, 6,* and *7,* summarized below, illustrate the point that the developing skeleton is neither the only nor the major site of expression of the BMPs.

Bmp-2 expression can be detected as early as 8.5 days post coitum (dpc) in mesodermal cells of the amnion and chorion cells of the visceral endoderm, the allantois, and the lateral plate mesoderm underlying the head fold (29,30). From 8.5 to 9.5 dpc, *Bmp-2* is also expressed in the dorsal surface ectoderm underlying the neural tube (31). Around 9.5 to 10.5 dpc, its expression can be detected in the outer myocardial layer of the heart, the apical ectodermal ridge, and the zone of polarizing activity of the developing limb (29–32). Starting at 12.5 dpc, *Bmp-2* expression is also observed in the mesenchymal condensation that will give rise to the ribs and vertebrae, tooth buds, developing eye, and whisker follicles (31–33). Later during development, *Bmp-2* transcript can be observed in hypertrophic chondrocytes of long bones and in forming digits (34).

Bmp-4, which encodes a protein closely related to BMP-2, starts to be expressed as early as 6.5 dpc, around the time of gastrulation (35–37). At 7.5 dpc, *Bmp-4* becomes widely expressed in the embryo, marking the allantois, the amnion, and the posterior part of the primitive streak (30,35). At that stage, expression is restricted to ectodermal tissues in the chicken embryo (30). Between 8.5 and 9.5 dpc, a strong *Bmp-4* expression can be observed in the neural tube area, principally localized in the posterior

mesoderm and prospective diencephalon but also present in the dorsal surface ectoderm and the presumptive neural crest cells (31). As development proceeds, *Bmp-4* transcripts become detectable in the mesoderm around the developing gut, the myocardium, the branchial arches, the developing eye, the otic vesicles, the neuroepithelium that is destined to associate with Rathke's pouch, and the dorsomedial telencephalon region that will give rise to the choroid plexus (31,35,37–39). As for *Bmp-2, Bmp-4* transcripts can be found in both the epithelium and mesenchyme tissues of the developing limb bud (mesoderm and apical ectodermal ridge) and tooth bud, suggesting that it also plays a role in the epithelial–mesenchymal interactions that characterize skeletal and tooth development as well as many other organogenesis processes (35,37).

Bmp-5 is expressed in the mesenchymal cells of the developing lung starting at 10.5 dpc. Thereafter, it is expressed in the ureter and connective tissue–producing cells underlying the bladder in the presumptive gut, the ventricular chamber of the heart, the meninges, and transiently in the telencephalon (31,39,40). During skeletal development, *Bmp-5* expression marks some of the mesenchymal condensations, such as the genital tubercle, the sternum, the thyroid cartilage, the cartilage rings of the trachea, and in the cells forming part of the vertebrae (34, 40,41).

Bmp-6 also has a broad pattern of expression. At 8.5 dpc, it is expressed in the branchial pouch and in the endodermal component of the visceral yolk sac (39,42). By 9.5 dpc, *Bmp-6* transcripts can be detected in the roof plate of the neural tube (39). In the developing heart, *Bmp-6* expression is restricted to the epithelium of the branchial pouch (29,35). Moreover, *Bmp-6* is expressed in the developing kidney, where it marks the stromal cells surrounding the developing and mature tubercles, and in the developing skin (33,35). In the developing skeleton, *Bmp-6* is expressed preferentially in hypertrophic chondrocytes (34,43).

Bmp-7 is another member of the family whose broad expression has been extensively studied. It starts to be expressed during early gastrulation, localizing in the ectoderm of the periphery of the embryo (29,30). At 8.5 and 9.5 dpc, *Bmp-7* is strongly expressed in the surface ectoderm and the notochord, the neuroepithelium extending toward the prospective forebrain, and the developing gut (29,31). *Bmp-7* is also expressed in the atrial and ventricular chambers; this heart expression will continue throughout development (31). During eye development, *Bmp-7* expression is detected in the surface ectoderm, the lens placode, and the optic vesicle (29, 31,44,45). *Bmp-7* is expressed in many cells of the developing kidney, including the metanephric mesenchymal nephrogenic tubules and glomeruli (31,44,45). In the developing skeleton, *Bmp-7* is expressed in the developing limb, the mesenchymal cells localized between the developing digits, and the chondrogenic zones (31,40,44,45).

From this long enumeration, a few common themes emerge: BMP expression is widespread and dynamic as development proceeds, it is frequently localized at areas of epithelial–mesenchymal interaction, it precedes by many days the earliest event of skeletogenesis, it is found in many more tissues and organs than the future skeleton, and sometimes it interests the developing skeleton only marginally. Thus from these few examples one could predict that the various BMPs could have a broad range of physiological functions during embryonic development and beyond development.

SKELETAL ABNORMALITIES IN BONE MORPHOGENETIC PROTEIN-DEFICIENT ANIMALS

Through identification of the mutated genes in classical mouse mutants or through conventional gene targeting approaches, many BMP-encoding genes have been inactivated. The chronology of publication of the molecular elucidation of these various mutations led initially to the belief that the BMPs act mostly on skeletal development. However, a careful review of all of the mutants available today clearly indicates that this is not the case. We first review skeletal abnormalities in mice carrying a mutation in BMP-encoding genes and subsequently the nonskeletal phenotype.

The recessive *short ear (se/se)* mouse is a classical skeleton patterning mutant that has been very well studied over the last 60 years (46,51). The *short ear* mouse has many anatomical abnormalities: reduced size of the ear, reduction in body size, reduction in the number of ribs, misshaping or absence of the xiphoid appendix, hydronephrosis, medial misplacement of the left gonad, giant cell granulomas of the liver, and lung abnormalities. Green (48,50,51), in a series of landmark studies, hypothesized that it was possible to relate the variety of the skeletal phenotypes observed in the *short ear* mouse to a single function of the *short ear* gene during chondrocyte differentiation. This hypothesis was supported by the finding, among others, that the abnormal shape or absence of the xiphoid appendix was due to a delay in the formation of the mesenchymal condensation prefiguring it. The original hypothesis proved to be extremely accurate as it stated that the *short ear* gene causes "a slight reduction in the rate of formation of cartilage" but not an arrest of differentiation, as chondrocytes and osteoblasts are present, even in affected skeletal structures. This hypothesis could extend to the nonskeletal phenotypes only if one assumes that the *short ear* gene acts in multiple organs where it is expressed.

In another landmark study, it was hypothesized that the *short ear* gene controlled cartilage formation. Kingsley et al. (52) demonstrated that the gene mutated or deleted in the *short ear* mouse was the *Bmp-5* gene. These authors went on to show that *Bmp-5* is expressed in the mesenchymal condensation outlining the future skeletal elements that are affected as well as in the periosteum (40). They showed subsequently that *Bmp-5* is also expressed in lung, liver, bladder, and intestines, all organs that are affected in the *short ear* mouse (40,51). A recent histomorphometric analysis revealed that the absence of BMP-5 led to a marginal increase in growth plate height and growth rate but no change in the number of proliferative and hypertrophic chondrocytes (53).

Brachypodism (bp) is another classical mouse mutation that appeared spontaneously on an outbred mouse strain in 1952 (54). Affected animals are characterized by a reduction in length of several long bones and the replacement of two bones in most digits by a single skeletal element (54,55). The product of the *bp* gene was thought for a long time to act cell non-autonomously and to control the formation of mesenchymal condensations (56,57). A similar approach was taken by the same group that uncovered the involvement of *Bmp-5* in the *short ear* mutation, demonstrating that the brachyphodism phenotype was due to frameshift mutations causing early termination in the *Gdf-5* gene (58). *Gdf-5* is a member of the BMP subfamily that does not have bone-forming activity but induces formation of tendon and ligament structures in the classical subcutaneous implantation assay used to identify the BMPs (23). Consistent with this pharmacological ability, *Gdf-5* is expressed during joint formation *in vivo* (41,59). However, mutations in the human GDF-5 gene called CDMP-1 have been implicated in two recessive chondrodysplasias, Hunter Thompson chondrodysplasia and chondrodysplasia-Grebe type (60–62). Mutations in the CDMP-1 gene also cause autosomal dominant brachydactyly type C (63). In *in vitro* studies, it was clear that overexpression of GDF-5 increased the size of the mesenchymal condensations without major effect on chondrocyte proliferation (56,57,64). This example illustrates the need to perform *in vivo* experiments to accurately understand the physiological function of a particular molecule.

Another remarkable fact is that for both *Bmp-5* and *Gdf-5*, mutations in the same gene cause recessive phenotypes in mice and dominant ones in humans. This seems to be a recurrent theme in the BMP field. Indeed, mice heterozygous for a deletion of noggin, an inhibitor of BMP action, have no overt phenotype, whereas humans heterozygous for a similar mutation develop a multiple synostosis phenotype (65,66).

Mutations in *Bmp-5* and *Gdf-5* were the first to be identified in BMP-encoding genes, and they seemed to indicate that the biological function of all BMPs could take place primarily, if not only, in the developing skeleton. As reported below, subsequent mutagenesis experiments in other genes showed that this was not the case. In fact, the mutations published in BMP-encoding

genes other than *Bmp-5* or *Gdf-5* have at best mild skeletal abnormalities. Homozygous *Bmp-2* or *Bmp-4* deletions in mice are embryonically lethal before the onset of skeletogenesis (29,37). Twelve percent of heterozygous *Bmp-4*-deficient mice have a preaxial polydactyly (37). Homozygous *Bmp-6*-deficient mice have no skeletal patterning defect and a mild delay of sternum ossification that could be traced to the formation of the mesenchymal condensation (34). Homozygous *Bmp-7*-deficient mice have patterning abnormalities of the ribs and a preaxial polydactyly in the hind limbs (44,45). As is the case for *short ear* mice, histological examination failed to detect any other abnormalities in chondrocyte and osteoblast differentiation in *Bmp-7*-deficient mice (45).

A generation of mice harboring mutations in two different BMP-encoding genes adds little to this picture. *Bmp-5/6* double mutant mice display only a slight exacerbation of the sternal defect present in single mutants (34). Mice carrying null mutations in both *Gdf-5* and *Bmp-5* have skeletal patterning defects that are not seen in any of the single mutants, but these abnormalities are extremely localized and do not disturb the differentiation of osteoblasts or chondrocytes (67). Likewise, mice carrying heterozygous mutations in both *Bmp-7* and *Bmp-4* have a higher frequency of rib cage and digit abnormalities than do single heterozygotes, suggesting that BMP-7 and BMP-4 may act jointly in the formation of the affected mesenchymal condensations (68). Lastly, *Bmp-5/7* double mutant mice die early during embryogenesis, before the beginning of skeletogenesis (69).

The mild and/or extremely localized skeletal defects observed in all of these mutant mice contrast strongly with the severity of the phenotype observed in other organs (see below). It indicates that the physiological functions of these proteins are different from their pharmacological abilities in two critical ways. Physiologically, they control mesenchymal condensation, i.e., skeletal patterning, but not cell differentiation, at least in the skeleton, and their actions in soft tissues appear to be more important than their actions in the skeleton.

EXTRASKELETAL ABNORMALITIES IN BONE MORPHOGENETIC PROTEIN-DEFICIENT ANIMALS

Consistent with their wide pattern of expression, mutations in BMP-encoding genes can affect many tissues and organogenesis processes. Some of these mutations cause early embryonic lethality, precluding for now analysis of the role of these proteins during skeletal development. We briefly review some of these phenotypes. Again, the purpose of this enumeration is to highlight the difference between the wealth of biological functions and the remarkable pharmacology of this group of molecules.

Inactivating mutation in some *Bmps* can result in early embryonic lethality or in perinatal lethality, caused by profound extraskeletal defects. For instance, *Bmp-2*-deficient mice died between 7.0 and 10.5 dpc, the mutant phenotype being evident at 7.75 dpc (29). The mutant embryo retained an open preamniotic canal and/or abnormal heart development. The maintenance of the preamniotic canal in an open state caused malformation of the amnion and the chorion. Heart development occurred abnormally in the exocoelonic cavity. Other abnormalities included delay in allantois development, open neural tubes, and overall slower growth of these embryos.

Inactivating mutations in *Bmp-4* also cause embryonic lethality, this time between 6.5 and 9.5 dpc with a variable phenotype (37). Most of the mutant embryos show virtually no mesodermal differentiation. Some embryos develop beyond 6.5 dpc and present with disorganized posterior structures, a reduction in extraembryonic mesoderm, and overall developmental retardation. More recently, it was shown that they contain no primordial germ and that lens induction does not occur (69–71). *Bmp-4* heterozygote-deficient mice present with a variable penetrance craniofacial malformation, microphthalmia, and preaxial polydactyly, indicating that *Bmp-4* gene dosage is essential for normal organogenesis. The extent and the severity of the abnormalities recorded in the *Bmp-4* homozygous or heterozygous mutant embryo mice emphasize the pleiotropic function of the BMPs *in vivo*.

Another BMP-encoding gene whose deletion causes a perinatal lethality in mice is *Bmp-7* (44,45). In the absence of *Bmp-7,* there is a failure of epithelial–mesenchymal interaction during metanephros development, leading eventually to a near absence of glomerular formation. Moreover, there is, with incomplete penetrance, an absence of lens induction and eye formation. This latter phenotype is reminiscent of what is observed in *Bmp-4*-deficient embryos. This is important as it suggests that, at least during lens formation, redundancy between BMPs may not prevent abnormalities. The argument of functional redundancy to explain the mild skeletal phenotype observed in single *Bmp*-deficient mice cannot be denied as long as appropriate genetic experiments have not been performed.

As Green (51) pointed out, *Bmp-5*-deficient mice also have many nonskeletal phenotypes, although none is life-threatening. These can include medial displacement of the left gonad, ventralization of the right renal artery, hydronephrosis, giant cell granuloma on the ventral surface of the liver, and cysts of the lung. These defects are in agreement with the pattern of expression of *Bmp-5* (40,51).

Lastly, one cannot ignore the increasing number of BMP-encoding genes whose inactivation in mice did not give any visible skeletal abnormalities while other organs or functions were profoundly affected. For instance, deficiency in GDF-7, a close relative of GDF-5 (58), blocks the generation of a particular class of neurons (71). Considering the ligament/tendon-forming activity of GDF-7 in the subcutaneous implantation assay (23), such a role was unexpected. This result, along with the expression of *Bmps 2, 4, and 7* and *Gdf-1* and *Gdf-11* in the developing brain (31,39,72,73), indicates that BMPs may play an important yet poorly understood role in the morphogenesis of the central nervous system. Inactivation of *Gdf-8*, also called myostatin, induced in mice or spontaneous in bovine, results in muscular hypertrophy, implicating BMPs in the control of skeletal muscle growth (74,75). Germ cell proliferation and maturation are other functions in which BMPs seem to play a critical role. *Bmp-8a* and *Bmp-8b* are tightly linked on mouse chromosome 4 and have similar patterns of expression. Inactivation of *Bmp-8a* leads to germ cell degeneration in nearly 50% of adult males (76). Likewise, *Bmp-8b*-deficient mice have as a sole reported phenotype a male germ cell deficiency and sterility (77). These two studies identified these two BMPs as critical proteins in germ cell development, maintenance of spermatogenesis, and fertility in male mice. BMPs are also involved in maintenance of the female reproductive system. Female mice null for *Gdf-9,* an oocyte-specific gene, exhibit primary infertility due to failed ovarian follicular development (78–80).

In summary, genetic and molecular studies have helped define the paramount importance of the BMPs in multiple physiological processes. In fact, it is now clear that most of the BMPs studied so far have, *in vivo,* profound and specific effects on organogenesis processes outside the skeleton. Because some of these effects lead to embryonic lethality before the onset of skeletogenesis, it is possible that roles in this latter process may have been underestimated. The possibility now exists to perform cell-specific and time-specific analyses of genes at will. Most likely, these studies will determine the extent of the physiological role of the BMPs during skeletal development. Regardless of what the genetics taught us, some BMPs have the unique pharmacological ability, not shared with other members of the TGF-β superfamily, to induce *de novo* bone formation. The domain responsible for this action remains a critical question to answer.

ACKNOWLEDGMENTS

Gerard Karsenty is indebted to Patricia Ducy, Ph.D., for her help in preparing this chapter.

REFERENCES

1. Wozney JM, Rosen V, Celeste AJ, et al. Novel regulators of bone formation: molecular clones and activities. *Science* 1988;242:1528–1534.
2. Rosen V, Thies RS. BMPs in bone formation and repair. *Trends Genet* 1992;8:97–102.
3. Kinglsey DM. The TGF-β superfamily: new members, new receptors, and genetic tests of function in different organisms. *Genes Dev* 1994b;8:133–146.
4. Urist MR. Bone: formation by autoinduction. *Science* 1965;150:893–899.
5. Urist MR, Iwata H, Ceccotti PL, et al. Bone morphogenesis in implants of insoluble bone gelatin. *Proc Natl Acad Sci USA* 1973;70:3511–3515.
6. Urist MR, Mikulski A, Lietze A. Solubilized and insolubilized bone morphogenetic protein. *Proc Natl Acad Sci USA* 1979;76:1828–1832.
7. Reddi AH. Regulation of cartilage and bone differentiation by bone morphogenetic proteins. *Curr Opin Cell Biol* 1992;4:850–855.
8. Horton WA. Morphology of connective tissue: cartilage. In: Royce PM, Steinmann B, eds. *Connective tissue and its heritable disorders.* New York: Wiley-Liss. 1993: 73–84.
9. Reddi AH. Bone and cartilage differentiation. *Curr Opin Genet Dev* 1994;4:737–744.
10. Sampath TK, Muthukumaran N, Reddi AH. Isolation of osteogenin, an extracellular matrix–associated bone-inductive protein, by heparin affinity chromatography. *Proc Natl Acad Sci USA* 1987;84:7109–7113.
11. Wang EA, Rosen V, Cordes P, et al. Purification and characterization of other distinct bone-inducing factors. *Proc Natl Acad Sci USA* 1988;85:9484–9488.
12. Luxenberg DP, McQuaid D, Moustatsos IK, et al. Recombinant human bone morphogenetic protein induces bone formation. *Proc Natl Acad Sci USA* 1990;87: 2220–2224.
13. Wang EA, Wozney JM. Identification of transforming growth factor β family members present in bone-inductive protein purified from bovine bone. *Proc Natl Acad Sci USA* 1990;87:9843–9847.
14. Sampath TK, Ozkaynak E, Jones WK, et al. Recombinant human osteogenic protein-1 (hOP1) induces new bone formation with a specific activity comparable to that of natural bovine osteogenic protein. *J Bone Miner Res* 1991;6:S155.
15. Wozney JM. The bone morphogenetic protein family and osteogenesis. *Mol Reprod Dev* 1992;32:160–167.
16. Kingsley DM. What do BMPs do in mammals? Clues from the mouse short-ear mutation. *Trends Genet* 1994; 10:16–21.
17. Harland RM. The transforming growth factor β family and induction of the vertebrate mesoderm: bone morphogenetic proteins are ventral inducers. *Proc Natl Acad Sci USA* 1994;91:10243–10246.
18. Hogan BLM. Bone morphogenetic proteins: multifunctional regulators of vertebrate development. *Genes Dev* 1996;10:1580–1594.
19. Reddi AH. Bone morphogenetic proteins: an unconventional approach to isolation of first mammalian morphogens. *Cytokine Growth Factor Rev* 1997;8:11–20.
20. Graff JM. Embryonic patterning: to BMP or not to BMP, that is the question. *Cell* 1997;89:171–174.
21. Ebendal T, Bengtsson H, Soderstrom S. Bone morphogenetic proteins and their receptors: potential functions in the brain. *J Neurosci Res* 1998;51:139–146.
22. Wozney JM. The bone morphogenetic protein family: multifunctional cellular regulators in the embryo and adult. *Eur J Oral Sci* 1998;106:160–166.
23. Wolfman NM, Hattesley G, Cox K, et al. Ectopic induction of tendon and ligament in rats by growth and differentiation factors 5, 6, and 7, members of the TGF-β gene family. *J Clin Invest* 1997;100:321–330.
24. Hammonds RG Jr, Schwall R, Dudley A, et al. Bone-inducing activity of mature BMP-2b produced from a

hybrid BMP-2a/2b precursor. *Mol Endocrinol* 1991;5: 149–155.

25. Cox K, Holtrop M, D'Alessandro JS, et al. Histological and ultrastructural comparison of the *in vivo* activities of rhBMP-2 and rhBMP-5. *J Bone Miner Res* 1991;6: S155.

26. D'Alessandro JS, Cox KA, Israel DI, et al. Purification, characterization and activities of recombinant bone morphogenetic protein 5. *J Bone Miner Res* 1991;6:S153.

27. Gitelman SE, Kobrin MS, YE J-Q, et al. Recombinant Bgr-1 BMP-6-expressing tumors induce fibrosis and endochondral bone formation *in vivo. J Cell Biol* 1994; 126:1595–1609.

28. Sampath TK, Maliakal JC, Hauschka PB, et al. Recombinant human osteogenic protein-1 (hOP-1) induces new bone formation *in vivo* with a specific activity comparable with natural bovine osteogenic protein and stimulates osteoblast proliferation and differentiation *in vitro. J Biol Chem* 1992;267:20352–20362.

29. Lyons KM, Hogan BL, Robertson EJ. Colocalization of BMP 7 and BMP 2 RNAs suggests that these factors cooperatively mediate tissue interactions during murine development. *Mech Dev* 1995;50:71–83.

30. Schultheiss TM, Burch JBE, Lassar AB. A role for bone morphogenetic proteins in the induction of cardiac myogenesis. *Genes Dev* 1997;11:451–462.

31. Dudley AT, Robertson EJ. Overlapping expression domains of bone morphogenetic protein family members potentially account for limited tissue defects in BMP7 deficient embryos. *Dev Dyn* 1997;208:349–362.

32. Lyons KM, Pelton RW, Hogan BL. Organogenesis and pattern formation in the mouse: RNA distribution patterns suggest a role for bone morphogenetic protein-2A (BMP-2A). *Development* 1990;109:833–844.

33. Lyons KM, Pelton RW, Hogan BL. Patterns of expression of murine Vgr-1 and BMP-2a RNA suggest that transforming growth factor-beta-like genes coordinately regulate aspects of embryonic development. *Genes Dev* 1989;3:1657–1668.

34. Solloway MJ, Dudley AT, Bikoff EK, et al. Mice lacking Bmp6 function. *Dev Genet* 1998;22:321–339.

35. Jones CM, Lyons KM, Hogan BL. Involvement of bone morphogenetic protein-4 (BMP-4) and Vgr-1 in morphogenesis and neurogenesis in the mouse. *Development* 1991;111:531–542.

36. Johansson BM, Wiles MV. Evidence for involvement of activin A and bone morphogenetic protein 4 in mammalian mesoderm and haematopoietic development. *Mol Cell Biol* 1995;15:141–151.

37. Winnier G, Blessing M, Labosky PA, et al. Bone morphogenetic protein-4 is required for mesoderm formation and patterning in the mouse. *Genes Dev* 1995;9: 2105–2116.

38. Oh SH, Johnson R, Wu DK. Differential expression of bone morphogenetic proteins in the developing vestibular and auditory sensory organs. *J Neurosci* 1996;16: 6463–6475.

39. Furuta Y, Piston DW, Hogan BL. Bone morphogenetic proteins (BMPs) as regulators of dorsal forebrain development. *Development* 1997;124:2203–2212.

40. King JA, Marker PC, Seung KJ, et al. BMP5 and the molecular, skeletal, and soft-tissue alterations in short ear mice. *Dev Biol* 1994;166:112–122.

41. Storm EE, Kingsley DM. GDF5 coordinates bone and joint formation during digit development. *Dev Biol* 1999;209:11–27.

42. Farrington SM, Belaoussoff M, Baron MH. Winged-helix, Hedgehog and BMP genes are differentially expressed in distinct cell layers of the murine yolk sac. *Mech Dev* 1997;62:197–211.

43. Iwasaki M, Le AX, Helms JA. Expression of *Indian hedgehog, bone morphogenetic protein 6* and *gli* during skeletal morphogenesis. *Mech Dev* 1997;69:197–202.

44. Dudley A, Lyons K, Robertson EJ. A requirement for bone morphogenetic protein-7 during development of the mammalian kidney and eye. *Genes Dev* 1995;9: 2795–2807.

45. Luo G, Hofmann C, Bronckers ALJ, et al. BMP-7 is an inducer of nephrogenesis, and is also required for eye development and skeletal patterning. *Genes Dev* 1995; 9:2808–2820.

46. Lynch CJ. Short ears, an autosomal mutation in the house mouse. *Am Nat* 1921;55:421–426.

47. Green EL, Green MC. The development of three manifestations of the short ear gene in the mouse. *J Morphol* 1942;70:1–19.

48. Green EL, Green MC. Effect of the short ear gene on number of ribs and presacral vertebrae in the house mouse. *Am Nat* 1946;80:619–625.

49. Green MC. Further morphological effects of the short ear gene in the house mouse. *J Morphol* 1951;88:1–22.

50. Green MC. Effects of the short ear gene in the mouse on cartilage formation in healing bone fractures. *J Exp Zool* 1958;137:75–88.

51. Green MC. Mechanism of the pleiotropic effects of the short ear mutant gene in the mouse. *J Exp Zool* 1968; 167:129–150.

52. Kingsley DM, Bland AE, Grubber JM, et al. The mouse short ear skeletal morphogenesis locus is associated with defects in a bone morphogenetic member of the TGF beta superfamily. *Cell* 1992;71:399–410.

53. Mikic B, Van der Meulen MC, Kingsley DM, et al. Mechanical and geometric changes in the growing femora of BMP-5 deficient mice. *Bone* 1996;18:601–617.

54. Landauer W. Brachypodism, a recessive mutation of house mice. *J Hered* 1952;43:293–298.

55. Gruneberg H, Lee AJ. The anatomy and development of brachypodism in the mouse. *J Embryol Exp Morphol* 1973;30:119–141.

56. Malinina NA, Kindiakov BN, Koniukhov BV. Mutant gene expression in mouse aggregation chimeras. 3. Brachypodism -H gene. *Ontogenez* 1984;15:514–521.

57. Owens EM, Solursh M. Cell–cell interaction by mouse limb cells during *in vitro* chondrogenesis: analysis of the brachypod mutation. *Dev Biol* 1982;91:376–388.

58. Storm EE, Huynh TV, Copeland NG, et al. Limb alterations in *brachypodism* mice due to mutations in a new member of the TGFβ-superfamily. *Nature* 1994;368: 639–643.

59. Merino R, Macias D, Ganan Y, et al. Expression and function of Gdf-5 during digit skeletogenesis in the embryonic chick leg bud. *Dev Biol* 1999;206:33–45.

60. Langer Lo Jr, Cervenka J, Camargo M. A severe autosomal recessive acromesomelic dysplasia, the Hunter-Thompson type, and comparison with the Grebe type. *Hum Genet* 1989;81:323–328.

61. Thomas JT, Lin K, Nandedkar M, et al. A human chondrodysplasia due to a mutation in a TGF-beta superfamily member. *Nat Genet* 1996;12:315–317.

62. Thomas JT, Kilpatrick MW, Keming L, et al. Disruption of human limb morphogenesis by a dominant negative mutation in CDMP1. *Nat Genet* 1997;17:58–64.

63. Polinkovsky A, Robin NH, Thomas JT, et al. Mutations in CDMP1 cause autosomal dominant brachydactyly type C. *Nat Genet* 1997;17:18–19.

64. Francis-West PH, Abdelfattah A, Chen P, et al. Mechanisms of GDF-5 action during skeletal development. *Development* 1999;126:1305–1315.

65. Brunet LJ, McMahon JA, McMahon AP, et al. Noggin, cartilage morphogenesis, and joint formation in the mammalian skeleton. *Science* 1998;280:1455–1457.

66. Gong Y, Krakow D, Marcelino J, et al. Heterozygous mutations in the gene encoding noggin affect human joint morphogenesis. *Nat Genet* 1999;21:302–304.

67. Storm EE, Kingsley DM. Joint patterning defects caused by single and double mutations in members of the bone morphogenetic protein (BMP) family. *Development* 1996;122:3969–3979.

68. Takenobu K, Boorla S, Frewndo J-L, et al. Skeletal abnormalities in doubly heterozygous *Bmp4* and *Bmp7* mice. *Dev Genet* 1998;22:340–348.

69. Furuta Y, Hogan BLM. BMP4 is essential for lens induction in the mouse embryo. *Genes Dev* 1998;12:3764–3775.

70. Lawson KA, Dunn NR, Roelen BA, et al. Bmp4 is required for the generation of primordial germ cells in the mouse embryo. *Genes Dev* 1999;13:424–436.

71. Lee KJ, Mendelsohn M, Jessell TM. Neuronal patterning by BMPs: a requirement for GDF7 in the generation of a discrete class of commissural interneurons in the mouse spinal cord. *Genes Dev* 1998;12:3394–3407.

72. Lee SJ. Expression of growth/differentiation factor 1 in the nervous system: conservation of a bicistronic structure. *Proc Natl Acad Sci USA* 1991;88:4250–4254.

73. Nakashima M, Toyono T, Akamine A, et al. Expression of growth/differentiation factor 11, a new member of the BMP/TGFβ superfamily during mouse embryogenesis. *Mech Dev* 1999;80:185–189.

74. McPherron AC, Lawler AM, Lee SJ. Regulation of skeletal muscle mass in mice by a new TGF-beta superfamily member. *Nature* 1997;387:83–90.

75. Kambadur R, Sharma M, Smith TP, et al. Mutations in myostatin (GDF8) in double-muscled Belgian blue and piedmontese cattle. *Genome Res* 1997;7:910–916.

76. Zhao GQ, Liaw L, Hogan BL. Bone morphogenetic protein 8A plays a role in the maintenance of spermatogenesis and the integrity of the epididymis. *Development* 1998;125:1103–1112.

77. Zhao GQ, Deng K, Labosky PA, et al. The gene encoding bone morphogenetic protein 8B is required for the initiation and maintenance of spermatogenesis in the mouse. *Genes Dev* 1996;10:1657–1669.

78. Dong J, Albertini DF, Nishimori K, et al. Growth differentiation factor-9 is required during early ovarian folliculogenesis. *Nature* 1996;383:531–535.

79. Fitzpatrick SL, Sindoni DM, Shughrue PJ, et al. Expression of growth differentiation factor-9 messenger ribonucleic acid in ovarian and nonovarian rodent and human tissues. *Endocrinology* 1998;139:2571–2578.

80. Carabatsos MJ, Elvin J, Matzuk MM, et al. Characterization of oocyte and follicle development in growth differentiation factor-9-deficient mice. *Dev Biol* 1998;204:373–384.

Skeletal Growth Factors,
edited by Ernesto Canalis.
Lippincott Williams & Wilkins, Philadelphia, © 2000.

21

Bone Morphogenetic Proteins and the Adult Skeleton

Vicki Rosen and *John M. Wozney

Genetics Institute, Cambridge, Massachusetts 02140
*Genetics Institute, Andover, Massachusetts 01310

The discovery of bone morphogenetic proteins (BMPs) and their roles as embryonic patterning and cell differentiation factors have been highlighted in the previous two chapters. Here, we focus on the adult skeleton, where the requirement for endogenously produced BMPs during normal bone remodeling and in bone repair is just beginning to be understood. We present an update on current ideas about the roles of BMPs in skeletal homeostasis and summarize recent data on the clinical utility of osteogenic BMPs in a wide variety of settings. Taken together, these data strengthen the idea that the signaling molecules required for embryonic skeletal development are also important for adult skeletal homeostasis and confirm that our understanding of the target cells for BMPs will allow us to design successful bone-regeneration therapies.

OSTEOGENESIS IN THE ADULT SKELETON

Formation of new bone by the adult skeleton occurs during bone remodeling and is activated when bones undergo trauma or surgical lenthening procedures. Each of these instances provides us with an opportunity to evaluate the role of BMPs.

Bone Remodeling

While determination of the size, shape, and location of skeletal elements is an embryonic event, the adult skeleton undergoes continuous turnover, a process known as bone remodeling. Removal of existing bone and its replacement by new bone is carried out in a highly controlled manner and requires the differentiation of both osteoblasts (bone-forming cells) and osteoclasts (bone-resorbing cells) from precursors located in the bone marrow environment (1). The exact nature of the signals that control remodeling remains to be established, but it is likely that both osteoblast and osteoclast precursors are affected by systemic and local signals and by mechanical stimuli (2). BMPs have been proposed to be the local signaling molecules that induce commitment of mesenchymal stem cells (MSCs) resident in bone marrow into osteoprogenitors and osteoblasts (3). Several lines of evidence make this hypothesis an attractive one. Much data exists to show that BMPs are present in bone matrix in a form that allows for their release or presentation to marrow stromal MSCs, cells that differentiate into osteoblasts *in vitro* in the presence of BMPs (4). Osteoblasts have also been shown to synthesize and secrete BMPs both *in vivo* and *in vitro,* suggesting that once BMPs initiate MSC differentiation, a positive-feedback loop is created, allowing for the production of additional BMP signals (5). Interestingly, the BMP antagonist noggin is also present in bone and made by osteoblasts, suggesting that local activation of MSCs may be highly controlled (6). It has also recently been reported that BMP-1, the procollagen C propeptide, is able to release

BMPs from collagenous matrix, providing another way that endogenous BMPs may be made available in a site-specific manner during the remodeling process (7). Finally, bone formation and bone resorption during remodeling may be linked through BMPs, as BMPs regulate the transcription of Cbfal, an osteoblast-specific transcription factor, which in turn may regulate transcription of receptor activator of NFκB (RANK) ligand, a signal important for the differentiation of hematopoietic progenitors into osteoclasts (3). If this is indeed the case, BMPs may be involved, directly or indirectly, in every step of the remodeling process.

These tantalizing links between BMPs and bone remodeling have become the focus of much research and may lead to new therapeutic approaches to osteopenia. Of fundamental importance in designing treatments that utilize site-specific activation of endogenous BMPs is the identification of which BMPs are available to affect bone remodeling and which cell types at each step of the remodeling process are the targets of these signals. Once the BMPs necessary for remodeling are identified, it will be interesting to determine whether factors that are known to change the balance in remodeling toward formation or resorption do so through effects on these BMPs. *In vitro* studies have shown that estrogens and glucocorticoids, two agents known to affect remodeling, increase BMP-6 synthesis by osteoblasts (8,9). However, mice in which the BMP-6 gene has been removed through homologous recombination in embryonic stem cells have no apparent skeletal defects and do not develop osteopenia, suggesting that BMP regulation of remodeling is likely to be complex (10). It will also be of great interest to determine whether the decrease in MSCs present in bone marrow that occurs with aging is related to the changes in levels of specific BMPs found in bone matrix of older animals (11). If BMPs are required for MSC survival as well as for MSC differentiation, changing the BMP content of bone matrix and bone marrow may have important clinical benefits.

Bone Morphogenetic Protein and Fracture Repair

New bone formation occurs in the adult skeleton during the process of fracture repair, when osteoblast progenitor cells resident in marrow and periosteum differentiate into osteoblasts in a highly regulated manner (12). BMPs have been shown to be present at fracture repair sites, and several lines of evidence support the role of BMPs in this process. First, all of the cell types that synthesize new bone during fracture healing have been shown to be targets for BMPs *in vitro* and to possess BMP receptors *in vivo* (13). In addition, immunohistochemical identification of BMPs 2 and 4 at the fracture site in rats suggests that BMPs may be released from bone matrix at the time of fracture and are then able to act on target cells in the area or recruit cells to the fracture site, where they differentiate into osteoblasts (14,15). Alternatively, BMPs may be synthesized by osteoblasts resident in bone and activated by other cytokines released during the fracture-healing process. While we still do not know which BMPs are absolutely required for fracture repair, data from the *short ear* mouse, a naturally occurring null for the BMP-5 gene, show that mice lacking BMP-5 have a reduced capacity to repair rib fractures as adults (16). The availability of animal models in which specific BMPs, BMP antagonists, and BMP receptors have been removed should allow us to address this issue and to begin to understand what regulates endogenous BMP production during fracture healing.

Bone Morphogenetic Proteins and Distraction Osteogenesis

A third circumstance in which the adult skeleton produces new bone is during distraction osteogenesis, a method of bone lengthening that takes advantage of the inherent capacity of bone to repair after breaking (17). In a clinically controlled setting, the bone to be lengthened is broken and the two opposing ends are increasingly separated from each other over the course of days or weeks. The end result of this engineered trauma is bone regeneration tailored to the distance of bone separation (18). We are just beginning to understand the molecular and cellular events that form the basis of distraction osteogenesis, and from these initial studies, it seems likely that BMPs are important mediators of bone formation at the distraction site. Recent data demonstrate temporal and spatial localization of mRNAs for BMPs in a rat model of distraction osteogenesis and link the mechanical stress/tension needed for successful distraction osteogenesis with BMP gene expression (19). It is likely that mechanical forces influence BMP gene expression at sites of distraction osteogenesis through a yet-to-be understood process and that BMPs are components of the complex signals required during several of the repair stages. The precise link between mechanical stress and BMP gene expression remains to be discovered, as do the other signaling pathways that must interact with BMPs to produce the cascade of events that results in temporally delayed bone formation. Understanding what regulates the temporal differences in bone formation seen between distraction osteogenesis and normal fracture healing, both thought to be BMP-mediated events, should provide insight into how BMPs affect the rate of repair.

THERAPEUTIC APPLICATIONS OF EXOGENOUS BONE MORPHOGENETIC PROTEINS

BMPs are currently being explored as bone-inductive agents in a wide range of therapeutic settings (Table 21.1). Among the most promising of these are the use of BMPs with specialty carriers to replace bone grafts, to regenerate bone at sites of osteonecrosis and periodontal disease, and to provide bone and augment integration and fixation of orthopedic prosthetic devices and dental implants. While fewer preclinical data exist on the ability of exogenously added BMPs to change the rate of fracture healing and the consolidation of bone during distraction osteogenesis, it is likely that BMPs will affect these important bone-formation events. The studies described in this section are limited to those conducted with recombinant, and thus pure, BMPs. Other reviews on some of these applications are also available (20–24).

Bone-Grafting Materials

The potent osteoinductive activity of BMPs provides an opportunity for development of novel bone-grafting materials able to create significant quantities of new bone *in vivo*. In this setting, a matrix/carrier material is used for BMP delivery. Components of bone matrix are obvious choices for such carriers, and demineralized bone matrix, growth factor–extracted demineralized bone matrix, and mineralized bone matrix from which the protein and cell components have been removed are each able to support BMP-induced bone formation. Purified collagen, applied in particulate, sponge, and gel forms, has also shown efficacy for BMP delivery in bone grafting. Additionally, calcium phos-

TABLE 21.1. *Applications of bone morphogenetic proteins (BMPs): preclinical study publications*

Application	rhBMP-2	rhBMP-7/OP-1
Orthopedics		
Long bone segmental defect repair	25–27,29–36	28,37–39
Fracture repair	92,94–97	93
Spinal fusion (intertransverse process)	53–61,67	62,68
Spinal fusion (interbody)	63–65	66
Implant fixation	69,70	71–73
Osteonecrosis	99,100	
Distraction osteogenesis	98	
Oral/maxillofacial		
Calvarial reconstruction	43–50	42
Mandibular reconstruction	40,41	89
Cleft palate repair	51,52	
Dental		
Periodontal repair	84–88	90,91
Alveolar augmentation/dental implant osseointegration	78–82	83
Subantral augmentation	74,75	76,77
Endodontic indications	104,105	101–103

OP-1, osteogenic protein-1; rh, recombinant human.

phate materials have been used to successfully deliver BMPs, as have other calcium salts. More recently, synthetic polymer materials made of polylactic acid and copolymers of polylactic acid and polyglycolic acid (PLGA) have been used to deliver BMPs at sites normally requiring bone grafting. The wide range of bone-derived and synthetic materials useful for BMP delivery allows for development of site- and application-specific bone graft replacements.

Preclinical Studies with Bone Morphogenetic Proteins in Bone Grafting

Large segmental long bone defects in several species have been used to evaluate the ability of BMPs to augment or replace bone grafts. These critical-sized defect models do not heal without surgical intervention, making it relatively easy to evaluate BMP-mediated bone induction using standard histological and radiographic techniques. The quality of the new bone and its ability to integrate into the preexisting bone can also be easily evaluated through simple biomechanical testing.

Early studies in which BMPs were combined with allogeneic demineralized bone revealed the osteoinductive capability of these molecules in small and large animals and highlighted the usefulness of BMPs in healing substantial defects. Bone union was evident in rat (25) and sheep (26) femur defects treated with recombinant human (rh) BMP-2, as assessed by radiography, histology, and biomechanics. In addition, longer-term evaluation showed the ability of the bone produced by rhBMP-2 to remodel in a manner similar to the host bone or bone graft, including reformation of the medullary cavity and cortex (27). A similar study in rabbit ulnae showed that osteogenic protein-1 (OP-1)/BMP-7 induced defect healing by 8 weeks (28). Remodeling of the new bone was apparent from the formation of new cortices and the appearance of marrow elements.

Subsequent studies have evaluated BMPs with more defined matrix materials. rhBMP-2 has been tested with bioerodible particles made of copolymers of PLGA formulated with autologous blood or carboxymethylcellulose (29–32),

porous polylactic acid rigid sponges (33), PLGA/gelatin composite sponges (PGS) (34), and an absorbable collagen sponge (ACS) (35,36). In these trials, rhBMP-2 successfully induced new bone formation with each matrix used. rhBMP-7/OP-1 has also successfully induced new bone formation in combination with demineralized extracted bovine bone matrix carrier in dog ulnar defects (37,38) and ulnar and tibial defects in nonhuman primates (39). In the latter study, 1 mg of BMP-7/OP-1 was shown to heal four out of five ulnar defects in African green monkeys. Comparing all of these long bone critical-sized defect models, it is apparent that the amount of BMP needed for healing varies with the species. For example, while 0.05 mg of BMP-7/OP-1 per gram of matrix was sufficient to heal ulnar defects in rabbits, 1.2 mg per gram provided superior efficacy in the canine study and 2.5 mg per gram was needed in nonhuman primates. The difference in BMP dose requirements in higher animals may relate to the available numbers of responsive mesenchymal cells or to the responsiveness of these cells. The characteristics of the carrier used to deliver BMPs in each of these studies may also affect the dose required for healing.

Similar to the orthopedic models, many studies have evaluated BMPs in critical-sized defects in the maxillofacial or cranial areas. The earliest report of the use of a recombinant BMP is the healing of 3-cm, full-thickness segmental defects in the mandibles of dogs (40). This study evaluated implantation of rhBMP-2 with demineralized extracted allogeneic bone matrix or the matrix alone compared with untreated defects. In the BMP-treated defects, bone was visible radiographically and palpable clinically by 4 weeks after implantation; the reconstruction plates could be removed by 3 months, and function was restored. None of the carrier-treated defects or untreated defects were bridged by bone at any time point. Histology revealed bone throughout the defects in the BMP-treated animals, with evidence of remodeling and recorticalization at later time points. The control and carrier defects healed with fibrous scar. This study highlighted the ability of BMP to induce substantial volumes of bone in the maxillofacial area, which can integrate and function with the original host bone.

The ability of BMPs to heal full-thickness defects in nonhuman primate mandibles has also been demonstrated. Bone-derived BMP in combination with a hydroxyapatite/collagen composite and rhBMP-2 with ACS have healed mandibular defects. In the latter study, following complete regeneration of the alveolar ridge with rhBMP-2/ACS, root-form dental implants were placed in the regenerated bone (41). The implants were then successfully brought into function 4 months after placement.

Critical-sized cranial defects have also been used to evaluate BMPs. BMP-7/OP-1 combined with bovine collagenous bone matrix successfully repaired large cranial defects in adult baboons (42). rhBMP-2 combined with PLGA matrices, collagens, and gelatin has been used to promote healing of rat and rabbit cranial defects (43–48). In addition, the ability of BMP to overcome the radiation-induced inhibition of bone healing has been demonstrated in rodent models (49,50).

Another application for BMPs is in the reconstruction of cleft palate defects. Current clinical practice suggests reconstruction at an early age, when bone graft procedures are debilitating and often yield suboptimal quantities of bone graft. rhBMP-2 has been successfully used to reconstruct induced cleft defects in dogs (51) and monkeys (52). One study demonstrated reconstruction of defects in young (18 months old) rhesus monkeys by rhBMP-2, which led to superior osseous reconstruction with thicker cortical bone than with autograft. Additional support for the use of BMPs in cleft palate repair comes from the demonstration that tooth eruption occurs normally in the presence of rhBMP-2 and BMP-induced bone.

Spinal fusion procedures require large amounts of bone-grafting materials, making the availability of an osteogenic bone graft quite attractive. The ability of BMPs to replace autograft has been extensively tested in animal models of spinal fusion. BMP-2 combined with carriers such as a collagen sponge or a polylactic acid porous rigid sponge has yielded solid fusions in rabbit (53,54), canine (55–61), and non-

human primate (54) models of intertransverse process spinal fusion. In general, these studies showed BMP-2 treatment to be superior to autograft, yielding a higher frequency of fusions, faster fusions, and larger fusion masses. Similar results have been seen with BMP-7/OP-1 in dog models (62). BMPs have also been evaluated in anterior spinal column fusion models and shown to induce bone repair in the presence of titanium fusion cages (63–66). Computed tomographic (CT) scans indicated bone growth in the BMP-treated animals both around and through the center of the cages; bone growth was confirmed by histological analysis.

Safety studies have been performed to evaluate the potential concerns using growth and differentiation factors such as the BMPs for spinal fusion procedures. No bone formation outside of the implant site or in the intrathecal environment was found following implantation of rhBMP-2/ACS on the dura after laminectomy and intentional creation of a dural tear in a canine model (67). Another study evaluated BMP-7/OP-1 placed within the subarachnoid space (68). While bone developed in the subarachnoid space, no clinical features of neurotoxicity were observed.

Fixation of Prosthetic Devices and Dental Implants

Conceptually, BMPs may be used to augment the quantity of bone present for fixation and to accelerate or augment the apposition of bone to the implant surface. Thus, BMPs may be useful in the fixation of prosthetic implants either at the time of placement (thus accelerating or augmenting fixation) or during revision surgery. While BMPs have been extensively tested with dental implants (see below), fewer studies are available that assess their efficacy in orthopedic settings. Initial studies in rats and dogs have been performed with BMP-2 (69,70) and BMP-7/OP-1 (71–73). Lind et al. (72) found an increase in mechanical strength at 6 weeks following implantation of BMP-7/OP-1 around uncoated and hydroxyapatite-coated titanium implants in dogs. Interestingly, an additional study by the same group (73) suggested a decrease in strength when BMP was applied with autograft in a primary fixation setting, whereas an increase in strength was accomplished in a revision setting. The ability of BMPs to increase the rate of bone remodeling or resorption may account for the differential effect.

The studies using critical-sized defect models suggest that BMP can induce significant amounts of bone, which then remodels consistently with its biological environment. In the dental area, bony augmentation is often required for the placement of dental implants. For maxillary augmentation, one procedure is augmentation of the floor of the maxillary sinus. The ability of rhBMP-2 to stimulate bone formation in the sinus has been demonstrated in goats, and bone induction followed by successful dental implant placement has been shown in monkeys (74,75). These studies have led to a clinical evaluation of rhBMP-2 in subantral augmentation procedures (see below). Similarly, rhBMP-7/OP-1 has been compared with a deproteinized cancellous bone grafting material in sinus floor augmentation procedures in monkeys (76,77). In the latter study, rhBMP-7/OP-1, as expected, resulted in sufficient bone formation; however, some inflammatory response was noted, which appeared to relate to the carrier material used.

Alveolar ridge augmentation and periimplant bone formation have also been accomplished using rhBMP-2/ACS in a stringent canine model (78). In this model, minimal new vertical bone height is gained without treatment. Thus, an average of 4.2 mm of bone was gained in BMP-treated sites, whereas only 0.5 mm formed in the controls. Of particular note is the demonstration that rhBMP-2 can regenerate bone and result in osseointegration of implants in periimplantitis defects in nonhuman primates (79). Thus, BMP is able to function in defects with a microbiological profile similar to that of human periodontal disease. Additional studies have investigated the bone-forming ability of BMP in conjunction with barrier membranes. One such study evaluated rhBMP-2 in combination with one of two carriers with and without barrier membranes in a canine model where defined defects were created surrounding implants (80,81). BMP-treated sites demonstrated two to three times as much bone regeneration and osseointegration (bone-to-implant contact) as did control sites. While the use of membranes helped to define the shape and area of bone that formed, BMP-induced bone formed more slowly, resulting in less bone, especially at the earlier time point. Presumably this resulted from occlusion of responsive mesenchymal cells. Similar observations have been made in other models using BMP and barrier membranes (82). rhBMP-7/OP-1 was also tested in extraction sockets in canines with concomitant implant placement (83). While all extraction sockets filled with bone at the end of this study, the amount and density of the bone formed, as well as the degree of remodeling, were greater at the BMP-treated sites. This suggested that BMP accelerated the bone-regeneration process.

Periodontal Regeneration

Another possible application for BMP is to regenerate bone which has been lost due to periodontal disease. This is a more complex application since bone and the correct interface between bone and tooth must be regenerated for optimal results. Partially purified bone-derived BMP was shown to regenerate bone, ligament, and cementum in baboon furcation defects. Subsequent studies have used recombinant proteins and proven that application of a single BMP can result in development of bone with the associated attachment tissues in a variety of models. For example, rhBMP-2 combined with bleomycin, etoposide, and cisplatin (Platinol) (BEP)/blood clot induced bone, cementum, and ligament formation in intrabony defects in dogs (84). Similar results were obtained in the stringent supra-alveolar ridge augmentation critical-sized defect model using the same material (85). Interestingly, additional studies using this model have suggested that the type of matrix material used to apply the BMPs affects the quality of the bone and periodontal regeneration (86–88). Similar observations have been made when applying rhBMP-7/OP-1 in mandibular defects (89). BMP-7/OP-1 combined with a bovine collagenous carrier also has shown substantial periodontal regeneration in furcation defects in dog and baboon models (90,91). The question remains as to whether regeneration of these multiple tissue types is due to a direct or an indirect effect of these BMPs.

Fracture Repair

The potent osteoinductive capacity of BMPs may allow for accelerating the rate of fracture repair, assuring that severe fractures heal and providing successful treatment of nonunion fractures. Fewer preclinical studies are available which test this potential application directly. Using the classic rat fracture model, a single percutaneous injection of rhBMP-2 in an aqueous vehicle was shown to accelerate fracture repair assessed biomechanically (92). Torsional stiffness of the BMP-treated limbs was found to be significantly higher by 3 weeks after fracture and strength increased by 4 weeks. Interestingly, histological analysis suggested that the acceleration observed biomechanically resulted from a combination of biological processes. In addition to producing more callus, maturation of the callus appeared to be accelerated by BMP. Application of BMP-7/OP-1 without a carrier material has also been demonstrated to accelerate fracture repair using a canine osteotomy model (93). Additional studies have demonstrated that surgical implantation of BMP in combination with matrix materials accelerates repair. For example, rhBMP-2/ACS has been shown to accelerate healing using a rabbit ulnar osteotomy model (94,95) and a goat closed fracture model (96). An additional case report suggests the successful treatment of a nonunion fracture with rhBMP-2/PGS implant (97).

Other Applications of Bone Morphogenetic Proteins

BMPs might also be used to accelerate the bone-formation phase in distraction osteogenesis procedures. Using a rabbit model, one study indicated that injection or implantation of rhBMP-2 in the regenerate following distraction can accelerate the rate of bone consolidation (98).

The ability of BMPs to induce bone, concomi-tantly leading to neovascularization, and to stimulate bone remodeling suggests that they could be ideal agents in the treatment of osteonecrosis. Animal modeling of osteonecrosis is difficult due to the idiopathic nature of the condition and to its complex etiology. rhBMP-2 combined with a blood clot has been evaluated following placement into core decompression channels in the femoral heads of normal pigs (99). BMP was found to dramatically accelerate the filling of the defects with bone. BMP has also been evaluated in combination with vascularized fibular grafts in a canine femoral head model where necrosis is induced by freezing (100). While differences in bone formation were not detectable radiographically in this model, increased revascularization did appear at the BMP-treated sites.

Endodontic applications for BMP have also been investigated in several models. Rutherford et al. (101–103) have led the efforts to evaluate the effects of application of BMP-7/OP-1. In several studies, including those using monkey models, BMP-7/OP-1 has been shown to result in formation of osteodentin and tubular dentin. Similar studies have shown similar results with rhBMP-2 in dog models (104,105). These results suggest that BMPs may be useful as capping agents for surgically exposed dental pulp, as well as in other endodontic procedures.

CLINICAL STUDIES USING BONE MORPHOGENETIC PROTEINS

Several reports of the use of bone-derived BMP preparations in clinical studies are available. Human bone-derived BMPs, applied with PLGA or bone matrix materials, have shown promising results in the treatment of nonunion fractures and segmental defects (106–111). As these are not controlled studies, however, it has been difficult to prove the efficacy of BMP in humans. A similar bone-derived preparation was also used to treat periodontal defects (112). Applied with demineralized bone matrix, significant regeneration was observed, though the amount of regeneration was similar to that of the matrix alone. A more recent study evaluated human BMP-containing bone extracts in the healing of tooth extraction sockets compared with a standard therapy of demineralized freeze-dried bone allograft (DFDBA) (113). Histological analysis indicated substantially more new bone formation in the BMP-treated defects; the DFDBA-treated defects exhibited residual bone matrix material with fibrous ingrowth.

Several controlled clinical studies using recombinant BMPs are now under way or have been completed. rhBMP-7/OP-1 combined with bovine collagenous bone matrix has been tested in the treatment of established tibial nonunions (114,115). This prospective, randomized, 122-patient study compared rhBMP-7/OP-1 with autograft. Follow-up at 9 and 24 months indicated that both groups had similar clinical outcomes, and the reoperation rate was similar in both groups (16% to 18%). Unfortunately, as no untreated control group was enrolled, it is difficult to determine the impact of either treatment group. A small, open-label study using rhBMP-2/ACS in the treatment of open tibial diaphysial fractures has also been reported (116). No safety issues related to the use of either recombinant BMP molecule were reported in these studies.

rhBMP-2 combined with autologous blood clot was tested in patients with osteonecrosis of the femoral head. In this 43-patient study, patients received either core decompression of the femoral head/neck (standard of care) or core decompression plus the rhBMP-2/blood material. Magnetic resonance imaging (MRI), commonly used to evaluate osteonecrosis, indicated that the volume of necrotic area decreased in the BMP-treated patients at 16 weeks posttreatment, whereas it increased in the control patients. The use of MRI to evaluate osteonecrosis is controversial; however, the results clearly suggest an effect of BMP in this setting.

The bone-inductive capacity of rhBMP-2 in humans has been demonstrated in a clinical study of sinus floor augmentation (117). In this 12-patient study, rhBMP-2/ACS was evaluated with a single concentration of rhBMP-2. Bone induction was clearly visible in all patients by CT scan at 16 weeks. Histological analysis of core biopsies, taken at the time of dental implant placement (approximately 6 months previously), confirmed the formation of new bone. The newly formed bone appeared to be remodeling normally. An additional study evaluated the same BMP material in alveolar ridge augmentation or preservation (tooth extraction socket repair). While significant bone augmentation could not be demonstrated, extraction sockets healed without reduction in alveolar ridge height, and analysis of dental implant fixation is ongoing (118).

rhBMP-2/ACS was also evaluated in a pilot study of interbody spinal fusion, in conjunction with a fusion cage (119). Fourteen patients received either rhBMP-2/ACS or autograft placed within the fusion cages. CT scans revealed the presence of bridging bone in all patients at 6 months. Comparison with autograft suggests that rhBMP-2/ACS yielded faster bridging and a higher frequency of bridging. Noteworthy is the substantial decrease in operative time and length of hospital stay when the BMP is used, due to the lack of surgical procedure to harvest autograft.

These studies demonstrate the safety of using recombinant human BMPs in several clinical procedures. Additional ongoing clinical evaluation will reveal the breadth of applications for these osteoinductive proteins.

REFERENCES

1. Manolagas SC, Jilka RL. Bone marrow, cytokines, and bone remodeling: emerging insights into the pathophysiology of osteoporosis. *N Engl J Med* 1995;332:305–311.
2. Rodan GA. Control of bone formation and resorption: biological and clinical perspective. *J Cell Biochem* 1998;30/31:55–61.
3. Manolagas SC, Weinstein RS. New developments in the pathogenesis and treatment of steroid-induced osteoporosis. *J Bone Miner Res* 1999;14:1061–1066.
4. Rosen V, Cox K, Hattersley G. Bone morphogenetic proteins. In: Bilezikian JP, Raisz LG, Rodan GA, eds. *Principles of bone biology.* New York: Academic Press, 1996:661–671.
5. Suzawa M, Takeuchi Y, Fukumoto S, et al. Extracellular matrix–associated bone morphogenetic proteins are essential for differentiation of murine osteoblastic cells *in vitro. Endocrinology* 1999;140:2125–2133.
6. Gazzerro E, Gangi V, Canalis E. Bone morphogenetic proteins induce the expression of noggin, which limits their activity in cultured rat osteoblasts. *J Clin Invest* 1998;102:2106–2114.
7. Wardle FC, Angerer LM, Angerer RC, Dale L. Regulation of BMP signaling by the BMP1/TLD-related metalloprotease, SpAN. *Dev Biol* 1999;206:63–72.
8. Ricard DJ, Hofbauer LC, Bonde SK, et al. Bone mor-

phogenetic protein 6 production in human osteoblastic cell lines. Selective regulation by estrogen. *J Clin Invest* 1998;101:413–422.

9. Boden SD, Hair G, Titus L, et al. Glucocorticoid-induced differentiation of fetal rat calvarial osteoblasts is mediated by bone morphogenetic protein 6. *Endocrinology* 1997;138:2820–2828.

10. Solloway MJ, Dudley AT, Bikoff EK, et al. Mice lacking BMP6 function. *Dev Genet* 1998;22:321–339.

11. D'Ippolito G, Schiller PC, Ricordi C, et al. Age-related osteogenic potential of mesenchymal stromal stem cells from human vertebral bone marrow. *J Bone Miner Res* 1999;14:1115–1122.

12. Rosen V, Thies RS. The BMP proteins in bone formation and repair. *Trends Genet* 1992;8:97–102.

13. Bostrom MPG, Lane JM, Berberian WS, et al. Immunolocalization and expression of bone morphogenetic proteins 2 and 4 in fracture healing. *J Orthop Res* 1995;13:357–367.

14. Nakase T, Noruma S, Yoshikawa H, et al. Transient and localized expression of bone morphogenetic protein 4 messenger RNA during fracture healing. *J Bone Miner Res* 1994;9:651–659.

15. Ishidou Y, Kitajama I, Obama H, et al. Enhanced expression of type I receptors for bone morphogenetic proteins during bone formation. *J Bone Miner Res* 1995;10:1651–1659.

16. Green MC. Effects of the short ear gene in the mouse on cartilage formation in healing bone fractures. *J Exp Zool* 1958;137:75–88.

17. Paley D. Current techniques of limb lengthening. *J Pediatr Orthop* 1988;8:73–92.

18. Yasui N, Sato M, Ochi T, et al. Three modes of ossification during distraction osteogenesis in the rat. *J Bone Joint Surg Br* 1997;79:824–830.

19. Sato M, Ochi T, Nakase T, et al. Mechanical tension-stress induces expression of bone morphogenetic protein (BMP)-2 and BMP-4 but not BMP-6, BMP-7, and GDF-5 mRNA, during distraction osteogenesis. *J Bone Miner Res* 1999;14:1084–1095.

20. Cook SD, Rueger DC. Osteogenic protein-1: biology and applications. *Clin Orthop* 1996;324:29–38.

21. Sandhu HS, Boden SD. Biologic enhancement of spinal fusion. *Orthop Clin North Am* 1998;29:621–631.

22. Wozney JM, Rosen V. Bone morphogenetic protein and bone morphogenetic protein gene family in bone formation and repair. *Clin Orthop* 1998;346:26–37.

23. Sakou T. Bone morphogenetic proteins: from basic studies to clinical approaches. *Bone* 1998;22:591–603.

24. Cochran DL, Wozney JM. Biological mediators for periodontal regeneration. *Periodontol 2000* 1999;19:40–58.

25. Yasko AW, Lane JM, Fellinger EJ, et al. The healing of segmental bone defects, induced by recombinant human bone morphogenetic protein (rhBMP-2). A radiographic, histological, and biomechanical study in rats. *J Bone Joint Surg Am* 1992;74A:659–670.

26. Gerhart TN, Kirker-Head CA, Kriz MJ, et al. Healing segmental femoral defects in sheep using recombinant human bone morphogenetic protein. *Clin Orthop* 1993;293:317–326.

27. Kirker-Head CA, Gerhart TN, Schelling SH, et al. Long-term healing of bone using recombinant human

bone morphogenetic protein 2. *Clin Orthop* 1995;318:222–230.

28. Cook SD, Baffes GC, Wolfe MW, et al. The effect of recombinant human osteogenic protein-1 on healing of large segmental bone defects. *J Bone Joint Surg Am* 1994;76-A:827–838.

29. Lee SC, Shea M, Battle MA, et al. Healing of large segmental defects in rat femurs is aided by rhBMP-2 in PLGA matrix. *J Biomed Mater Res* 1994;28:1149–1156.

30. Smith JL, Jin L, Parsons T, et al. Osseous regeneration in preclinical models using bioabsorbable delivery technology for recombinant human bone morphogenetic protein 2 (rhBMP-2). *J Control Release* 1995;36:183–195.

31. Bostrom M, Lane JM, Tomin E, et al. Use of bone morphogenetic protein-2 in the rabbit ulnar nonunion model. *Clin Orthop* 1996;327:272–282.

32. Kirker-Head CA, Gerhart TN, Armstrong R, et al. Healing bone using recombinant human bone morphogenetic protein 2 and copolymer. *Clin Orthop* 1998;349:205–217.

33. Zegzula HD, Buck DC, Brekke J, et al. Bone formation with use of rhBMP-2 (recombinant human bone morphogenetic protein-2). *J Bone Joint Surg Am* 1997;79A:1778–1790.

34. Itoh T, Mochizuki M, Nishimura R, et al. Repair of ulnar segmental defect by recombinant human bone morphogenetic protein-2 in dogs. *J Vet Med Sci* 1998;60:451–458.

35. Hollinger JO, Schmitt JM, Buck DC, et al. Recombinant human bone morphogenetic protein-2 and collagen for bone regeneration. *J Biomed Mater Res* 1998;43:356–364.

36. Sciadini MF, Johnson KD. Evaluation of recombinant human BMP-2 as a bone graft substitute in a canine segmental defect model. *J Orthop Res* 2000 (in press).

37. Cook SD, Baffes GC, Wolfe MW, et al. Recombinant human bone morphogenetic protein-7 induces healing in a canine long-bone segmental defect model. *Clin Orthop* 1994;301:302–312.

38. Cook SD, Salkeld SL, Brinker MR, et al. Use of an osteoinductive biomaterial (rhOP-1) in healing large segmental bone defects. *J Orthop Trauma* 1998;12:407–412.

39. Cook SD, Wolfe MW, Salkeld SL, et al. Effect of recombinant human osteogenic protein-1 on healing of segmental defects in non-human primates. *J Bone Joint Surg Am* 1995;77A:734–750.

40. Toriumi DM, Kotler HS, Luxenberg DP, et al. Mandibular reconstruction with a recombinant bone inducing factor. *Arch Otolaryngol Head Neck Surg* 1991;117:1101–1112.

41. Boyne PJ. Animal studies of the application of rhBMP-2 in maxillofacial reconstruction. *Bone* 1996;19:S83–S92.

42. Ripamonti U, van den Heever B, Sampath TK, et al. Complete regeneration of bone in the baboon by recombinant human osteogenic protein-1 (hOP-1, bone morphogenetic protein-7). *Growth Factors* 1996;13:273–289.

43. Kenley R, Marden L, Turek T, et al. Osseous regeneration in the rat calvarium using novel delivery systems for recombinant human bone morphogenetic protein-2 (rhBMP-2). *J Biomed Mater Res* 1994;28:1139–1147.

44. Marden LJ, Hollinger JO, Chaudhari A, et al. Recombinant human bone morphogenetic protein-2 is superior to demineralized bone matrix in repairing craniotomy defects in rats. *J Biomed Mater Res* 1994;28: 1127–1138.

45. Duggirala SS, Rodgers JB, DeLuca PP. The evaluation of lyophilized polymer matrices for administering recombinant human bone morphogenetic protein-2. *Pharm Dev Technol* 1996;1:165–174.

46. Rodgers JB, Vasconez HC, Wells MD, et al. Two lyophilized polymer matrix recombinant human bone morphogenetic protein-2 carriers in rabbit calvarial defects. *J Craniofac Surg* 1998;9:147–153.

47. Koempel JA, Patt BS, O'Grady K, et al. The effect of recombinant human bone morphogenetic protein-2 on the integration of porous hydroxyapatite implants with bone. *J Biomed Mater Res* 1998;41:359–363.

48. Zellin G, Linde A. Bone neogenesis in domes made of expanded polytetrafluoroethylene: efficacy of rhBMP-2 to enhance the amount of achievable bone in rats. *Plast Reconstr Surg* 1999;103:1229–1237.

49. Howard BK, Brown KR, Leach JL, et al. Osteoinduction using bone morphogenic protein in irradiated tissue. *Arch Otolaryngol Head Neck Surg* 1998;124: 985–988.

50. Wurzler KK, DeWeese TL, Sebald W, et al. Radiation-induced impairment of bone healing can be overcome by recombinant human bone morphogenetic protein-2. *J Craniofac Surg* 1998;9:131–137.

51. Mayer M, Hollinger J, Ron E, et al. Maxillary alveolar cleft repair in dogs using recombinant human bone morphogenetic protein-2 and a polymer carrier. *Plast Reconstr Surg* 1996;98:247–259.

52. Boyne PJ, Nath R, Nakamura A. Human recombinant BMP-2 in osseous reconstruction of simulated cleft palate defects. *Br J Oral Maxillofac Surg* 1998;36: 84–90.

53. Schimandle JH, Boden SD, Hutton WC. Experimental spinal fusion with recombinant human bone morphogenetic protein-2. *Spine* 1995;20:1326–1337.

54. Boden SD, Moskovitz PA, Morone MA, et al. Video-assisted lateral intertransverse process arthrodesis: validation of a new minimally invasive lumbar spinal fusion technique in the rabbit and nonhuman primate (rhesus) models. *Spine* 1996;21:2689–2697.

55. Muschler GF, Hyodo A, Manning T, et al. Evaluation of human bone morphogenetic protein 2 in a canine spinal fusion model. *Clin Orthop* 1994;308:229–240.

56. Sandhu HS, Kanim LEA, Kabo JM, et al. Evaluation of rhBMP-2 with an OPLA carrier in a canine posterolateral (transverse process) spinal fusion model. *Spine* 1995;20:2669–2682.

57. Sandhu HS, Kanim LEA, Kabo JM, et al. Effective doses of recombinant human bone morphogenetic protein-2 in experimental spinal fusion. *Spine* 1996;21: 2115–2122.

58. Helm GA, Sheehan JM, Sheehan JP, et al. Utilization of type I collagen gel, demineralized bone matrix, and bone morphogenetic protein-2 to enhance autologous bone lumbar spinal fusion. *J Neurosurg* 1997;86: 93–100.

59. Sheehan JP, Kallmes DF, Sheehan JM, et al. Molecular methods of enhancing lumbar spine fusion. *Neurosurgery* 1996;39:548–554.

60. Sandhu HS, Kanim LEA, Toth JM, et al. Experimental spinal fusion with recombinant human bone morphogenetic protein-2 without decortication of osseous elements. *Spine* 1997;22:1171–1180.

61. David SM, Gruber HE, Meyer RA Jr, et al. Lumbar spinal fusion using recombinant human bone morphogenetic protein (rhBMP-2) in the canine: a comparison of three dosages and two carriers. *Spine* 1999;24: 1973–1979.

62. Cook SD, Dalton JE, Tan EH, et al. *In vivo* evaluation of recombinant human osteogenic protein (rhOP-1) implants as a bone graft substitute for spinal fusions. *Spine* 1994;19:1655–1663.

63. Zdeblick TA, Ghanayem AJ, Rapoff AJ, et al. Cervical interbody fusion cages. An animal model with and without bone morphogenetic protein. *Spine* 1998;23: 758–766.

64. Boden SD, Martin GJ Jr, Horton WC, et al. Laparoscopic anterior spinal arthrodesis with rhBMP-2 in a titanium interbody threaded cage. *J Spinal Disord* 1998;11:95–101.

65. Hecht BP, Fischgrund JS, Herkowitz HN, et al. The use of recombinant human bone morphogenetic protein 2 (rhBMP-2) to promote spinal fusion in a nonhuman primate anterior interbody fusion model. *Spine* 1999; 24:629–636.

66. Cunningham BW, Kanayama M, Parker LM, et al. Osteogenic protein versus autologous interbody arthrodesis in the sheep thoracic spine. A comparative endoscopic study using the Bagby and Kuslich interbody fusion device. *Spine* 1999;24:509–518.

67. Meyer RA Jr, Gruber HE, Howard BA, et al. Safety of recombinant human bone morphogenetic protein-2 after spinal laminectomy in the dog. *Spine* 1999;24: 747–754.

68. Paramore CG, Lauryssen C, Rauzzino MI, et al. The safety of OP-1 for lumbar fusion with decompression—a canine study. *Neurosurgery* 1999;44:1151–1156.

69. Cole BJ, Bostrom MPG, Pritchard TL, et al. Use of bone morphogenetic protein 2 on ectopic porous coated implants in the rat. *Clin Orthop* 1997;345:219–228.

70. Sumner DR, Turner TM, Urban RM, et al. rhBMP-2 enhances bone ingrowth and gap healing. *Trans Orthop Res Soc* 1998;23:599.

71. Jensen TB, Overgaard S, Lind M, et al. Osteogenic protein-1 device in combination with bone allograft and Pro-Osteon 200 around noncemented implants. *Trans Orthop Res Soc* 1998;23:5.

72. Lind M, Overgaard S, Song Y, et al. Osteogenic protein-1 enhances mechanical fixation of implants in trabecular bone. *Trans Orthop Res Soc* 1998;23:339.

73. Soballe K, Bechtold JE, Bunger C, et al. Differential response to OP-1 in primary and revision implants. *Trans Orthop Res Soc* 1999;24:865.

74. Nevins M, Kirker-Head C, Wozney JM, et al. Bone formation in the goat maxillary sinus induced by absorbable collagen sponge implants impregnated with recombinant human bone morphogenetic protein-2. *Int J Periodont Restor Dent* 1996;16:9–19.

75. Hanisch O, Tatakis DN, Rohrer MD, et al. Bone formation and osseointegration stimulated by rhBMP-2 following subantral augmentation procedures in nonhuman primates. *Int J Oral Maxillofac Implants* 1997; 12:785–792.

76. Margolin MD, Cogan AG, Taylor M, et al. Maxillary

sinus augmentation in the non-human primate: a comparative radiographic and histologic study between recombinant human osteogenic protein-1 and natural bone mineral. *J Periodontol* 1998;69:911–919.

77. McAllister BS, Margolin MD, Cogan AG, et al. Residual lateral wall defects following sinus grafting with recombinant human osteogenic protein-1 or Bio-Oss in the chimpanzee. *Int J Periodont Restor Dent* 1998; 18:227–239.

78. Sigurdsson TJ, Fu E, Tatakis DN, et al. Bone morphogenetic protein-2 for peri-implant bone regeneration and osseointegration. *Clin Oral Implant Res* 1997;8: 367–374.

79. Hanisch O, Tatakis DN, Boskovic MM, et al. Bone formation and reosseointegration in peri-implantitis defects following surgical implantation of rhBMP-2. *Int J Oral Maxillofac Implants* 1997;12:604–610.

80. Cochran DL, Nummikoski PV, Jones AA, et al. Radiographic analysis of regenerated bone around endosseous implants in the canine using recombinant human bone morphogenetic protein-2. *Int J Oral Maxillofac Implants* 1997;12:739–748.

81. Cochran DL, Schenk R, Buser D, et al. Recombinant human bone morphogenetic protein-2 stimulation of bone formation around endosseous dental implants. *J Periodontol* 1999;70:139–150.

82. Zellin G, Linde A. Importance of delivery systems for growth-stimulatory factors in combination with osteopromotive membranes. An experimental study using rhBMP-2 in rat mandibular defects. *J Biomed Mater Res* 1997;35:181–190.

83. Cook SD, Salkeld SL, Rueger DC. Evaluation of recombinant human osteogenic protein-1 (rhOP-1) placed with dental implants in fresh extraction sites. *J Oral Implantol* 1995;21:281–289.

84. Ishikawa I, Oda S, Roongruanphol T. Regenerative therapy in periodontal diseases—histological observations after implantation of rhBMP-2 in the surgically created periodontal defects in dogs. *Dent Jpn* 1994;31: 141–146.

85. Sigurdsson TJ, Lee MB, Kubota K, et al. Periodontal repair in dogs: recombinant human bone morphogenetic protein-2 significantly enhances periodontal regeneration. *J Periodontal* 1995;66:131–138.

86. Sigurdsson TJ, Nygaard L, Tatakis DN, et al. Periodontal repair in dogs: evaluation of rhBMP-2 carriers. *Int J Periodont Restor Dent* 1996;16:525–537.

87. Kinoshita A, Oda S, Takahashi K, et al. Periodontal regeneration by application of recombinant human bone morphogenetic protein-2 to horizontal circumferential defects created by experimental periodontitis in beagle dogs. *J Periodontol* 1997;68:103–109.

88. Wikesjö UME, Guglielmoni P, Promsudthi A, et al. Periodontal repair in dogs: effect of rhBMP-2 concentration on regeneration of alveolar bone and periodontal attachment. *J Clin Periodontol* 1999;26:392–400.

89. Terheyden H, Jepsen S, Vogeler S, et al. Recombinant human osteogenic protein 1 in the rat mandibular augmentation model: differences in morphology of the newly formed bone are dependent on the type of carrier. *Mund Kiefer Gesichtschir* 1997;1:272–275.

90. Ripamonti U, Heliotis M, Rueger DC, et al. Induction of cementogenesis by recombinant human osteogenic protein-1 (hOP-1/BMP-7) in the baboon *(Papio ursinus)*. *Arch Oral Biol* 1996;41:121–126.

91. Giannobile WV, Ryan S, Shih MS, et al. Recombinant human osteogenic protein-1 (OP-1) stimulates periodontal wound healing in class III furcation defects. *J Periodontol* 1998;69:129–137.

92. Einhorn TA, Majeska RJ, Ghadir O, et al. Enhancement of experimental fracture healing with a local percutaneous injection of rhBMP-2. *Trans Orthop Res Soc* 1997.

93. Popich LS, Salkeld SL, Rueger DC, et al. Critical and noncritical size defect healing with OP-1. *Trans Orthop Res Soc* 1997;22:600.

94. Turek TJ, Bostrom MPG, Camacho N, et al. Acceleration of bone healing in a rabbit ulnar osteotomy model with rhBMP-2. *Trans Orthop Res Soc* 1997;22:526.

95. Bouxsein ML, Turek TJ, Blake C, et al. rhBMP-2 accelerates healing in a rabbit ulnar osteotomy model. *Trans Orthop Res Soc* 1999;24:138.

96. Welch RD, Jones AL, Bucholz RW, et al. Effect of recombinant human bone morphogenetic protein-2 on fracture healing in a goat tibial fracture model. *J Bone Miner Res* 1998;13:1483–1490.

97. Itoh T, Mochizuki M, Fuda K, et al. Femoral nonunion fracture treated with recombinant human bone morphogenetic protein-2 in a dog. *J Vet Med Sci* 1998;60: 535–538.

98. Li G, Luppen C, Li XI, et al. Bone consolidation is enhanced by rhBMP-2 during distraction osteogenesis in rabbits. *Trans Orthop Res Soc* 1999;24:320.

99. Mazières B. Bone morphogenetic protein and bone necrosis: a perspective. *ARCO News Lett* 1994;6:3–5.

100. Scully SP, Rizk WAS, Seaber AV, et al. Augmentation of subchondral bone formation in AVN with rhBMP-2. *Trans Orthop Res Soc* 1995;20:495.

101. Rutherford B, Spangberg L, Tucker M, et al. Transdentinal stimulation of reparative dentine formation by osteogenic protein-1 in monkeys. *Arch Oral Biol* 1995; 40:681–683.

102. Rutherford RB, Spangberg L, Tucker M, et al. The time-course of the induction of reparative dentine formation in monkeys by recombinant human osteogenic protein-1. *Arch Oral Biol* 1994;39:833–838.

103. Rutherford RB, Wahle J, Tucker M, et al. Induction of reparative dentine formation in monkeys by recombinant human osteogenic protein-1. *Arch Oral Biol* 1993;38:571–576.

104. Nakashima M. Induction of dentin formation on canine amputated pulp by recombinant human bone morphogenetic proteins (BMP)-2 and -4. *J Dent Res* 1994;73: 1515–1522.

105. Nakashima M. Induction of dentine in amputated pulp of dogs by recombinant human bone morphogenetic proteins-2 and -4 with collagen matrix. *Arch Oral Biol* 1994;39:1085–1089.

106. Johnson EE, Urist MR. One-stage lengthening of femoral nonunion augmented with human bone morphogenetic protein. *Clin Orthop* 1998;347:105–116.

107. Johnson EE, Urist MR. Preliminary explorations of reconstructive surgery with implants of autolyzed antigen-extracted allogeneic (AAA) bone supercharged with bone morphogenetic protein (BMP). 1994; 363–376.

108. Johnson EE, Urist MR, Finerman GAM. Bone morphogenetic protein augmentation grafting of resistant femoral nonunions: a preliminary report. *Clin Orthop* 1988;230:257–265.

109. Johnson EE, Urist MR, Finerman GAM. Distal metaphyseal tibial nonunion: deformity and bone loss treated by open reduction, internal fixation, and human bone morphogenetic protein (hBMP). *Clin Orthop* 1990;250:234–240.

110. Johnson EE, Urist MR, Finerman GAM. Repair of segmental defects of the tibia with cancellous bone grafts augmented with human bone morphogenetic protein. *Clin Orthop* 1988;236:249–257.

111. Johnson EE, Urist MR, Schmalzried TP, et al. Autogeneic cancellous bone grafts in extensive segmental ulnar defects in dogs. *Clin Orthop* 1989;243:254–265.

112. Bowers G, Felton F, Middleton C, et al. Histologic comparison of regeneration in human intrabony defects when osteogenin is combined with demineralized freeze-dried bone allograft and with purified bovine collagen. *J Periodontol* 1991;62:690–702.

113. Becker W, Clokie C, Sennerby L, et al. Histologic findings after implantation and evaluation of different grafting materials and titanium micro screws into extraction sockets: case reports. *J Periodontol* 1998;69:414–421.

114. Muschler GF, Perry CR, Cole JD, et al. Treatment of established tibial nonunions using human recombinant osteogenic protein-1. *Trans Am Acad Orthop Surg* 1998;172–173.

115. Cook SD, Salkeld SL, Armstrong DL, et al. Osteogenic protein-1 (OP-1) heals tibial nonunion fractures. *Trans Orthop Res Soc* 1998;24:602.

116. Swiontkowski MF, Goulet JA, Paiement G, et al. Safety and feasibility of implanting recombinant human bone morphogenetic protein-2 (rhBMP-2)/absorbable collagen sponge (ACS) in patients with open tibial shaft fractures. *J Orthop Trauma* 2000 *(in press).*

117. Boyne PJ, Marx RE, Nevins M, et al. A feasibility study evaluating rhBMP-2/absorbable collagen sponge for maxillary sinus floor augmentation. *Int J Periodont Restor Dent* 1997;17:10–25.

118. Howell TH, Fiorellini J, Jones A, et al. A feasibility study evaluating rhBMP-2/absorbable collagen sponge device for local alveolar ridge preservation or augmentation. *Int J Periodont Restor Dent* 1997;17:125.

119. Boden SD. *Spine* 2000 *(in press).*

Skeletal Growth Factors,
edited by Ernesto Canalis.
Lippincott Williams & Wilkins, Philadelphia, © 2000.

22

Role of Growth Factors in Fracture Healing

Leslie S. Beasley and *Thomas A. Einhorn

*Department of Orthopedic Surgery, Boston University School of Medicine,
Boston, Massachusetts 02118-2393*
°Boston Medical Center, Boston, Massachusetts 02118-2393

Growth factors, a class of small protein molecules which act as signaling agents for cells, provide a principal mechanism for altering cell behavior, including effects on cell division, matrix synthesis, and tissue differentiation (1). They elicit their cellular actions by binding to large transmembrane receptors on their target cells, which are linked, by a cascade of chemical reactions in the cytoplasm, to specific gene sequences in the nucleus. Commonly, this cascade activates several genes at once; thus, specific growth factors may generate multiple effects, even within a single cell type. Moreover, growth factors have pleiotropic effects on cells, eliciting different effects in different cell types or even in the same cell type at different stages of development.

In fracture healing, growth factors play a central role in mediating skeletal tissue reparative responses. Bone is unique in its response to structural damage in that it is capable of true tissue regeneration, leading to cellular, morphological, and functional restoration. This is in contrast to the type of healing seen in most tissues, in which repair involves the formation of a fibrous scar. Among the known growth factors which participate in fracture healing and may lead to this unique type of response are the transforming growth factors-β (TGF-β), bone morphogenetic proteins (BMPs), fibroblast growth factors (FGFs), insulin-like growth factors (IGFs), and platelet-derived growth factors (PDGFs) (1) (Table 22.1). This chapter reviews the current knowledge on the roles of these factors in normal fracture healing and their potential use as therapeutic agents to enhance this reparative process.

TRANSFORMING GROWTH FACTOR-β

The TGF-β family of polypeptides has been studied extensively. It is composed of at least five molecules and is a member of a growth factor superfamily which includes the BMPs as well as many other growth and differentiation factors (1). Most members of this family are recognized as multifunctional signaling molecules that can act as both inhibitors and stimulators of cell replication. Relative to the skeleton, TGF-β is known to regulate proliferation and expression of the differentiated phenotype of chondrocytes, osteoblasts, and osteoclasts. Studies have shown that, during endochondral ossification, chondrocytes and osteoblasts synthesize TGF-β (2), which then accumulates in the extracellular matrix, forming the largest source of TGF-β in the body. Additional data suggest that a fracture activates the genes for TGF-β, increasing the concentrations of TGF-β mRNA and, thus, the synthesis and release of TGF-β itself (3,4). Joyce et al. (5) investigated the endogenous expression of TGF-β in organ cultures of fracture callus *in vitro*. Using immunohistochemistry, they evaluated fresh femur fractures in male rats at four time intervals: (a) immediately after fracture, (b) during intramembranous bone formation, (c) during chondrogenesis, and (d) during endo-

TABLE 22.1. *Selected growth factors that regulate skeletal tissue*

Growth factor[a]	Principal actions
IGFs (somatomedins)	
IGF-I[b], somatomedin-C	Mitogenic, anabolic, mediates some growth hormone actions
IGF-II[b], multiplication stimulating activity, skeletal growth factor	Mitogenic, anabolic, generally less potent than IGF-I
FGFs	
FGF-1[c] (acidic fibroblast growth factor)	Mitogenic, angiogenic, regulates cell differentiation
FGF-2[c] (basic fibroblast growth factor)	Mitogenic, angiogenic, regulates cell differentiation
TGF-β[d]	Context-dependent, multifunctional
BMPs[d]	Prototypes induce bone formation
PDGF[e]	Mitogenic

[a] IGF, insulin-like growth factor; BMP, bone morphogenetic protein; FGF, fibroblast growth factor; PDGF, platelet-derived growth factor; TGF, transforming growth factor.
[b] IGF-I and IGF-II are structurally and biologically related to insulin.
[c] FGF-1 and FGF-2 are the prototypes of the FGF family, of which there are at least nine members.
[d] The TGF-β and BMP families are representatives of a large superfamily that includes at least five TGF-βs, 15 BMPs, the activins, the inhibins, and other factors involved in morphogenesis.
[e] PDGF occurs as a dimer of subunits, termed A and B, and may therefore take three forms: AA, AB, or BB. From Ref. 48, with permission.

chondral ossification. The appearance of TGF-β in the fracture hematoma was observed within 24 hours after fracture and persisted for up to 10 days. Within the region of intramembranous bone formation, TGF-β was seen both intracellularly, in mesenchymal cells and osteoblasts specifically, and in the extracellular matrix. Early in chondrogenesis, TGF-β was seen in mesenchymal cells and in young and mature chondrocytes. During endochondral ossification, the surrounding extracellular matrix stained intensely for TGF-β, while the ossified matrix on the bone side of the ossification front no longer stained. TGF-β gene expression was then quantitated in the fracture calluses by Northern analysis performed at 3-day intervals in both the soft (cartilaginous) and hard (calcified) calluses. The soft callus showed a peak in TGF-β mRNA concentrations at day 13, corresponding with mesenchymal cell proliferation and the histological progression of chondrogenesis. In the hard callus, peaks were observed at 5 and 15 days after fracture, corresponding to osteoblast activity associated with intramembranous ossification and then endochondral ossification, respectively. These investigators concluded that TGF-β is first localized to the fracture hematoma, being released by platelets, and then synthesized by osteoblasts and chondrocytes within the callus during the entire healing process.

Exogenously administered TGF-β has been studied as well. Findings from several animal studies suggest that exogenously applied recombinant human TGF-β stimulates recruitment and proliferation of osteoblasts, enhances rapid deposition of bone matrix, increases maximum bending strength and callus formation, and augments healing (6–8). The potential role of TGF-β in fracture healing was reviewed by Rosier et al. (9). These authors concluded that TGF-β isoforms and receptors are normally expressed in specific patterns in fracture callus. It has not been shown definitively that fracture healing is defective or impaired in the absence of TGF-β or TGF-β receptor. Experiments involving subperiosteal injections of TGF-β demonstrated that this factor can act as a morphogen, inducing the full cascade of events in endochondral ossification; however, the *in vitro* actions of TGF-β seem to be contradictory, as it has been shown to both stimulate and inhibit target cells (10). Overall, the majority of *in vitro* studies indicate that TGF-β increases the expression of osteoblast differentiation markers, such as alkaline phosphatase, type I collagen, and osteonectin, and acts in synergy with 1,25-dihydroxyvitamin D_3 to increase alkaline phosphatase concentrations (11,12). Additionally, TGF-β may enhance the proliferation of osteoblasts and fibroblasts by increasing production of the PDGF B chain

(13). While some studies have shown a decrease in rat osteoblast differentiation and mineralization (14), the net effect of TGF-β appears to be an increase in extracellular bone matrix synthesis and regulation of bone and cartilage formation.

Studies attempting to demonstrate the TGF-β stimulation of fracture healing have shown increased callus volume and improved biomechanical properties; however, they lack consistency in terms of fracture models, dose ranges, exogenously applied isoforms, delivery methods, and end points, making analysis difficult (9). Similarly, work done on critical-sized defect healing models suggests efficacy of locally delivered TGF-β in accelerated healing, although the same experimental variables are encountered. Overall, the enhancing effects of TGF-β on bone healing seem to be of lesser magnitude than those of some other growth factors, particularly BMP; however, it is not clear that optimization of study parameters has been achieved, making it difficult to truly evaluate the potential of TGF-β to enhance fracture healing.

TABLE 22.2. *Bone morphogenetic protein (BMP)[a] superfamily in mammals[b]*

BMP subfamily	Christened name	BMP
BMP-2/4	BMP-2A	BMP-2
	BMP-2B	BMP-4
BMP-3	Osteogenin	BMP-3
	GDF-10	BMP-3b
OP-1/BMP-7	BMP-5	BMP-5
	Vgr 1	BMP-6
	OP-1	BMP-7
	OP-2	BMP-8
	OP-3	BMP-8b
Miscellaneous	GDF-2	BMP-9
	BMP-10	BMP-10
	GDF-11	BMP-11
CDMP/GDF	CDMP-3 or GDF-7	BMP-12
	CDMP-2 or GDF-6	BMP-13
	CDMP-1 or GDF-5	BMP-14
Others	BMP-15	BMP-15
	BMP-16	BMP-16

[a] BMP-1 is not a bone morphogenetic protein family member with seven canonical cysteines. It is a procollagen C proteinase related to *Drosophila* tolloid.
[b] CDMP, cartilage-derived morphogenetic protein; GDF, growth and differentiation factor; OP, osteogenic protein; Vgr, vegetal related.
From ref. 15, with permission.

BONE MORPHOGENETIC PROTEINS

BMPs, which are part of the TGF-β superfamily of proteins, comprise a group of at least 15 growth factors known to be highly osteoinductive (15) (Table 22.2). Bostrom et al. (16), using a monoclonal antibody against BMPs 2 and 4, determined the presence, location, and chronology of expression of BMPs 2 and 4 in fracture healing by immunohistochemistry. The study showed that a small number of primitive cells stained positively in the fracture callus during the early stages of fracture healing; however, as the process of endochondral ossification proceeded, the primitive mesenchymal cells and chondrocytes showed a dramatic increase in staining. With maturation of the cartilaginous component of the callus, the number of primitive cells decreased, as did the number of positively staining cells. The osteoblasts also stained strongly positive as they began to deposit woven bone. The intensity of the staining then decreased as the woven bone was replaced by lamellar bone. The areas of the callus undergoing intramembranous ossification showed similar staining patterns. Several days after fracture, periosteal cells and osteoblasts stained strongly positive for BMPs 2 and 4. Then, as the lamellar bone replaced the woven bone, the staining decreased. These data clearly demonstrate the endogenous expression of BMPs 2 and 4 in fracture healing. The investigators concluded that BMPs 2 and 4 may be important regulators of cell differentiation and fracture repair, specifically playing a role in the formation of intramembranous bone and in the differentiation of mesenchymal cells into chondrocytes.

Nakase et al. (17) studied the temporal and spatial distribution of BMP-4 in fracture healing. They used reverse-transcriptase polymerase chain reaction (RT-PCR) and *in situ* hybridization in a mouse rib model to localize a gene-encoding murine BMP-4 (mBMP-4). Using a digoxigenin-11 uridine triphosphate (UTP)–labeled probe, they compared concentrations of mBMP-4 in fractured ribs and surrounding tissues to those in ribs without fracture. In mice with fractured ribs, mBMP-4 mRNA was detected in the early phase of fracture healing, at 12 to 72 hours postfracture, in three distinct regions: (a) proliferating periosteum, (b) medullary cavity, and (c) surrounding muscles. mBMP-4 mRNA was not detected at all in the ribs without fracture. Moreover, RT-PCR also demonstrated a transient increase of mBMP-4 in the early phase of fracture repair. These authors concluded that the BMP-4 gene is produced by the less-differentiated osteoprogenitor cells, as it is present in the very early stages of fracture healing. They also concluded that the BMP-4 gene is enhanced by the impact of fracture healing and that it is localized in callus-forming tissue, suggesting that the BMP-4 gene product is one of the local contributing factors in callus formation in the early phase of fracture healing.

Two BMP type I receptors have been defined, type IA (BMPR-IA) and type IB (BMPR-IB). They are transmembrane serine/threonine kinase receptors that are known to bind BMP-4 and BMP-7 and may bind other BMPs with different affinities (18). Using antibodies specific to BMPRs IA and IB and immunostaining in a rat femoral fracture model, Ishidou et al. (18) investigated the expression of these two type I receptors during bone formation. They demonstrated that, in normal rat bone, osteoblasts in the periosteum express BMPR-IA but not BMPR-IB. Three days after fracture, both the BMPR-IA and BMPR-IB receptors were upregulated at the proliferating osteogenic layer of the periosteum. On the seventh day, both receptors were seen in chondrocytes at the sites of endochondral ossification, in osteoblasts in the newly formed trabecular bone, and in fibroblast-like spindle cells. On day 14, both receptors were seen at the same sites where they were observed on day 7, though at lower levels of expression. These investigators concluded that expression of BMP type I receptors is upregulated in various cell types from the early to the late stages of fracture healing, suggesting that they play a role in bone morphogenesis. Moreover, expression BMPR-IA in osteoblasts at the periosteum in normal intact femurs suggests that BMPs may also play a role in the maintenance and stabilization of bone.

Many investigators have tested the ability of different BMPs and BMP preparations to enhance the healing of fractures and bone defects (15,19–27). Stevenson et al. (19) investigated the effects of partially purified BMP-3 (osteogenin) on the formation of bone in rats. Segmental femoral defects were created and then filled either with an osteogenin/hydroxyapatite/tricalcium phosphate ceramic or a hydroxyapatite/tricalcium phosphate ceramic alone. They found that the total area of bone, the area of bone outside the implant, and the amount of bone within the pores of the implant were significantly greater in the osteogenin-implanted femora than in controls.

Cook et al. (20) used a rabbit ulnar nonunion model to evaluate the effect of recombinant human osteogenic protein-1 (rhOP-1, also known as BMP-7) on the healing of a large segmental osteoperiosteal defect. Ulnar defects were filled with an implant containing either rhOP-1 (which consisted of a carrier of 125 mg of demineralized, guanidine-extracted, insoluble bone matrix reconstituted with 3.13, 6.25, 12.5, 25, 50, 100, 200, 300, or 400 μg of rhOP-1) or 250 μg of naturally occurring bovine osteogenic protein (bOP). Controls received either the collagen carrier alone or no implant. Healing was assessed by mechanical testing. The results showed that all of the implants containing at least 6.25 μg of rhOP-1 as well as those receiving bOP induced complete radiographic osseous union within 8 weeks. Additionally, the average torsional strength and energy-absorption capacity of rhOP-1-implanted bones was comparable to that of intact bone. These investigators concluded that highly purified rhOP-1 is capable of inducing healing in a large bone defect in an animal model.

Similarly, a study investigating the use of rhBMP in segmental femoral defect in sheep was performed by Gerhart et al. (21). These investigators studied the healing of sheep femora treated with either no implant, inactive bone matrix, rhBMP-2, or autogenous bone graft. They found that femora treated with rhBMP-2 showed union of all defects, while there was a lack of union in both the no-implant group and the inactive bone matrix group. They concluded that rhBMP-2 is able to heal large segmental defects in a challenging and clinically relevant model.

Yasko et al. (22) demonstrated similar results in their study evaluating subcutaneous implants of rhBMP-2. Three groups were created in a segmental defect model involving rat femora. Two groups were implanted with varying doses of lyophilized rhBMP-2 (either 1.4 or 11.0 μg) in a guanidine-hydroxychloride–extracted demineralized bone matrix carrier or guanidine-hydroxychloride–extracted demineralized rat bone matrix alone. The results showed that rhBMP-2 induced formation of endochondral bone in the osseous defects in a dose-related manner. Implantation of 11.0 μg of rhBMP-2 yielded bone formation and osseous union, while the femora receiving 1.4 μg of rhBMP-2 demonstrated bone formation without evidence of union.

While it is known that implantation of rhBMP-2 can lead to the bridging of critical-sized defects in rat femora and the induction of spinal fusion, the development of a convenient delivery system has been lacking. Einhorn et al. (23) investigated the response of closed mid-diaphyseal femoral fractures in retired breeder Sprague-Dawley rats to a local percutaneous injection of rhBMP-2. Six hours after fracture, the rats were divided into three groups: one group received no treatment, one received an injection of aqueous buffer only, and one received an injection of buffer plus 80 μg of rhBMP-2. They were then divided further into four groups, which were euthanized on days 7, 14, 21, and 28 after fracture, at which time the femora underwent biomechanical testing. A parallel experiment evaluated the histological response of fractures to rhBMP-2 injections. The results showed no statistical difference in stiffness or strength at any time between the fracture-only group and the buffer-treated fractures; however, by day 14, the rhBMP-2 group showed an increase in stiffness that was sustained throughout the experiment. Also, by day 28, the rhBMP-2-treated fractures showed a statistically significant increase in strength. A robust subperiosteal membranous bone response, greater than that seen in either of the control groups, was demonstrated histologically. Furthermore, there was relative maturation in the appearance of the os-

teochondrogenic cell types in the rhBMP-2-treated group. The rhBMP-2-treated fractures also demonstrated significant amounts of peripheral woven bone bridging the gaps as early as day 14. The investigators concluded that a local percutaneous injection of rhBMP-2 may enhance fracture healing by accelerating the rate of the healing response. It was also noted that the rhBMP-2-treated fractures had the appearance of woven bone, resembling that seen after autogenous bone graft implantation, suggesting that rhBMP-2 may have a bone graft-like effect. The therapeutic potential for rhBMP-2 injections may thus range from enhancement of fresh fracture healing to stimulating or preventing delayed healing to possibly inducing a bone graft-like response in other orthopedic applications.

Bostrom et al. (24,25) tested the use of BMP-2 in an absorbable collagen sponge in a rabbit ulnar osteotomy model. They studied 60 rabbits divided into three groups: (a) BMP-2 with collagen carrier, (b) collagen carrier alone, and (c) untreated surgical control limbs. Healing was assessed biomechanically and radiographically at 2, 3, 4, and 6 weeks. Radiographically, at week 2, the BMP-2-treated group showed slightly more callus formation than did the control limbs. By week 3, the callus cross-sectional area in this group tended to be larger than that of the control group and bony bridging was seen in seven of ten limbs receiving BMP-2, although the difference was not statistically significant. By week 6, there was no difference among the three treatment groups in terms of overall fracture callus area or hard callus area. Biomechanically, the stiffness and strength values increased over time for all three groups. At week 3, limbs treated with BMP-2 showed greater energy and strength values (statistically significant) than either the collagen-treated or surgical control limbs. Also at 3 weeks, the mean values of strength, energy to failure, and stiffness for the BMP-2-treated group were not significantly different from the values for the intact controls. The fractures were additionally assessed by the Lane modification of White's classification (22,28) at three time points. At 2 weeks, the fracture scores indicated that most fractures occurred through the soft callus in all three groups. At 3 weeks, the integrity of all fractures was improved, most notably in the BMP-2-treated group. At 4 weeks, the fracture scores of the BMP-2-treated limbs were greater than those of the surgical control limbs and equivalent to the scores of all groups at week 6. These authors concluded that the local application of BMP-2 on a collagen carrier can accelerate bony repair, leading to equivalent strength of the calluses in treated and control limbs as early as 6 weeks after osteotomy.

Although various preparations of demineralized bone matrix had been used in the past, the first clinical use of BMPs in fracture repair was by Urist and colleagues (26,27), who treated difficult-to-heal nonunions with composites of bone grafts and purified human BMP. These investigators have reported the long-term results of using purified human BMP for the treatment of severely resistant nonunions and healing defects (26). Between 1983 and 1994, these investigators treated five tibias, 14 femurs, seven humeri, one radius, and one ulna (28 patients total) with composites of allogenic bone graft, noncollagenous proteins, and purified human BMP. Twenty-six of the 28 (93%) of the nonunions achieved successful union after the first BMP aiplautation. Two of the hun unions (7%) required reoperation, subsequently resulting in successful union. No cases of tumor induction, allergic reaction, or postoperative infection were reported. Although their study was small, the results suggested that BMP composite induces bone in humans.

Only preliminary results are available for the clinical application of rhBMP-2. Recently described is an open-label safety and feasibility trial using an absorbable collagen sponge carrier (25). Twelve patients with grade II or greater open tibial fractures from four major trauma centers were treated with either 3.4 or 6.8 mg of BMP-2. One or two Helistat (Colla-tec, Plainsboro, NJ) absorbable collagen sponges were used as delivery vehicles and applied to the fracture site at the time of definitive wound closure. Eight of the 12 patients were treated with a nonreamed tibial rod, and the other four were treated with an external fixator. Four months postoperatively, the radiographs were reviewed. Nine (75%) of the fractures healed without additional interventions, while three (25%) required a secondary bone-graft procedure. No patients suffered significant changes in vital signs, hematology, or blood chemistry, although two developed transient serum antibodies toward BMP-2. The investigators concluded that, although the use of BMP-2 in these patients appeared safe and feasible, the efficacy of BMP-2 at enhancing bone healing can be determined only by a larger prospective randomized clinical trial.

Preliminary results of a multicenter clinical trial using OP-1 (NOVOS; Stryker Biotech, Natick, MA), a BMP-7 with a bovine-derived collagen carrier, have been reported (25). In this trial, 122 patients with 124 tibial nonunions were evaluated in 18 centers. Inclusion criteria were nonunion of at least 9 months' duration and the surgeon's choice of intramedullary fixation with bone graft as the most appropriate method of treatment. These nonunions were not expected to heal if left untreated. Patients received either autograft or OP-1. Good results were defined as return to full weight bearing, reduction in pain, and radiographic union within 9 months. Preliminary results suggest that OP-1 is as effective at healing nonunions as autograft, although neither treatment group reached a healing rate of 100%.

Based on extensive preclinical animal studies, the potential uses of BMPs to enhance fracture healing are encouraging; however, despite their impressive theoretical potential, the therapeutic efficacy requires further investigation to be more completely defined (25).

FIBROBLAST GROWTH FACTORS

FGFs comprise a group of heparin-binding polypeptides that have mitogenic effects on fibroblasts and have been implicated in the regulation of chondrocyte and osteoblast function (29). Acidic fibroblast growth factor (aFGF) has been shown to act on osteoblasts and to be present in high concentrations in bone; therefore, it is hypothesized that it may be an important factor in the regulation of fracture healing (30). Basic fibroblast growth factor (bFGF) has been recognized as a critical regulator of bone cell function and is considered essential for bone formation in vitro. It is known to promote the proliferation of mesenchymal cells in vitro, while inhibiting the differentiation of chondrocytes, the expression of alkaline phosphatase activity, and the synthesis of type I collagen in osteoblasts. Additionally, it has been shown to stimulate bone resorption *in vitro,* although its biological activity *in vivo* has not yet been fully described. bFGF is synthesized by osteoblasts and stored in the bone matrix; it has been shown to stimulate the repair of fibular fractures in rats (31) and to increase bone mass following local injection into the rabbit ilium (32).

The effect of administration of aFGF on normal fracture healing was examined in a rat femoral fracture model by Jingushi et al. (33). Bilateral femur fractures were produced. Either every day or every other day for 9 days, one fracture was injected with 1 μg of rhaFGF in buffer, and the contralateral fracture was injected with buffer alone, serving as a control. The investigators found that the aFGF-injected calluses were significantly larger than those of the controls and remained so until 4 weeks after fracture. Histology of the aFGF-treated group showed a marked increase in the size of the cartilaginous soft callus. mRNA and collagen in the cartilaginous portion of the aFGF-injected calluses were also greater than those of the controls. Northern blot analysis of total cellular RNA showed a decrease in the expression of type II procollagen and proteoglycan core protein in the aFGF-treated calluses relative to controls. The authors concluded that administration of aFGF changed the fracture repair process and increased cartilage tissue, suggesting that aFGF treatment may be beneficial in abnormal fracture repair if chondrogenesis is impaired.

Nakamura et al. (34) have demonstrated the osteogenic activity of bFGF in fracture healing *in vivo* by showing that systemic injections of bFGF in rats stimulate endosteal bone formation by increasing the number of preosteoblasts. In a subsequent study, this group evaluated the role of bFGF in fracture healing in beagle dogs (34). A tibial fracture model was developed in which fractures are fixed with an intramedullary nail. The dogs were divided into two groups: one received a single injection of 200 μg of bFGF at the fracture site and the other, which served as the control group, was treated with an intramed-

ullary nail alone. Callus volume and morphology were evaluated at 2, 4, 8, 16, and 32 weeks, and mechanical strength was tested at weeks 16 and 32. Bone mineral content in the callus was measured at week 8. The results showed that, by the second week, the bFGF-treated fractures showed numerous periosteal mesenchymal cells that had been recruited to the fracture site and had begun to differentiate into both osteoblasts and chondrocytes. There was also abundant membranous ossification. This suggests that the essential effect of bFGF on callus formation is stimulation of mesenchymal cell proliferation in the periosteum. A remarkable increase in callus area was noted by weeks 4 and 8 in the bFGF-treated fractures, which was followed by a twofold increase in bone mineral content at the fracture site in control dogs. Moreover, by week 2, the number of osteoclasts in the bFGF group had increased to nearly threefold that of the control group; it reached a maximum at week 4. The role of bFGF in this increase is not completely clear; however, it has been shown that bFGF may enhance the expression of *in vivo.* TGF-β is a growth factor which has been shown previously to increase the number of osteoblasts after repeated injection into the periosteum of neonatal rat parietal bone (35). The osteoclastic index, defined as the number of osteoclasts per millimeter of callus perimeter, reached its peak at week 4 in the bFGF-treated group and reached an almost identical value at weeks 8 and 16 in the control group, indicating that resorption of the fracture callus was accelerated by bFGF treatment. These data suggest that bFGF accelerates callus remodeling both by increasing callus formation as a result of mitogenic effects on periosteal cells and by osteoclastic resorption. Evaluation of fracture strength showed a reduction in the callus volume at week 8 after fracture in the bFGF-treated group and recovery of fracture strength at week 16. The control group showed insufficient recovery of fracture strength at week 16. The more rapid recovery of fracture strength with bFGF treatment was likely the consequence of bFGF promotion of bone remodeling. The authors concluded that bFGF promotes fracture healing by stimulation of all stages of bone remodeling.

Recently, Radomsky et al. (36) investigated the effects of direct injection of bFGF in a hyaluronan gel into a freshly created fracture in a rabbit fibula. Hyaluronan gel was chosen because its viscosity allows it to serve as reservoir which holds the bFGF at the fracture site long enough to create an environment conducive to fracture healing. The results showed stimulation of callus formation, increased bone formation, and earlier restoration of mechanical strength at the fracture site. The investigators concluded that there is a synergistic relationship between the bFGF and the hyaluronan gel, serving to accelerate fracture healing, and this combination may be suitable for clinical evaluation as a therapy in fracture treatment.

INSULIN-LIKE GROWTH FACTORS

The two classes of IGF identified to date are IGF-I and IGF-II. While IGF-II is predominantly involved in fetal growth regulation, IGF-I may mediate the effects of growth hormone on the skeleton, stimulating cell division and matrix synthesis by cartilage, bone, tendon, and muscle cells (1). Recent data suggest that IGF-I may enhance the repair of bone defects (37,38); however, its role in endochondral fracture repair has not been carefully documented. Because IGF-I concentrations can be increased indirectly by the administration of growth hormone and because studies have shown stimulation of fracture healing with growth hormone (39,40), investigators have proposed that growth hormone may augment fracture repair through its effects on IGF-I expression.

IGF-II binds with a lower affinity and is generally less potent than IGF-I. It is present in bone in high concentrations, making it among the most abundant growth factors in the skeleton (41); however, its role in fracture healing is not well defined. Externally applied magnetic fields may stimulate the production of IGF-II in human osteoblast-like cell cultures (42), yet the clinical significance of this has yet to be elucidated.

PLATELET-DERIVED GROWTH FACTOR

PGDF is a potent regulator of bone cells, either alone or in combination with other factors.

Nash et al. (43) demonstrated that a single injection of PDGF increases the density and volume of callus formed in a rat tibial osteotomy model. Histological analysis suggested a more advanced stage of osteogenesis around the osteotomy sites in fractures treated with PDGF compared with controls; however, mechanical testing showed no improvement in strength in the PDGF-treated tibiae.

GENE THERAPY

Originally, the transfer of genes to individuals for therapeutic purposes was intended as a means of compensating for heritable genetic diseases. Gene therapy now is being considered for the treatment of acquired diseases, where it promises to function as a sophisticated type of drug-delivery system (44). The role of gene therapy is currently being investigated in the treatment of several orthopedic diseases, including poorly healing fractures. With few exceptions, naked DNA is not taken up well and expressed by cells; therefore, vectors which enable the cellular uptake and expression of genetic material must be employed. Viruses have proved to be effective vectors because part of their normal life cycle involves the entry into human cells and expression of virally encoded genes. Because the desired effect is not viral expression, these agents must be altered, removing certain elements of the genome, then providing the agents with the necessary proteins to enable replication. The resultant viral vectors are then able to deliver their genetic material to the nuclei of the target cells without permitting replication of the virus or development of pathological conditions caused by the virus. Some concerns with regard to safety still exist when generating large amounts of recombinant viruses; thus, nonviral delivery systems have also been developed.

Once in the nucleus of the host cell, the DNA may be integrated into the chromosomes or it may remain extrachromosomal (episomal). Chromosomal integration of the gene ensures that it will be transmitted to daughter cells during cellular division. Episomal DNA, although often initially expressed at high levels, tends to be lost with time as the cell divides. Retroviruses and adeno-associated viruses are two types of virus that integrate their genetic material into the DNA of the cells that they infect. Retroviruses are the best developed viruses for gene therapy and are currently being employed in several clinical trials. Advantages of retroviruses are that they are well developed as vectors and are obtained in useful titers of 100,000 or more per millimeter; however, most retroviruses used in gene therapy are limited to accepting only 8 kb of extraneous nucleic acid because of the size of the genome. While this is adequate for many applications, it is not well suited for genes encoding large proteins or for multiple genes. Additionally, because insertion of the retroviral genes into the host's DNA occurs at random locations, there is the potential for mutagenesis. Although this has not yet proven to be a problem, a more immediate concern is the inability of retroviruses to transduce nondividing cells, as they require mitosis for the viral DNA to enter the nucleus.

Adeno-associated viruses are less well developed; however, they may have the potential to circumvent some of the limitations of retroviruses. Adeno-associated viruses can be obtained in very high titers (up to twice that of retroviruses), are nonpathogenic, and insert their DNA into the genome of the host cell at a known specific location. Therefore, they have the ability to infect nondividing cells, which is an attractive property in certain applications. Limitations to the use of this viral line relate to the fact that their use is less well understood. Recombinant viruses appear to lose the ability to insert their DNA at a specific site in the host cell genome, and it is sometimes difficult to produce high titers of the recombinant virus. Additionally, the virus is small, permitting it to carry a maximum of 4 kb of extraneous DNA.

Adenovirus is the best developed of the nonintegrating viruses. Recombinant adenovirus can be produced readily at high titers and is highly infectious toward a wide range of dividing and nondividing cell types. While initial expression of the transferred gene is often very high, it tends to decrease rapidly with time. This phenomenon may be due to the fact that the DNA remains episomal or that the adenoviral vectors produce adenoviral proteins that are antigenic and provoke an immune response against the infected cells.

Nonviral vectors, such as liposomes, DNA–ligand complexes, and gene guns, are usually easier to produce than their viral counterparts and often have a greater chemical stability. Their advantages and disadvantages in gene therapy are currently being investigated.

There are two basic strategies for gene therapy. The first is direct, or *in vivo,* gene therapy, in which the vectors are introduced into the body. The second is indirect, or *ex vivo,* gene therapy, which requires the removal of target cells, followed by *in vitro* genetic alteration and subsequent reimplantation. The choice of strategy is based on the anatomy and physiology of the target organs, the pathophysiology of the disease, the chosen vector, relative safety, and other variables. While *in vivo* techniques are technically simpler, *ex vivo* gene therapy remains safer as the target cells are isolated and manipulated *in vitro.* Moreover, *ex vivo* methods permit the use of retroviral gene delivery to cells such as chondrocytes, synoviocytes, and bone marrow stromal cells, which do not normally divide rapidly *in vivo* yet undergo rapid mitoses *in vitro.*

In vivo or *ex vivo* techniques can be used to deliver genes locally to sites of disease, known as regional gene therapy, or to other sites, where the gene product can enter the systemic circulation, known as systemic delivery. Regional gene therapy has the potential to be used in humans to enhance the formation and repair of bone. This concept is attractive because genes can theoretically be delivered to the appropriate anatomic site, and the duration of protein expression can be controlled by selecting the appropriate vector. Lieberman et al. (45) demonstrated that regional gene therapy with continuous delivery of BMP-2 to a specific anatomic site can enhance the formation and repair of bone *in vivo* by developing a BMP-2-containing adenoviral vector. Using an *ex vivo* technique, a bone marrow stromal cell line was infected with an adenovirus expressing recombinant BMP-2 cDNA. Using Western blot, the infected cells were shown to secrete biologically active BMP-2. Histological analysis and serial radiographs demonstrated the induction of abundant heterotopic bone when the infected bone marrow stromal cells were implanted into the quadriceps muscles of severe combined immunodeficiency (SCID) mice. When implanted into a large segmental femoral defect in nude rats, the cells were able to produce sufficient quantities of bone to heal critical-sized defects.

Regional gene therapy offers several advantages over traditional treatment strategies, such as autologous or allogeneic bone grafting, and possibly over newer strategies using implanted recombinant growth factors. First, delivering an increased dose of therapeutic protein to the bone defect site would be possible. Second, this gene therapy may have the ability to control the duration of treatment by altering the vector selected. In addition, autologous bone marrow cells are osteoinductive, easy to harvest, and capable of responding in both an autocrine and a paracrine fashion (46). Finally, improved adenoviral vectors with increased capacity for multiple transgenes should allow for the delivery of multiple growth factors to a specific anatomic site. This may enhance the recruitment of pleuripotential cells.

Additional considerations regarding the use of gene therapy to enhance fracture healing and bone regeneration or to treat osteoporosis relate to the cost of therapy and efficiency. While recombinant growth factor therapies offer promising therapeutic advantages, they must be delivered in the microgram range. In gene therapy, localized delivery techniques with efficient targeting of cell surface receptors make for a more efficient delivery system overall by requiring less protein when compared to the systemic application of growth hormone.

In a study conducted by Fang et al. (47), the implantation of gene-activated matrices (GAMs) containing β-galactosidase or luciferase plasmids into 5-mm segmental gaps in the adult rat femur was evaluated. It was shown that implantation of the GAMs leads to DNA uptake and functional enzyme expression by host cells in the gap. Implantation of a GAM containing a BMP-4 plasmid or one that codes for a fragment of parathyroid hormone (PTH) (1–34) resulted in a biological response whereby bone formation

in the gap resulted in functional union. Furthermore, the implantation of a plasmid containing both BMP-4 and the PTH fragment led to a synergistic effect *in vivo,* causing new bone formation faster, at 4 weeks, than implantation of either agent alone. This led to the conclusion that delivery of plasmid DNA from a matrix is a simple means to stimulate mammalian bone growth following transient local overexpression of osteogenic factors. Moreover, the rate of bridging at 4 weeks surpassed, and at 9 weeks equaled, those results reported for the repair of similar defects treated with recombinant BMP-2, OP-1, or TGF-β1. This is the first study to demonstrate that host fibroblasts can be genetically manipulated *in vivo* to express and synthesize bone-active proteins.

SUMMARY

At the present time, the therapeutic potential of growth factors in the treatment of fractures has not been fully explored. Issues such as method of delivery, optimal dose, and the need to combine several factors as therapeutic cocktails remain unresolved. Like the application of other exogenous substances in a treatment regimen, growth factors must meet certain criteria. They must lack immunogenicity, side effects, and toxicity. They must be available in a delivery system that is easy to use. Most importantly, they must convincingly demonstrate their effectiveness and, in today's era of cost-conscious health care, must be cost-effective. While some growth factors have demonstrated exciting potential in controlled clinical trials, widespread therapeutic application will probably require several more years of careful research.

REFERENCES

1. Trippel SB. Growth factors as therapeutic agents. *Instr Course Lect* 1997;46:473–476.
2. Joyce ME, Roberts AB, Sporn MB, et al. Transforming growth factor-beta and the initiation of chondrogenesis and osteogenesis in the rat femur. *J Cell Biol* 1990;110: 2195–2207.
3. Andrew JG, Hoyland J, Andrew SM, et al. Demonstration of TGF-beta1 mRNA by *in situ* hybridization in normal human fracture healing. *Calcif Tissue Int* 1993; 52:74–78.

4. Campbell IK, Wojta J, Novak U, et al. Cytokine modulation of plasminogen activator inhibitor-1 (PAI-1) production by human articular cartilage and chondrocytes. Down-regulation by tumor necrosis factor α and up-regulation by transforming growth factor-β basic fibroblast growth factor. *Biochim Biophys Acta* 1994;1226: 277–285.

5. Joyce ME, Jingushi S, Bolander ME. Transforming growth factor-beta in the regulation of fracture repair. *Orthop Clin North Am* 1990;21:199–209.

6. Beck LS, Amento EP, Xu Y, et al. TGF-beta1 induces bone closure of skull defects: temporal dynamics of bone formation in defects exposed to rhTGF-beta1. *J Bone Miner Res* 1993;8:753–761.

7. Lind M, Schumacker B, Soballe K, et al. Transforming growth factor-beta enhances fracture healing in rabbit tibiae. *Acta Orthop Scand* 1993;64:553–556.

8. Nielsen HM, Andreassen TT, Ledet T, et al. Local injection of TGF-beta increases the strength of tibial fractures in the rat. *Acta Orthop Scand* 1994;65:37–41.

9. Rosier RN, O'Keefe RJ, Hicks DG. The potential role of transforming growth factor beta in fracture healing. *Clin Orthop* 1998;355[Suppl]:S294–S300.

10. Bostrom MP, Asnis P. Transforming growth factor beta in fracture repair. *Clin Orthop* 1998;355[Suppl]: S124–S131.

11. Ingram RT, Bonde SK, Riggs BL, et al. Effects of transforming growth factor beta (TGF beta) and 1,25 dihydroxyvitamin D3 on the function, cytochemistry and morphology of normal human osteoblast-like cells. *Differentiation* 1994;55:153–163.

12. Wergedal JE, Matsuyama T, Strong DD. Differentiation of normal human bone cells by transforming growth factor-beta and 1,25(OH)2 vitamin D3. *Metabolism* 1992;41:42–48.

13. Massague J. The transforming growth factor-beta family. *Annu Rev Cell Biol* 1990;6:597–609.

14. Talley-Ronsholdt DJ, Lajiness E, Nagodawithana K. Transforming growth factor-beta inhibition of mineralization by neonatal rat osteoblasts in monolayer and collagen gel culture. *In Vitro Cell Dev Biol Anim* 1995;31: 274–282.

15. Reddi AH. Initiation of fracture repair by bone morphogenetic proteins. *Clin Orthop* 1998;355[Suppl]:S66–S72.

16. Bostrom MP, Lane JM, Berberian WS, et al. Immunolocalization and expression of bone morphogenetic proteins 2 and 4 in fracture healing. *J Orthop Res* 1995; 13:357–367.

17. Nakase T, Nomura S, Yoshikawa H, et al. Transient and localized expression of bone morphogenetic protein 4 messenger RNA during fracture healing. *J Bone Miner Res* 1994;9:651–659.

18. Ishidou Y, Kitajima I, Obama H, et al. Enhanced expression of type I receptors for bone morphogenetic proteins during bone formation. *J Bone Miner Res* 1995;10: 1651–1659.

19. Stevenson S, Cunningham N, Toth J, et al. The effect of osteogenin (a bone morphogenetic protein) on the formation of bone in orthotopic segmental defects in rats. *J Bone Joint Surg Am* 1994;76:1676–1687.

20. Cook SD, Baffes GC, Wolfe MW, et al. The effect of recombinant human osteogenic protein-1 on healing of large segmental bone defects. *J Bone Joint Surg Am* 1994;76:827–838.

21. Gerhart TN, Kirker-Head CA, Kriz MJ, et al. Healing segmental femoral defects in sheep using recombinant human bone morphogenetic protein. *Clin Orthop* 1993; 293:317–326.

22. Yasko AW, Lane JM, Fellinger EJ, et al. The healing of segmental bone defects, induced by recombinant human bone morphogenetic protein (rhBMP-2). A radiographic, histological, and biomechanical study in rats [published erratum appears in *J Bone Joint Surg Am* 1992;74:1111]. *J Bone Joint Surg Am* 1992;74: 659–670.

23. Einhorn TA, Oloumi G, Mohaideen A, et al. Enhancement of experimental fracture healing with a local percutaneous injection of rhBMP-2. *Trans Am Acad Orthop Surg* 1997.

24. Bostrom M, Lane JM, Tomin E, et al. Use of bone morphogenetic protein-2 in the rabbit ulnar nonunion model. *Clin Orthop* 1996;327:272–282.

25. Bostrom MP, Camacho NP. Potential role of bone morphogenetic proteins in fracture healing. *Clin Orthop* 1998;355[Suppl]:S274–S282.

26. Johnson EE, Urist MR, Finerman GA. Bone morphogenetic protein augmentation grafting of resistant femoral nonunions. A preliminary report. *Clin Orthop* 1988; 230:257–265.

27. Johnson EE, Urist MR, Finerman GA. Resistant nonunions and partial or complete segmental defects of long bones. Treatment with implants of a composite of human bone morphogenetic protein (BMP) and autolyzed, antigen-extracted, allogeneic (AAA) bone. *Clin Orthop* 1992;277:229–237.

28. White AA, Panjabi MM, Southwick WO. The four biomechanical stages of fracture repair. *J Bone Joint Surg Am* 1977;59:188–192.

29. Bostrom MPG, Saleh DJ, Einhorn TA. Osteoinductive growth factors in pre-clinical fracture and long bone defects models. *Orthop Clin North Am* 1999;30: 647–658.

30. Einhorn TA. Enhancement of fracture-healing [see comments]. *J Bone Joint Surg Am* 1995;77:940–956.

31. Kawaguchi H, Kurokawa T, Hanada K, et al. Stimulation of fracture repair by recombinant human basic fibroblast growth factor in normal and streptozotocin-diabetic rats. *Endocrinology* 1994;135:774–781.

32. Nakamura K, Kurokawa T, Kato T, et al. Local application of basic fibroblast growth factor into the bone increases bone mass at the applied site in rabbits. *Arch Orthop Trauma Surg* 1996;115:344–346.

33. Jingushi S, Heydemann A, Kana SK, et al. Acidic fibroblast growth factor (aFGF) injection stimulates cartilage enlargement and inhibits cartilage gene expression in rat fracture healing. *J Orthop Res* 1990;8:364–371.

34. Nakamura T, Hara Y, Tagawa M, et al. Recombinant human basic fibroblast growth factor accelerates fracture healing by enhancing callus remodeling in experimental dog tibial fracture. *J Bone Miner Res* 1998;13: 942–949.

35. Tanaka T, Taniguchi Y, Gotoh K, et al. Morphological study of recombinant human transforming growth factor beta1–induced intramembranous ossification in neonatal rat parietal bone. *Bone* 1993;14:117–123.

36. Radomsky ML, Thompson AY, Spiro RC, et al. Potential role of fibroblast growth factor in enhancement of fracture healing. *Clin Orthop* 1998;355[Suppl]: S283–S293.

37. Thaller SR, Dart A, Tesluk H. The effects of insulin-like growth factor-1 on critical-size calvarial defects in Sprague-Dawley rats. *Ann Plast Surg* 1993;31:429–433.
38. Thaller SR, Hoyt J, Tesluk H, et al. Effect of insulin-like growth factor-1 on zygomatic arch bone regeneration: a preliminary histological and histometric study. *Ann Plast Surg* 1993;31:421–428.
39. Koskinen EVS, Lindholm RV, Nieminen RA, et al. Human growth hormone in delayed union and nonunion of fractures. *Int Orthop* 1978;1:317–322.
40. Northmore-Ball MD, Wood MR, Meggitt BF. A biomechanical study of the effects of growth hormone in experimental fracture healing. *J Bone Joint Surg Br* 1980; 62:391–396.
41. Frolik CA, Ellis LF, Williams DC. Isolation and characterization of insulin-like growth factor-II from human bone. *Biochem Biophys Res Commun* 1988;151: 1011–1018.
42. Ryaby JT, Fitzsimmons RJ, Khin NA, et al. A growth factor dependent model for magnetic field regulation of bone formation. *Trans Orthop Res Soc* 1994;19:518.
43. Nash TJ, Howlett CR, Martin C, et al. Effect of platelet-derived growth factor on tibial osteotomies in rabbits. *Bone* 1994;15:203–208.
44. Evans CH, Robbins PD. Possible orthopaedic applications of gene therapy. *J Bone Joint Surg Am* 1995;77: 1103–1114.
45. Lieberman JR, Le LQ, Wu L, et al. Regional gene therapy with a BMP-2-producing murine stromal cell line induces heterotopic and orthotopic bone formation in rodents. *J Orthop Res* 1998;16:330–339.
46. Gazit D, Turgerman G, Kelley P, et al. Engineered pluripotent mesenchymal cells integrate and differentiate in regenerating bone: a novel cell-mediated gene therapy. *J Gene Med* 1999;1:1–13.
47. Fang J, Zhu YY, Smiley E, et al. Stimulation of new bone formation by direct transfer of osteogenic plasmid genes. *Proc Natl Acad Sci USA* 1996;93:5753–5758.
48. Trippel SB, Coutts RD, Einhorn TA, et al. Growth factors as therapeutic agents. *J Bone Joint Surg Am* 1996; 78:1272–1286.

Skeletal Growth Factors,
edited by Ernesto Canalis.
Lippincott Williams & Wilkins, Philadelphia, © 2000.

23

Clinical Disorders Associated with Bone Morphogenetic Proteins

Frank P. Luyten, Frederick S. Kaplan,*† and Eileen M. Shore*‡

*Department of Rheumatology, University Hospitals Leuven, Belgium; Department of *Orthopaedic Surgery, †Medicine and ‡Genetics, The University of Pennsylvania School of Medicine, Philadelphia, Pennsylvania 19104*

The bone morphogenetic proteins (BMPs), a large group of morphogens belonging to the transforming growth factor-β (TGF-β) superfamily, were originally described as an *in vivo* bone-inducing activity isolated from demineralized bone matrix (1). Characterization of this activity by protein purification and cDNA cloning led to the discovery of several soluble, secreted, TGF-β-related molecules named BMP-2A (now BMP-2), BMP-2B (now BMP-4), BMP-3 or osteogenin, and osteogenic protein-1 (OP-1) or BMP-7 (2–7). Homology screening resulted in the identification of a substantial number of additional BMP-like genes, some of which also display *de novo* ectopic bone-induction activity. The existence of the homologous genes dpp and 60A in *Drosophila* and the embryonic expression patterns of BMPs at distinct stages of development and in many tissues suggested a much broader role than just bone formation for these potent morphogens. Mouse genetic approaches have revealed critical functions for BMPs in early embryonic patterning, organogenesis, and tissue differentiation, including formation of the heart, lungs, eye, kidney, and skeletal tissues (8).

Although one would expect similar functions for BMPs in humans, it was only recently that the first human clinical disorders associated with BMPs or attributable to mutations in BMP family members have been described. This chapter focuses on several illustrative chondrodysplasias caused by genetic mutations in BMP family members and on fibrodysplasia ossificans progressiva (FOP), a disabling disorder of ectopic osteogenesis and skeletal malformations associated with the overexpression of a BMP. It is through such studies that the molecular basis of an increasing number of diseases and disorders will be discovered, and understanding these processes will undoubtedly lead to the development of novel therapeutic approaches.

BONE MORPHOGENETIC PROTEINS AND HUMAN CHONDRODYSPLASIAS

Acromesomelic Dysplasias

The acromesomelic chondrodysplasias comprise a heterogeneous group of inherited disorders affecting the skeleton (9). The acromesomelic skeletal phenotype exhibits abnormalities predominantly in the middle and distal segments of the upper and lower limbs (10).

The association of a BMP with this heterogeneous group of osteochondrodysplasias evolved from the finding that murine brachypodism (*bp*) was due to null mutations in growth and differentiation factor-5 (Gdf-5), the mouse homologue of cartilage-derived morphogenetic protein-1 (hCDMP-1) (11,12). Gdf-5/CDMP-1 is a member of the TGF-β superfamily and belongs to a subfamily of three closely related morphogens, CDMPs 1–3/Gdfs 5–7 (11,12). Based on sequence identity and genomic structure, these morphogens are most closely related to BMPs 2 and 4. The CDMPs are not only structurally related to the BMP family members but also share a number of functional characteristics. Recombinant CDMPs induce ectopic cartilage and bone formation *in vivo* and promote chondrogenic and osteogenic differentiation *in vitro* (13–15). Interestingly, the bone-promoting activity of the CDMPs both *in vitro* and *in vivo* is fairly limited when compared with other BMPs/OPs in dose-response curves, with a preference for enhancement of the cartilage phenotype. This latter property may be related to the affinity of the CDMPs for the BMP receptor type IB (BMPR-IB)/activin receptor-like kinase-6 (ALK-6) receptor (14,16). In contrast to other BMP family members, the expression pattern of CDMP-1 predominated in and around the developing mouse and human limbs, with striking expression in the joint interzones (11,12,17). The *bp* phenotype and the restricted expression pattern of CDMP-1 in human embryonic development led us to identify the acromesomelic chondrodysplasias as potential disorders associated with mutations in the CDMP-1 gene.

Hunter-Thompson Chondrodysplasia

Some disorders in the acromesomelic group of chondrodysplasias exhibit striking similarities to the *bp* mutation in particular individuals from a previously described family from the Choco district in Colombia. Because of similarities with a sporadic case previously reported by Hunter and Thompson (18), this family was described as Hunter-Thompson type (HT) recessive acromesomelic dysplasia (19). HT is characterized by abnormalities restricted to the limbs, with no involvement of either the craniofacial or axial skeletal elements. The severity of the long bone shortening progresses in a proximodistal fashion (Fig. 23.1). In collaboration with the clinical geneticists who originally described this family, and not without considerable effort and adventures, we were able to obtain blood samples from both affected and nonaffected family members. Sequence differences

were observed between them within the mature protein-coding region of the CDMP-1 gene, and revealed a frameshift mutation resulting from a 22-bp insertion. The insertion was a tandem duplication leading to an altered open reading frame after the third cysteine, thereby disrupting the highly conserved seven-cysteine pattern so characteristic and functionally critical for the TGF-β superfamily members. As the altered reading frame led to a stop codon and the 43 out-of-frame amino acids did not share any homology to the normal protein sequence or any BMP family member, this mutation predicted loss of function. The affected individuals were homozygous for the mutation and therefore, we reported HT as the first human genetic disorder due to a mutation in a BMP family member (20). Clinical inspection of heterozygous family members did not reveal major skeletal abnormalities, but radiographs of upper or lower extremities could not be obtained due to the local conditions and the apparent lack of cooperativity of the involved individuals. Based on the findings in *bp* mice and in HT in humans, it is likely that the size, shape, and form of individual skeletal elements are probably controlled by the composite activity of a number of different morphogens.

CDMP-1, a member of the BMP family, is certainly a critical component in the formation of the appendicular skeleton, especially the distal elements of both the upper and lower limbs. The proximodistal gradient of the skeletal abnormalities may correspond to a gradient in expression of CDMP-1, although there is insufficient evidence to support this. Rather, a relatively higher expression level of other BMPs or involvement of other morphogens in the more proximal skeletal elements appears more likely. Interestingly, the long bone shortening in one affected family member was coupled to an apparent premature closure of some growth plates of the phalanges. Although seen only in this one individual, this finding suggested that signals from the joint interzone, where CDMP-1 is expressed most strikingly during long bone development, may interfere with and regulate, directly or indirectly, longitudinal bone growth.

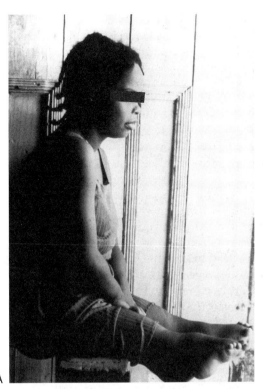

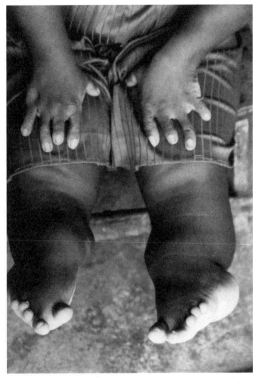

A   B

FIG. 23.1. Morphological characteristics of acromesomelic chondrodysplasia, Hunter-Thompson type. **A:** Abnormalities of the limbs, normal craniofacial and axial skeleton. **B:** Distal parts of limbs more severely affected than proximal parts, feet more affected than hands.

Grebe Syndrome

Grebe syndrome is a recessively inherited disorder exhibiting abnormal limb development in a proximodistal gradient, therefore classified as a form of acromesomelic dysplasia (9). The highest concentration of affected individuals was identified in the state of Bahia in Brazil (21,22). The rarity of the condition and the high frequency of consanguinity suggested a low mutation frequency in the general population. The similarities with HT are striking, most importantly the disproportionately short and deformed limbs and the normal craniofacial and axial skeleton. However, more detailed investigation and radiographic imaging revealed a much more severe phenotype than HT. Clinically, the findings were limited to the limbs with symmetrical defects of increasing severity in a proximodistal fashion. The fingers and toes appeared as globu-

lar appendages joined to hands or feet by bridges of soft tissue without apparent articulations. In some cases, postaxial polydactyly was present. A more detailed description of the phenotype has been published elsewhere (23). The severity of the Grebe phenotype became even more striking when evaluated by skeletal radiographs displaying a plethora of abnormalities (23,24).

As the pattern of malformations is similar to HT, we decided to pursue a possible link to the CDMP-1 gene. Genomic DNA from affected individuals was obtained and screened for possible mutations. A G-to-A transition at nucleotide 1199 was found in affected individuals, predicting a tyrosine-for-cysteine substitution at amino acid 400 (C400Y) in the mature region of CDMP-1 (24). The effect of this mutation on the synthesis and secretion of CDMP-1 was further analyzed in a series of *in vitro* experiments. The

results indicated that CDMP-1C400Y is not secreted and thus is most likely biologically inactive. In addition, the mutated protein appeared
to behave as a dominant-negative, not only suppressing the other CDMP-1 allele but also selectively interfering with the secretion of some
other BMPs, most likely through heterodimerization (24). These structure/function studies
provided a mechanistic basis for the much more
severe phenotype of the Grebe families as compared to HT and for the presence of a heterozygous phenotype. Indeed, and in contrast to HT,
obligate heterozygotes displayed a number of
minor anomalies, including short metacarpals
and middle phalanges, with considerable variation among subjects but surprising symmetry
within an individual.

Human CDMP-1 maps to chromosome
20q11.2, in a region on mouse chromosome 2
syntactic with the locus described for Gdf-5
(25). Interestingly, haplotype analysis of seven
affected individuals with polymorphic markers
demonstrated a common haplotype in 13 of the
14 chromosomes. One individual, a man indistinguishable clinically and radiographically
from the other affected cases, was a compound
heterozygote for the C400Y mutation and for
deletion of a G nucleotide at position 1144, predicting a frameshift and premature stop codon
(24). In this case, there is one null allele and
one CDMP-1C400Y allele. This exemplifies the
"potency" of the C400Y mutation at disrupting
the function of other BMPs, as half of the amount
of mutated CDMP-1 can produce the same phenotype.

The data from the HT and Grebe families provided strong evidence for the role of CDMPs
and associated BMP family members in the formation of the appendicular skeleton: symmetrical limb abnormalities with a proximodistal gradient of severity, postaxial polydactyly, and
abnormal joint formation. It is of interest that
these disorders also show abnormal endochondral ossification, resulting in bone aplasia and
hypoplasia, as well as delayed bone maturation,
establishing *in vivo* evidence that BMPs are, directly or indirectly, also involved in skeletal tissue differentiation. In addition, the Grebe syndrome points toward the possible consequences

of overlapping expression patterns of BMPs in
developing structures, that is, providing a degree
of biological redundancy but at the potential cost
of more severe phenotypes associated with dominant-negative mutations.

It should be noted that although the above-
mentioned *in vitro* findings very likely represent
the *in vivo* events in the patients, there is no
direct proof of this to date. Immunoprecipitation
experiments of endogenous CDMP/BMP heterodimers on samples from affected individuals
collected as biopsy material appear to be very
difficult to accomplish, as obtaining tissue specimens from patients during the developmental
phases when these molecular events are taking
place is obviously not possible. Proof of "natural" endogenous heterodimer formation could
be pursued on limbs from embryonic mice using
immunoaffinity columns, but the amounts of
heterodimers may be very limited; thus, large
quantities of limb material and additional purification steps might be needed. Finally, the production of Grebe-type mice using transgenic approaches to overexpress mutated CDMP-1 under
the control of an appropriate promotor, ideally
its own, should provide even more evidence.

Brachydactyly C

During the analysis of the obligate Grebe heterozygotes, we noted the occurrence of brachydactyly as a common feature. Brachydactylies
are disorders in which individual bones in the
hands and feet are altered in size and/or shape.
The inherited brachydactylies comprise a well-
documented and classified group of autosomal-
dominant disorders (26). Genetic studies in a
family with brachydactyly type C (Bd-C)
mapped the locus to an interval on chromosome
20 shown to contain CDMP-1 (27). In this family, 12 individuals across five generations displayed shortening of the second, third, and fifth
middle phalanges. Sequencing of CDMP-1
exons led to the identification of a heterozygous
C-to-T transition at nucleotide 901 of the mRNA
coding sequence, converting an arginine at position 301 to a stop codon. Additional screening
of other unrelated persons with Bd-C revealed
further CDMP-1 mutations (28). The mecha-

nism of the mutational effect in these families is most likely functional haploinsufficiency of CDMP-1. Previous data obtained from the findings in bp mice and the absence of a heterozygous phenotype in the HT family suggested no functional haploinsufficiency for CDMP-1. However, detailed clinical investigations and more extensive radiographic investigation of obligate carriers of the HT family were lacking for reasons mentioned above. Interestingly, heterozygous *bp* littermates revealed anomalous tendon insertions in hindlimbs, raising the possibility of a subtle heterozygous effect (29). Heterozygous phenotypes for BMP knockout mice have been observed (B. Hogan, personal communication). It is likely that the phenotypic variations in Bd-C families are at least partially due to the CDMP-1 mutational effect, as exemplified in the Grebe CDMP-1C400Y mutation, which causes a dominant-negative effect. Most importantly, the Bd-C findings suggest the existence of clinically apparent human heterozygous phenotypes associated with BMP family members, possibly affecting the development of various organ systems.

Perspectives on Bone Morphogenetic Protein–Associated Chondrodysplasias

It has been postulated that the molecular mechanisms of skeletal morphogenesis are highly conserved across species. Taking a candidate disorder approach, we hypothesized that the HT-type acromesomelic dysplasia was the human equivalent of murine *bp*. The identification of a frameshift mutation in the mature region of CDMP-1, the human homologue of Gdf-5, provides direct evidence for the involvement of a BMP family member in the formation of the human appendicular skeleton. The causative mutation in CDMP-1 and its proposed mechanism of action in chondrodysplasia Grebe-type are good evidence that a composite expression pattern of different BMPs dictates limb and digit morphogenesis. Haploinsufficiency may cause distinct and milder phenotypes, as exemplified in Bd-C.

A striking finding is also the restriction of the phenotypic changes involving CDMP-1 to the appendicular skeleton with no involvement of axial or craniofacial skeletal structures. The data indicate that CDMP-1 may be a predominant BMP in the more distal parts of the developing appendicular skeleton. In this regard, careful analysis of the chondrodysplastic phenotypes indicates that CDMP-1 is an excellent marker of the joint interzone as opposed to a factor directly involved in the joint formation or cavitation process. Indeed, especially the longitudinal growth of the distal skeletal elements and the shape and size of the epiphyses are affected and not the joint formation process itself. In addition, the proximodistal gradient of severity suggests that the ultimate shape and form of the skeletal elements and the process of joint formation are determined by the relative ratios, abundance, and thresholds of different BMPs. This biological principle is probably also critical in the formation of other organ systems. Therefore, one can predict the association of an increasing number of congenital multiorganic defects with mutations in BMP family members.

FIBRODYSPLASIA OSSIFICANS PROGRESSIVA

Clinical Features

FOP is a rare disabling genetic disorder of connective tissue characterized by congenital malformation of the toes and progressive postnatal heterotopic ossification in specific anatomic patterns. Although skeletal malformations may be detected radiologically at a number of sites, they are evident clinically only in the hands and feet (30). Characteristically, in 90% of patients, the big toes are short with malformations of the first metatarsals and contain only a single phalanx, which may be deviated laterally. Less commonly, in 10% of patients, the big toes are of normal length but stiff from early childhood or become rigid in adolescence due to early degenerative arthritis. The shortened, malformed big toes may be noted at birth but tend to be dismissed as isolated congenital hallux valgus. The child is otherwise asymptomatic until heterotopic ossification begins.

Heterotopic ossification in FOP usually begins as a series of lumps in the muscles of the

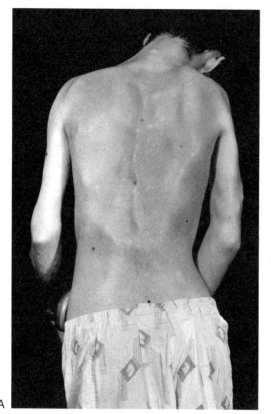
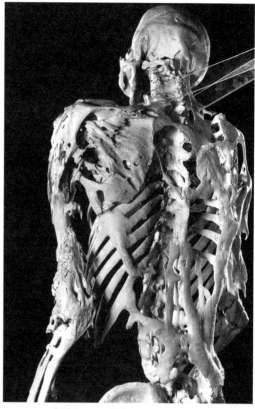

A

B

FIG. 23.2. Clinical photograph and skeleton of a man with fibrodysplasia ossificans progressiva (FOP): The rigid posture noted in this 25-year-old man with FOP is due to ankylosis of the spine, shoulders, and elbows. Plates and ribbons of ectopic bone contour the skin over the back and arms **(A)** and can be visualized directly on the skeleton **(B)** (following death from pneumonia at age 40 years). (Courtesy Mutter Museum, College of Physicians of Philadelphia. From ref. 55, with permission.)

neck or back (31,32). Typically, these lumps are first noted before 5 years of age (33–35). Soft tissue swellings that resemble tumors appear over several hours (36). The lumps themselves cause stiffness. When ectopic bone forms, irreversible limitation of movement becomes apparent (33). Mature heterotopic bone replaces skeletal muscle, tendon, ligament, and fascia, locking joints in place and rendering movement impossible (34) (Fig. 23.2). Most episodes of ectopic ossification occur spontaneously, although local trauma may induce ossification.

Ectopic bone in FOP has a predilection for certain sites. The axial musculature is most severely affected. In general, bone-induction events in axial regions precede appendicular in-

volvement and dorsal events precede ventral involvement (33). Bone formation in the limbs tends to be most marked proximally, with proximal muscles affected prior to distal muscles. Ankylosis of the jaw is common (37–40); however, involvement of the facial muscles is uncommon. Certain muscles, including the tongue, extraocular muscles, diaphragm, heart, sphincter muscles, and visceral smooth muscles, are not affected (31,33).

Routine biochemical and hematological investigations are normal in FOP, with the exception of transient elevations of serum alkaline phosphatase during disease flare-ups (41,42).

Erratic progression of disability is usual in FOP. Patients typically have long periods of apparent disease inactivity, but in general, limitation in movement of the spine and both shoulders occurs by 10 years of age. One or both hips are generally involved by 20 years of age, and most patients are chair-bound or bed-bound by 30 years of age (31,33,34). Episodes of new ectopic ossification, though generally less frequent in adults, do not stop completely but continue into old age (31,34). The ultimate level of disability does not appear to be related to the patient's gender, age of onset of heterotopic ossification, or type or extent of skeletal malformations. Once present, disability is permanent (34).

Although life span is reduced in FOP, most patients will reach adult age. The average age at death of 33 patients was 34.7 years, and several patients have survived into old age (>60 years) (35,43). Pneumonia has been reported to be the usual terminal illness, and this is promoted by severe chest wall restriction. There is no established medical treatment for FOP (44–46). The rarity of the disorder, its variable severity, and the fluctuating clinical course are substantial difficulties for evaluating potential therapies.

Ectopic bone is apparent radiographically as early as 4 weeks after the initial appearance of an ossifying lump. Ectopic bone matures through an endochondral process, develops normal trabecular architecture, and eventually develops secondary synostoses to the normotopic skeleton (47). Radionuclide bone scans show increased uptake at ossifying sites before new bone can be documented radiologically (48,49). Computerized tomograph (CT) scans showed swelling in the muscle fascial planes (corresponding to the active phase on the bone scan) during the initial stages of a flare-up and, subsequently, ectopic bone (50).

Pathological Studies

Since surgical trauma can induce heterotopic bone formation, tissue samples from FOP patients are available only rarely, from nonelective surgical procedures or from biopsies taken prior to the diagnosis of FOP.

Early FOP lesions exhibit an intense perivascular lymphocytic aggregation, followed by invasion of lymphocytes into the surrounding muscle with subsequent myocyte death. A role for hematopoietic cells in heterotopic osteogenesis had been suggested by Buring (51). Immunohistochemical evaluation of lymphocytic markers revealed a predominance of perivascular B lymphocytes and a mixed population of B lymphocytes and T lymphocytes weakly positive for BMP-4 invading the skeletal muscle (52). Whether the early lymphocytic infiltrate is a causative or reactive event, or both, cannot be determined from the observations in the small sample of patients examined. Interfascicular fibroproliferative tissue follows with extensive neovascularity (52). Levels of basic fibroblast growth factor (bFGF), a potent angiogenic peptide, are markedly elevated in the urine of patients with FOP during times of disease flare-up (53) and correlate with the appearance of the highly vascular fibroproliferative lesion.

Intermediate-stage FOP lesions cannot be distinguished histologically from aggressive juvenile fibromatosis, a condition which does not progress to form bone (36), but immunohistochemistry can be useful (32,54). BMP-4 expression has been detected in cultured fibroproliferative cells and in intact tissue specimens from preosseous FOP lesions but not in aggressive juvenile fibromatosis lesions (36,55). Later-stage FOP lesions show characteristic features of endochondral ossification, including chondrocyte hypertrophy, calcification of cartilage, and formation of lamellar bone with marrow elements, almost identical to the pattern seen in a normally developing growth plate or in fracture repair (32).

Inheritance

Most described cases of FOP result from new mutations, with the mutation rate estimated to be 1.8×10^{-6} (standard error 1.04) mutations per gene per generation (56). Reproductive fitness in FOP is low, and only a few examples of inheritance of FOP within a family have been documented (31,57–63). The inheritance pattern is autosomal-dominant. The rarity of FOP suggests the likelihood of a single mutated locus causing the disorder in all or most individuals, and recent genome-wide linkage analysis in four small multigenerational families suggests linkage to a region on the long arm of human chromosome 4 (64).

Molecular Genetics

Positional cloning was, until recently, impractical for FOP due to the small number of affected individuals and the lack of multigenerational families showing inheritance of the disease. The candidate gene approach has been pursued as an alternative method to identify the mutated gene. In selecting a candidate gene for FOP, the major diagnostic criteria (congenital malformations of the great toes, heterotopic endochondral ossification, temporal and spatial patterns of ectopic bone formation) must be considered.

The genes that best fit the criteria of FOP candidate genes are those that encode BMPs and other components in the BMP signal-transduction pathways (3,8,65–70). Many members of the BMP family, such as BMP-2 and BMP-4, can induce endochondral bone formation in a manner similar to the events observed in FOP lesion formation.

The BMP-2 and BMP-4 genes encode proteins that are about 90% similar to each other and are homologous to the *Drosophila* decapentaplegic (dpp) gene. The DPP protein shows ~75% amino acid identity to BMP-2 and BMP-4 in the mature carboxyl-terminal region, the mature functional domain of these proteins. In *Drosophila*, the dpp gene is essential for early embryonic development as well as in the later larval stage, when it provides necessary information for limb formation (65). The pattern of dpp expression is analogous to the expression of BMP-2 and BMP-4 in vertebrate development (8,65,68), although the dorsal–ventral axis is reversed. These BMPs play critical roles both in early embryogenesis and in skeletal formation, important criteria for FOP candidate genes.

BMP-4 and DPP both appear to function by directing cell fate (65,71). The absence of BMP-4 in a transgenic knockout mouse is lethal in early embryogenesis, showing little or no mesodermal differentiation and no hematopoiesis (69, 72). In later developmental stages and poten-

tially more directly relevant to the bone formation in FOP, BMP-4 has been implicated in patterning of the developing mouse and human limb and skeletal morphogenesis (11,20,73). Overexpression of BMP-4 in the chick embryonic limb bud is associated with ectopic osteogenesis and polarizing defects in limb formation (74).

Although early FOP lesions are histologically identical to those of aggressive juvenile fibromatosis, these two disorders can be distinguished by immunohistochemistry with BMP-2/4 antibodies (36). Tissues from aggressive juvenile fibromatosis lesions (which do not progress to form bone) show no binding of the BMP-2/4 antibody, while FOP lesional tissues bind the antibody, indicating the presence of BMPs within early-stage FOP lesions that will progress to endochondral ossification.

Cells derived from a preosseous FOP lesion and from immortalized lymphoblastoid cell lines established from FOP patients showed increased expression (by Northern analysis and ribonuclease protection assays) of BMP-4 but not BMP-2 when compared to controls. In addition, correlation of BMP-4 expression with FOP was observed in a family showing inheritance of FOP; the affected father and three affected children expressed detectable amounts of BMP-4, while the unaffected mother did not (55). Further studies have verified that BMP-4 is synthesized in cells from patients who have FOP (75,76).

Steady-state levels of mRNA for BMP-4 and the BMP receptors were evaluated using semiquantitative reverse-transcription polymerase chain reaction (RT-PCR), documenting the presence of type I and type II BMP-4 receptor mRNAs in FOP lesional tissue as well as in unaffected muscle tissue (76). In lymphoblastoid cell lines of affected individuals in a family that exhibited autosomal-dominant inheritance of FOP, the previous finding of elevated steady-state levels of BMP-4 mRNA were confirmed (76) but no differences in the steady-state levels of mRNA for either type I or type II BMP-4 receptors were observed between affected and unaffected individuals.

The increased levels of BMP-4 mRNA and protein in the cells of FOP patients could be due to a mutation within the BMP-4 gene itself or to a mutation in another genetic locus. While it is unlikely that a mutation in the protein coding region of the BMP-4 gene would produce higher protein levels, mutations in the RNA coding region or splice junctions could synthesize BMP-4 mRNA with increased stability. Alternatively, mutations in the transcriptional regulatory regions of the BMP-4 gene could enhance the rate of mRNA synthesis. Either possibility would result in greater accumulation of BMP-4 mRNA, leading to higher protein production. Recent results have indicated that the higher levels of BMP-4 mRNA in FOP cells are caused by an increased rate of transcription of the BMP-4 gene, not differences in BMP-4 mRNA stability (75). This is consistent with an examination of the RNA coding and splice junction sequences of BMP-4 genes from patients with FOP that has identified no mutations in these regions (77). Mutations in sequences within the BMP-4 gene promoter and enhancer regions as well as mutations within genes that encode transcriptional regulatory factors could result in an increased BMP-4 transcription rate. In order to identify the sequences within the BMP-4 gene promoter relevant to gene activation and the factors which stimulate promoter activity, transcriptional regulation of the human BMP-4 gene is being examined (78).

Recently, a genome-wide linkage analysis using four families showing inheritance of FOP revealed consistent linkage with the 4q27-31 region of chromosome 4 (64). The BMP-4 gene is not within this locus, supporting the hypothesis that the mutation causing FOP is not within the BMP-4 gene. However, genes involved in the BMP signaling pathway, in addition to other candidate genes that may affect BMP-4 signaling, have been identified in this interval and are being studied for possible mutations.

Genetic mutations in FOP could reside anywhere in the BMP-4 signaling pathway (64) or in other molecular pathways that affect the level of BMP-4 expression. Additional information about the cellular and molecular events that occur during progression of FOP lesion formation as well as better understanding of the events that induce bone formation during normal embryonic development and fracture healing will both expand the list of candidate genes and focus on the most likely causes of this disorder.

Animal Models

A FOP-like condition has been recognized in cats, with six cases reported (79–82). Unfortunately, all evaluations performed to date have been postmortem studies on pet cats, and no live animals are available for examination.

In a compelling transgenic animal model, murine embryonic overexpression of the c-fos protooncogene leads to postnatal heterotopic chondrogenesis and osteogenesis with phenotypic features similar to those seen in children who have FOP (83). The overexpression of Fos protein in embryonic stem cell chimeras leads to heterotopic endochondral osteogenesis mediated at least in part through a BMP-4 signal-transduction pathway. In contrast, early FOP lesions express abundant BMP-4 without overexpression of c-Fos, suggesting that the primary molecular defect in FOP may be independent of sustained Fos effects on chondrogenesis and osteogenesis (83,84).

Perspectives on Bone Morphogenetic Protein–Associated Heterotopic Ossification

Creative use of BMP technology will likely have important applications in the inhibition of heterotopic ossification in diseases such as FOP. Soluble BMP receptors, dominant-negative receptors, and BMP antagonists may be promising in binding and physiologically inactivating BMP where it is not needed or wanted (85,86). The hope for an effective treatment for FOP has been increased by the discovery of BMP-4 overexpression in the condition (55,87,88). ''With so much being discovered about how the BMPs act,'' says Brigid Hogan, a developmental geneticist at Vanderbilt University in Nashville, Tennessee, ''it might be possible to develop drugs that would block some part of the BMP-4 pathway—and therefore prevent the progression of what is a horrible nightmare disease'' (89).

CONCLUSIONS

The genetic data have convincingly established the physiological importance of BMPs in human skeletogenesis and have demonstrated that mutations in BMP genes may cause heritable disorders affecting the formation and repair of the skeleton. Based on these studies and our current understanding of the mechanisms of action of the BMP signaling pathways, many more human clinical syndromes are likely to be associated with abnormalities in BMP signaling in the future.

The role of the BMP signaling pathways in disease states is just beginning to be addressed. Such studies have led to an increased understanding of BMP biology and have broad implications for therapy of human diseases.

ACKNOWLEDGMENTS

The authors are indebted to Drs. J. Michael Connor, Judah Folkman, William Gelbart, Richard Harland, Victor McKusick, Maximilian Muenke, John Rogers, Vicki Rosen, Roger Smith, Neil Stahl, James Triffitt, Marshall Urist, John Wozney, and Michael Zasloff for their enduring intellectual contributions to this field and to the evolution of the work presented here. The authors also thank Drs. T. Thomas, M. Camargo, P. Tsipouras, and M. Warman for their critical contributions to the work on acromesomelic chondrodysplasias and brachydactyly. The authors dedicate this work to Jeannie Peeper (President of the International Fibrodysplasia Ossificans Progressiva Association) and to all of the patients worldwide affected with FOP, in appreciation for their continuous inspiration and in admiration of their steadfast courage. This work was supported in part by grants from the International Fibrodysplasia Ossificans Progressiva Association, The Ian Cali Fellowship, The Gund Foundation, The European Neuromuscular Center, The Isaac and Rose Nassau Professorship of Orthopaedic Molecular Medicine, the National Institutes of Health (R01-AR-41916), and the National Institute of Craniofacial and Dental Research, Intramural Program.

REFERENCES

1. Urist MR. Bone formation by autoinduction. *Science* 1965;150:893–899.
2. Wang EA, Rosen V, Cordes P, et al. Purification and characterization of other distinct bone-inducing factors. *Proc Natl Acad Sci USA* 1988;85:9484–9488.
3. Wozney JM, Rosen V, Celeste AJ, et al. Novel regulators of bone formation: molecular clones and activities. *Science* 1988;242:1528–1534.
4. Luyten FP, Cunningham NS, Ma S, et al. Purification and partial amino acid sequence of osteogenin, a protein initiating bone differentiation. *J Biol Chem* 1989;264:13377–13380.
5. Celeste AJ, Iannazzi JA, Taylor RC, et al. Identification of transforming growth factor beta family members present in bone-inductive protein purified from bovine bone. *Proc Natl Acad Sci USA* 1990;87:9843–9847.
6. Ozkaynak E, Rueger DC, Drier EA, et al. OP-1 cDNA encodes an osteogenic protein in the TGF-beta family. *EMBO J* 1990;9:2085–2093.
7. Sampath TK, Coughlin JE, Whetstone RM, et al. Bovine osteogenic protein is composed of dimers of OP-1 and BMP-2A, two members of the transforming growth factor-beta superfamily. *J Biol Chem* 1990;265:13198–13205.
8. Hogan BL. Bone morphogenetic proteins: multifunctional regulators of vertebrate development. *Genes Dev* 1996;10:1580–1594.
9. Spranger J. International classification of osteochondrodysplasias. The International Working Group on Constitutional Diseases of Bone. *Eur J Pediatr* 1992;151:407–415.
10. McKusick VA, ed. *Mendelian inheritance in man: a catalogue of human genes and genetic disorders.* Baltimore: Johns Hopkins University Press, 1994.
11. Storm EE, Huynh TV, Copeland NG, et al. Limb alterations in brachypodism mice due to mutations in a new member of the TGF beta-superfamily. *Nature* 1994;368:639–643.
12. Chang SC, Hoang B, Thomas JT, et al. Cartilage-derived morphogenetic proteins. New members of the transforming growth factor-beta superfamily predominantly expressed in long bones during human embryonic development. *J Biol Chem* 1994;269:28227–28234.
13. Hotten GC, Matsumoto T, Kimura M, et al. Recombinant human growth/differentiation factor 5 stimulates mesenchyme aggregation and chondrogenesis responsible for the skeletal development of limbs. *Growth Factors* 1996;13:65–74.
14. Erlacher L, McCartney J, Piek E, et al. Cartilage-derived morphogenetic proteins and osteogenic protein-1 differentially regulate osteogenesis. *J Bone Miner Res* 1998;13:383–392.
15. Erlacher L, Ng CK, Ullrich R, et al. Presence of cartilage-derived morphogenetic proteins in articular cartilage and enhancement of matrix replacement *in vitro.* *Arthritis Rheum* 1998;41:263–273.
16. Nishitoh H, Ichijo H, Kimura M, et al. Identification of type I and type II serine/threonine kinase receptors for growth/differentiation factor-5. *J Biol Chem* 1996;271:21345–21352.
17. Storm EE, Kingsley DM. Joint patterning defects caused by single and double mutations in members of the bone

morphogenetic protein (BMP) family. *Development* 1996;122:3969–3979.

18. Hunter AG, Thompson MW. Acromesomelic dwarfism: description of a patient and comparison with previously reported cases. *Hum Genet* 1976;34:107–113.

19. Langer LO Jr, Cervenka J, Camargo M. A severe autosomal recessive acromesomelic dysplasia, the Hunter-Thompson type, and comparison with the Grebe type. *Hum Genet* 1989;81:323–328.

20. Thomas JT, Lin K, Nandedkar M, et al. A human chondrodysplasia due to a mutation in a TGF-beta superfamily member. *Nat Genet* 1996;12:315–317.

21. Quelce-Salgado A. A new type of dwarfism with various bone aplasias and hypoplasias of the extremities. *Acta Genet* 1964;14:63–66.

22. Quelce-Salgado A. A rare genetic syndrome. *Lancet* 1968;1:1430.

23. Costa T, Ramsby G, Cassia F, et al. Grebe syndrome: clinical and radiographic findings in affected individuals and heterozygous carriers. *Am J Med Genet* 1998;75: 523–529.

24. Thomas JT, Kilpatrick MW, Lin K, et al. Disruption of human limb morphogenesis by a dominant negative mutation in CDMP1. *Nat Genet* 1997;17:58–64.

25. Lin K, Thomas JT, McBride OW, et al. Assignment of a new TGF-beta superfamily member, human cartilage-derived morphogenetic protein-1, to chromosome 20q11.2. *Genomics* 1996;34:150–151.

26. Fitch N. Classification and identification of inherited brachydactylies. *J Med Genet* 1979;16:36–44.

27. Robin NH, Gunay-Aygun M, Polinkovsky A, et al. Clinical and locus heterogeneity in brachydactyly type C. *Am J Med Genet* 1997;68:369–377.

28. Polinkovsky A, Robin NH, Thomas JT, et al. Mutations in CDMP1 cause autosomal dominant brachydactyly type C. *Nat Genet* 1997;17:18–19.

29. Gruneberg H, Lee AJ. The anatomy and development of brachypodism in the mouse. *J Embryol Exp Morphol* 1973;30:119–141.

30. Schroeder HW Jr, Zasloff M. The hand and foot malformations in fibrodysplasia ossificans progressiva. *Johns Hopkins Med J* 1980;147:73–78.

31. Connor JM, Evans DA. Fibrodysplasia ossificans progressiva. The clinical features and natural history of 34 patients. *J Bone Joint Surg Br* 1982;64:76–83.

32. Kaplan FS, Tabas JA, Gannon FH, et al. The histopathology of fibrodysplasia ossificans progressiva. An endochondral process. *J Bone Joint Surg Am* 1993;75: 220–230.

33. Cohen RB, Hahn GV, Tabas JA, et al. The natural history of heterotopic ossification in patients who have fibrodysplasia ossificans progressiva. A study of forty-four patients. *J Bone Joint Surg Am* 1993;75:215–219.

34. Rocke DM, Zasloff M, Peeper J, et al. Age- and joint-specific risk of initial heterotopic ossification in patients who have fibrodysplasia ossificans progressiva. *Clin Orthop* 1994;301:243–248.

35. Janoff HB, Tabas JA, Shore EM, et al. Mild expression of fibrodysplasia ossificans progressiva: a report of 3 cases. *J Rheumatol* 1995;22:976–978.

36. Gannon FH, Kaplan FS, Olmsted E, et al. Bone morphogenetic protein (BMP) 2/4 in early fibromatous lesions of fibrodysplasia ossificans progressiva. *Hum Pathol* 1997;28:339–343.

37. Renton P, Parkin SF, Stamp TCB. Abnormal temporo-

mandibular joints in fibrodysplasia ossificans progressiva. *Br J Oral Surg* 1982;20:31–38.

38. Nunnelly JF, Yussen PS. Computed tomographic findings in patients with limited jaw movement due to myositis ossificans progressiva. *J Oral Maxillofac Surg* 1986;44:818–821.

39. Janoff HB, Zasloff MA, Kaplan FS. Submandibular swelling in patients with fibrodysplasia ossificans progressiva. *Otolaryngol Head Neck Surg* 1996;114: 599–604.

40. Luchetti W, Cohen RB, Hahn GV, et al. Severe restriction in jaw movement after routine injection of local anesthetic in patients who have fibrodysplasia ossificans progressiva. *Oral Surg Oral Med Oral Pathol Oral Radiol Endod* 1996;81:21–25.

41. Smith R, Russell RG, Woods CG. Myositis ossificans progressiva. Clinical features of eight patients and their response to treatment. *J Bone Joint Surg Br* 1976;58: 48–57.

42. Smith R. Fibrodysplasia (myositis) ossificans progressiva: clinical lessons from a rare disease. *Clin Orthop* 1998;346:7–14.

43. Connor JM. *Soft tissue ossification.* Berlin: Springer, 1983:54–74.

44. Beighton P. Fibrodysplasia ossificans progressiva. In: Beighton P, ed. *McKusick's heritable disorders of connective tissue,* 5th ed. St. Louis: C.V. Mosby, 1993: 501–518.

45. Connor JM. Fibrodysplasia ossificans progressiva. In: Royce PM, Steinmann B, eds. *Connective tissue and its heritable disorders.* New York: Wiley-Liss, 1993: 603–611.

46. Whyte MP, Kaplan FS, Shore EM. Fibrodysplasia ossificans progressiva. In: Favus MJ, ed. *Primer on the metabolic bone diseases and disorders of mineral metabolism,* 3rd ed. Philadelphia: Lipincott-Raven, 1996: 428–430.

47. Kaplan FS, Strear CM, Zasloff MA. Radiographic and scintigraphic features of modeling and remodeling in the heterotopic skeleton of patients who have fibrodysplasia ossificans progressiva. *Clin Orthop* 1994;304:238–247.

48. Holan J, Galanda V, Buchanec J. Isotopenuntersuchungen bei der fibrodysplasia ossificans progressiva in kindersalter mittels radiostrontium. *Radiol Diagn (Berl)* 1973;14:719–726.

49. Fang MA, Reinig JW, Hill SC, et al. Technetium-99m MDP demonstration of heterotopic ossification in fibrodysplasia ossificans progressiva. *Clin Nucl Med* 1986; 11:8–9.

50. Reinig JW, Hill SC, Fang MA, et al. Fibrodysplasia ossificans progressiva: CT appearance. *Radiology* 1986; 159:153–157.

51. Buring K. On the origin of cells in heterotopic bone formation. *Clin Orthop* 1975;110:293–302.

52. Gannon FH, Valentine BA, Shore EM, et al. Acute lymphocytic infiltration in extremely early lesions of fibrodysplasia ossificans progressiva. *Clin Orthop* 1998; 346:19–25.

53. Kaplan FS, Sawyer J, Connors S, et al. Urinary basic fibroblast growth factor: a biochemical marker for preosseous fibroproliferative lesions in patients who have fibrodysplasia ossificans progressiva. *Clin Orthop* 1998; 346:59–65.

54. Smith R, Athanasou NA, Vipond SE. Fibrodysplasia

(myositis) ossificans progressiva: clinicopathological features and natural history. *Q J Med* 1996;89:445–446.

55. Shafritz AB, Shore EM, Gannon FH, et al. Overexpression of an osteogenic morphogen in fibrodysplasia ossificans progressiva. *N Engl J Med* 1996;335:555–561.

56. Connor JM, Evans DA. Genetic aspects of fibrodysplasia ossificans progressiva. *J Med Genet* 1982;19:35–39.

57. Kaplan FS, McCluskey W, Hahn G, et al. Genetic transmission of fibrodysplasia ossificans progressiva. Report of a family. *J Bone Joint Surg Am* 1993;75:1214–1220.

58. Lutwak L. Myositis ossificans progressiva. Mineral, metabolic and radioactive calcium studies of the effects of hormones. *Am J Med* 1964;37:269–293.

59. McKusick VA. *Heritable disorders of connective tissue,* 4 ed. St. Louis: C.V. Mosby, 1972.

60. Koontz AR. Myositis ossificans progressiva. *Am J Med Sci* 1927;174:406–412.

61. Fox S, Khoury A, Mootabar H, et al. Myositis ossificans progressiva and pregnancy. *Obstet Gynecol* 1987;69:453–455.

62. Thornton YS, Birnbaum SJ, Lebowitz N. A viable pregnancy in a patient with myositis ossificans progressiva. *Am J Obstet Gynecol* 1987;156:577–578.

63. Connor JM, Evans CC, Evans DA. Cardiopulmonary function in fibrodysplasia ossificans progressiva. *Thorax* 1981;36:419–423.

64. Feldman G, Li M, Urtizberea JA, et al. Genome-wide linkage analysis of families with fibrodysplasia ossificans progressiva (FOP). *Bone* 1998;23:S379.

65. Kaplan FS, Tabas JA, Zasloff MA. Fibrodysplasia ossificans progressiva: a clue from the fly? *Calcif Tissue Int* 1990;47:117–125.

66. Reddi AH, Cunningham NS. Initiation and promotion of bone differentiation by bone morphogenetic proteins. *J Bone Miner Res* 1993;8[Suppl 2]:S499–S502.

67. Vainio S, Karavanova I, Jowett A, et al. Identification of BMP-4 as a signal mediating secondary induction between epithelial and mesenchymal tissues during early tooth development. *Cell* 1993;75:45–58.

68. Kingsley DM. The TGF-beta superfamily: new members, new receptors, and new genetic tests of function in different organisms. *Genes Dev* 1994;8:133–146.

69. Winnier G, Blessing M, Labosky PA, et al. Bone morphogenetic protein-4 is required for mesoderm formation and patterning in the mouse. *Genes Dev* 1995;9:2105–2116.

70. Urist MR. Bone morphogenetic protein: the molecularization of skeletal system development. *J Bone Miner Res* 1997;12:343–346.

71. Jones CM, Lyons KM, Hogan BL. Involvement of bone morphogenetic protein-4 (BMP-4) and Vgr-1 in morphogenesis and neurogenesis in the mouse. *Development* 1991;111:531–542.

72. Johansson BM, Wiles MV. Evidence for involvement of activin A and bone morphogenetic protein 4 in mammalian mesoderm and hematopoietic development. *Mol Cell Biol* 1995;15:141–151.

73. Kingsley DM, Bland AE, Grubber JM, et al. The mouse short ear skeletal morphogenesis locus is associated with defects in a bone morphogenetic member of the TGF beta superfamily. *Cell* 1992;71:399–410.

74. Francis-West PH, Richardson MK, Bell E, et al. The effect of overexpression of BMP-4 and GDF-5 on the development of limb skeletal elements. *Ann NY Acad Sci* 1996;785:254–255.

75. Olmsted EA, Liu C, Haddad JG, et al. Characterization of mechanisms controlling bone morphogenetic protein-4 message expression in fibrodysplasia ossificans progressiva. *J Bone Miner Res* 1996;11:S164.

76. Lanchoney TF, Olmsted EA, Shore EM, et al. Characterization of bone morphogenetic protein-4 receptors in fibrodysplasia ossificans progressiva. *Clin Orthop* 1998;346:38–45.

77. Xu M, Shore EM. Mutational screening of the bone morphogenetic protein 4 gene in a family with fibrodysplasia ossificans progressiva. *Clin Orthop* 1998;346:53–58.

78. Shore EM, Xu M, Shah PB, et al. The human bone morphogenetic protein 4 (BMP-4) gene: molecular structure and transcriptional regulation. *Calcif Tissue Int* 1998;63:221–229.

79. Warren HB, Carpenter JL. Fibrodysplasia ossificans in three cats. *Vet Pathol* 1984;21:495–499.

80. Waldron D, Pettigrew V, Turk M, et al. Progressive ossifying myositis in a cat. *J Am Vet Med Assoc* 1985;187:64–65.

81. Valentine BA, George C, Randolph JF, et al. Fibrodysplasia ossificans progressiva in the cat. A case report. *J Vet Intern Med* 1992;6:335–340.

82. Valentine BA, Kaplan FS. Fibrodysplasia ossificans progressive in cats: a potentially important animal model of the human disease. *Feline Pract* 1996;24:6.

83. Olmsted EA, Gannon FH, Wang Z-Q, et al. Embryonic over-expression of the c-fos proto-oncogene: a murine stem cell chimera applicable to the study of fibrodysplasia ossificans progressiva in humans. *Clin Orthop* 1998;346:81–94.

84. Wang ZQ, Grigoriadis AE, Mohle-Steinlein U, et al. A novel target cell for c-fos-induced oncogenesis: development of chondrogenic tumours in embryonic stem cell chimeras. *EMBO J* 1991;10:2437–2450.

85. Kimble RB, Liu X, Gannon FH, et al. Noggin inhibits bone formation in a model of heterotopic ossification. *Bone* 1998;23:S244.

86. Graff JM. Embryonic patterning: to BMP or not to BMP, that is the question. *Cell* 1997;89:171–174.

87. Kaplan FS, Shore EM, Zasloff MA. Fibrodysplasia ossificans progressiva: searching for the skeleton key. *Calcif Tissue Int* 1996;59:75–78.

88. Connor JM. Fibrodysplasia ossificans progressiva—lessons from rare maladies. *N Engl J Med* 1996;335:591–593.

89. Roush W. Protein builds second skeleton. *Science* 1996;273:1170.

Skeletal Growth Factors,
edited by Ernesto Canalis.
Lippincott Williams & Wilkins, Philadelphia, © 2000.

24

Parathyroid Hormone–related Protein

T. John Martin, Mark H. C. Lam, Vicky Kartsogiannis,
and Matthew T. Gillespie

*St. Vincent's Institute of Medical Research and the Department of Medicine, The University of
Melbourne, Fitzroy, 3065, Australia*

The discovery of parathyroid hormone–related protein (PTHrP) resulted from investigations of the mechanisms by which certain cancers cause hypercalcemia without metastasizing to bone. This syndrome, humoral hypercalcemia of malignancy (HHM), had for a long time been ascribed to inappropriate production of parathyroid hormone (PTH) by cancers. However, when studies throughout the 1970s indicated that the tumor product differed from PTH immunochemically but nevertheless was associated with very similar clinical effects to those resulting from PTH excess, the existence of a previously uncharacterized factor seemed most likely. This suspicion led to a number of excellent clinical studies, which put the question beyond doubt (1,2). By that time, biological assays of PTH had improved to the point that rapid, sensitive, robust assays were available which lent themselves to the identification of PTH-like activity. Extracts of hypercalcemic tumors from humans and other species and of culture supernatant from hypercalcemic tumor were found to contain PTH-like activity, assayed as adenylate cyclase responses in the PTH targets of osteoblasts or kidney.

PROTEIN AND GENE

The molecular cloning of PTHrP revealed it to be substantially larger than PTH, the cDNA clones predicting PTHrP to be 141 amino acids in length, with a prepro peptide of 36 amino acids (3). The deduced primary amino acid sequence revealed that eight of the first 13 amino acids are identical to those of PTH, with the remainder of the two sequences being unique (Fig. 24.1) (3). Shortly after the cloning of PTHrP, other reports predicted additional PTHrP proteins of 173 (4–6) and 139 (7) amino acids in length. All PTHrP isoforms were identical up to amino acid 139; however, the 173–amino acid isoform possessed a unique C-terminal sequence of an additional 35 amino acids (4,6).

The marked conservation of the PTHrP amino acid sequence in human, rat, mouse, chicken, and canine up to position 111 indicates that important functions are likely to reside in this region. Indeed, this region contains the known biological activities of PTHrP, which include PTH/PTHrP receptor binding, transplacental calcium transport, renal bicarbonate excretion, and *in vitro* osteoclast inhibition (8,9). The gene for human PTHrP is complex, with nine exons and three promoters, and together with the 3' alternate splicing is able to generate multiple mRNA transcripts (6,10). The structural organization of the rat, mouse, and chicken PTHrP genes has been resolved (Fig. 24.2) (11–13). The rat and mouse PTHrP genes have a much simpler structure than does to the human PTHrP gene and do not undergo alternative 3' splicing, producing only one form of PTHrP cDNA (Fig. 24.2). The conservation of the exons equivalent to human exons IV, V, VI, and IX among the rat, mouse, and chicken PTHrP genes implies that these exons constitute the minimum

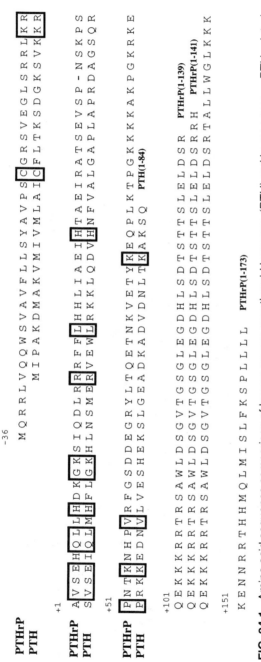

FIG. 24.1. Amino acid sequence comparison of human prepro-parathyroid hormone (*PTH*) and human prepro-PTH-related protein (*PTHrP*). The different isoforms of PTHrP (139, 141, and 173 amino acids) are provided from amino acid 101 onward. Residues of identity between PTH and PTHrP are *boxed*, and *gaps* have been introduced to maximize the alignment.

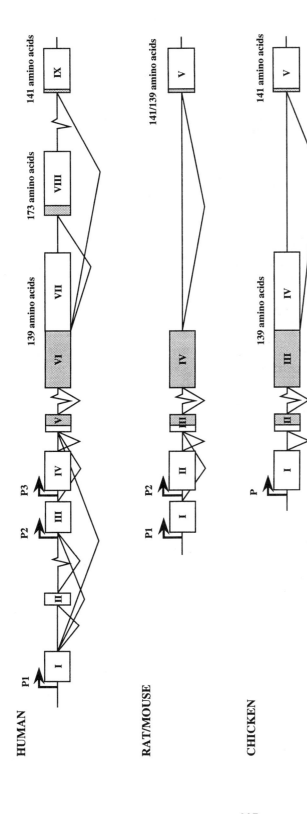

FIG. 24.2. Comparison of the structural organization of the human, rat, mouse, and chicken parathyroid hormone–related protein *(PTHrP)* genes. The coding regions and untranslated sequences are indicated by the *closed* and *open boxes*, respectively. Splicing events are denoted below each map. Indicated above the maps are the identified promoter regions: P1 and P3 of the human gene are TATA promoters and P2 is a GC-rich promoter; P1 of the rat and murine genes is a GC-rich promoter and P2 is a TATA promoter; P of the chicken gene is a TATA promoter.

PTHrP gene structure. Moreover, the TATA promoter region 5' to human exon IV appears to be the major promoter for the PTHrP gene because it is conserved among the rat, mouse, chicken, and canine genes. Similarly, the 141–amino acid isoform encoded by human PTHrP exon IX appears to be the major molecular form of the protein.

In the human gene, the presence of several promoters suggests the potential use of different promoter regions, which may result in tissue-specific and/or developmentally regulated expression of PTHrP. A comprehensive analysis of tissue-specific or developmental regulation of PTHrP promoters or 3' alternative splicing has not been undertaken. These analyses have been hindered since rodent PTHrP genes do not display the alternative splicing or the multiple promoters of their human counterpart. Apart from specifying different isoforms of PTHrP, the alternative transcripts confer different properties as mRNA species. While three different isoforms of human PTHrP have different 3'-untranslated regions, they all contain multiple copies of an AUUUA instability motif (3–7,14). This motif is associated with the rapid turnover of mRNA from cytokines and oncogenes (15, 16), and PTHrP mRNA has been found to have a short half-life of approximately 90 to 120 minutes. Expression of the PTHrP gene is subject to regulation by many growth factors, cytokines, and hormones (Table 24.1), some acting by transcriptional and others by posttranscriptional mechanisms. The facts that PTHrP mRNA is unstable and that its expression is regulated by so many growth factors and cytokines with which it is coexpressed during development and in various tissues ideally equips PTHrP to function as a cytokine. Indeed, although discovered as a hormone produced in excess by certain cancers, PTHrP seems to exert its physiological functions by acting locally in several tissues, including bone.

STRUCTURE AND BIOLOGICAL ACTIVITIES OF PARATHYROID HORMONE-RELATED PROTEIN

On the basis of its primary amino acid sequence, PTHrP can be divided into different re-

TABLE 24.1. *Factors that regulate parathyroid hormone–related protein expression and production*

Positive regulators	Negative regulators
Angiotensin II	Androgens
Bradykinin	Chromogranin A
Calcitonin	Dexamethasone
Calcium	$1,25(OH)_2D_3$
Cyclic adenosine	p53 gene product
monophosphate	Retinoic acid
Cycloheximide	Testosterone
$1,25(OH)_2D_3$	
Endothelin	
Epidermal growth factor	
Estradiol	
Forskolin	
3-Isobutyl-1-methylxanthine	
Insulin	
Insulin-like growth factor	
Interleukins (IL-1β, IL-2, IL-4, IL-6)	
Mechanical stretch	
Norepinephrine	
Phorbol ester	
Prolactin	
Prostaglandin E_1	
Retinoic acid	
Serotonin	
Serum	
Sodium butyrate	
tax gene product	
Thrombin	
Transforming growth factor-β	
Tumor necrosis factor-α	

gions. The first 36 amino acids (-36 to -1) code for the intracellular "prepro" and "pro" precursors of the mature peptide, which are important for intracellular trafficking. The next region includes the first 13 residues of the mature protein, which is the region showing primary sequence homology with PTH. This region is critical for most of the agonist effects of PTH on its classical target tissues (bone, kidney) to regulate calcium metabolism (17). PTHrP residues 14 to 36 are interesting in that, although they have almost no homology with PTH in primary sequence, they nevertheless appear to be critical for binding of PTHrP to the classical PTH/PTHrP receptor (18,19). Competitive binding assays show that PTH-(1–34) and PTHrP-(1–36) bind the receptor with approximately equal affinity, while shorter N-terminal fragments of either PTH or PTHrP do not (18, 20). This reflects the strong similarity of the secondary/tertiary structure of PTH and PTHrP, despite the differences in primary amino acid sequence in this region.

The significance of the next region, extending from amino acids 36 to 139, is less well established. This region is encoded by all three isoforms of human PTHrP mRNA, and the primary sequence is highly conserved across species through amino acid 111. The midmolecule portion, between residues 35 and 84, has been shown to be responsible for promoting calcium transport across the placenta, making calcium available for fetal skeletal development (21,22). A portion of the midmolecule beyond residue 84 is responsible for inhibiting bicarbonate excretion by the kidney (23). In addition, residues 107 to 111 at the carboxy terminus of the midmolecule have been reported to inhibit osteoclast activity and bone resorption *in vitro* (24,25) and *in vivo* (26) and to be mitogenic for osteoblasts (27).

The final tail region of PTHrP, from amino acids 142 to 173, is encoded by only one of the three isoforms of human PTHrP mRNA. Its significance in terms of tissue distribution, processing, or function is unknown, although Burtis et al. (28) have reported PTHrP(141–173) immunoreactivity in plasma and Brandt et al. (29) have shown that PTHrP(140–173) immunoreactivity is present in human amnion. It is presumed that the actions ascribed to regions of the molecule beyond the N-terminal 34 amino acids are mediated by unique PTHrP receptors, although these have yet to be discovered.

The posttranslational processing of PTHrP has been reviewed by Orloff et al. (9,30). In summary, the steps which have been documented include (a) signal peptide pro peptide cleavage at Arg^{-2} Lys^{-1} (presumably in all tissues), (b) Arg^{37} cleavage [thus far in keratinocytes, rat insulinoma (RIN) cells, Chinese hamster ovary (CHO) cells, and renal carcinoma cells], (c) *O*-glycosylation in keratinocytes and (d) generation of a carboxy-terminal PTHrP containing immunoreactivity at residues 109 to 138 in CHO and RIN cells, keratinocytes, and renal carcinomas. Additionally, with respect to pro-peptide endoproteolytic processing of PTHrP, efficient cleavage by the subtilisin-like prohormone convertase furin has been reported (31–35). The above steps lead to the secretion of (a) an amino-terminal fragment, PTHrP-(1–36) (36–39); (b) a midregion fragment beginning at position 38 and extending approximately 70 to 80 amino acids (38,39), although subsequent findings by Wu et al. (40), defined the presence of three midregion secretory forms of PTHrP, all beginning at Ala^{38} and each terminating at a different amino acid (94,95, and 101); (c) a larger amino-terminal *O*-glycosylation form of the peptide (41); and (d) a carboxy-terminal PTHrP species (39,42–44).

Two secretory pathways exist in eukaryotic cells: the regulated pathway, where the proteins are packaged into secretory granules, and the constitutive pathway, where the secretory peptides are found in the endoplasmic reticulum (45). Recent studies have shown that all forms of PTHrP are secreted via the regulated pathway in neuroendocrine cell types and via the constitutive pathway in nonendocrine cell types (46). This is unusual in the sense that PTHrP is both a neuroendocrine peptide and a growth factor or cytokine. It is neuroendocrine in the sense that it undergoes extensive posttranslational processing in a fashion analogous to chromogranin A or somatostatin, and it is a product of a broad variety of neuroendocrine cell types (e.g., pancreatic islet cells, parathyroid cells, adrenal medullary cells, pituitary cells, central nervous system neurons, etc.) (reviewed in 8,47). In these cells, it is packaged into secretory granules. On the other hand, PTHrP is also produced by a broad range of constitutively secreting cell types (e.g., vascular smooth muscle cells, hepatocytes, osteoblasts, keratinocytes, chondrocytes, and renal tubular cells) (reviewed in 8,47). In these cells, which do not contain the neuroendocrine machinery. PTHrP is secreted in a constitutive fashion, analogous to the cytokines and growth factors whose actions it so closely resembles. Interestingly, Matsushita et al. (48) have recently shown that in parathyroid adenoma cells, which are classical endocrine cells, PTHrP is secreted through both the regulated and the constitutive pathways. This duality of secretory mechanisms has not been documented for other peptides, including PTH, which is secreted only via the regulated pathway.

For the most part, PTHrP is viewed as having an autocrine or paracrine role. Only three circumstances have been identified in which PTHrP species are convincingly present in the circulation and act in an endocrine manner (28,49–54): (a) HHM syndrome, in which PTHrP is secreted by tumors and targeted to bone and kidney; (b) lactation, in which PTHrP is made in the breast and reaches the circulation; and (c) fetal life, during which PTHrP is made by the fetal parathyroids to regulate maternal-to-fetal placental calcium transport.

Defining the circulating forms of PTHrP has proved to be extremely difficult because of the low amount of PTHrP and the need for assays with greater sensitivity. Although N-terminal PTHrP cannot be detected in the circulation of normal subjects using current assays, there is evidence from patients with renal failure (in whom C-terminal epitopes can be identified in the absence of detectable N-terminal epitopes) that PTHrP may normally circulate and that a C-terminal fragment is disposed of by the kidney (42,54,55). Further, the ability to detect C-terminal PTHrP in urine supports this notion (56–60).

TISSUE DISTRIBUTION OF PARATHYROID HORMONE–RELATED PROTEIN AND ITS FUNCTIONS AS A CYTOKINE

The widespread expression of PTHrP in the developing embryo, particularly in epithelia at many locations and in a number of adult tissues, has supported the hypothesis that PTHrP is a cellular cytokine whose actions involve both cell growth and differentiation. Indeed, there is a growing body of evidence, particularly in epithelial cells, cancer cells, smooth muscle cells, and bone, to support this notion, although its precise roles are not established. PTHrP mRNA and protein have been detected in the following human tissues: adrenal, bone, brain, heart, intestine, kidney, liver, lung, mammary gland, ovary, parathyroid, placenta, prostate, skeletal muscle, skin, spleen, stomach, and smooth muscle (reviewed in 8).

Although its role is yet to be defined, there is a growing body of evidence supporting a role for PTHrP in epithelial growth and differentiation in the embryo and in the adult (61,62). It may function as an autocrine and/or paracrine factor, contributing to keratinocyte growth and differentiation, but may also be part of a paracrine interaction between keratinocytes and fibroblasts, for which it may have a role in the normal physiology or development of skin.

The role of PTHrP as a local paracrine regulator of smooth muscle tone has been one of its most clearly defined physiological actions. PTHrP is produced in the vascular smooth muscle cells, where its levels appear to be upregulated in response to mechanical distension of the arterial wall, to increases in arterial pressure, and to vasoconstrictors such as angiotensin II (63–66). PTHrP-(1–34) is a potent vasodilator of cardiac and smooth muscle from many locations, such as blood vessels, uterus, and gastrointestinal tract (67–70). Its vasodilatory effects are thought to be the result of its interaction with the classical receptor PTH1R, which is also expressed in vascular smooth muscle cells (71). In addition, it has been speculated that PTHrP may play a role in vascular smooth muscle cell proliferation and may therefore exert important roles in arterial modeling and remodeling in response to injury (63,71,72).

Recent work has focused on the heart and peripheral vasculature as important sites for PTHrP action in the control of blood flow. From a localization standpoint, the work has documented the presence of PTHrP in fetal and adult heart, at both the mRNA and the protein levels (43,73). From a functional point of view, several investigators have reported that PTHrP has effects on the intact heart, the isolated perfused heart, and the coronary artery (65,67,74). PTHrP is also thought to exert inotropic effects *in vivo* and in the isolated perfused heart, possibly as a consequence of increased coronary blood flow due to the vasodilatory action of PTHrP on the coronary circulation, as discussed above (74). Despite evidence of a role for PTHrP as a cardiac hormone, a vasodilatory agent, and a local paracrine regulator of smooth muscle tone, PTHrP-null mutant mice develop normal cardiovascular systems (75). It is clear, therefore, that PTHrP is not essential for cardiovascular development; however, because the animals die at birth of skeletal and perhaps other defects, the role of PTHrP in vascular remodeling, local regulation of vascular flow, and the vascular response to injury in adult animals remains undefined.

In the myometrium, it is proposed that PTHrP plays a role in expansion of the uterus to accommodate fetal growth (76,77). Moreover, pretreatment of rats with 17β-estradiol was demonstrated to increase the sensitivity of the uterus to the effects of exogenous PTHrP and to induce PTHrP mRNA expression (78,79). Angiotensin II, a potent vasoconstrictor, has been shown to produce a marked induction of PTHrP mRNA (63) in vascular smooth muscle cells. The detection of PTHrP in human amnion and amniotic fluid is suggested to relate to the ability of PTHrP to act as a vasorelaxant (29,80–82). In the amnion, PTHrP is thought to play a role in the modulation of fetal vessel tone and thereby fetal–placental blood flow (80). After rupture of the fetal membranes, PTHrP mRNA in the amnion decreased by 78%, leading to the proposal that PTHrP may have a role in the onset of labor (81). In the chicken, PTHrP mRNA expression was detected in smooth muscle of the oviduct as the egg moved through the oviduct (82). PTHrP was also detected in the vascular smooth muscle of vessels in the shell gland, where it is thought that PTHrP is responsible for the increased blood flow to the shell gland during the calcification phase of egg laying (82). Thus, PTHrP-(1–34) is proposed to function as a relaxant of both ductal and vascular smooth muscle.

PARATHYROID HORMONE–RELATED PROTEIN AND PLACENTAL CALCIUM TRANSPORT

The concentration of ionized calcium in mammalian fetal plasma is greater than that in maternal plasma and is maintained by active placental calcium transport. These are properties necessary for normal fetal skeletal growth. Thyroparathyroidectomy of fetal lamb abolished the placental calcium gradient, which could be restored by extracts of fetal parathyroid glands or partially purified PTHrP (21) but not by PTH infusion (21). This and the demonstration that PTHrP is produced by fetal parathyroid glands (21,83–85) implied that production of PTHrP by fetal parathyroids could contribute to the relative hypercalcemia of the fetal lamb (21).

PTHrP-(1–141), -(1–108), and -(1–84) stimulated calcium transport in the placenta of thyroparathyroidectomized lambs, but PTHrP-(1–34) was without effect (21,22). This implies that the effect is not mediated by the PTH-like N-terminal region of PTHrP but by a midmolecular region. Some evidence in sheep indicates that the region of PTHrP responsible for stimulating placental calcium transport was contained within PTHrP (67–86).

Although the role of PTHrP in placental calcium transport has not been established in human subjects, evidence supporting it in another species comes from studies in PTHrP-knockout mice (87), showing that fetuses homozygous for PTHrP gene deletion have a lower blood calcium and a reduced fetal–maternal calcium gradient, thereby providing direct evidence that PTHrP is required for placental calcium transport. Most interestingly, the same group of workers further investigated the placental calcium gradient in mothers and fetuses deficient for PTH1R, noting once again that the receptor-null fetuses were hypocalcemic (lacking the skeletal and renal responses to PTH and amino-terminal PTHrP), yet placental calcium transport was more efficient than normal. These findings highlight the importance of midregion PTHrP in placental calcium transport and provide additional evidence suggestive of a separate receptor that recognizes the midportion of PTHrP.

PARATHYROID HORMONE–RELATED PROTEIN IN LACTATION AND BREAST DEVELOPMENT

The presence of PTHrP in pregnant (88) and lactating (89) breast and in milk (90–92) indicates several possible roles for PTHrP, both endocrine and paracrine, in lactation and milk production and in breast development.

There is direct evidence in goats and humans

(87,92–94) and indirect evidence in rats (95) that significant levels of PTHrP circulate in lactating mothers. This raises the possibility that PTHrP has an endocrine role in the mother, to mobilize skeletal calcium for milk production. In support of this hypothesis, clinical studies have shown that lactation is associated with maternal bone loss and renal calcium retention (94,96), and in light of the current evidence, PTHrP would be the most likely mediator. There are no convincing data, however, with regard to the role of PTHrP in milk formation or in the transport of calcium into milk or whether it serves as a nutrient to the neonate, despite evidence of induction of PTHrP mRNA expression in rat lactating mammary tissue in response to suckling (89) and the fact that there are high levels of PTHrP in breast milk (90–92). Nevertheless, further evidence to support an endocrine role of PTHrP during lactation comes from the demonstration of increased maternal renal excretion of cAMP and phosphate in the rat in response to suckling (95), indicating that PTHrP may reach the circulation to act on the kidney.

Alternatively, PTHrP may play a local role in the mammary gland, perhaps influencing growth and development and/or blood flow to and within the gland. PTHrP is readily detectable in mammary tissue, being demonstrated predominantly in epithelial and myoepithelial cells (88,97–100). When PTHrP(−/−) mice were "rescued" by expressing PTHrP in cartilage using the collagen type II promoter, among the striking, persistent abnormalities in the rescued mice was complete failure of breast ductal development (101); PTHrP overexpression in the mouse results in abnormal differentiation and impaired ductal formation, suggesting an imbalance between the growth and differentiation phases (102) and, hence, further supporting the view of PTHrP acting as a cellular cytokine in cell growth and differentiation.

PARATHYROID HORMONE–RELATED PROTEIN IN FETAL DEVELOPMENT

Multiple studies using immunohistochemistry, *in situ* hybridization, or Northern blot analyses have shown early embryonic detection of PTHrP in mouse (103), chicken (13), rat (104), and human (105,106) tissues.

In the mouse, PTHrP has been identified immunohistochemically as early as the eight-cell stage during embryogenesis, primarily in developing trophoectoderm cells and in cells lining the blastocoelic cavity, which are likely to be primitive endoderm cells (103). Using immunohistology and *in situ* hybridization, we have delineated the temporal and spatial distribution of PTHrP expression in fetal and adult skeletal and extraskeletal mouse tissues, such as brain, kidney, lung, heart, liver, small intestine, skin, and skeletal muscle (107; Kartsogiannis, unpublished data, 1999). The expression of PTHrP was highest in tissues where active growth and differentiation occurred, such as renal tubules, bronchioles, and intestine, thus favoring the idea that PTHrP may be closely associated with the regulation of fetal and perhaps neonatal cellular growth and differentiation.

In the rat, PTHrP mRNA is first detected by *in situ* hybridization in polar and mural trophoblast cells at 7.5 days of gestation, and is not seen in the embryo proper before 15.5 days (104). Strong hybridization is apparent in ectoderm-derived tissues such as the epithelial cells of the dental lamina and hair follicles (by day 18.5), as well as in endoderm- and mesoderm-derived tissues such as the lung (at day 15.5) and perichondrium (at days 16.5 to 19) (104). Immunohistochemical studies have essentially provided similar results, with PTHrP immunopositivity being largely confined to the placental decidua and trophoblast layer in rat fetal tissues at days 8 to 12 (108). At days 13 to 14, protein expression is found in the epidermis and skin appendages, skeletal and cardiac muscle, vascular smooth muscle, liver, and the epithelial layers of the renal tubules, bronchioles, and the gastrointestinal tract (108). By day 18, expression is prominently localized in the choroid plexus, salivary ducts, pancreatic ducts and islets, and the seminiferous tubules of the testis (108). In the nervous system, strong PTHrP staining is seen in the brain, spinal cord, dorsal root ganglia, peripheral nerves, and developing eye (73). Additionally, in the skeletal system, PTHrP mRNA and protein are detected in the early mesenchyme and immature cartilage of the vertebral column, tail, and long bones. The intensity of PTHrP expression, however, gradually decreases until the onset of ossification, when chondrocytes and osteoblasts become positive (73,109).

Analogous profiles of PTHrP expression have also been reported in the human fetus (105,106, 110). Early expression of PTHrP mRNA is observed in both the syncytiotrophoblastic and the cytiotrophoblastic layers in first-trimester chorionic villi (105). Both the peptide and the mRNA are also expressed in the ectodermal cells of the avascular amnion. In the fetus at 7 to 8 weeks of gestation, ectodermal structures that are strongly positive for PTHrP expression include the epidermis, the otic placode, and the tooth bud (105). PTHrP-expressing tissues of endodermal origin include the lung, liver, pancreas, stomach, intestine, and hindgut, while those of mesodermal origin include the perichondrium and the developing kidney (105). In most of these tissues, the PTHrP peptide seems to be confined to the epithelial layer, while the mRNA is sometimes seen in mesenchymal components (105,106). Later in embryonic development (18 to 20 weeks of gestation), PTHrP expression is also apparent in cardiac and skeletal muscle, vascular smooth muscle, neural tissues, and areas of both endochondral and intramembranous osteogenesis in the limb buds and calvarium, respectively (105,106,110).

The spatial and temporal distribution of PTHrP correlates highly with that of PTH1R (111,112), which can be detected in the parietal endoderm from day 5.5 in the mouse and at sites of epithelial–mesenchymal interactions in the rat embryo from day 9.5 (111). The relative expression levels of PTHrP and its receptor are often inversely correlated within a tissue or in certain locales along a border of apposition. Such a tight inverse coupling of expression would seem to imply either feedback downregulation of the receptor or a precise coordinate regulation of the two genes during the course of fetal development (112).

Finally, functional evidence of a role for PTHrP and its receptor in mammalian fetal development comes from studies of animals which are transgenic or have gene-targeted knockouts (102,112–115). Homozygous deletion of the *PTHrP* gene is lethal; neonatal mice die shortly after birth and display a multitude of skeletal defects (75,116) (discussed below).

PARATHYROID HORMONE–RELATED PROTEIN AS A REGULATOR OF CELL GROWTH AND DIFFERENTIATION

The widespread expression of PTHrP in the developing embryo supports the hypothesis that it is a cytokine involved in the paracrine, and possibly intracrine, regulation of epithelial cell growth and differentiation, with a potential function in intracellular calcium control and cell cycle events.

A number of studies on cultured keratinocytes have shown an inhibitory effect of PTHrP on cell growth (61,117). The introduction of antisense mRNA for PTHrP into a stable human keratinocyte cell line by Kaiser et al. (61) resulted in loss of PTHrP production and a subsequent increase in cell growth, suggesting that endogenous PTHrP acts as an inhibitor of cell growth in this keratinocyte cell line. In contrast, PTHrP has also been shown to promote differentiation of keratinocytes, as indicated in follow-up experiments by Kaiser et al. (62). They found that interference with PTHrP production further inhibited expression of maturation-specific keratinocyte indices, indicating that PTHrP enhances differentiation in this cell line and that the effect of PTHrP on cellular differentiation may be dependent on cell type. Similarly, epidermal proliferation was inhibited by PTHrP-(1–34) and increased by a PTH/PTHrP receptor antagonist *in vivo* (117). In addition, experiments in mice overexpressing PTHrP targeted to skin cells by use of the keratin 14 promoter resulted in abnormal differentiation of hair follicles (115), hence further supporting the role for PTHrP in regulating cellular differentiation in skin. In a subsequent study by Wysolmerski et al. (102), using the same model in the mammary gland, PTHrP overexpression in breast myoepithelial cells delayed and profoundly diminished the extent of ductal proliferation and branching morphogenesis. Thus, evidence from antisense and targeted overexpression studies clearly indicates that PTHrP is an important factor in keratinoyte and mammary epithelial growth and differentiation (61,62,102,115).

Other evidence for the involvement of PTHrP in differentiation comes from observations of chondrocytes in *PTHrP* and *PTH1R* gene knockout mice (75,113,114,118). During normal endochondral bone formation, chondrocytes undergo differentiation into hypertrophic cells and apoptose as capillaries and bone-forming cells invade the region. In the absence of PTHrP, as observed in *PTHrP* gene knockout mice (see following), chondrocytes differentiate prematurely, resulting in a reduced number of proliferating chondrocytes, early hypertrophy, and subsequent death of chondrocytes, leading to premature bone formation (75,112–114). Consistent with these observations, *PTH1R* gene knockout mice, although having more severe effects, similarly exhibited accelerated chondrocyte differentiation (119). Alternatively, in transgenic mice with targeted overexpression of PTHrP in proliferating and prehypertrophic chondrocytes using the mouse collagen (α_1) type II promoter (101), delays in chondrocyte differentiation and ossification were observed, hence confirming the findings of the PTHrP knockout model (75), in which PTHrP was shown to have an important role in regulating the correct sequence of events in endochondral bone formation.

Henderson et al. (120) carried out further studies into the role of PTHrP in chondrocyte growth and differentiation. A unique role for the C terminus of PTHrP was proposed, whereby PTHrP promoted its effects by translocating to the nucleolus. Residues 87 to 107 of PTHrP bear homology to the nucleolar localization sequence identified in human immunodeficiency virus type I (HIV-I) (121,122) and human leukemia virus type I regulatory proteins (123). PTHrP-(1–141) transiently expressed in African green monkey kidney cells (COS-7) was shown to be targeted to the nucleolus (120). Additional experimental evidence localized endogenous PTHrP to the nucleolus of murine bone cells *in vitro* and *in situ* (120). These findings provided

evidence for a nuclear site of PTHrP action (reviewed in 124). Subsequent studies confirmed these initial observations in a human keratinocyte cell line (HaCaT) (125) and in cultured vascular smooth muscle cells (66), although in the latter case the intranuclear localization of endogenous PTHrP was diffuse within the nucleoplasm and not exclusively nucleolar, suggestive of alternative intranuclear effects by this protein.

Recent findings have further implicated a nuclear function for PTHrP at the G_1 phase of the cell cycle. Lam et al. (125) have reported that in the human keratinocyte cell line HaCaT PTHrP localizes to the nucleolus at G_1 and is excluded from the nucleus from the start of the S phase to mitosis, hence supporting a cell cycle–dependent nuclear exclusion of PTHrP. In vascular smooth muscle cells, nuclear PTHrP has been observed in cells that are dividing or are in the process of completing cell division, suggesting that nuclear translocation is associated with activation of the cell cycle (66).

Finally, a growing body of evidence has provided strong support for a role for PTHrP as a key factor involved in the orderly program of cell growth, differentiation, and apoptosis. Henderson et al. (120) showed that localization of PTHrP to the nucleolus enhanced chondrocyte survival under conditions such as serum deprivation that normally promote programmed cell death (120). Amizuka et al. (126) further reported that chondrocytes in mice with a homozygous deletion of PTHrP underwent apoptosis while chondrocytes in wild-type littermates did not. More recently, PTHrP has also been reported to be a downstream target for the antiapoptosis gene *Bcl-2* (127).

While previously the effects of PTHrP were considered to result mostly from interaction with the amino-terminal receptor, the capacity of PTHrP to influence normal cellular function must now also be considered in terms of its effects at the level of the nucleus. Further clarification of the mechanisms involved would add significantly to our present understanding of this protein as a signaling molecule during embryonic development.

PARATHYROID HORMONE–RELATED PROTEIN IN BONE

With its identification in tumors associated with the syndrome of HHM, PTHrP was recognized as a potent bone-resorbing agent *in vivo* and *in vitro,* and the pathogenesis of hypercalcemia in HHM in large part reflects the bone-resorbing properties of PTHrP (1,128–131). The finding that PTHrP exerts a number of additional actions on bone and bone-derived cells suggests a physiological role of PTHrP in bone. The distinct PTH-like and PTH-unlike domains of the PTHrP molecule are responsible for eliciting multiple and opposing actions.

The anabolic effects of intermittent PTH administration on bone and its therapeutic potential in osteoporosis have been extensively studied (reviewed in 132). With the recognition that PTHrP is the endogenous ligand for PTH1R in osteoblasts, its use as an anabolic agent has also been investigated. PTHrP-(1–74) was shown to increase bone mass in rats (133). PTHrP-(1–36), one of the authentic secretory forms of PTHrP (30), has been reported to have potency equivalent to PTH-(1–34) in its actions (134). PTHrP-(1–34) appeared to be less potent than PTH-(1–34) at producing an anabolic response in bone (135), although that could be partly attributed to its higher clearance rate (136). In a recent study by Rihani-Bisharat et al. (137), N-terminal fragments of both PTH and PTHrP were also reported to have anabolic effects on neonatal mouse bones.

Evidence for skeletal production of PTHrP comes from several sources. PTHrP protein has been identified by immunological detection in normal human and rat fetal bone and cartilage (106,138,139) and its immunological activity has been demonstrated in fetal rat long bones in culture (140). Furthermore, PTHrP mRNA has been shown by reverse-transcription polymerase chain reaction to be expressed in human and rat osteoblastic sarcoma cell lines (141,142), rat osteoblast-rich cultures and pre-osteoblastic cell lines (142), primary cultures of human bone-derived cells (143), and heterogeneous populations of bone cells (144). *In situ* hybridization analyses have localized PTHrP to active osteoblasts on the bone surface of newborn rat calvarial sections (142) and to spindle-shaped cells of the periosteum, which may represent immature pre-osteoblasts (112,137,142). In areas of endochondral bone formation, PTHrP mRNA has been detected by *in situ* hybridization in the perichondrium and maturing chondrocytes in a cell–type and stage-specific manner during fetal rat development (112). Using a model of intramembranous bone formation in the rabbit, we showed that PTHrP mRNA and protein are strongly expressed in osteoblastic cells throughout the bone-formation process, including in mature, actively synthetic osteoblasts (107).

The first evidence of a physiological role for PTHrP in chondrocyte biology was provided by the generation of mice missing the PTHrP gene using homologous recombination (75,112,113, 116). Neonatal mice homozygous for PTHrP gene ablation exhibit severe skeletal abnormalities at birth and die within 24 hours, most likely from respiratory failure as a consequence of widespread abnormalities of endochondral bone development. The PTHrP homozygous mutant mice had a distinct phenotype at birth, characterized by a domed skull, short snout and mandible, protruding tongue, and disproportionately short limbs, whereas their nonskeletal organs and tissues appeared normal. These abnormalities were evident throughout the endochondral skeleton (axial as well as appendicular), while in contrast, no abnormality was noted in skeletal structures that develop entirely by intramembranous ossification.

Microscopic examination of the growth plates of bones in the PTHrP($-/-$) mutant mice revealed a marked reduction in the height of the zones of resting and proliferating chondrocytes as a result of the decreased number of cell divisions, disorganization of the cartilage columns in the hypertrophic zone, and altered deposition of matrix molecules such as type II collagen (116). PTHrP thus proved to be necessary for normal proliferation of chondrocytes, and the untimely maturation of the skeleton was presumably a consequence of the reduced proliferation and accelerated differentiation/premature hypertrophy and apoptosis of chondrocytes within the growth plate. These findings have been substantiated by another recent study (101), in which transgenic mice overexpressing PTHrP in chondrocytes (by means of the mouse collagen type II promoter) were found to have a form of short-limbed dwarfism, where the rate of endochondral ossification is significantly delayed as a result of persistent chondrocyte proliferation and spatially and temporally abnormal chondrocyte hypertrophy. This form of chondrodysplasia mirrors the PTHrP-null phenotype, and the delay in endochondral ossification is initially so profound that mice are born with cartilaginous endochondral skeletons. However, by 7 weeks of age, this delay in chondrocyte differentiation and ossification has been largely corrected, leaving foreshortened and misshapen but histologically near-normal bones. It should be noted that, just as PTHrP and PTH1R localize to the growth plate region of long bones, so too does Indian hedgehog (IHH) (119,145). IHH belongs to the hedgehog family of genes, which also includes Sonic, Desert, Tiggy-winkle, and Echidna (146,147). These genes in *Drosophila* are involved in the regulation of segment polarity and in many organisms they regulate correct embryonic patterning during development (148). The studies by Lanske et al. (119) and Vortkamp et al. (145) show that PTHrP and PTH1R are downstream effectors of the IHH pathway, which regulates the correct spatial and temporal progression of chondrocyte differentiation that determines the rate and extent of long bone formation. In this instance, the role of PTHrP is proposed as a paracrine one, making use of PTH1R. A similar paracrine mechanism has been proposed for the skin, where it was shown that PTH1R is expressed in fibroblasts but not in keratinocytes (149).

Interestingly, the sequence of the chondrocyte maturation program and this ultimate histological healing are reminiscent of that seen in patients with Jansen's metaphyseal chondrodysplasia, a condition arising from constitutive activation of PTH1R (150–152), and in transgenic mice in which expression of a constitutively active PTH1R was targeted to the growth plate (153). In the latter study, targeted expression of constitutively active PTH1R corrected the growth plate abnormalities of PTHrP(−/−) mice at birth and allowed for their prolonged survival. These "rescued" animals lacked tooth eruption and showed premature epiphyseal closure, indicating the requirement of PTHrP in both processes. Therefore, overexpression of PTHrP or constitutive activation of PTH1R in the growth plate ultimately results in a similar pattern of abnormalities in endochondral bone formation.

Further investigations of PTHrP mutant mice provided evidence to suggest that PTHrP is equally important for the orderly commitment of precursor cells toward the osteogenic lineage and their subsequent maturation and/or function. Firstly, in PTHrP(−/−) mice, osteoblastic progenitor cells (as with chondrocytes) were observed to contain inappropriate accumulations of glycogen, which is indicative of a defect, metabolic or otherwise, in cells of the osteogenic lineage arising as a consequence of PTHrP deficiency (113). Secondly, heterozygous PTHrP(+/−) mice, while phenotypically normal at birth, by 3 months of age exhibited a form of osteopenia characterized by a marked decrease in trabecular thickness and connectivity (154). Moreover, their bone marrow contained an abnormally high number of adipocytes. Since the same pluripotent stromal cells in the bone marrow compartment can give rise to adipocytes and osteoprogenitor cells (155), the increased number of adipocytes and osteopenia in these mice could be attributed to altered stem cell differentiation as a consequence of PTHrP haploinsufficiency. Alternatively, alterations in the mechanism of programmed cell death, or apoptosis, which is known to be modulated by PTHrP (120), may also have important implications in the development of the osteopenic state in these animals. Future investigations with targeted ablation of *PTHrP* or *PTH1R* gene sequences, specifically in osteoblasts, will undoubtedly provide a better understanding of the role played by PTHrP in adult bone metabolism under physiological and pathological conditions.

NUCLEAR/NUCLEOLAR PARATHYROID HORMONE–RELATED PROTEIN, AN EXTRA DIMENSION TO PHYSIOLOGY

Although PTHrP was discovered as a hormone causing hypercalcemia by virtue of its excessive production by certain cancers, it became clear over the next few years that its physiological functions are manyfold and derive from its functioning as a cytokine in many tissues throughout development and in adulthood. As is the case with similar multifunctional cytokines, the effects of PTHrP vary depending on the tissue in which it is produced.

We have drawn attention to the evidence that PTHrP exerts actions mediated by portions of the molecule which do not require the participation of PTH1R, implying that other receptors and signaling pathways exist for these motifs within PTHrP. Taken together with the obvious susceptibility of PTHrP to posttranslational modification through proteolysis and the generation of several constituent peptides, this increases the complexities in understanding the paracrine role of PTHrP. This is even more so now, with the compelling evidence that PTHrP attains a nuclear/nucleolar location through a specific transport process and is likely to exert some of its functions from that site.

Henderson et al. (120) first noted the nucleolar localization of PTHrP in chondrocytes and concluded that this localization resulted in en-

hanced chondrocyte survival following prolonged periods of serum starvation. Deletion of the nucleolar localization motif within PTHrP prevented the molecule from entering the nucleus, maintaining it as a cytoplasmic protein. Nucleolar localization of PTHrP also increased smooth muscle cell proliferation (66). Studies in both smooth muscle cells (156) and keratinocytes (125) have shown that PTHrP expression is cell cycle–dependent, with the highest expression of PTHrP mRNA occurring in response to mitogenic factors only at the G_1 phase of the cell cycle, and that it is localized to the nucleolus at the G_1 phase (125).

We obtained evidence that phosphorylation of T^{85} in PTHrP by the cyclin-dependent kinases $p33^{cdk2}$ and $p34^{cdc2}$ resulted in exclusion of PTHrP from the nucleus. It is a known consequence of protein phosphorylation by these kinases that there is increased affinity for the cytoplasm of some molecules containing a nuclear localization signal. Within the PTHrP sequence, there are putative nucleus (CcN) and nucleolus localization motifs, with the former being similar to that described for the archetypal CcN-containing protein SV40 T antigen (Fig. 24.3), com-

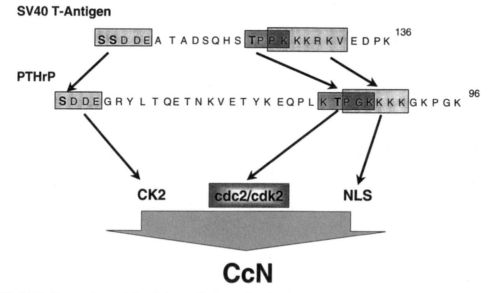

FIG. 24.3. Comparison of the CcN motif of parathyroid hormone–related protein *(PTHrP)* with that of SV40 T antigen. The CK2 (Ser) and CDC2/CDK2 (Thr) phosphorylation sites are *bold.* NLS, nuclear localization signal.

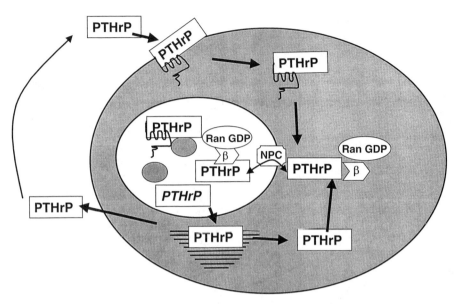

FIG. 24.4. Proposed trafficking pathways of parathyroid hormone–related protein *(PTHrP)* synthesis and action. PTHrP can be synthesized as a prepro molecule, targetted to the trans-Golgi network destined for secretion from the cell. Alternatively, PTHrP remains intracellular as a result of translation from an alternate translational initiation codon. As a consequence of intracellularly targetted PTHrP binding to importin *β,* PTHrP can attain a nuclear localization. Additionally, exogenous PTHrP can bind to the receptor PTH1R, be internalized, and escape degradation to localize to the nucleus and nucleolus. For exogenous PTHrP to be internalized and directed to the nucleus, the PTH1R binding region (amino acids 1–34) and the nuclear localization signal *(NLS,* amino acids 85–91) must be contiguous.

prising also consensus protein kinase CK2 and confirmed cyclin-dependent kinase phosphorylation sites (157,158).

This similarity in structure led to experiments showing specific import of PTHrP into the nucleus, brought about by binding to importin *β,* which together with the guanosine triphosphate–binding protein Ran was able to mediate efficient nuclear accumulation in the absence of importin *α,* whereas addition of nuclear transport factor-2 reduced transport. This novel nuclear import mechanism for PTHrP might arise as a result either of an intracrine pathway in a cell expressing PTHrP or in a target cell as a result of binding of PTHrP to PTH1R and internalization of the complex. We have evidence that each of these pathways can operate (159, 160) (Fig. 24.4).

PTHrP appears so far to be the only protein classed, at least in some circumstances, as a hormone which possesses a CcN motif and displays differential cellular localization (nuclear) nucleolar vs. cytoplasm). Most proteins that possess a CcN motif are of large molecular weight, usually greater than 45 kDa. The findings of the CcN motif, the redistribution within the cell as a result of phosphorylation of T^{85}, the resulting striking cell cycle dependence of PTHrP location, and the participation of PTHrP with importin *β* in a specific, regulated nuclear import process come together to indicate that PTHrP is likely to exert important functions from its nuclear site. In the many tissues in which PTHrP is considered to play a local role, including bone and cartilage, this possibility will need to be considered in further studies.

ACKNOWLEDGMENTS

Work from the authors' laboratory was supported by an National Health and Medical Research Council, Australia (NHMRC) program grant (963211), the Anti-Cancer Council of Victoria, and Chugai Pharmaceutical Company, Japan.

REFERENCES

1. Stewart AF, Horst L, Deftos LJ, et al. Biochemical evaluation of patients with cancer-associated hypercalcemia: evidence for humoral and nonhumoral groups. *N Engl J Med* 1980;303:1377–1383.
2. Kukreja SC, Rosol TJ, Wimbiscus SA, et al. Tumor resection and antibodies to parathyroid hormone–related protein cause similar changes on bone histomorphometry in hypercalcemia of cancer. *Endocrinology* 1990;127:305–310.
3. Suva LJ, Winslow GA, Wettenhall REH, et al. A parathyroid hormone–related protein implicated in malignant hypercalcemia: cloning and expression. *Science* 1987;237:893–896.
4. Mangin M, Webb AC, Dreyer BE, et al. Identification of a cDNA encoding a parathyroid hormone-like peptide from a human tumor associated with humoral hypercalcemia of malignancy. *Proc Natl Acad Sci USA* 1988;85:597–601.
5. Mangin M, Ikeda K, Dreyer BE, et al. Two distinct tumor-derived, parathyroid hormone-like peptides result from alternative ribonucleic acid splicing. *Mol Endocrinol* 1988;2:1049–1055.
6. Mangin M, Ikeda K, Dreyer BE, et al. Isolation and characterization of the human parathyroid hormone-like peptide gene. *Proc Natl Acad Sci USA* 1989;86: 2408–2412.
7. Thiede MA, Strewler GJ, Nissenson RA, et al. Human renal carcinoma expresses two messages encoding a parathyroid hormone-like peptide: evidence for the alternative splicing of a single-copy gene. *Proc Natl Acad Sci USA* 1988;85:4605–4609.
8. Moseley JM, Gillespie MT. Parathyroid hormone–related protein. *Crit Rev Clin Lab Sci* 1995;32:299–343.
9. Orloff JJ, Stewart AF. Parathyroid hormone–related protein as a prohormone: postranslational processing and receptor interactions: update 1995. *Endocr Rev* 1995;4:207–210.
10. Gillespie MT, Martin TJ. The parathyroid hormone–related protein gene and its expression. *Mol Cell Endocrinol* 1994;100:143–147.
11. Karaplis AC, Yasuda T, Hendy GN, et al. Gene-encoding parathyroid hormone-like peptide: nucleotide sequence of the rat gene and comparison with the human homologue. *Mol Endocrinol* 1990;4:441–446.
12. Mangin M, Ikeda K, Broadus AE. Structure of the mouse gene encoding parathyroid hormone–related peptide. *Gene* 1990;95:195–202.
13. Schermer DT, Chan SD, Bruce R, et al. Chicken parathyroid hormone–related protein and its expression during embryologic development. *J Bone Miner Res* 1991;6:149–155.
14. Yasuda T, Banville D, Rabbani SA, et al. Rat parathyroid hormone-like peptide: comparison with the human homologue and expression in malignant and normal tissue. *Mol Endocrinol* 1989;3:518–525.
15. Shaw G, Kamen R. A conserved AU sequence from the 3′ untranslated region of GM-CSF mRNA mediates selective mRNA degradation. *Cell* 1986;46:659–667.
16. Ikeda K, Lu C, Weir EC, et al. Regulation of parathyroid hormone–related peptide gene expression by cycloheximide. *J Biol Chem* 1990;265:5398–5402.
17. Habener JF, Rosenblatt M, Potts JT Jr. Parathyroid hormone: biochemical aspects of biosynthesis, secretion, action, and metabolism. *Physiol Rev* 1984;64: 985–1053.
18. Kemp BE, Moseley JM, Rodda CP, et al. Parathyroid hormone–related protein of malignancy: active synthetic fragments. *Science* 1987;238:1568–1570.
19. Jüppner H, Abou-Samra AB, Uneno S, et al. The parathyroid hormone-like peptide associated with humoral hypercalcemia of malignancy and parathyroid hormone bind to the same receptor on the plasma membrane of ROS 17/2.8 cells. *J Biol Chem* 1988;263: 8557–8560.
20. Orloff JJ, Wu TL, Stewart AF. Parathyroid hormone-like proteins: biochemical responses and receptor interactions. *Endocr Rev* 1989;10:476–495.
21. Rodda CP, Kubota M, Heath JA, et al. Evidence for a novel parathyroid hormone–related protein in fetal lamb parathyroid glands and sheep placenta: comparisons with a similar protein implicated in humoral hypercalcemia of malignancy. *J Endocrinol* 1988;117: 261–271.
22. Abbas SK, Pickard DW, Rodda CP, et al. Stimulation of ovine placental calcium transport by purified natural and recombinant parathyroid hormone–related protein (PTHrP) preparations. *O J Exp Physiol* 1989;74: 549–552.
23. Ellis AG, Adam WR, Martin TJ. Comparison of the effects of parathyroid hormone (PTH) and recombinant PTH-related protein on bicarbonate excretion by the isolated perfused rat kidney. *J Endocrinol* 1990;126: 403–408.
24. Fenton AJ, Kemp BE, Kent GN, et al. A carboxy-terminal fragment of parathyroid hormone–related protein inhibits bone resorption by osteoclasts. *Endocrinology* 1991;129:1762–1768.
25. Fenton AJ, Kemp BE, Hammonds RG Jr, et al. A potent inhibitor of osteoclastic bone resorption within a highly conserved pentapeptide region of parathyroid hormone–related protein; PTHrP[107–111]. *Endocrinology* 1991;129:3424–3426.
26. Cornish J, Callon KE, Nicholson GC, et al. Parathyroid hormone–related protein-(107–139) inhibits bone resorption *in vivo. Endocrinology* 1997;138:1299–1304.
27. Cornish J, Callon KE, Lin C, et al. Stimulation of osteoblast proliferation by C-terminal fragments of parathyroid hormone–related protein. *J Bone Miner Res* 1999;14:915–922.
28. Burtis WJ, Debeyssey M, Philbrick WM, et al. Evidence for the presence of an extreme carboxy-terminal parathyroid hormone–related peptide in biological specimens. *J Bone Miner Res* 1992;7:S225(abst).
29. Brandt DW, Bruns ME, Bruns DW, et al. PTH-like protein production in human amnion. *J Bone Miner Res* 1992;7:S236(abst).

30. Orloff JJ, Reddy D, De Papp AE, et al. Parathyroid hormone–related protein as a prohormone: posttranslational processing and receptor interactions. *Endocr Rev* 1994;15:40–60.

31. Hendy GN, Bennett HP, Gibbs BF, et al. Proparathyroid hormone is preferentially cleaved to parathyroid hormone by the prohormone convertase furin. A mass spectrometric study. *J Biol Chem* 1995;270:9517–9525.

32. Liu B, Goltzman D, Rabbani SA. Regulation of parathyroid hormone–related peptide production *in vitro* by the rat hypercalcemic Leydig cell tumor H-500. *Endocrinology* 1993;132:1658–1664.

33. Liu B, Amizuka N, Goltzman D, et al. Inhibition of processing of parathyroid hormone–related peptide by anti-sense furin: effect *in vitro* and *in vivo* on rat Leydig (H-500) tumor cells. *Int J Cancer* 1995;63:276–281.

34. Liu B, Goltzman D, Rabbani SA. Processing of pro-PTHrP by the prohormone convertase, furin: effect on biological activity. *Am J Physiol* 1995;268:E832–E838.

35. Lazure C, Gauthier D, Jean F, et al. *In vitro* cleavage of internally quenched fluorogenic human proparathyroid hormone and proparathyroid-related peptide substrates by furin. Generation of a potent inhibitor. *J Biol Chem* 1998;273:8572–8580.

36. Brandt DW, Burton DW, Gazdar AF, et al. All major lung cancer cell types produce parathyroid hormone-like protein: heterogeneity assessed by high performance liquid chromatography. *Endocrinology* 1991;129:2466–2470.

37. Rabbani SA, Haq M, Goltzman D. Biosynthesis and processing of endogenous parathyroid hormone–related peptide (PTHrP) by rat Leydig cell tumor H-500. *Biochemistry* 1993;32:4931–4937.

38. Soifer ND, Dee KE, Insogna KL, et al. Parathyroid hormone–related protein. Evidence for secretion of a novel mid-region fragment by three different cell types. *J Biol Chem* 1992;267:18236–18243.

39. Yang KH, DePapp AE, Soifer NE, et al. Parathyroid hormone–related protein: evidence for isoform- and tissue-specific posttranslational processing. *Biochemistry* 1994;33:7460–7469.

40. Wu TL, Vasavada RC, Yang K, et al. Structural and physiologic characterization of the mid-region secretory species of parathyroid hormone–related protein. *J Biol Chem* 1996;271:24371–24381.

41. Wu TL, Soifer NE, Burtis WJ, et al. Glycosylation of parathyroid hormone–related peptide secreted by human epidermal keratinocytes. *J Clin Endocrinol Metab* 1991;73:1002–1007.

42. Burtis WJ, Brady TG, Orloff JJ, et al. Immunochemical characterization of circulating parathyroid hormone–related protein in patients with humoral hypercalcemia of cancer. *N Engl J Med* 1990;322:1106–1112.

43. Deftos LJ, Burton DW, Brandt DW. Parathyroid hormone-like protein is a secretory product of atrial myocytes. *J Clin Invest* 1993;92:727–735.

44. Pilbeam CC, Alander CB, Simmons HA, et al. Comparison of the effects of various lengths of synthetic human parathyroid hormone–related peptide (hPTHrP) of malignancy on bone resorption and formation in organ culture. *Bone* 1993;14:717–720.

45. Kelly RB. Pathways of protein secretion in eukaryotes. *Science* 1985;230:25–32.

46. Plawner LL, Philbrick WM, Burtis WJ, et al. Cell type-specific secretion of parathyroid hormone–related protein via the regulated versus the constitutive secretory pathway. *J Biol Chem* 1995;270:14078–14084.

47. Philbrick WM, Wysolmerski JJ, Galbraith S, et al. Defining the roles of parathyroid hormone–related protein in normal physiology. *Physiol Rev* 1996;76:127–173.

48. Matsushita H, Usui M, Hara M, et al. Co-secretion of parathyroid hormone and parathyroid-hormone-related protein via a regulated pathway in human parathyroid adenoma cells. *Am J Pathol* 1997;150:861–871.

49. Stewart AF, Broadus AE. Clinical review 16: parathyroid hormone–related proteins: coming of age in the 1990s. *J Clin Endocrinol Metab* 1990;71:1410–1414.

50. Stewart AF, Broadus AE. Parathyroid hormone–related protein and humoral hypercalcemia of malignancy. In: Isselbacher KJ, Braunwald E, Wilson JD, et al. eds. *Harrison's principles of internal medicine (supplement 10)*. Chicago: McGraw-Hill, 1994:1–10.

51. Strewler GJ, Nissenson RA. Hypercalcemia in malignancy. *West J Med* 1990;153:635–640.

52. Bilezikian JP. Parathyroid hormone–related peptide in sickness and in health. *N Engl J Med* 1990;322:1151–1153.

53. Broadus AE, Stewart AF. Parathyroid hormone–related protein: structure, processing and physiological actions. In: Bilezikian JP, Levine MA, Marcus R, eds. *The parathyroids: basic and clinical concepts*. New York: Raven Press, 1993:259–294.

54. Burtis WJ, Fodero JP, Gaich G, et al. Preliminary characterization of circulating amino- and carboxy-terminal fragments of parathyroid hormone–related peptide in humoral hypercalcemia of malignancy. *J Clin Endocrinol Metab* 1992;75:1110–1114.

55. Orloff JJ, Soifer NE, Fodero JP, et al. Accumulation of carboxy-terminal fragments of parathyroid hormone–related protein in renal failure. *Kidney Int* 1993;43:1371–1376.

56. Kashahari H, Tsuchiya M, Adachii R. Development of a C-terminal-region specific radioimmunoassay of parathyroid hormone–related protein. *Biomed Res* 1992;13:155–161.

57. Dodwell DJ, Abbas SK, Morton AR, et al. Parathyroid hormone–related protein (50–69) and response to pamidronate therapy for tumor-induced hypercalcemia. *Eur J Cancer* 1991;27:1629–1633.

58. Imamura H, Sato K, Shizume K, et al. Urinary excretion of parathyroid hormone–related protein fragments in patients with humoral hypercalcemia of malignancy and hypercalcemic tumor-bearing nude mice. *J Bone Miner Res* 1991;6:77–84.

59. Grill V, Martin TJ. Hypercalcemia of malignancy. In: Grossman A, ed. *Clinical endocrinology* (2nd ed). Oxford: Blackwell Science, 1998:1018–1033.

60. Grill V, Rankin W, Martin TJ. Parathyroid hormone–related protein (PTHrP) and hypercalcemia. *Eur J Cancer* 1998;34:222–229.

61. Kaiser SM, Laneuville P, Bernier SM, et al. Enhanced growth of a human keratinocyte line by antisense RNA for PTHrP. *J Biol Chem* 1992;267:13623–13628.

62. Kaiser SM, Sebag M, Rhim JS, et al. Antisense-mediated inhibition of parathyroid hormone–related pep-

tide production in a keratinocyte cell line impedes differentiation. *Mol Endocrinol* 1994;8:139–147.

63. Pirola CJ, Wang HM, Kamyar A, et al. Angiotensin II regulates parathyroid hormone–related protein expression in cultured rat aortic smooth muscle cells through transcriptional and post-transcriptional mechanisms. *J Biol Chem* 1993;268:1987–1994.

64. Pirola CJ, Wang HM, Strgacich MI, et al. Mechanical stimuli induce vascular parathyroid hormone–related protein gene expression *in vivo* and *in vitro*. *Endocrinology* 1994;134:2230–2236.

65. Massfelder T, Helwig JJ, Stewart AF. Parathyroid hormone–related protein as a cardiovascular regulatory peptide. *Endocrinology* 1996;137:3151–3153.

66. Massfelder T, Dann P, Wu TL, et al. Opposing mitogenic and anti-mitogenic actions of parathyroid hormone–related protein in vascular smooth muscle cells: a critical role for nuclear targeting. *Proc Natl Acad Sci USA* 1997;94:13630–13635.

67. Mok LL, Ajiwe E, Martin TJ, et al. Parathyroid hormone–related protein relaxes rat gastric smooth muscle and shows cross-desensitization with parathyroid hormone. *J Bone Miner Res* 1989;4:433–439.

68. Winquist RJ, Baskin EP, Vlasuk GP. Synthetic tumor-derived human hypercalcemic factor exhibits parathyroid hormone-like vasorelaxation in renal arteries. *Biochem Biophys Res Commun* 1987;149:227–232.

69. Shew RL, Yee JA, Kliewer DB, et al. Parathyroid hormone–related protein inhibits stimulated uterine contraction *in vitro*. *J Bone Miner Res* 1991;6:955–959.

70. Crass MF III, Scarpace PJ. Vasoactive properties of a parathyroid hormone–related protein in the rat aorta. *Peptides* 1993;14:179–183.

71. Maeda S, Wu S, Jüeppner H, et al. Cell-specific signal transduction of parathyroid hormone (PTH)–related protein through stably expressed recombinant PTH/PTHrP receptors in vascular smooth muscle cells. *Endocrinology* 1996;137:3154–3162.

72. Massfelder T, Fiaschi-Taesch N, Stewart AF, et al. Parathyroid hormone–related peptide-A smooth muscle tone and proliferation regulatory protein. *Curr Opin Nephrol Hypertens* 1998;7:27–32.

73. Burton PB, Moniz C, Quirke P, et al. Parathyroid hormone–related peptide: expression in fetal and neonatal development. *J Pathol* 1992;167:291–296.

74. Ogino K, Burkhoff D, Bilezikian JP. The hemodynamic basis for the cardiac effects of parathyroid hormone (PTH) and PTH-related protein. *Endocrinology* 1995;136:3024–3030.

75. Karaplis AC, Luz A, Glowacki J, et al. Lethal skeletal dysplasia from targeted disruption of the parathyroid hormone–related peptide gene. *Genes Dev* 1994;8:277–289.

76. Thiede MA, Daifotis AG, Weir EC, et al. Intrauterine occupancy controls expression of the parathyroid hormone–related peptide gene in preterm rat myometrium. *Proc Natl Acad Sci USA* 1990;87:6969–6973.

77. Daifotis AG, Weir EC, Dreyer BE, et al. Stretch-induced parathyroid hormone–related peptide gene expression in the rat uterus. *J Biol Chem* 1992;267:23455–23458.

78. Paspaliaris V, Vargas SJ, Gillespie MT, et al. Oestrogen enhancement of the myometrial response to exogenous parathyroid hormone–related protein (PTHrP), and tissue localization of endogenous PTHrP and its

mRNA in the virgin rat uterus. *J Endocrinol* 1992;134:415–425.

79. Thiede MA, Harm SC, Hasson D, et al. *In vivo* regulation of parathyroid hormone–related peptide messenger ribonucleic acid in the rat uterus by 17 beta-estradiol. *Endocrinology* 1991;128:2317–2323.

80. Germain AM, Attaroglu H, MacDonald PC, et al. Parathyroid hormone–related protein mRNA in avascular human amnion. *J Clin Endocrinol Metab* 1992;75:1173–1175.

81. Ferguson JE, Gorman JV, Bruns DE, et al. Abundant expression of parathyroid hormone–related protein in human amnion and its association with labor. *Proc Natl Acad Sci USA* 1992;89:8384–8388.

82. Thiede MA, Harm SC, McKee RL, et al. Expression of the parathyroid hormone–related protein gene in the avian oviduct: potential role as a local modulator of vascular smooth muscle tension and shell gland motility during the egg-laying cycle. *Endocrinology* 1991;129:1958–1966.

83. Loveridge N, Caple IW, Rodda C, et al. Further evidence for a parathyroid hormone–related protein in fetal parathyroid glands of sheep. *Q J Exp Physiol* 1988;73:781–784.

84. Abbas SK, Pickard DW, Rodda CP, et al. Measurement of parathyroid hormone–related protein in extracts of fetal parathyroid glands and placental membranes. *J Endocrinol* 1990;124:319–325.

85. MacIsaac RJ, Heath JA, Rodda CP, et al. Role of the fetal parathyroid glands and parathyroid hormone–related protein in the regulation of placental transport of calcium, magnesium and inorganic phosphate. *Reprod Fertil Dev* 1991;3:447–457.

86. Care AD, Abbas SK, Pickard DW, et al. Stimulation of ovine placental transport of calcium and magnesium by mid-molecule fragments of human parathyroid hormone–related protein. *Exp Physiol* 1990;75:605–608.

87. Kovacs CS, Chik CL. Hyperprolactinemia caused by lactation and pituitary adenomas is associated with altered serum calcium, phosphate, parathyroid hormone (PTH), and PTH-related peptide levels. *J Clin Endocrinol Metab* 1995;80:3036–3042.

88. Rakopoulos M, Vargas SJ, Gillespie MT, et al. Production of parathyroid hormone–related protein by the rat mammary gland in pregnancy and lactation. *Am J Physiol* 1992;263:E1077–E1085.

89. Thiede MA, Rodan GA. Expression of a calcium-mobilizing parathyroid hormone-like peptide in lactating mammary tissue. *Science* 1988;242:278–280.

90. Budayr AA, Halloran BP, King JC, et al. High levels of a parathyroid hormone-like protein in milk. *Proc Natl Acad Sci USA* 1989;86:7183–7185.

91. Law FM, Moate PJ, Leaver DD, et al. Parathyroid hormone–related protein in milk and its correlation with bovine milk calcium. *J Endocrinol* 1991;128:21–26.

92. Ratcliffe WA, Thompson GE, Care AD, et al. Production of parathyroid hormone–related protein by the mammary gland of the goat. *J Endocrinol* 1992;133:87–93.

93. Grill V, Hillary J, Ho PM. Parathyroid hormone–related protein: a possible endocrine function in lactation. *Clin Endocrinol (Oxf)* 1992;37:405–410.

94. Dobnig H, Kainer F, Stepan V, et al. Elevated parathyroid hormone–related peptide levels after human gestation: relationship to changes in bone and mineral me-

tabolism. *J Clin Endocrinol Metab* 1995;80:3699–3707.

95. Yamamoto M, Duong LT, Fisher JE, et al. Suckling-mediated increases in urinary phosphate and 3',5'-cyclic adenosine monophosphate excretion in lactating rats: possible systemic effects of parathyroid hormone–related protein. *Endocrinology* 1991;129:2614–2622.

96. Kent GN, Price RI, Gutteridge DH, et al. Human lactation: forearm trabecular bone loss, increased bone turnover, and renal conservation of calcium and inorganic phosphate with recovery of bone mass following weaning. *J Bone Miner Res* 1990;5:361–369.

97. Ferrari SL, Rizzoli R, Bonjour JP. Parathyroid hormone–related protein production by primary cultures of mammary epithelial cells. *J Cell Physiol* 1992;150:304–311.

98. Seitz PK, Cooper KM, Ives KL, et al. Parathyroid hormone–related peptide production and action in a myoepithelial cell line derived from normal human breast. *Endocrinology* 1993;133:1116–1124.

99. Grone A, Werkmeister JR, Steinmeyer CL, et al. Parathyroid hormone–related protein in normal and neoplastic canine tissues: immunohistochemical localization and biochemical extraction. *Vet Pathol* 1994;31:308–315.

100. Sebag M, Henderson J, Goltzman D, et al. Regulation of parathyroid hormone–related peptide production in normal human mammary epithelial cells *in vitro*. *Am J Physiol* 1994;267:C723–C730.

101. Weir EC, Philbrick WM, Amling M, et al. Targeted overexpression of parathyroid hormone–related peptide in chondrocytes causes chondrodysplasia and delayed endochondral bone formation. *Proc Natl Acad Sci USA* 1996;93:10240–10245.

102. Wysolmerski JJ, McCaughern-Carucci JF, Daifotis AG, et al. Overexpression of parathyroid hormone–related protein or parathyroid hormone in transgenic mice impairs branching morphogenesis during mammary gland development. *Development* 1995;121:3539–3547.

103. Van De Stolpe A, Karperien M, Löwik CW, et al. Parathyroid hormone–related peptide as an endogenous inducer of parietal endoderm differentiation. *J Cell Biol* 1993;120:235–243.

104. Senior PV, Heath DA, Beck F. Expression of parathyroid hormone–related protein mRNA in the rat before birth: demonstration by hybridization histochemistry. *J Mol Endocrinol* 1991;6:281–290.

105. Dunne FP, Ratcliffe WA, Mansour P, et al. Parathyroid hormone related protein (PTHrP) gene expression in fetal and extra-embryonic tissues of early pregnancy. *Hum Reprod* 1994;9:149–156.

106. Moseley JM, Hayman JA, Danks JA, et al. Immunohistochemical detection of parathyroid hormone–related protein in human fetal epithelia. *J Clin Endocrinol Metab* 1991;73:478–484.

107. Kartsogiannis V, Moseley JM, McKelvie B, et al. Temporal expression of PTHrP during endochondral bone formation in mouse and intramembranous bone formation in an *in vivo* rabbit model. *Bone* 1997;21:385–392.

108. Campos RV, Asa SL, Drucker DJ. Immunocytochemical localization of parathyroid hormone-like peptide in the rat fetus. *Cancer Res* 1991;51:6351–6357.

109. Lee K, Deeds JD, Segre GV. Expression of parathyroid hormone–related peptide and its receptor messenger ribonucleic acids during fetal development of rats. *Endocrinology* 1995;136:453–463.

110. Moniz C, Burton PB, Malik AN, et al. Parathyroid hormone–related peptide in normal human fetal development. *J Mol Endocrinol* 1990;5:259–266.

111. Karperien M, van Dijk TB, Hoeijmakers T, et al. Expression pattern of parathyroid hormone/parathyroid hormone related peptide receptor mRNA in mouse postimplantation embryos indicates involvement in multiple developmental processes. *Mech Dev* 1994;47:29–42.

112. Lee K, Lanske B, Karaplis AC, et al. Parathyroid hormone–related peptide delays terminal differentiation of chondrocytes during endochondral bone development. *Endocrinology* 1996;137:5109–5118.

113. Amizuka N, Warshawsky H, Henderson JE, et al. Parathyroid hormone–related peptide–depleted mice show abnormal epiphyseal cartilage development and altered endochondral bone formation. *J Cell Biol* 1994;126:1611–1623.

114. Amizuka N, Warshawsky H, Karaplis AC, et al. Localization of gene expression of PTHrP and of the PTH/PTHrP receptor in normal adult bone tissues: consequences for bone formation in PTHrP-deficient animals. *J Bone Miner Res* 1994;9:S128.

115. Wysolmerski JJ, Broadus AE, Zhou J, et al. Overexpression of parathyroid hormone–related protein in the skin of transgenic mice interferes with hair follicle development. *Proc Natl Acad Sci USA* 1994;91:1133–1137.

116. Karaplis AC, Kronenberg HM. Physiological roles for parathyroid hormone–related protein: lessons from gene knockout mice. *Vitam Horm* 1996;52:177–193.

117. Holick MF, Ray S, Chen TC, et al. A parathyroid hormone antagonist stimulates epidermal proliferation and hair growth in mice. *Proc Natl Acad Sci USA* 1994;91:8014–8016.

118. Lanske B, Karaplis AC, Luz A, et al. Characterization of mice homozygous for the PTH/PTHrP receptor gene null mutation. *J Bone Miner Res* 1994;9:S121.

119. Lanske B, Karaplis AC, Lee K, et al. PTH/PTHrP receptor in early development and Indian hedgehog–regulated bone growth. *Science* 1996;273:663–666.

120. Henderson JE, Amizuka N, Warshawsky H, et al. Nucleolar localization of parathyroid hormone–related peptide enhances survival of chondrocytes under conditions that promote apoptotic cell death. *Mol Cell Biol* 1995;15:4064–4075.

121. Dang CV, Lee WM. Nuclear and nucleolar targeting sequences of c-erb-A, c-myb, N-myc, p53, HSP70, and HIV tat proteins. *J Biol Chem* 1989;264:18019–18023.

122. Cochrane AW, Perkins A, Rosen CA. Identification of sequences important in the nucleolar localization of human immunodeficiency virus Rev: relevance of nucleolar localization to function. *J Virol* 1990;64:881–885.

123. Siomi H, Shida H, Nam SH, et al. Sequence requirements for nucleolar localization of human T cell leukemia virus type I pX protein, which regulates viral RNA processing. *Cell* 1988;55:197–209.

124. Nguyen MT, Karaplis AC. The nucleus: a target site for parathyroid hormone–related peptide (PTHrP) action. *J Cell Biochem* 1998;70:193–199.

125. Lam MHC, Olsen SL, Rankin WA, et al. PTHrP and

cell division: expression and localization of PTHrP in a keratinocyte cell line (HacaT) during the cell cycle. *J Cell Physiol* 1997;173:433–446.

126. Amizuka N, Henderson JE, Hoshi K, et al. Programmed cell death of chondrocytes and aberrant chondrogenesis in mice homozygous for parathyroid hormone–related peptide gene deletion. *Endocrinology* 1996;137:5055–5067.

127. Amling M, Neff L, Tanaka S, et al. Bcl-2 lies downstream of parathyroid hormone–related peptide in a signaling pathway that regulates chondrocyte maturation during skeletal development. *J Cell Biol* 1997;136: 205–213.

128. Stewart AF, Vignery A, Silverglate A, et al. Quantitative bone histomorphometry in humoral hypercalcemia of malignancy: uncoupling of bone cell activity. *J Clin Endocrinol Metab* 1982;55:219–227.

129. Stewart AF, Insogna KL, Broadus AE. Malignancy-associated hypercalcemia. In: De Groot LJ, ed. *Endocrinology* (3rd ed). Philadelphia: Saunders, 1995: 1061–1074.

130. Martin TJ, Suva LJ. Parathyroid hormone–related protein in hypercalcemia of malignancy. *Clin Endocrinol (Oxf)* 1989;31:631–647.

131. Stewart AF. Humoral hypercalcemia of malignancy. In: Favus M, ed. *Primer on the metabolic bone diseases and disorders of mineral metabolism.* New York: Lippincott-Raven Press, 1993:169–173.

132. Reeve J. PTH: a future role in the management of osteoporosis? *J Bone Miner Res* 1996;11:440–445.

133. Weir EC, Terwilliger G, Sartori L, et al. Synthetic parathyroid hormone-like protein (1–74) is anabolic for bone *in vivo. Calcif Tissue Int* 1992;51:30–34.

134. Everhart-Caye M, Inzucchi SE, Guinness-Henry J, et al. Parathyroid hormone (PTH)–related protein (1–36) is equipotent to PTH(1–34) in humans. *J Clin Endocrinol Metab* 1996;81:199–208.

135. Hock JM, Fonseca J, Gunness-Hey M, et al. Comparison of the anabolic effects of synthetic parathyroid hormone–related protein (PTHrP) 1–34 and PTH 1–34 on bone in rats. *Endocrinology* 1989;125:2022–2027.

136. Fraher LJ, Klein K, Marier R. Comparison of the pharmacokinetics of parenteral parathyroid hormone-(1–34) [PTH-(1–34)] and PTH-related peptide-(1–34) in healthy young humans. *J Clin Endocrinol Metab* 1995;80:60–64.

137. Rihani-Bisharat S, Maor G, Lewinson D. *In vivo* anabolic effects of parathyroid hormone (PTH) 28–48 and N-terminal fragments of PTH and PTH-related protein on neonatal mouse bones. *Endocrinology* 1998;139: 974–981.

138. Karmali R, Schiffmann SN, Vanderwinden J, et al. Expression of mRNA of parathyroid hormone–related peptide in fetal bones of the rat. *Cell Tissue Res* 1992; 270:597–600.

139. Tsukazaki T, Ohtsuru A, Enomoto H, et al. Expression of parathyroid hormone–related protein in rat articular cartilage. *Calcif Tissue Int* 1995;57:196–200.

140. Nijs-de Wolf N, Pepersack T, Corvilain J, et al. Adenylate cyclase stimulating activity immunologically similar to parathyroid hormone–related peptide can be extracted from fetal rat long bones. *J Bone Miner Res* 1991;6:921–927.

141. Rodan SB, Wesolowski G, Ianacone J, et al. Production of parathyroid hormone-like peptide in a human osteo-

142. Suda N, Gillespie MT, Traianedes K, et al. Expression of parathyroid hormone–related protein in cells of osteoblast lineage. *J Cell Physiol* 1996;166:94–104.

143. Walsh CA, Birch MA, Fraser WD, et al. Expression and secretion of parathyroid hormone–related protein by human bone-derived cells *in vitro:* effects of glucocorticoids. *J Bone Miner Res* 1995;10:17–25.

144. Guenther HL, Hofstetter W, Moseley JM, et al. Evidence for the synthesis of parathyroid hormone–related protein (PTHrP) by nontransformed clonal rat osteoblastic cells *in vitro. Bone* 1995;16:341–347.

145. Vortkamp A, Lee K, Lanske B, et al. Regulation of rate of cartilage differentiation by Indian hedgehog and PTH-related protein. *Science* 1996;273:613–622.

146. Marigo V, Davey RA, Zuo Y, et al. Biochemical evidence that patched is the Hedgehog receptor. *Nature* 1996;384:176–179.

147. van den Heuvel M, Ingham PW. Smoothened encodes a receptor-like serpentine protein required for hedgehog signalling. *Nature* 1996;382:547–551.

148. Goodrich LV, Johnson RL, Milenkovic L, et al. Conservation of the hedgehog/patched signaling pathway from flies to mice: induction of a mouse patched gene by hedgehog. *Genes Dev* 1996;10:301–312.

149. Hanafin NM, Chen TC, Heinrich G, et al. Cultured human fibroblasts and not cultured human keratinocytes express a PTH/PTHrP receptor mRNA. *J Invest Dermatol* 1995;105:133–137.

150. Schipani E, Kruse K, Jüeppner H. A constitutively active mutant PTH-PTHrP receptor in Jansen-type metaphyseal chondrodysplasia. *Science* 1995;268:98–100.

151. Schipani E, Langman CB, Parfitt A, et al. Constitutively activated receptors for parathyroid hormone and parathyroid hormone–related peptide in Jansen's metaphyseal chondrodysplasia. *N Engl J Med* 1996;335: 708–714.

152. Schipani E, Jensen GS, Pincus J, et al. Constitutive activation of the cyclic adenosine 3′,5′-monophosphate signaling pathway by parathyroid hormone (PTH)/ PTH-related peptide receptors mutated at the two loci for Jansen's metaphyseal chondrodysplasia. *Mol Endocrinol* 1997;11:851–858.

153. Schipani E, Lanske B, Hunzelman J, et al. Targeted expression of constitutively active receptors for parathyroid hormone and parathyroid hormone–related peptide delays endochondral bone formation and rescues mice that lack parathyroid hormone–related peptide. *Proc Natl Acad Sci USA* 1997;94:13689–13694.

154. Amizuka N, Karaplis AC, Henderson JE, et al. Haploinsufficiency of parathyroid hormone–related peptide (PTHrP) results in abnormal postnatal bone development. *Dev Biol* 1996;175:166–176.

155. Owen M, Friedenstein AJ. Stromal stem cells: marrow-derived osteogenic precursors. *Ciba Found Symp* 1988; 136:42–60.

156. Okano K, Pirola CJ, Wang HM, et al. Involvement of cell cycle and mitogen-activated pathways in induction of parathyroid hormone–related protein gene expression in rat aortic smooth muscle cells. *Endocrinology* 1995;136:1782–1789.

157. Jans DA, Ackerman MJ, Bischoff JR, et al. p34cdc2-

mediated phosphorylation at T124 inhibits nuclear import of SV-40 T antigen proteins. *J Cell Biol* 1991; 115:1203–1212.

158. Jans DA. The regulation of protein transport to the nucleus by phosphorylation. *Biochem J* 1995;311: 705–716.

159. Lam MHC, Briggs LJ, Hu W, et al. Importin β recognizes parathyroid hormone–related protein (PTHrP)

with high affinity and mediates its nuclear import in the absence of importin α. *J Biol Chem* 1999;274: 7391–7398.

160. Lam MHC, House CM, Tiganis T, et al. Phosphorylation at the cyclin dependent kinases p34^{cdc2} and p33^{cdc2} site (Thr^{65}) of parathyroid hormone–related protein (PTHrP) negatively regulates its nuclear localization. *J Biol Chem* 1999;274:18559–18566.

Skeletal Growth Factors,
edited by Ernesto Canalis.
Lippincott Williams & Wilkins, Philadelphia, © 2000.

25

Role of Parathyroid Hormone–related Protein and Indian Hedgehog in Skeletal Development

Ung-il Chung and Henry M. Kronenberg

Endocrine Unit, Massachusetts General Hospital, Boston, Massachusetts 02114

ENDOCHONDRAL BONE FORMATION

The bones of the developing limb form through the process of endochondral bone formation (1–3) (Fig. 25.1). This process is characterized by replacement of a cartilage mold by bone. First, undifferentiated mesenchymal cells condense and form a model of the future skeleton; cells in the core of these condensations differentiate into chondrocytes that produce a characteristic matrix and spindle-shaped cells at the periphery that differentiate into the perichondrium. Then, chondrocytes in the central portion stop proliferating, further differentiate into prehypertrophic and then hypertrophic chondrocytes, induce mineralization of the surrounding matrix, and undergo apoptosis. Concomitantly, perichondrial cells near prehypertrophic and hypertrophic chondrocytes become osteoblasts and form a bone collar; this bone collar is the precursor of cortical bone. Subsequently, blood vessels invade the mineralized cartilage and, in association with vascular invasion, osteoblasts, and hematopoietic cells, replace the mineralized cartilage with bone and bone marrow. The mineralized cartilaginous matrix provides a scaffold for the organization of osteoblasts. The remaining chondrocytes at both ends of bone continue to divide, then hypertrophy, mineralize matrix, and die, thus forming the growth plates that contribute to longitudinal growth of bone.

Thus, differentiation and proliferation of various types of cell must be temporally and spatially coordinated for normal bone growth. Parathyroid hormone–related protein (PTHrP), its receptor, the PTH/PTHrP receptor, and Indian hedgehog (Ihh) participate in this coordination.

PARATHYROID HORMONE–RELATED PROTEIN AND THE GROWTH PLATE

Ablation of the Parathyroid Hormone–related Protein and the Parathyroid Hormone/Parathyroid Hormone–related Protein Receptor Genes

PTHrP was first identified as a factor with PTH-like activity responsible for humoral hypercalcemia of malignancy, a common paraneoplastic syndrome (4–7). The amino-terminal sequence of PTHrP is highly homologous to that of PTH, perhaps because the genes for both molecules derived from a common precursor gene by chromosomal duplication. While PTH is synthesized and secreted almost exclusively by the parathyroid gland and regulates calcium homeostasis as an endocrine factor, PTHrP is synthesized in a wide variety of tissues and usually functions as a paracrine/autocrine factor. Like PTH, PTHrP binds to the PTH/PTHrP receptor and activates both adenylate cyclase and phospholipase C (8,9). In many nonskeletal tissues, such as the mammary gland, the lung, and the tooth bud, PTHrP is expressed principally in the

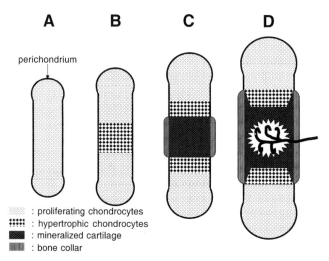

FIG. 25.1. Fetal endochondral bone development. **A:** Formation of a cartilage mold by mesenchymal condensations and differentiation of mesenchymal cells into chondrocytes and perichondrium. **B:** Differentiation of chondrocytes, first in the central region (hypertrophy). **C:** Appearance of a periosteal bone collar and mineralization of cartilaginous matrix surrounding hypertrophic chondrocytes. **D:** Vascular invasion of mineralized cartilage and replacement of cartilage by bone and bone marrow.

epithelium whereas the PTH/PTHrP receptor is expressed in adjacent mesenchymal tissues; PTHrP signaling is suggested to play an important role in epithelial–mesenchymal interactions (10–14).

In the growth plate, PTHrP is synthesized by perichondrial cells and proliferating chondrocytes in the periarticular region (15), and PTH/PTHrP receptor mRNA is expressed in growth plate chondrocytes, modestly in proliferating chondrocytes, and at high levels in prehypertrophic chondrocytes (16). This relationship of ligand and receptor expression suggested that PTHrP might function as a paracrine factor in the growth plate.

Ablation of the *PTHrP* gene through homologous recombination in embryonic stem cells (gene "knockout") and subsequent generation of mice missing both copies of the *PTHrP* gene established the essential role of PTHrP signaling in endochondral bone development. Mice missing both copies of the *PTHrP* gene died shortly after birth and showed striking abnormalities of endochondral bone development (17). Chondrocytes in the growth plates of these mice differentiated prematurely and in a poorly coordinated

manner, yielding a short proliferating layer in association with accelerated cartilage and bone mineralization (11,18) (Fig. 25.2). Mice missing both copies of the *PTH/PTHrP receptor* gene were smaller than wild-type or *PTHrP*(−/−) mice, even before bones were formed, and died early in gestation in some genetic backgrounds. In other backgrounds, however, the *PTH/PTHrP receptor*(−/−) mice, though still small, lived throughout gestation and thus allowed assessment of endochondral bone formation (19). These mice exhibited abnormalities in growth plate chondrocytes strongly resembling those of the *PTHrP*(−/−) mice, including poorly coordinated, accelerated differentiation of chondrocytes (Fig. 25.2). Humans with Blomstrand chondrodysplasia have mutant *PTH/PTHrP receptor* genes and die before birth with a bone disorder that resembles that of the *PTH/PTHrP receptor*(−/−) mice (20,21). The similarity of the *PTHrP*(−/−) and the *PTH/PTHrP receptor*(−/−) mice phenotypes suggests that, in the growth plate, PTHrP acts through the PTH/PTHrP receptor to slow the pace and increase the coordination of differentiation of growth plate chondrocytes.

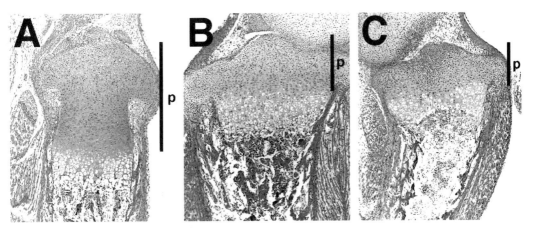

FIG. 25.2. Microscopic sections of tibiae from wild-type **(A)**, PTHrP($-/-$) **(B)**, and PTH/PTHrP receptor($-/-$) **(C)** embryos at embryonic day 17.5. Note the dramatic shortening of the layer of proliferating chondrocytes in PTHrP($-/-$) and PTH/PTHrP receptor($-/-$) growth plates. Sections were stained with hematoxylin–eosin. *p,* length of the proliferating layer. PTH, parathyroid hormone; PTHrP, PTH-related protein.

Effects of Increased Activation of the Parathyroid Hormone/Parathyroid Hormone–related Protein Receptor

Increased PTHrP signaling results in abnormalities of the growth plate opposite to those of gene ablation. Patients with activating mutations in the *PTH/PTHrP receptor* gene have a metaphyseal chondrodysplasia (Jansen type) due to abnormal chondrocyte differentiation (22). Studies of transgenic mice overexpressing PTHrP in the chondrocytes using the α1(II) collagen promoter demonstrate that excess activation of PTHrP signaling slows the differentiation of growth plate chondrocytes *in vivo* (23). Transgenic expression of a constitutively active PTH/PTHrP receptor found in patients with Jansen-type metaphyseal chondrodysplasia led to an analogous slowing of differentiation of growth plate chondrocytes in mice (24). These studies showed that inappropriate activation of the PTH/PTHrP receptor delayed both the transition from chondrocyte proliferation to hypertrophy and the apoptotic death of hypertrophic chondrocytes.

Further, in a mouse limb explant system, treatment with PTHrP(1–34) delayed the differentiation of wild-type growth plate chondrocytes and reversed accelerated differentiation of *PTHrP*($-/-$) chondrocytes but did not affect accelerated differentiation of *PTH/PTHrP receptor*($-/-$) chondrocytes (19,25). These *in vitro* experiments support the idea that in the growth plate PTHrP acts directly on chondrocytes and confirm that these actions are mediated by the PTH/PTHrP receptor. Moreover, they emphasize either both too little or too much PTHrP action leads to abnormal differentiation of growth plate chondrocytes.

Rescue and Chimeric Analysis

Although the data obtained from the conventional gene ablation technique are very useful, they have several limitations. First, mice generated by this technique lack the *PTHrP* gene or the *PTH/PTHrP receptor* gene in all cells. Thus, it is possible that the phenotypes seen in the growth plates of these mice might be influenced by the gene ablation in some other tissues. Second, the specific target cell of PTHrP signaling is not defined. Proliferating chondrocytes, the cells most affected in *PTHrP*($-/-$) or *PTH/PTHrP receptor*($-/-$) mice, synthesize little PTH/PTHrP receptor mRNA, whereas more differentiated prehypertrophic chondrocytes, which are little affected morphologically, express large amounts of PTH/PTHrP receptor mRNA. This expression pattern suggests that PTHrP may use a complicated pathway to regulate chondrocyte differentiation: PTHrP may act directly on prehypertrophic cells, which then secrete a factor that slows the differentiation of proliferating chondrocytes. Ablation of the PTH/PTHrP receptor from all chondrocytes, however, does not allow definition of the relevant target cell. Third, early lethality of $PTHrP(-/-)$ and especially $PTH/PTHrP$ $receptor(-/-)$ mice precludes detailed study of the postnatal functions of PTHrP signaling.

To overcome these problems, so far two strategies have been successfully employed. The first strategy is to overexpress the PTHrP transgene or the constitutively active PTH/PTHrP receptor transgene in the $PTHrP(-/-)$ growth plate under the control of the $\alpha 1(II)$ collagen promoter (12,24). Accelerated differentiation of growth plate chondrocytes in these mice was reversed, and they lived beyond the perinatal period. These data demonstrate that the perinatal lethality of the $PTHrP(-/-)$ mice results from abnormal skeletal development. Since the expression of the transgene only in chondrocytes reversed the growth plate defects in $PTHrP(-/-)$ mice, it follows that effects of the gene knockout in other tissues are not required for the abnormal differentiation of chondrocytes in $PTHrP(-/-)$ mice. The survival of these rescued mice opens opportunities to study postnatal roles of PTHrP signaling in nonskeletal tissues. The second strategy is to generate chimeric mice containing both wild-type and $PTH/PTHrP$ $receptor(-/-)$ cells (26). Embryonic stem cell lines were established from early $PTH/PTHrP$ $receptor(-/-)$ embryos (blastocysts). These cells were marked with a β-galactosidase transgene to allow their detection in chimeric mice. The mutant embryonic stem cells were then introduced into wild-type blastocysts; the resultant mice were chimeras with organs populated by cells of both wild-type and $PTH/PTHrP$ $receptor(-/-)$ genotypes. This technique thus allows the examination of cell–cell interactions between cells of different genotypes in an *in vivo* setting. The

chimeric growth plates provided a way to define the direct cellular target of PTHrP. If PTHrP primarily acts on prehypertrophic chondrocytes, which then secrete a factor that slows differentiation of proliferating chondrocytes, the wild-type prehypertrophic chondrocytes in the chimeric growth plate should be able to reverse the accelerated differentiation of *PTH/PTHrP receptor*$(-/-)$ chondrocytes in the chimeric growth plate. The actual result was quite different: *PTH/PTHrP receptor*$(-/-)$ chondrocytes differentiated rapidly even when greatly outnumbered by wild-type chondrocytes in the proliferating layer (Fig. 25.3). Since the absence of the PTH/PTHrP receptors from proliferating chondrocytes makes them ignore all other signals and differentiate quickly, PTHrP must normally act directly on these cells to slow differentiation.

INDIAN HEDGEHOG AND THE GROWTH PLATE

The Hedgehog Family of Genes

Indian hedgehog (Ihh) is one of the vertebrate homologues of the *Drosophila* segment polarity gene, *hedgehog (hh)* (27–29). In *Drosophila*, *hh* plays an essential role in the early differentiation within segments, as well as multiple roles in later processes such as differentiation of appendages and of the retina (30,31). Hh protein exerts its effect by binding to its cell surface receptor, Patched (Ptc) (32,33). Ptc forms a functional heterodimer with another membrane protein, Smoothened (Smo) (34–36). Ptc is an inhibitor of the activity of Smo; Hh binding to Ptc releases this inhibition. Smo activity triggers a cascade that leads to the activation of the transcription factor Cubitus interruptus (Ci) (37–39). Activated Ci upregulates the transcription of the *hh* target genes such as *wingless (wg), ptc,* and *decapentaplegic (dpp)* (Fig. 25.4).

Effects of Signaling on Bone Development

While only one *hh* gene has been identified in *Drosophila,* several *hh* genes have been found in vertebrates. One of them, *Ihh,* is strongly ex-

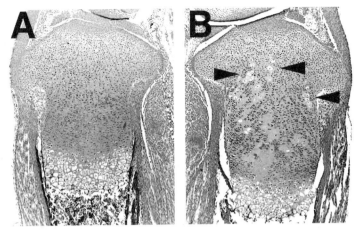

FIG. 25.3. Microscopic sections of tibiae from wild-type embryo **(A)** and chimeric embryo containing both wild-type and PTH/PTHrP receptor(−/−) cells **(B)** at embryonic day 17.5. PTH/PTHrP receptor(−/−) cells prematurely differentiate into hypertrophic chondrocytes in the middle of the layers of wild-type proliferating chondrocytes *(arrowheads)*. Sections were stained with hematoxylin–eosin. PTH, parathyroid hormone; PTHrP, PTH-related protein.

pressed in prehypertrophic and hypertrophic chondrocytes of the mouse embryo (40). Overexpression of Ihh protein through injection of a recombinant retrovirus into embryonic chicken

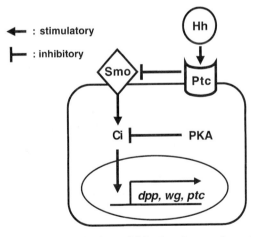

FIG. 25.4. Hedgehog (Hh) signaling pathway. Activity of Smoothened *(Smo)* is inhibited by Patched *(Ptc)*. When Hh binds to Ptc, this inhibition is released and Smo starts a cascade that activates the downstream transcription factor Cubitus interruptus *(Ci)*. Activated Ci then stimulates the expression of *hh* target genes such as *decapentaplegic (dpp)*, *wingless (wg)*, and *ptc*. Activity of Ci is blocked by protein kinase A *(PKA)*.

limbs delayed differentiation of growth plate chondrocytes. The phenotype resembled that of PTHrP overexpression (25). Mice missing both copies of the *Ihh* gene had extremely short limbs and died right after birth (B. St-Jacques, M. Hammerschmidt, and A.P. McMahon, manuscript in preparation). The proliferation of chondrocytes was severely reduced in these mice, an abnormality much greater than that found in *PTHrP*(−/−) or *PTH/PTHrP receptor*(−/−) mice. As predicted from the Ihh overexpression experiment, hypertrophic chondrocytes predominate in the *Ihh*(−/−) limbs late in fetal development.

INTERACTIONS BETWEEN PARATHYROID HORMONE–RELATED PROTEIN AND INDIAN HEDGEHOG

The action of Ihh to slow chondrocyte differentiation in the chick overexpression system resembled the action of PTHrP and raised the possibility that these two signaling systems might interact. This hypothesis was supported when Ihh overexpression was shown to increase PTHrP mRNA dramatically in the perichondrial region at the ends of chicken long bones. An analogous overexpression system was then established using embryonic mouse limbs. These limbs were placed in chemically defined medium and exposed to an active recombinant fragment of sonic hedgehog (Shh), a relative of Ihh known to mimic Ihh actions in the chick limb system. As expected, the Shh fragment upregulated PTHrP mRNA expression in the periarticular growth plate and delayed differentiation of growth plate chondrocytes in the mouse limbs. In contrast, the Shh fragment had no effect on either *PTHrP*(−/−) or *PTH/PTHrP receptor*(−/−) limbs (19,25). These data strongly suggest that Ihh slows chondrocyte differentiation by stimulating the production of PTHrP. On the other hand, PTHrP indirectly inhibits Ihh production by delaying the differentiation of proliferating chondrocytes into Ihh-producing prehypertrophic and hypertrophic chondrocytes. These interactions suggest that PTHrP and Ihh might control a negative-feedback loop that serves to regulate the rate and synchrony of the differentiation of growth plate chondrocytes. As chondrocytes differentiate into prehypertrophic cells, they synthesize Ihh. Ihh then directly or indirectly signals to the PTHrP-producing cells at the ends of bones, which increase their production of PTHrP. PTHrP then slows the differentiation of chondrocytes and delays the production of cells making Ihh (Fig. 25.5).

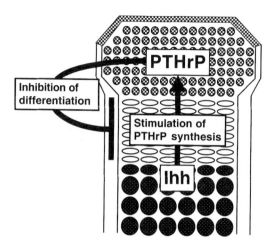

FIG. 25.5. Indian hedgehog (Ihh)-parathyroid hormone-related protein (PTHrP) negative-feedback loop. As proliferating chondrocytes differentiate into prehypertrophic chondrocytes, they synthesize Ihh. Ihh directly or indirectly stimulates the synthesis of PTHrP at the periarticular region. PTHrP then slows the differentiation of proliferating chondrocytes and consequently slows production of the prehypertrophic chondrocytes that make Ihh. Thus, Ihh and PTHrP participate in a negative-feedback loop that serves to regulate the rate of chondrocyte differentiation.

ANALYSIS OF BONES FROM CHIMERIC MICE

The responses to overexpression of hh proteins in chicken and mouse limbs suggested the existence of an Ihh–PTHrP feedback loop, but the design of such experiments made it difficult to assess whether physiologically relevant amounts of these paracrine factors could act in the manner postulated in the hypothesis. The chimeric growth plates containing both wild-type and *PTH/PTHrP receptor*(−/−) cells provided an opportunity to more stringently test the hypothesis (26). As already noted, the *PTH/PTHrP receptor*(−/−) chondrocytes differentiated more quickly than did the wild-type ones, even when surrounded by wild-type proliferating chondrocytes. Further, the wild-type

cells did not behave normally; instead, their differentiation was slowed, leading to abnormally long columns of them. Somehow, the wild-type cells "sensed" the rapid differentiation of the *PTH/PTHrP receptor*(−/−) chondrocytes and responded by slowing their own differentiation. The Ihh–PTHrP pathway might control this response. Supporting this possibility was the observation that the *PTH/PTHrP receptor*(−/−) chondrocytes produced Ihh much closer to the periarticular region than did wild-type cells since the proliferating columns of the *PTH/PTHrP receptor*(−/−) cells are short. This ectopic Ihh expression leads to abnormal Ptc expression in surrounding wild-type proliferating chondrocytes and an increase in PTHrP mRNA in the periarticular growth plate (26). This increase in PTHrP expression is expected to slow the differentiation of wild-type chondrocytes and may explain the elongated columns of them observed in chimeric mice (Fig. 25.6). Thus, rather modest perturbation in the location

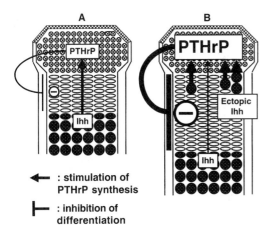

← : stimulation of
PTHrP synthesis

⊢ : inhibition of
differentiation

FIG. 25.6. Possible mechanism for elongation of columns of wild-type proliferating chondrocytes in chimeric mice. **A:** Wild-type growth plate. **B:** Chimeric growth plate containing both wild-type cells and *PTH/PTHrP receptor(−/−)* cells. In the wild-type growth plate, the Indian hedgehog *(Ihh)* stimulus for parathyroid hormone–related protein *(PTHrP)* synthesis and the PTHrP inhibition of production of Ihh-making prehypertrophic and hypertrophic chondrocytes strike a balance when Ihh-producing cells in the prehypertrophic layer and PTHrP-producing cells at the periarticular region are placed at a certain distance. In the chimeric growth plate, this balance is disturbed since *PTH/PTHrP receptor(−/−)* cells prematurely hypertrophy and produce Ihh much closer to PTHrP-producing cells at the periarticular region. This ectopic Ihh expression results in an increase in PTHrP synthesis. Increased PTHrP abnormally slows the differentiation and causes elongation of columns of wild-type proliferating chondrocytes.

of Ihh-expressing cells leads to activation of PTHrP production; this is a key prediction from the hypothesis that Ihh and PTHrP interact to determine the rate of differentiation of growth plate chondrocytes.

ACTIONS OF INDIAN HEDGEHOG THAT ARE INDEPENDENT OF PARATHYROID HORMONE–RELATED PROTEIN

The interactions between Ihh and PTHrP mentioned above are an incomplete description of the actions of Ihh on the growth plate. As

noted earlier, the chondrocytes of the *Ihh(−/−)* mice proliferate much more slowly than those of the *PTHrP(−/−)* mice. The *Ihh(−/−)* mice synthesize little, if any, PTHrP mRNA in their growth plate, and hypertrophic chondrocytes predominate late in fetal development. To clarify which of the abnormalities in the *Ihh(−/−)* mice could be explained by the effects of PTHrP, the transgene that expresses the constitutively active PTH/PTHrP receptor in the growth plate was introduced into knockout mice by appropriate matings. When this constitutively active PTH/PTHrP receptor transgene was introduced into the *PTHrP(−/−)* background, the transgene virtually restored the normal anatomy of the growth plate at birth (24). Further, when this transgene was introduced into the *Ihh(−/−)* background, the increased number of hypertrophic chondrocytes was no longer seen. In contrast, the constitutively active PTH/PTHrP receptor had no effect on the defect in proliferation in the *Ihh(−/−)* growth plate (41). These data demonstrate that effects of Ihh on differentiation of growth plate chondrocytes are mediated by PTHrP, while effects of Ihh on proliferation of growth plate chondrocytes are independent of PTHrP.

CONCLUSION AND FUTURE DIRECTIONS

In the growth plate, PTHrP is synthesized by periarticular chondrocytes, directly acts on proliferating chondrocytes, and inhibits their differentiation into hypertrophic chondrocytes. By doing so, PTHrP delays the expression of Ihh protein, which is synthesized mainly by prehypertrophic and hypertrophic chondrocytes. On the other hand, Ihh protein directly or indirectly stimulates PTHrP production by periarticular chondrocytes. Thus, PTHrP and Ihh control a negative-feedback loop that serves to regulate the pace and synchrony of differentiation of growth plate chondrocytes.

The existence of the Ihh–PTHrP feedback loop raises a host of unanswered questions. First, how does Ihh regulate PTHrP synthesis? It is possible that Ihh target cells respond directly and increase PTHrP synthesis, but several cell layers separate the periarticular cells that synthesize PTHrP from the prehypertrophic cells that secrete Ihh. This separation raises the question of whether Ihh protein can diffuse sufficiently far to directly activate *PTHrP* gene expression. Ihh is covalently bound to cholesterol; this may limit the diffusion of the molecule. Further, Ptc, the hh receptor, absorbs substantial amounts of Ihh and limits its diffusion. In *Drosophila,* diffusion of hh protein is also regulated by the *tout-velu* gene (42). The *tout-velu* gene encodes an integral membrane protein that belongs to the *EXT* gene family. This gene family is implicated in the human multiple exostoses syndrome, which affects bone morphogenesis. One member of the gene family, *EXT1,* encodes an endoplasmic reticulum–resident type II transmembrane glycoprotein and is required for the synthesis and cell surface display of heparan sulfate glycosaminoglycans (43,44). The syndrome of multiple exostoses may well be caused by abnormal diffusion of Ihh, in analogy with the effects of the *tout-velu* gene in *Drosophila.* Further, a recently characterized Hedgehog-binding protein may regulate the diffusion of Ihh protein as well (45).

Thus, multiple mechanisms may limit the ability of Ihh to reach the periarticular cells that synthesize PTHrP. Therefore, Ihh may instead trigger a cascade that leads to PTHrP synthesis. In some settings in *Drosophila,* the *hh* gene amplifies its signal by stimulating the synthesis of other ligands such as Dpp and Wg, vertebrate homologues of which are bone morphogenetic proteins (BMPs) and Wnts, respectively. These proteins may mediate the actions of Ihh to increase PTHrP synthesis.

Second, how does PTHrP slow the differentiation of growth plate chondrocytes? PTHrP activates the PTH/PTHrP receptor. The activated PTH/PTHrP receptor then activates both adenylate cyclase and phospholipase C (8,9). It is not yet known which of these two pathways mediates PTHrP signaling in chondrocyte differentiation, but there are some data suggesting a major role of the adenylate cyclase pathway. Mice carrying the constitutively active PTH/PTHrP receptor transgene, which signals only through the adenylate cyclase pathway *in vitro,* showed delayed differentiation of growth plate chondrocytes. Moreover, the introduction of the same transgene rescued the accelerated differentiation of growth plate chondrocytes in *PTHrP*(−/−) mice (24). By controlling the differentiation of growth plate chondrocytes, this feedback loop also serves to control other important processes in endochondral bone development. In the chimeric analysis, individual *PTH/PTHrP receptor*(−/−) cells were able to differentiate into hypertrophic cells in the normal proliferating layer, but these individual hypertrophic cells were not able to mineralize their surrounding matrix (26). In contrast, when a larger number of *PTH/PTHrP receptor*(−/−) cells, as a group, differentiated into hypertrophic chondrocytes prematurely, this critical mass of cells was able to mineralize the surrounding matrix. This requirement for a critical mass of synchronously differentiating cells may explain the importance of the normal orderly wave of differentiation as cells progress through the growth plate. The Ihh–PTHrP feedback loop serves to increase this synchrony.

Finally, Ihh may help regulate the development of the bone collar surrounding the differentiating chondrocytes. Ihh can induce osteogenic differentiation of mesenchymal cell lines *in vitro* (46), and Shh induces ectopic bone formation *in vivo* (47). Overexpression of Ihh protein through injection of a recombinant retrovirus into embryonic chicken limbs not only delays differentiation of growth plate chondrocytes but also leads to an increase in bone collar formation in the adjacent perichondrium despite the absence of hypertrophic chondrocytes. Judging from these data, Ihh is a candidate molecule that might control bone collar formation, but further study is required. One can expect that multiple signaling pathways are required to coordinate the proliferation and differentiation of cells in developing bone.

REFERENCES

1. Erlebacher A, Filvarof EH, Gitelman SE, et al. Toward a molecular understanding of skeletal development. *Cell* 1995;80:371–378.
2. Marks SC, Hermey DC. The structure and development of bone. In: Bilezikian JP, Raisz LG, Rodan GA, eds.

Principles of bone biology. San Diego: Academic Press, 1996:3–14.

3. Ianotti JP, Goldstein S, Kuhn J, et al. Growth plate and bone development. In: Simon SR, ed. *Orthopaedic basic science.* Rosemont, Illinois: American Academy of Orthopaedic Surgeons, 1994:185–217.

4. Stewart AF, Horst R, Deftos LJ, et al. Biochemical evaluations of patients with cancer-associated hypercalcemia: evidence for humoral and nonhumoral groups. *N Engl J Med* 1980;303:1377–1383.

5. Suva LJ, Winslow GA, Wettenhall RE, et al. A parathyroid hormone–related protein implicated in malignant hypercalcemia: cloning and expression. *Science* 1987;237:893–896.

6. Mangin M, Webb AC, Dreyer BE, et al. Identification of a cDNA encoding a parathyroid hormone-like peptide from a human tumor associated with humoral hypercalcemia of malignancy. *Proc Natl Acad Sci USA* 1988;85:597–601.

7. Thiede MA, Strewler GJ, Nissenson RA, et al. Human renal carcinoma expresses two messages encoding a parathyroid hormone-like peptide: evidence for the alternative splicing of a single-copy gene. *Proc Natl Acad Sci USA* 1988;85:4605–4609.

8. Jüppner H, Abou-Samra A-B, Freeman M, et al. A G-protein-linked receptor for parathyroid hormone and parathyroid hormone–related peptide. *Science* 1991;254:1024–1026.

9. Abou-Samra A-B, Jüppner H, Force T, et al. An expression cloning of a common receptor for parathyroid hormone and parathyroid hormone–related peptide from rat osteoclast-like cells: a single receptor stimulates intracellular accumulation of both cAMP and inositol triphosphates and increases intracellular free calcium. *Proc Natl Acad Sci USA* 1992;89:2723–2726.

10. Wysolmerski JJ, Broadus AE, Zhou J, et al. Overexpression of parathyroid hormone–related protein in the skin of transgenic mice interferes with hair follicle development. *Proc Natl Acad Sci USA* 1994;91:1133–1137.

11. Lee K, Lanske B, Karaplis AC, et al. Parathyroid hormone–related peptide delays terminal differentiation of chondrocytes during endochondral bone development. *Endocrinology* 1996;137:5109–5118.

12. Philbrick WM, Dreyer BE, Nakchbandi LA, et al. Parathyroid hormone–related protein is required for tooth eruption. *Proc Natl Acad Sci USA* 1998;95:11846–11851.

13. Wysolmerski JJ, Philbrick WM, Dunbar ME, et al. Rescue of the parathyroid hormone–related protein knockout mouse demonstrates that parathyroid hormone–related protein is essential for mammary gland development. *Development* 1998;125:1285–1294.

14. Dunbar ME, Young P, Zhang J-P, et al. Stromal cells are critical targets in the regulation of mammary ductal morphogenesis by parathyroid hormone–related protein. *Dev Biol* 1998;203:75–89.

15. Lee K, Deeds JD, Segre GV. Expression of parathyroid hormone–related peptide and its receptor messenger ribonucleic acids during fetal development of rats. *Endocrinology* 1995;136:453–463.

16. Lee K, Deeds JD, Chiba S, et al. Parathyroid hormone induces sequential c-fos expression in bone cells *in vivo: in situ* localization of its receptor and c-fos messenger ribonucleic acids. *Endocrinology* 1994;134:441–450.

17. Karaplis AC, Luz JA, Glowacki JR, et al. Lethal skeletal dysplasia from targeted disruption of the parathyroid hormone–related peptide gene. *Genes Dev* 1994;8:277–289.

18. Amizuka N, Henderson JE, Warshawsky H, et al. Parathyroid hormone–related peptide (PTHrP)–depleted mice show abnormal epiphyseal cartilage development and altered endochondral bone formation. *J Cell Biol* 1994;126:1611–1623.

19. Lanske B, Karaplis AC, Lee K, et al. PTH/PTHrP receptor in early development and Indian hedgehog–regulated bone growth. *Science* 1996;273:102–106.

20. Jobert AS, Zhang P, Couvineau A, et al. Absence of functional receptors for parathyroid hormone and parathyroid hormone–related peptide in Blomstrand chondrodysplasia. *J Clin Invest* 1998;102:34–40.

21. Zhang P, Jobert AS, Couvineau A, et al. A homozygous inactivating mutation in the parathyroid hormone/parathyroid hormone–related peptide receptor causing Blomstrand chondrodysplasia. *J Clin Endocrinol Metab* 1998;83:3365–3368.

22. Schipani E, Kruse K, Jüppner H. A constitutively activated mutant PTH/PTHrP receptor in Jansen-type metaphyseal chondrodysplasia. *Science* 1995;268:98–100.

23. Weir EC, Philbrick WM, Amling M, et al. Targeted overexpression of parathyroid hormone–related peptide in chondrocytes causes chondrodysplasia and delayed endochondral bone formation. *Proc Natl Acad Sci USA* 1996;93:10240–10245.

24. Schipani E, Lanske B, Hunzelman J, et al. Targeted expression of constitutively active receptors for parathyroid hormone and parathyroid hormone–related peptide delays endochondral bone formation and rescues mice that lack parathyroid hormone–related peptide. *Proc Natl Acad Sci USA* 1997;94:13689–13694.

25. Vortkamp A, Lee K, Lanske B, et al. Regulation of rate of cartilage differentiation by Indian hedgehog and PTH-related protein. *Science* 1996;273:613–622.

26. Chung U, Lanske B, Lee K, et al. The parathyroid hormone/parathyroid hormone–related peptide receptor coordinates endochondral bone development by directly controlling chondrocyte differentiation. *Proc Natl Acad Sci USA* 1998;95:13030–13035.

27. Riddle RD, Johnson RL, Laufer E, et al. *Sonic hedgehog* mediates the polarizing activity of the ZPA. *Cell* 1993;75:1401–1416.

28. Echelard Y, Epstein DJ, St-Jacques B, et al. Sonic hedgehog, a member of a family of putative signaling molecules, is implicated in the regulation of CNS polarity. *Cell* 1993;75:1417–1430.

29. Krauss S, Concordet J-P, Ingham PW. A functionally conserved homolog of the *Drosophila* segment polarity gene hh is expressed in tissues with polarizing activity in zebrafish embryos. *Cell* 1993;75:1431–1444.

30. Nüsslein-Volhard C, Wieshaus E. Mutations affecting segment number and polarity in *Drosophila. Nature* 1980;287:795–801.

31. Hammerschmidt M, Brook A, McMahon AP. The world according to *hedgehog. Trends Genet* 1997;13:14–21.

32. Stone DM, Hynes M, Armanini M, et al. The tumor-suppressor gene *patched* encodes a candidate receptor for sonic hedgehog. *Nature* 1996;384:129–134.

33. Marigo V, Davey RA, Zuo Y, et al. Biochemical evidence that patched is the hedgehog receptor. *Nature* 1996;384:176–179.

34. Chen Y, Struhl G. Dual roles for patched in sequestering and transducing hedgehog. *Cell* 1996;87:553–563.

35. Alcedo J, Ayzenton M, Von Ohlen T, et al. The *Drosophila smoothened* gene encodes a seven-pass membrane protein, a putative receptor for the hedgehog signal. *Cell* 1996;86:221–232.

36. Van den Heuvel M, Ingham PW. *Smoothened* encodes a receptor-like serpentine protein required for hedgehog signaling. *Nature* 1996;382:547–551.

37. Von Ohlen T, Lessing D, Nusse R, et al. Hedgehog signaling regulates transcription through Cubitus interruptus, a sequence-specific DNA binding protein. *Proc Natl Acad Sci USA* 1997;94:2404–2409.

38. Chen Y, Gallagher N, Goodman RH, et al. Protein kinase A directly regulates the activity and proteolysis of Cubitus interruptus. *Proc Acad Natl Sci USA* 1998;95:2349–2354.

39. Ohlmeyer JT, Kalderon D. Hedgehog stimulates maturation of Cubitus interruptus into a labile transcriptional factor. *Nature* 1998;396:749–753.

40. Bitgood MJ, McMahon AP. *Hedgehog* and *bmp* genes are coexpressed at many diverse sites of cell–cell interaction in the mouse embryo. *Dev Biol* 1995;172:126–138.

41. Karp SJ, Schipani E, St-Jacques B, et al. Activation of the PTHrP signaling pathway rescues the accelerated chondrocyte hypertrophy but not the short limb dwarfism of Ihh mutants. *J Bone Miner Res* 1998;23:S162.

42. Bellaiche Y, The I, Perrimon N. *Tout-velu* is a *Drosophila* homologue of the putative tumour suppressor *EXT-1* and is needed for Hh diffusion. *Nature* 1998;394:85–88.

43. McCormick C, Leduc Y, Martindale D, et al. The putative tumour suppressor EXT1 alters the expression of cell-surface heparan sulfate. *Nat Genet* 1998;19:158–161.

44. Lin X, Gan L, Klein WH, et al. Expression and functional analysis of mouse *EXT1*, a homolog of the human multiple exostoses type 1 gene. *Biochem Biophy Res Commun* 1998;243:61–66.

45. Chuang P, McMahon AP. Vertebrate hedgehog signaling modulated by induction of a hedgehog-binding protein. *Nature* 1999;397:617–621.

46. Nakamura T, Aikawa T, Iwamoto-Enomoto M, et al. Induction of osteogenic differentiation by hedgehog proteins. *Biochem Biophys Res Commun* 1997;237:465–469.

47. Kinto N, Iwamoto M, Enomoto-Iwamoto M, et al. Fibroblasts expressing sonic hedgehog induce osteoblast differentiation and ectopic bone formation. *FEBS Lett* 1997;404:319–323.

Skeletal Growth Factors,
edited by Ernesto Canalis.
Lippincott Williams & Wilkins, Philadelphia, © 2000.

26

Osteoprotegerin

William J. Boyle and *David L. Lacey

*Departments of Cell Biology and *Pathology, Amgen, Inc., Thousand Oaks, California 91320-1799*

Osteoprotegerin (OPG) is a newly described protein that appears to have an emerging role as a major factor that affects the metabolism of the skeleton (1). It is a member of the tumor necrosis factor receptor (TNFR) superfamily, with special properties. OPG is a secreted protein and not a traditional surface membrane-associated receptor, which transmits signals that regulate cell functions. The primary structure of OPG suggests that it functions in the extracellular milieu as a receptor-like protein that binds to, and regulates, the activity of a TNF-related ligand (see 2, 3 for reviews). The term ''osteoprotegerin'' simply refers to a protein that protects or guards against the destruction of bone. Based on *in vitro* and *in vivo* analyses of this protein, OPG has been found to negatively regulate osteoclastogenesis and osteoclast activation and, in doing so, to control bone remodeling and bone density homeostasis.

Bone remodeling is a physiological process that occurs throughout life and involves the resorption of bone by osteoclasts and the synthesis of bone matrix by osteoblasts (4–6). Osteoclasts are of hematopoietic origin and degrade bone matrix and mineral by fusing to bone surfaces and secreting lytic enzymes. The production of bone (and its removal) is a highly regulated process, under the control of various growth factors, hormones, and cytokines (6–8). Osteoclast recruitment and activation can be accelerated in certain disease processes, leading to inappropriate increases in bone resorption and, subsequently, net loss of bone mass. Increased osteoclast activity is seen in many osteopenic

disorders, including primary osteoporosis, hypercalcemia associated with malignancy, and osteolytic arthritis. The biology of the osteoclast is an important field of study, carrying with it implications that may lead to the development of effective therapies to treat bone loss.

This chapter reviews the discovery and characterization of the OPG gene, mRNA, and polypeptide and recent advancements in our understanding of its role as a key determinant in the regulation of bone mass. OPG does not act alone; it effects a pathway of hematopoietic cell development that is dependent on a key ligand–receptor interaction found to be essential for osteoclast maturation and activation. OPG has been useful as a reagent to probe the nature of this regulatory pathway, and combined biochemical, cell biological, and molecular genetic analyses in mice have provided a clear mechanism-based view of how osteoclastogenesis is regulated.

DISCOVERY AND MOLECULAR CLONING OF OSTEOPROTEGERIN

Osteoprotegerin was first identified as a novel expressed sequence tag (EST) from a cDNA library prepared from fetal rat intestine, independent of any perceived biological function, i.e., via genomics (9). Computational analysis of this sequence revealed that it encoded a homologue of the TNFR superfamily. Using this sequence information, full-length rat cDNA clones were isolated, and the amino acid sequence of its protein product (OPG) was deduced (Fig. 26.1).

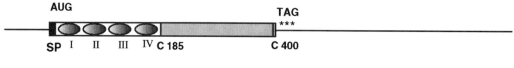

**TNFR Homology   Dimerization
Domain   Domain**

FIG. 26.1. Structure of rat osteoprotegerin *(OPG)* mRNA and protein. The rat OPG mRNA is a 2.4-kb transcript, represented by the *thin line.* The 401–amino acid long open reading frame encoding the rat OPG product is represented by the *coded box.* The first 21 amino acids *(black)* indicate the position of the signal peptide sequence. The N-terminal half of OPG contains four tandem cysteine-rich repeat sequences *(shaped ellipses).* The C-terminal dimerization domain is indicated by a *gray box.* The coding frame begins at a methionine codon (AUG) and terminates at a stop codon (TAG) following leucine-401. *C185* represents the last cysteine residue of the tumor necrosis factor receptor homology domain. The mouse and human OPG cDNA sequences also encode 401–amino acid polypeptides that are approximately 89% to 94% identical to the rat protein shown here.

This same protein was also identified by purification of secreted protein activity known as osteoclastogenesis inhibitory factor (OCIF) (10–11). The OPG/OCIF protein was found to be a 401-residue polypeptide with two functional regions. The N-terminal half of OPG (aa residues 22–185) consists of four tandem cysteine-rich repeat sequences and bears striking homology to the ligand-binding domain of all TNFR family members (12). The C-terminal half of the protein (aa residues 186–401) bears no obvious homology to other known proteins but appears to contain minimal sequence identity to a portion of the intracellular protein death domain motif (11,13). This region has been shown to be involved in OPG homodimerization and extracellular matrix binding (1,10,11,13). At the extreme N terminus of the protein lies a functional 21–amino acid hydrophobic signal peptide that directs secretion and is cleaved during biosynthesis (1,11). Further analysis of the entire OPG amino acid sequence failed to reveal any potential hydrophobic transmembrane domain seen in other TNFR family members (12) and was an early indication that it was a secreted protein. Pulse-chase studies in mammalian cell lines that overexpress the murine OPG cDNA revealed that it is indeed a secreted protein that is proteolytically processed, modified by glycosylation, and exported into conditioned medium (1). Analysis of the biosynthetic product under nonreducing conditions also revealed that the

primary OPG polypeptide self-associates during secretion and is secreted from the cell both as a disulfide-linked dimer and as a monomer. Structural analysis of the C-terminal region indicates that the cysteine residue at position 400 is critical for the formation of secreted homodimer (13). Dimerization and oligomerization of TNFR-related proteins are associated with high affinity for ligand (12). Formation of a secreted dimer is a unique property for members of the TNFR superfamily and suggests that OPG is biosynthesized as a high-affinity cytokine antagonist.

Structure and function analyses of OPG reveal that the biological activity domain resides within the N-terminal 185 amino acids, which harbor the four tandem cysteine-rich repeat sequences (Fig. 26.1) (1,11,13). All four domains are required for biological activity, as well as each of the 18 individual cysteine residues that help form the tertiary structure of these motifs (1,13). This region of all TNFR-related proteins comprises the ligand-binding domain of this family of receptors, implying that OPG activity is mediated via binding to a TNF-related protein. The C-terminal domain of the protein can be deleted, and OPG molecules retain biological activity *in vitro* and *in vivo* (1,11,13), further suggesting that OPG functions via binding to a TNF-related cytokine.

The rat, mouse, and human OPG cDNAs have been cloned and sequenced and their protein products compared (1,11,14,15). OPG sequences are highly conserved during evolution at the DNA and protein levels. The rat and mouse proteins are about 94% identical, whereas the mouse and human proteins are about 89% identical, without sequence gaps. All of the cysteine residues located in the full-length mature proteins (residues 22–401) are conserved and in identical positions. The mouse OPG transcript is expressed in the cartilaginous primordia of bone during embryonic development, then later is expressed in the intestine, kidney, and lung (1). In humans, OPG expression is detected at relatively high levels in the lung, kidney, and heart (1,11). OPG expression can be detected in osteoblastic stromal cells and is regulated by cytokines, growth factors, and steroid hormones, suggesting a role as a factor that regulates osteoblast and osteoclast coupling during bone development and remodeling (14–22). Members of the transforming growth factor-β (TGF-β) superfamily, such as TGF-β1 and bone morphogenetic protein-2 (BMP-2), can induce expression of OPG (18–20). Calciotropic agents known to induce bone resorption, such as vitamin D_3, prostaglandin E_2 (PGE$_2$), and hydrocortisone, can also downregulate OPG/OCIF expression in osteoblasts (17,18,20). OPG transcripts have also been detected in cell lines from various sources, including the intestine, T cells, dendritic cells, and osteoblastic sarcomas (1,14,16). Expression in some lymphoid cells is upregulated by the ligation of CD40 receptor, a TNFR protein that is closely related to OPG (14). Cytokines such as TNF-α and TNF-β, as well as interleukin-1 (IL-1), upregulate the production of OPG in an osteosarcoma cell line and in osteoblast-like stromal cells (19,21,22), indicating a possible link or coupling of immune system responses to effects on bone remodeling.

MOLECULAR GENETIC ANALYSIS OF OSTEOPROTEGERIN IN MOUSE

The biological activity of OPG was determined *in vivo* by analyzing the effects of systemic administration of OPG via transgenic delivery of the rat and mouse cDNA into mouse. This system employed the apolipoprotein E (ApoE) promoter and hepatocyte control element to produce high levels of OPG protein in the liver beginning around day 1 of postnatal development and continuing throughout adulthood (1,23). Overexpression of OPG in this way is designed to mimic the chronic systemic administration of protein and, therefore, to perturb any OPG-regulated process and lead to an identifiable phenotype.

Transgenic OPG founder mice expressing varying levels of OPG were found to be healthy and appeared of normal size and weight (1). They had no abnormalities in blood cell levels or in serum chemistry. They were able to breed and readily gave rise to transgenic mouse lines. However, they all had a noticeable phenotype that correlated in severity with the level of exogenous OPG measured in their circulation. OPG transgenics had increased bone density (osteopetrosis), resulting from the accumulation of newly synthesized bone. The bones were of normal length and shape, suggesting that bone growth and modeling were not adversely affected. The increase in bone mass detected in transgenic animals was restricted to the endosteal regions of the trabecular, or marrow-containing, bones. Within the endosteal region, there were few, if any, tartrate-resistant acid phosphatase (TRAP)-positive multinucleated osteoclasts observed, suggesting a defect in bone resorption (1). Comparison of bone sections obtained from OPG transgenic mice and control littermates showed that OPG transgenics lacked mature osteoclasts within the endosteal regions of the affected bones. Normal osteoclast progenitor cells can be detected in the spleens of these mice using *in vitro* osteoclast formation assays, and immunohistochemistry of the spleen indicated normal expression of the myelomonocytic cell surface marker F4/80 (1). F4/80 is a surface antigen associated with macrophage and osteoclast precursors, and its abundant expression in the spleens of these animals indicates normal development in the myeloid cell lineages. This would indicate that the OPG transgenic phenotype is not due to alterations in hematopoiesis leading to the production of the osteoclast progenitor but rather that these mice harbor a defect in the later stages of osteoclast maturation. This led to the early hypothesis that OPG served as a negative regulator of osteoclast development and could act as a humoral factor regulating bone metabolism.

The murine and human OPG gene has been isolated and partially characterized (24–27). Using the murine gene, OPG knockout mice have been generated and analyzed to further characterize the function of OPG (26,27). OPG($-/-$) mice were born live and found to primarily have early-onset osteoporosis that increases in severity with aging. These mice have extremely fragile bones, and multiple long bone fractures can be readily observed upon x-ray examination of mice maintained with normal handling. Histological examination of the bones of OPG($-/-$) mice shows a dramatic decrease in trabecular and cortical bone mass. The cortical region of the long bones degenerates over time into a trabecularized structure with woven matrix, indicating a very weak form of bone in these animals. Interestingly, the heterozygous OPG($-/+$) mice also have decreased bone mass, at a level intermediate to ($+/+$) and ($-/-$) mice (26). If one compares the OPG gene dosing level seen in OPG transgenic, wildtype, and OPG($-/+$) and ($-/-$) mice, one can readily conclude that the level of OPG directly determines the level of bone mass, implying that OPG is a secreted molecule that regulates bone density. OPG($-/-$) mice have also been shown to have calcifications in the vessel walls of major arteries in the heart and kidney (26). The mechanism of this is not known but may be related to secondary events that occur following losses in bone mineral density. The knockout of the OPG actually provided a phenotype in mice that is diametrically opposite that of OPG overexpression, reinforcing the concept that it regulates bone mass as a negative regulator of osteoclast activity.

OSTEOPROTEGERIN REGULATES AN IMPORTANT STEP IN OSTEOCLAST MATURATION

Osteoclasts are specialized macrophage cells that develop from hematopoietic precursors in the bone marrow and spleen. They stem from a common monocyte/macrophage precursor that can give rise to several mature macrophage cell types, including alveolar macrophages and hepatic Kupffer cells (28). At the time OPG was first identified and characterized, little was actually known about the various steps involved in the commitment to the osteoclast lineage and the processes that control osteoclast maturation (osteoclastogenesis). However, using *in vitro* culture systems, mature osteoclasts could be formed from bone marrow and spleen cells (29). The polypeptide factor macrophage colony-stimulating factor (M-CSF, also called CSF-I) along with stromal cells, vitamin D_3, and dexamethasone are required for osteoclastogenesis to occur in these *in vitro* systems.

A vitamin D_3-dependent bone marrow and stromal cell coculture system was used to determine the effects of OPG on osteoclast development (29,30). This assay system was used to purify the native human OPG polypeptide to homogeneity from conditioned media produced by a normal human diploid lung fibroblast cell line (10). The purified protein product included both homodimeric and monomeric OPG polypeptide chains, similar to the expression product characterized in the circulation of OPG transgenic mice (1). Native OPG and recombinant OPG protein have been shown to block *in vitro* osteoclastogenesis in a dose-dependent manner, with a half-maximal effective concentration in the range of 1 to 2 ng/ml (1,10,11,13). OPG blocks the formation of large multinucleated osteoclasts that express TRAP activity, the calcitonin receptor, and the integrin $\alpha V \beta 3$, all markers of the mature osteoclast (Fig. 26.2). This indicated that in OPG transgenic mice the increases in bone mass observed are likely due to failure to resorb newly synthesized bone, leading to accumulation of trabecular bone matrix within regions normally filled with bone marrow. Only the N-terminal half of the protein, which resembles a ligand-binding domain, is required for biological activity in this *in vitro* system (1,11).

OPG transgenic mice still produce and harbor osteoclast progenitor cells that could differentiate *in vitro* after being removed from exogenous OPG exposure *in vivo* (1). This means that hematopoiesis leading to the production of os-

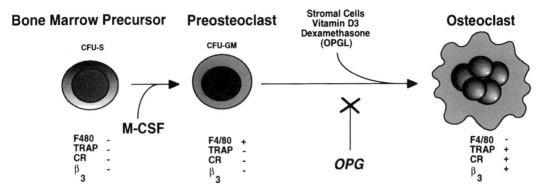

FIG. 26.2. Osteoprotegerin *(OPG)* effect on osteoclastogenesis *in vitro*. Diagram depicting the hypothetical action of OPG on osteoclast development *in vitro* using the bone marrow and stromal cell coculture system (1,30). Bone marrow precursor cells treated with macrophage colony-stimulating factor (*M-CSF*, CSF-I) give rise to bone marrow macrophage cells capable of differentiating into mature osteoclasts. Coculture of bone marrow macrophages with ST-2 stromal cells (8,9) in the presence of $1\alpha,25$-dihydroxyvitamin D_3 and dexamethasone differentiate into mature osteoclasts. Prostaglandin E_2 (PGE_2) increases osteoclast formation in this system. OPG blocks osteoclast development at the stage which requires stromal cells, vitamin D_3, and dexamethasone. *F4/80*, a monocyte/macrophage surface marker; *TRAP*, artrate-resistant acid phosphatase; *CR*, calcitonin receptor; $\alpha V\beta3$, osteoclast-specific integrin $\alpha V\beta3$; *CFU-S*, colony-forming unit-stem cells; *CFU-GM*, colony-forming unit-granulocyte/macrophage.

teoclast precursors is unaffected by OPG, and these precursor cells are blocked in their ability to differentiate along the terminal osteoclast maturation pathway (Fig. 26.2). From this work, we now know that OPG impacts a crucial regulatory step during osteoclast development and that further study of this novel protein will lead to a better understanding of this process and physiological cues that help to regulate bone density.

ANTIRESORPTIVE EFFECTS OF OSTEOPROTEGERIN IN ANIMAL MODELS

The early hypothesis that OPG functions as a secreted osteoclastogenesis inhibitor *in vivo* was tested by administration of recombinant OPG in neonate animals. Young, growing mice were injected with recombinant murine OPG protein daily for 3 to 7 days, and its effects on bone were measured by radiography and quantitative histology (1,11). In growing mice, newly synthesized bone is actively generated at the growth plates of the long bones, particularly at the proximal tibial metaphysis. Injection of OPG leads to the rapid accumulation of bone at this site,

coincident with the decreased numbers of TRAP-positive osteoclasts. Microscopic analysis of this area shows the accumulation of newly synthesized bone-encased cartilage, or osteoid. This is the same histological picture seen in OPG transgenic mice and indicates that the phenotypic effects seen in transgenics can be recapitulated in normal mice when given intravenous recombinant protein. The effects of recombinant OPG in young, growing mice were similar to those seen in mice treated with bisphosphonates (31), small-molecule antiresorptive therapeutics useful for the treatment of osteoporosis. The effects of OPG and the bisphosphonate pamidronate (Aredia; Ciba-Geigy, Summit, NJ) were tested in this *in vivo* model, and both compounds were found to lead to equivalent changes in the accumulation of bone mass (1). Thus, the biological activity of OPG on osteoclast maturation acts like an antiresorptive agent in normal animals.

OPG can also block bone resorption in a disease model characterized by increased osteoclast numbers and/or activity. A rat model for osteoporosis associated with the loss of estrogen was used to compare the effects of OPG with those of pamidronate. In this model, ovariectomy leads to rapid loss of bone mass due to increased osteoclast activity (32). OPG and pamidronate both blocked increases in osteoclast numbers and activity and prevented bone loss in untreated ovariectomized rat controls. OPG has also been analyzed in the thyroparathyroidectomized rat model (33). In this model, serum calcium levels are raised by the exogenous addition of either PTH or vitamin D_3 via induction of osteoclast-mediated bone resorption. OPG can block the induction of, or reverse once established, serum hypercalcemia in a rapid manner, suggesting an immediate effect on osteoclast function and/or survival. These data indicate that OPG bioactivity translates into a protection that may be useful for the treatment of osteopenic disorders characterized by excessive bone loss due to elevated osteoclast numbers or activity and may have important implications for the clinic.

OSTEOPROTEGERIN LIGAND AND THE OSTEOCLASTOGENESIS PATHWAY

The biological activity of OPG strongly suggests that it negatively regulates a cytokine that stimulates osteoclast maturation and activation. It had been known for many years that osteoblastic cells could be stimulated by calciotropic agents to produce a factor that stimulates osteoclasts (2–4). The ligand for OPG (OPGL) was a likely candidate for this factor, but it had not yet been identified and its biological activities remained elusive. Using OPG/OCIF as a probe, a putative ligand was expression-cloned from cDNA libraries made from osteoblastic stromal cells induced with vitamin D_3 (34) or from the murine myelomonocytic cell line 32D (35). Both clones encoded an identical 316–amino acid mouse protein that was termed osteoclast differentiation factor (ODF) and OPGL. This novel protein was predicted to be a type II transmembrane surface protein with the clear structural motifs found in TNF family members. OPGL can be cleaved from the surface of expressing cells (35) and released in a soluble, biologically active form. It is not yet clear whether the soluble form of OPGL plays a role in regulating os-

teoclast functions *in vivo,* although recombinant forms of soluble OPGL have potent bioactivity when administered to animals (see below). ODF/OPGL cDNA had previously been isolated by two different approaches that suggested a role for this cytokine in the regulation of immune responses. The first report of this sequence was the differential cloning of a T-cell protein induced by calcineurin-regulated transcription factors and named TNF-related activation-induced (TRANCE) cytokine (36). It was subsequently also identified as RANKL, a ligand for the novel TNFR-related protein RANK (receptor activator of NFκB), a dendritic cell surface protein. Some T-cell clones express TRANCE/RANKL, suggesting a role in co-stimulatory processes during antigen processing by regulating dendritic cell survival (36,37).

Several lines of evidence support the role of ODF/OPGL/TRANCE/RANKL as the key factor that regulates osteoclastogenesis (referred to herein as OPGL for contuinity). First, recombinant OPGL binds specifically and with high affinity to biologically active forms of OPG but not inactive OPG mutants (34,35). Second, either native cell surface–expressed OPGL (34,38,39) or recombinant soluble OPGL (34,35, 38,39) acts as a potent ODF *in vitro* using either murine or human hematopoietic precursors. Osteoclastogenesis is dependent on coadministration of CSF-I (35,39), and is characterized by induction of expression of key markers that typify the osteoclast cell lineage (such as TRAP, cathepsin K, $\alpha V \beta 3$) and the formation of large multinucleated cells that are capable of resorbing bone. OPGL stimulates not only osteoclast differentiation but also activation of bone resorption *in vitro* (38,40) and survival in cell culture (41). Furthermore, OPGL was found to stimulate rapid induction of bone resorption and to elevate serum calcium when administered to mice and rats (35). Third, using fluoresceinated OPGL as a probe, all of the hematopoietic progenitors capable of giving rise to osteoclasts during *in vitro* culture could be isolated and purified from bone marrow cells by flow cytometry (35). Finally, agents that increase osteoclast development *in vitro,* such as vitamin D_3, IL-1, IL-11, PGE_2, and PTH (34,39,41,42), induced expression of OPGL in osteoblasts. Interestingly, some of these agents also appear to simultaneously downregulate or inhibit OPG expression in osteoblasts (20). This raises the possibility that coordinate regulation of OPG and OPGL expression by osteotropic and calciotropic hormones may be a mechanism used to couple osteoblast and osteoclast development and activation during bone remodeling. Thus, the combination of cell biological data measuring osteoclast differentiation and activation activity, its ability to tightly bind to OPG, and its relatedness to TNF family members indicate that OPGL is a critical factor that regulates osteoclastogenesis.

Clear evidence as to the role of this protein during osteoclastogenesis and in regulating bone metabolism was derived from the analysis of knockout mice that lack OPGL (43). OPGL (−/−) mice were born with severe osteopetrosis that did not resolve with age and other characteristic hallmarks seen in other rodent osteopetrosis models, such as lack of tooth eruption, club-shaped bones, and splenomegaly (44). At the histological level, increases in bone mass were due to accumulation of newly synthesized bone, suggesting a defect in resorption and remodeling. These mice completely lack osteoclasts, although normal osteoclast progenitors are present in spleen as detected by *in vitro* culture assays in the presence of CSF-I and OPGL (43). These mice were found to have an intrinsic defect in the ability of stromal cells to promote osteoclastogenesis via OPGL, suggesting that OPGL is the sole factor that initiates the osteoclast differentiation program. OPGL(−/−) mice also lack lymph nodes and have hematopoietic cell intrinsic defects in the early stages of T-cell and B-cell development. Dendritic cells appear normal in these mice, and circulating levels of B and T cells are observed in the circulation. OPGL can act as a dendritic cell survival factor *in vitro,* an activity that can be complemented by CD40L (36). These data provide a biological link between the role of OPGL in both bone and immune homeostasis and raise the intriguing possibility of a functional link between these two critical organ systems.

A putative osteoclast cell surface receptor for

OPGL had previously been identified as the TNFR-related protein RANK (37). RANK was first characterized as a dendritic cell surface protein proposed to function in T cell and dendritic cell interactions during the immune response. In contrast, the finding that OPGL had a critical role in bone metabolism suggested a role for RANK in regulating a key osteoclast signaling pathway. RANK mRNA was found to be expressed at very high levels in osteoclast precursors isolated by binding to recombinant OPGL (35,45,46). Soluble RANK–Fc fusion protein, delivered transgenically or via administration of recombinant protein, blocked OPGL-induced osteoclastogenesis, leading to increases in bone mass similar to native OPG (45). As further proof of the role of RANK in eliciting osteoclastogenic signal transduction, polyclonal antibodies to the extracellular domain of the receptor were found to have agonistic activity (45,46). In the presence of CSF-I, anti-RANK antibodies stimulate osteoclast development and induction of osteoclast-specific gene expression, suggesting that ligation of this receptor is sufficient for initiating osteoclastogenesis. Finally, recent analysis of RANK(−/−) mice revealed that it is absolutely required for osteoclast formation (47), as is OPGL (43). Hematopoietic precursors isolated from RANK(−/−) mice are unable to form osteoclasts in the presence of CSF-I and OPGL, but retroviral delivery of wild-type murine RANK cDNA restores osteoclastogenic potential (47). Together these data indicate that RANK is the critical hematopoietic surface determinant that controls differentiation into the osteoclast lineage via binding to OPGL.

The RANK protein is a 625–amino acid transmembrane protein with homology to other TNFR family members. The extracellular domain contains four cysteine-rich motifs, while the C-terminal cytoplasmic domain contains no obvious structural features that imply a signaling mechanism (35,37). Other members of the TNFR family are known to mediate signal transduction via cytoplasmic factors belonging to the TNFR-associated factor (TRAF) family of proteins (48). In addition to activating the transcription factor NFκB, RANK stimulates Jun N-terminal kinase (JNK) activity (37,41,45,49–52), presumably by coupling with cytoplasmic factors. TRAF family members 2, 5, and 6 were found to interact with the cytoplasmic domain of RANK (37,41,42). TRAFs 2 and 5 bind to the same region at the very C terminus of the protein, while TRAF-6 binds to a small region lying between amino acid residues 336 and 454 (45,52). This same internal region of the RANK cytoplasmic domain was also found to be required for induction of NFκB and JNK activity, suggesting that TRAF-6 is an important signal transducer during induction of osteoclastogenesis. A knockout mouse lacking TRAF-6 has recently been analyzed and found to have an osteopetrotic phenotype (osteosclerosis and failure in tooth eruption), confirming a biological role for this protein in osteoclast function and in bone metabolism (53). *In vivo*, TRAP-positive osteoclasts are observed, but ultrastructural analysis indicates that there is a defect in the ability of osteoclasts lacking TRAF-6 to adhere to bone surface and to form proper resorption lacunae (44).

MOLECULAR MODEL FOR THE REGULATION OF OSTEOCLASTOGENESIS

OPG/OCIF, OPGL/ODF/TRANCE/RANKL, and RANK have been implicated as the key proteins that coordinately interact to regulate osteoclast differentiation and activation. Each of these proteins has been evaluated in mouse molecular genetic models, and their interrelated functions during osteoclastogenesis have been confirmed. A mechanistic model for regulation of osteoclastogenesis can be derived that invokes binding of these proteins in a selective fashion to produce negative or positive regulation of bone mass (Fig. 26.3). OPGL is a pathway agonist that activates the RANK receptor on osteoclast precursors or on mature osteoclasts, resulting in bone resorption. OPG is a cytokine antagonist that acts as a negative regulator of osteoclast development and activation by sequestering OPGL. The resulting effect *in vivo* is to block bone resorption, leading to accumulation of bone mass. Differential expression of OPG and OPGL by the osteoblast is under the control of

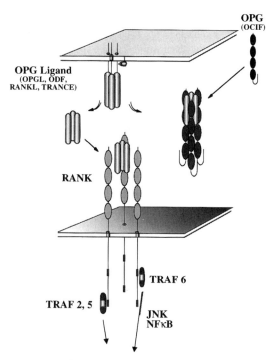

FIG. 26.3. Molecular mechanism for the regulation of osteoclast differentiation and activation via osteoprotegerin *(OPG)* and its ligand *(OPGL)* on osteoclast precursors. OPGL is represented as a transmembrane and soluble protein as previously described (35) and is also known as osteoclast differentiation factor *(ODF)*, TNF-related, activation-induced cytokine *(TRANCE)*, and receptor activator of NFκB ligand *(RANKL)*. OPGL binds to and activates the osteoclast receptor RANK, stimulating signal transduction, leading to the induction of osteoclast-specific gene expression. OPG, also known as osteoclast inhibitory factor (OCIF), is a secreted neutralizing or decoy receptor. OPG functions by binding to and sequestering OPGL, thus rendering it unable to activate RANK and thereby preventing the induction of osteoclastogenesis. The membrane-bound arrowhead complex represents the putative OPGL convertase activity detected in human 293 fibroblasts that liberates soluble OPGL (35). TNFR, tumor necrosis factor receptor; TRAF, TNFR-associated factor [TRAFs 2, 5, and 6 are TNFR-associated cytoplasmic factors (48)]; *TRAP,* tartrate-resistant acid phosphatase; *CTR,* calcitonin receptor; $\alpha V\beta 3$, osteoclast-specific integrin $\alpha V\beta 3$; *CatK,* osteoclast-specific protease cathepsin K.

a diverse collection of hormones and cytokines that influence the rate of bone remodeling and can control the numbers and activity of osteoclasts. At the level of the bone, OPGL appears to control the coupling of osteoblast and osteoclast coordinate functions during remodeling, while OPG can uncouple this process and block bone remodeling. There is still much to learn about this pathway, and OPGL can produce changes in gene expression patterns in hematopoietic progenitors that yield an osteoclast cell phenotype. Further study of this pathway should provide great insight as to how bone density is regulated by cytokines and hormones during normal development and during disease.

ACKNOWLEDGMENTS

We acknowledge the support of several colleagues who made available reprints and information that have contributed to the models presented in this chapter, including Hisataka Yasuda, Kanji Higashio, Tatsuo Suda, Josef Penninger, Yun-Young Kong, Ji Li, and Colin Dunstan. D.L.L. is Senior Director of Pathology and W.J.B. is Associate Director of Cell Biology at Amgen, Inc.

REFERENCES

1. Simonet WS, Lacey DL, Dunstan CR, et al. Osteoprotegerin: a novel secreted protein involved in the regulation of bone density. *Cell* 1997;89:309–319.
2. Suda T, Takahashi N, Udagawa N, et al. Modulation of osteoclast differentiation and function by the new members of the tumor necrosis factor receptor and ligand families. *Endocr Rev* 1999;20:345–357.
3. Takahashi N, Udagawa N, Suda T. A new member of tumor necrosis factor ligand family, ODF/OPGL/TRANCE/RANKL, regulates osteoclast differentiation and function. *Biochem Biophys Res Commun* 1999;256:449–455.
4. Suda T, Takahashi N, Martin TJ. Modulation of osteoclast differentiation. *Endocr Rev* 1992;13:66–80.
5. Roodman GD. Advances in bone biology: the osteoclast. *Endocr Rev* 1996;17:308–332.
6. Rodan GA, Martin TJ. Role of osteoblasts in hormonal control of bone resorption—a hypothesis. *Calcif Tissue Int* 1981;95:13361–13362.
7. Martin TJ, Udagawa N. Hormonal regulation of osteoclast function. *Endocrinol Metab* 1998;9:6–12.
8. Mundy GR. Cytokines and local factors which affect osteoclast function. *Int J Cell Clon* 1993;10:215–222.
9. Adams MD, Kelley JM, Gocayne JD, et al. Complimentary DNA sequencing: expressed sequence tags and human genome project. *Science* 1991;252:1651–1656.
10. Tsuda E, Goto M, Mochizuki S-I, et al. Isolation of a novel cytokine from human fibroblasts that specifically inhibits osteoclastogenesis. *Biochem Biophys Res Commun* 1997;234:137–142.
11. Yasuda H, Shima N, Nakagawa N, et al. Identity of osteoclastogenesis inhibitory factor (OCIF) and osteoprotegerin (OPG): a mechanism by which OPG inhibits osteoclastogenesis *in vitro*. *Endocrinology* 1998;139:1329–1337.
12. Smith CA, Farrah T, Goodwin RG. The TNF receptor superfamily of cellular and viral proteins: activation, costimulation, and death. *Cell* 1994;76:959–962.
13. Yamaguchi K, Kinosaki M, Goto M, et al. Characterization of structural domains of human osteoclastogenesis inhibitory factor (OCIF)/OPG. *J Biol Chem* 1998;273:5117–5123.
14. Yun TJ, Chaudhary PM, Shu GL, et al. OPG/FDCR-1, a TNF receptor family member, is expressed in lymphoid cells and is up-regulated by ligating CD40. *J Immunol* 1998;161:6113–6121.
15. Kwon BS, Wang S, Udagawa N, et al. TR1, a new member of the tumor necrosis factor superfamily, induces fibroblast proliferation and inhibits osteoclastogenesis and bone resorption. *FASEB J* 1998;12:845–854.
16. Tan KB, Harrop J, Reddy M, et al. Characterization of a novel TNF-like ligand and recently described TNF ligand and TNF receptor superfamily gene and their constitutive and inducible expression in hematopoietic and non-hematopoietic cells. *Gene* 1997;204:35–46.
17. Vidal NO, Brandstrom H, Jonsson KB, et al. Osteoprotegerin mRNA is expressed in primary human osteoblast-like cells: down-regulation by glucocorticoids. *J Endocrinol* 1998;159:191–195.
18. Hofbauer LC, Dunstan CR, Spelsberg TC, et al. Osteoprotegerin production by human osteoblast lineage cells is stimulated by vitamin D, bone morphogenetic protein-2, and cytokines. *Biochem Biophys Res Commun* 1998;250:776–781.
19. Takai H, Kanematsu M, Yano K, et al. Transforming growth factor-beta stimulates the production of osteoprotegerin/osteoclastogenesis inhibitory factor by bone marrow stromal cells. *J Biol Chem* 1998;273:27091–27096.
20. Horwood NJ, Elliott J, Martin TJ, et al. Osteotropic agents regulate the expression of osteoclast differentiation factor and osteoprotegerin in osteoblastic stromal cells. *Endocrinology* 1998;139:4743–4746.
21. Vidal ON, Sjogren K, Eriksson BI, et al. Osteoprotegerin mRNA is increased by interleukin-1 alpha in the human osteosarcoma cell line MG-63 and in human osteoblast-like cells. *Biochem Biophys Res Commun* 1998;248:696–700.
22. Brandstrom H, Jonsson KB, Vidal O, et al. Tumor necrosis factor-alpha and -beta upregulate the levels of osteoprotegerin mRNA in human osteosarcoma MG-63 cells. *Biochem Biophys Res Commun* 1998;248:454–457.
23. Simonet WS, Hughes TM, Nguyen HQ, et al. Long-term impaired neutrophil migration in mice overexpressing human interleukin-8. *J Clin Invest* 1994;94:1310–1319.
24. Austyn JM, Gordon S. F4/80, a monoclonal antibody directed specifically against the mouse macrophage. *Eur J Immunol* 1981;11:805–815.

25. Morinaga T, Nakagawa N, Yasuda H, et al. Cloning and characterization of the gene encoding human osteo-protegerin/osteoclastogenesis inhibitory factor. *Eur J Biochem* 1998;254:685–691.

26. Bucay N, Sarosi I, Dunstan CR, et al. Osteoprotegerin-deficient mice develop early onset osteoporosis and arterial calcifications. *Genes Dev* 1998;12:1260–1268.

27. Mizuno A, Amizuka N, Irie K, et al. Severe osteoporosis in mice lacking osteoclastogenesis inhibitory factor/osteoprotegerin. *Biochem Biophys Res Commun* 1998; 237:610–615.

28. Chambers TJ. Regulation of osteoclast development and functions. In: Rifkin BR, Gay CV, eds. *Biology and physiology of the osteoclast.* Boca Raton, FL: CRC Press, 1992:105–128.

29. Udagawa N, Takahashi N, Akatsu T, et al. The bone marrow–derived stromal cell lines MC3T3/PA6 and ST2 support osteoclast-like cell differentiation in cocultures with mouse spleen cells. *Endocrinology* 1989;125: 1805–1813.

30. Lacey DL, Erdmann JM, Teitelbaum SL, et al. Interleukin-4, interferon-γ, and prostaglandin E impact the osteoclastic cell-forming potential of murine bone marrow macrophages. *Endocrinology* 1995;136:2367–2376.

31. Sietsema WK, Ebetino FH, Salvagno AM, et al. Antiresorptive dose-response relationships across three generations of bisphosphonates. *Drugs Exp Clin Res* 1989; 15:389–396.

32. Kalu DN, Liu CC, Hardin RR, et al. The aged rat model of ovarian deficiency bone loss. *Endocrinology* 1989; 124:7–16.

33. Yamamoto M, Murakami T, Nishikawa M, et al. Hypocalcemic effect of osteoclastogenesis inhibitory factor/osteoprotegerin in the thyroparathryoidectomized rat. *Endocrinology* 1998;139:4012–4015.

34. Yasuda H, Shima N, Nakagawa N, et al. Osteoclast differentiation factor is a ligand for osteoprotegerin/osteoclastogenesis inhibitory factor and is identical to TRANCE/RANKL. *Proc Natl Acad Sci USA* 1998;95: 3597–3602.

35. Lacey DL, Timms E, Tan H-L, et al. Osteoprotegerin ligand is a cytokine that regulates osteoclast differentiation and activation. *Cell* 1998;93:165–176.

36. Wong BR, Rho J, Arron J, et al. TRANCE is a novel ligand of the tumor necrosis factor receptor family that activates c-Jun N-terminal kinase in T cells. *J Biol Chem* 1997;272:25190–25194.

37. Anderson DM, Maraskovsky E, Billingsley WL, et al. A homologue of the TNF receptor and its ligand enhance T-cell growth and dentritic-cell function. *Nature* 1997; 390:175–179.

38. Fuller K, Wong B, Fox S, et al. TRANCE is necessary and sufficient for osteoblast-mediated activation of bone resorption in osteoclasts. *J Exp Med* 1998;188:977–1001.

39. Tsuki K, Shima N, Nakagawa N, et al. Osteoclast differentiation factor mediates an essential signal for bone

resorption induced by 1α, 25-dihydroxyvitamin D_3, prostaglandin E_2 or parathyroid hormone in the microenvironment of the bone. *Biochem Biophys Res Commun* 1998;246:337–341.

40. Burgess TL, Qian Y-X, Kaufman S, et al. The ligand for osteoprotegerin (OPGL) directly activates mature osteoclasts. *J Cell Biol* 1999;145:527–538.

41. Jimi E, Akiyama S, Tsurukai T, et al. Osteoclast differentiation factor acts as a multifunctional regulator in murine osteoclast differentiation and punction. *J Immunol* 1999;163:434–442.

42. Martin TJ, Romas E, Gillespie MT. Interleukins in the control of osteoclast differentiation. *Crit Rev Eukaryot Gene Expr* 1998;8:107–123.

43. Kong Y-Y, Yoshida H, Sarosi I, et al. OPGL is a key regulator of osteoclastogenesis, lymphocyte development and lymph-node organogenesis. *Nature* 1999;397: 315–323.

44. Marks SC Jr. Osteoclast biology, lessons from mammalian mutations. *Am J Med Genet* 1989;34:43–53.

45. Hsu H, Lacey DL, Dunstan CR, et al. Tumor necrosis factor receptor family member RANK mediates osteoclast differentiation and activation induced by osteoprotegerin ligand. *Proc Natl Acad Sci USA* 1999;96: 3540–3545.

46. Nakagawa N, Kinosaki M, Yamaguchi K, et al. RANK is the essential signaling receptor for osteoclast differentiation in osteoclastogenesis. *Biochem Biophys Res Commun* 1998;253:395–400.

47. Li J, Yan X-Q, McCabe S, et al. TNFR-related protein RANK is the intrinsic hematopoietic cell surface determinant that controls osteoclastogenesis, and regulation of bone mass and calcium metabolism 1999 *(submitted.)*

48. Arch RH, Gedrich RW, Thompson CB. Tumor necrosis factor receptor–associated factors (TRAFs)—a family of adapter proteins that regulates life and death. *Genes Dev* 1998;12:2821–2830.

49. Darney BG, Haridas V, Ni J, et al. Characterization of the intracellular domain of receptor activator of NF-κB (RANK). *J Biol Chem* 1999;273:20551–20555.

50. Galibert L, Tometsko ME, Anderson DM, et al. The involvement of multiple tumor necrosis factor receptor (TNFR)–associated factors in the signaling mechanisms of receptor activator of NF-κB, a member of the TNFR superfamily. *J Biol Chem* 1998;273:34120–34127.

51. Wong BR, Josien R, Lee SY, et al. The TRAF family of signal transducers mediates NF-κB activation by the TRANCE receptor. *J Biol Chem* 1998;273:28355–28359.

52. Darney BG, Ni J, Moore PA, et al. Activation of NFκB by RANK requires tumor necrosis factor receptor associated factor (TRAF) 6 and NFκB-inducing kinase. *J Biol Chem* 1999;274:7724–7731.

53. Lomaga MA, Yeh W-C, Sarosi I, et al. TRAF 6 deficiency results in osteopetrosis and defective interleukin-1, CD40, and LPS signaling. *Genes Dev* 1999;13:1015–1024.

Skeletal Growth Factors,
edited by Ernesto Canalis.
Lippincott Williams & Wilkins, Philadelphia, © 2000.

27

Nonskeletal Effects of Cytokines Secreted by Bone Cells

*Melissa Alsina and †G. David Roodman

*Department of Medicine, Division of Hematology, University of Texas Health Science Center,
San Antonio, Texas 78284-7880; †Research Service, Audie L. Murphy Veterans Administration
Hospital, San Antonio, Texas 78284

Skeletal cells produce a great number of cytokines and growth factors that can affect their own growth and differentiation, in terms of their effects on both bone formation and osteoclastic bone resorption. In addition, these cytokines and growth factors can have a major impact on immune cell function, cell growth, and hematopoiesis. In this chapter, we discuss the non-skeletal effects of cytokines and growth factors produced by bone cells and focus especially on their effects on hematopoiesis. The effects of these cytokines on osteoclast and osteoblast function will be discussed in the next chapter. Cytokines produced by skeletal cells are secreted locally in the bone microenvironment or expressed on the cell surface and influence hematopoiesis via cell-to-cell interactions. These cytokines are also released into the systemic circulation, where they can have far-reaching effects on immune cell function and glucose and lipid metabolism.

FACTORS PRODUCED BY OSTEOBLASTS

Osteoblasts, in addition to their important role in laying down new bone during the process of bone remodeling, produce factors that are critical for maintaining hematopoiesis. The factors produced by osteoblasts include hematopoietic growth factors, such as granulocyte-macrophage colony-stimulating factor (GM-CSF), macro-phage colony-stimulating factor (M-CSF), hepatocyte growth factor (HGF), transforming growth factor-β (TGF-β), and insulin-like growth factors (IGFs), as well as cytokines such as interleukin-1 (IL-1), IL-6, and IL-11 (Table 27.1).

Hematopoiesis occurs in direct proximity to osteoblasts within the bone marrow. Taichman et al. (1) demonstrated that osteoblasts can support the development of hematopoietic precursor colonies as well as maintaining more primitive hematopoietic stem cells *in vitro*. These authors showed clearly that osteoblasts stimulated the development of hematopoietic colonies to a level that was at least tenfold greater than control cultures containing progenitor cells alone. Furthermore, treatment of more primitive hematopoietic precursors with conditioned media from osteoblasts expanded the number of these progenitors three- to fourfold.

Both human and murine osteoblasts can support the expansion of hematopoietic progenitors (CD34$^+$ cells) *in vitro*. This occurs through close cell-to-cell contact between CD34$^+$ bone marrow cells and osteoblasts *in vitro*, suggesting that osteoblasts may play an important role in stem cell regulation. Taichman et al. (2) have shown that close contact between osteoblasts and CD34$^+$ hematopoietic progenitor cells upregulates IL-6 production by the osteoblasts. These data demonstrate an important role for osteoblasts in maintaining hematopoiesis.

TABLE 27.1. *Factors produced by osteoblasts*

Factor	Effects on hematopoiesis
GM-CSF	Enhances hematopoiesis
G-CSF	Enhances granulopoiesis
M-CSF	Enhances growth of macrophage precursors
SCF	Enhances survival of hematopoietic stem cells
EGF	Enhances growth of fibroblasts
LIF	Induces maturation of megakaryocytes
HGF	Enhances erythropoiesis
TNF-α	Inhibits erythropoiesis
PDGF	Enhances growth of fibroblasts
TGF-β	Inhibits hematopoiesis
Oncostatin M	Enhances megakaryocyte colony formation
IL-8	Activates neutrophils
IL-6	Increases platelet production
IL-11	Increases growth of CFU-GM
IL-18	Induces T-cell production of GM-CSF
IGF	Enhances erythropoiesis
RANK ligand	Enhances dendritic cell capacity to stimulate T-cell growth

CFU-GM, Colony-forming unit-granulocyte macrophage; EGF, epidermal growth factor; GM-CSF, granulocyte-macrophage colony-stimulating factor; HGF, hepatocyte growth factor; IgF, insulin-like growth factor; IL, interleukin; LIF, leukemia inhibitory factor; PDGF; platelet-derived growth factor; RANK, receptor activator of NFκB; SCF, stem cell factor; TGF β, transforming growth factor β; TNF-2, tumor necrosis factor-2.

Several observations suggest that intimate interactions between osteoblasts and hematopoietic stem cells are required *in vivo* as well as *in vitro* to sustain hematopoiesis. First, hematopoiesis in adults occurs almost exclusively within the bone. Second, after bone marrow transplantation, donor stem cells initially circulate to all organs but home specifically to the bone marrow. Furthermore, hematopoiesis is not sustained in other tissues even if the infused marrow cells lodge in these sites, e.g., the lungs. Third, Steel (Sl/Sl^d) mice have impaired hematopoiesis due to a stromal cell defect in which they do not produce stem cell factor (3,4).

Therefore, these data suggest that bone cells play an important role in sustaining hematopoietic stem cell proliferation and differentiation and that osteoblasts mediate this important function by secreting hematopoietic growth factors or expressing them on their surfaces. However, because osteoblasts produce such a large array

of factors that can either enhance hematopoietic cell growth and differentiation or inhibit it, the exact role of the osteoblast in hematopoiesis has not been clearly defined. For example, isolated human osteoblasts synthesize mRNAs for hematopoietic stimulatory factors such as granulocyte colony-stimulating factor (G-CSF), GM-CSF, M-CSF, IGF-1, platelet-derived growth factor-α (PDGF-α), stem cell factor (SCF), epidermal growth factor (EGF), and leukemia inhibitory factor (LIF). In addition, osteoblasts express TGF-β and oncostatin M mRNAs, factors that inhibit hematopoiesis.

Growth Factors Produced by Osteoblasts that Stimulate Hematopoiesis

Granulocyte-Macrophage Colony-Stimulating Factor

GM-CSF stimulates the growth of multipotent hematopoietic progenitors, which give rise to monocytes, macrophages, eosinophils, neutrophils, megakaryocytes, and erythrocytes, and enhances the growth of both erythroid and megakaryocyte precursors (5). In addition to stimulating the growth and differentiation of progenitors for cells in the neutrophil-macrophage lineage, it activates macrophages, neutrophils, and eosinophils that are postmitotic (6–8). GM-CSF can induce release of prostaglandin E_2 and phagocytosis by mature neutrophils and induce chemotaxis and migration of neutrophils to inflammatory sites. Furthermore, GM-CSF can induce production of tumor necrosis factor-α (TNF-α) by mature monocyte-macrophages at sites of inflammation (9). In addition, GM-CSF can mediate antibody-dependent cellular cytotoxicity against bacteria as well as tumor cells (10), suggesting that it is a multifunctional cytokine with important effects on both cellular proliferation and differentiation of hematopoietic progenitors as well as activation of mature cells for host defenses.

GM-CSF is encoded by a single gene located on the long arm of chromosome 5 (11). This region of the chromosome contains genes for several other growth factors, including PDGF and M-CSF, as well as their receptors. The receptor for GM-CSF has been recently cloned and is located on the X chromosome (12). The molecular weight of the GM-CSF gene products varies between 14 and 35 kDa, resulting from a differential glycosylation of the peptide. The GM-CSF receptor is expressed on malignant myeloid cells and normal myeloid progenitor cells (13); it is also expressed on some nonhematopoietic cells, such as lung fibroblasts, although it is unclear if it has any effects on the growth of nonhematopoietic cells. Receptors for GM-CSF are relatively rare, numbering between 100 and 300 per cell, which is a common feature for most hematopoietic growth factor receptors including erythropoietin (14). Once GM-CSF binds to its receptor, it signals through a guanosine triphosphate (GTP)-binding protein, which results in the release of inositol triphosphates and diacylglycerol. Release of inositol triphosphates and diacylglycerol induces mobilization of intracellular calcium stores, which then induce protein synthesis and cell growth and differentiation (15).

In summary, GM-CSF is a multilineage hematopoietic growth factor that stimulates the growth of less committed, as well as more differentiated, hematopoietic progenitor cells and at very high levels enhances the growth of erythroid and megakaryocyte progenitor cells and expands the number of circulating monocyte-macrophage progenitor cells (16). GM-CSF also prevents programmed cell death (apoptosis) of granulocytes and macrophages as well as their progenitors and activates mature monocytes and neutrophils.

Granulocyte Colony-Stimulating Factor

G-CSF stimulates the growth and differentiation of granulocytic progenitor cells, activates neutrophil function by increasing the respiratory burst and phagocytosis, and prevents neutrophil apoptosis (17,18). In addition, G-CSF has been implicated in the differentiation of more primitive hematopoietic precursors, stimulating quiescent pluripotent hematopoietic progenitors to enter the G_1/S phase. Infusion of G-CSF or GM-CSF to normal subjects can increase neutrophil counts to levels as high as 70,000 to 80,000 per microliter (19). Although G-CSF can have effects on more primitive hematopoietic precursors, its biological activity appears to be relatively restricted to the more mature committed progenitor cells of the neutrophil lineage and their products. In addition to its effects on neutrophil function, it can enhance antibody-dependent cellular cytotoxicity and induce neutrophil migration (20).

Macrophage Colony-Stimulating Factor

M-CSF, or CSF-I, occurs as both a membrane-bound and a soluble protein. It stimulates the growth of macrophage progenitor cells as well as inducing macrophage proliferation and activating of phagocytic cells in the monocyte-macrophage lineage (21). M-CSF also prevents apoptosis of cells in the monocyte-macrophage lineage. Osteopetrotic *(op/op)* mice, which have a null mutation in the M-CSF gene in addition to lacking osteoclasts, have markedly decreased marrow monocyte-macrophages, although they do have monocyte-macrophages in other organs (22). These data suggest that M-CSF plays an important role in monocyte-macrophage differentiation in the marrow but may not be absolutely required for monocyte-macrophage production at extramedullary sites.

Stem Cell Factor

SCF, also known as kit ligand or mast cell growth factor, is an important hematopoietic growth factor that promotes the differentiation and proliferation of very primitive hematopoietic precursors (23). Absence of SCF is responsible for the hematopoietic abnormalities present in the $S1/S1^d$ mouse (4). It binds to the c-kit receptor, which is missing in the W/W^v mouse, which also has impaired hematopoiesis. SCF occurs as both a soluble and a membrane-bound protein and, in combination with IL-3 and IL-6, promotes the differentiation and proliferation of the most primitive hematopoietic progenitor cells to become committed progenitor cells (24). It acts synergistically with IL-3, GM-CSF, and IL-1 to induce the growth of more committed hematopoietic progenitor cells *in vitro*. SCF also promotes the growth and differentiation of mast cells, and treatment of animals with SCF results in marked mast cell hyperplasia (25). In addition, SCF in combination with other hematopoietic growth factors stimulates the growth of myeloid, erythroid, and megakaryocyte colonies in both mouse and human bone marrow (26–28).

Platelet-Derived Growth Factor

PDGF is a glycoprotein produced by osteoblasts that is also produced by megakaryocytes. It enhances the growth of marrow fibroblasts. PDGF is thought to play a role in the development of marrow fibrosis in agnogenic myeloid metaplasia. PDGF is released by the increased numbers of megakaryocytes derived from the abnormal hematopoietic stem cell clone responsible for agnogenic myeloid metaplasia and induces fibroblast proliferation.

PDGF binds to an intrinsic receptor that has tyrosine kinase activity. When the receptor is activated, there is also activation of a signaling cascade that includes mitogen-activated protein (MAP) kinase (29), activation of the Jak-STAT signaling pathway (30), and activation of protein kinase C (31). PDGF also upregulates expression of the IGF-I receptor in vascular smooth muscle (32). PDGF, like fibroblast growth factor (FGF), induces progression of cells from the G_0 into the G_1 phase of the cell cycle (33).

Hepatocyte Growth Factor

HGF is a glycoprotein that is involved in cell proliferation and differentiation, and it has been proposed to have a role in hematopoiesis and macrophage activation. Takai et al. (34) have shown that HGF enhances the growth of primitive erythroid progenitor cells and multipotent hematopoietic progenitors in vitro but does not enhance the growth of granulocyte-macrophage progenitors. It also has no effect on colony formation by highly purified $CD34^+$ cells. These data suggest that HGF indirectly promotes hematopoiesis. In addition, Bezerra et al. (35) examined the effects of knocking out the HGF gene in mice. They found that these animals had abnormalities in their livers but no defects in hematopoiesis, although macrophage activation was delayed.

Growth Factors Produced by Osteoblasts that Inhibit Hematopoiesis

Tumor Necrosis Factor-α

TNF-α can inhibit the growth of colony-forming unit–granulocyte macrophage (CFU-GM), the granulocyte-macrophage progenitor cell, as well as erythroid precursors (36,37). TNF-α is also produced by activated, but not resting, macrophages. TNF-α has been implicated in the pathogenesis of the anemia of chronic disease through its capacity to inhibit the growth of primitive erythroid progenitors (36). In addition to its inhibitory effects, TNF-α can stimulate granulopoiesis by inducing the production of G-CSF and GM-CSF by endothelial cells and macrophages (38,39). TNF-α also induces prostaglandin synthesis by monocyte-macrophages, which in turn further enhances GM-CSF production. TNF-α can also induce IL-1 and IL-6 expression in fibroblasts (40) and endothelial cells and enhance GM-CSF expression by T cells.

Transforming Growth Factor-β

TGF-β significantly inhibits myeloid, erythroid, megakaryocytic, and multilineage progenitor cell growth in vitro when assayed in semisolid culture systems (41). TGF-β inhibits the growth of very primitive hematopoietic progenitors and acts synergistically with monocyte chemoattractant protein-1 (MCP-1) to inhibit the growth of these primitive precursors (42). TGF-β appears to inhibit the growth of hematopoietic progenitor cells by signaling through the Smad5 gene because antisense constructs to Smad5 block the inhibitory effects of TGF-β on human hematopoietic progenitor cell growth (43). Furthermore, TGF-β appears to induce cell cycle arrest of hematopoietic stem cells.

Cytokines Secreted by Osteoblasts that Regulate Hematopoiesis

Interleukin-6

IL-6 is a pleotropic cytokine that is produced by a variety of cell types, including osteoblasts and marrow stromal cells (44). IL-6, in addition to its effects on bone cells, enhances megakaryocytopoiesis and platelet production *in vitro* and *in vivo* (44). IL-6 can act synergistically with IL-3 or GM-CSF (or CSF) to induce pluripotent and macrophage or granulocytic colony formation, respectively (45), and can act synergistically with IL-4 to induce T-cell proliferation and immunoglobulin synthesis (46). IL-6 induces its effects by binding to the IL-6 receptor, which is coupled to GP130, and then signals through the GP130 signaling cascade (44). IL-6 is also a potent stimulator of the growth of myeloma cells in bone marrow, and its production is upregulated when myeloma cells bind to marrow stromal cells and/or osteoblasts (47). This enhanced production of IL-6 may explain the propensity for myeloma cells to grow in bone marrow rather than solid organs. IL-6 also inhibits the growth of murine M1 leukemia cells, induces their macrophage differentiation (48), enhances the survival of cholinergic neurons, and stimulates secretion of pituitary hormones (49). IL-6 also induces production of acute-phase proteins by hepatocytes (50).

Interleukin-11

IL-11 has many of the biological effects of IL-6 and signals through the GP130 signaling cascade. IL-11, like IL-6, stimulates production of acute-phase reacting proteins by hepatocytes (51) and enhances hematopoietic recovery following treatment with cytotoxic agents or ionizing radiation (52). IL-11 can also enhance the growth of myeloma cells as well as the proliferation of hematopoietic progenitors. IL-11 has been shown to induce neural differentiation of hippocampal progenitors (53).

Leukemia Inhibitory Factor

LIF was originally identified as a peptide that inhibited the growth of murine leukemic cells and induced their differentiation to more mature cells (54). More recently, it has been learned that LIF also plays an essential role in regulating the self-renewal capacity of hematopoietic stem cells as well as their progenitors. LIF enhances

thrombopoiesis (55) and promotes the growth of myeloma cells. LIF also increases acetylcholinesterase expression and increases ploidy in megakaryocytes in mouse bone marrow cultures but does not enhance megakaryocytic colony formation (55). These data suggest that LIF can promote megakaryocytic maturation. In addition, LIF induces the production of acute-phase proteins by hepatocytes and cholinergic nerve differentiation, as well as the survival of cholinergic neurons (53). LIF has also been implicated in astrocyte differentiation, as well as the differentiation of adipocytes, hepatocytes, and kidney epithelial cells, and in the maintenance of embryonic stem cell pluripotentiality (56). LIF has many biological functions that are similar to those of IL-6, oncostatin M, ciliary neurotrophic factor (CNTF), IL-11, and cardiotrophin-1 because the LIF receptor signals through the GP130 family of receptors, as do these other cytokines.

Oncostatin M

Oncostatin M is another of the peptides, including IL-6, IL-11, and LIF, that signal through GP130. Oncostatin M can increase splenic megakaryocytes in nude mice implanted with oncostatin M–secreting cell lines but by itself does not induce megakaryocytic colony formation (57). However, in combination with IL-3, oncostatin M enhances megakaryocytic colony formation. Furthermore, administration of oncostatin M to normal mice increases platelet counts. Oncostatin M also inhibits the growth of melanoma cells and can inhibit growth and induce macrophage differentiation of murine M1 leukemia cells (53). Similar to IL-6 and LIF, oncostatin M can also induce production of acute-phase proteins by hepatocytes and cholinergic nerve differentiation.

Interleukin-8

IL-8, although named an interleukin, is really a chemoattractant similar to chemokines and is also called neutrophil-activating peptide. IL-8 induces neutrophil chemotaxis (58) and exocytosis of storage granules in neutrophils (59). It also enhances the respiratory burst; is chemotactic for endothelial cells, basophils, and lymphocytes; and is a potent angiogenic agent (60). IL-8 plays a critical role in host defenses by promoting neutrophil activation, as well as acting as a chemoattractant for neutrophils. IL-8 blocks the growth of primitive normal hematopoietic progenitor cells. IL-8 as well as macrophage inflammatory protein-1α (MIP-1α) have previously been shown to inhibit normal human primitive progenitor cell growth in semisolid culture assays and to act as negative regulators of hematopoiesis when added to long-term marrow cultures (61). Chemokines appear to have important effects on hematopoiesis and to act as chemoattractants for monocyte-macrophages. Although these chemokines can inhibit hematopoiesis, they have stimulatory effects on osteoclastogenesis, suggesting that factors that inhibit hematopoiesis may have stimulatory effects on bone cells.

Interleukin-18

IL-18 is a novel proinflammatory cytokine initially described as interferon-γ (IFN-γ)-inducing factor. It induces both C-C and CXC chemokines and activates NFκB and Fas ligand expression (62). IL-18 is thought to be related to the IL-1 family of proteins and is structurally similar to IL-1β. In addition, Gillespie and coworkers (63) have shown that IL-18 can induce production of GM-CSF, a potent hematopoietic growth factor, by T cells.

Interleukin-1

IL-1 is a cytokine that has a variety of activities on hematopoiesis. During an inflammatory response, IL-1 can induce production of G-CSF and GM-CSF by other cells, including fibroblasts, endothelial cells, and T cells (64,65). IL-1 has been shown to be an inhibitor of erythropoiesis (66,67), but its effects appear to be mediated through induction of TNF-α production by macrophages. IL-1 has two high-affinity receptors, an 80-kDa type 1 receptor and a 68-kDa type 2 receptor, which show different patterns of expression depending on the tissue type examined. The IL-1 receptors are members of the immunoglobulin superfamily. Once IL-1 binds its receptor, it regulates expression of many of the genes that encode mediators of the inflammatory response. IL-1 by itself probably has no direct effects on hematopoiesis but only indirect effects (64–68).

Other Factors Produced by Osteoblasts that Affect Cell Growth and Differentiation

Insulin-like Growth Factor

In addition to the cytokines and growth factors that affect hematopoiesis, osteoblasts produce IGF-I, IGF-II, FGF, EGF, and endothelial cell growth factor. IGF-I has been shown to mediate most of the growth-promoting actions of growth hormone. It may also play a role in local tissue growth. Its activity is regulated by binding to a family of IGF binding proteins. IGF-I appears to play a role in maintaining the proliferation of hematopoietic progenitor cells (69). IGF-I binds a receptor that is a membrane tyrosine kinase which also binds IGF-II. The IGF receptor has an affinity that is 100-fold less for insulin than for IGF-I and IGF-II. IGF-I can promote cell growth and differentiation, enhance protein synthesis, and stimulate cell migration, as well as prevent apoptosis of hematopoietic precursors and is induced by hematopoietic growth factors (70). IGF-I also stimulates the growth of vascular smooth muscle cells and may play a role in the development of atherosclerotic lesions (32).

Receptor Activator of NFκB Ligand

Receptor activator of NFκB (RANK) ligand, also known as osteoclast differentiation–inducing factor or TNF-related, activation-induced cytokine (TRANCE), is a recently identified member of the TNF family that has profound effects on osteoclast differentiation and survival (71). RANK ligand is expressed as a membrane-bound protein on the surface of marrow stromal cells and osteoblasts in response to a variety of osteotropic factors, including 1,25-dihydroxyvitamin D_3, parathyroid hormone, IL-11, and prostaglandin E_2. In addition to its effects on osteoclastogenesis, RANK ligand enhances the ability of dendritic cells to stimulate T-cell growth and increase the survival of T cells (72). RANK ligand induces its effects through the RANK receptor, which activates NFκB (72).

CYTOKINES AND GROWTH FACTORS SECRETED BY OSTEOCLASTS

Osteoclasts are hematopoietic in origin and formed by fusion of mononuclear precursors from cells in the monocyte-macrophage lineage. In addition to their capacity to secrete hydrolytic enzymes and degrade both bone matrix and bone, osteoclasts have recently been identified as secretory cells that release multiple factors that regulate their own formation and activity. In addition, these factors have effects on nonskeletal cells. Cytokines produced by osteoclasts include IL-6, TNF-α, IL-1β, TGF-β, annexin II, IFN-γ, and MIP-1α (Table 27.2). Mills and Frausto (73) have used immunocytochemical techniques to demonstrate expression of EGF, PDGF, basic FGF, and IGF-I in addition to the cytokines mentioned above. IL-1, IL-6, TNF-α, PDGF, IGF-I, and TGF-β have been discussed under "Cytokines Produced by Osteoblasts" and are not discussed further in this section.

Annexin II

The annexins are a family of structurally related proteins that bind phospholipids in a calcium-dependent fashion (74). All contain highly conserved sequences. Diversity and specificity of the different annexins are carried by the N-terminal domains, which are unique for each of the annexins. Annexins have predominantly been considered intracellular proteins and have been assayed as phospholipase A_2 inhibitors. They have been implicated in such diverse processes as anticoagulation, antithrombosis, mitogenesis, and membrane trafficking (74). Annexin II has also been thought to play a role in exocytosis, endocytosis, and cell-to-cell adhesion. We have recently shown that annexin II can induce production of GM-CSF by CD4$^+$ T cells (75). T cells express a putative receptor for annexin II, as do marrow stromal cells.

Macrophage Inflammatory Protein-1-α

MIP-1α is a low-molecular-weight chemokine of the RANTES family. It induces osteoclast formation and migration (76,77), and we have recently shown that it is expressed in an osteoclast cDNA expression library. MIP-1α induces migration of granulocytes and macrophages, enhancing the immune response. It also inhibits proliferation of CD34$^+$ hematopoietic stem cells, while enhancing proliferation of more committed hematopoietic precursors (78). MIP1-α has been implicated in the pathogenesis of anemia in multiple myeloma, and we have recently shown it to be overexpressed in the bone marrow cells and plasma of myeloma patients (79).

Interferon-γ

IFN-γ differs from IFN-α and IFN-β in its protein structure and binds to its own receptor (80). IFN-γ is made primarily by T cells and natural killer cells in response to foreign antigens and mitogens and acts mainly as an immunomodulator rather than as an antiviral agent, in contrast to IFN-α and IFN-β. IFN-γ inhibits the proliferation of hematopoietic precursors (81,82) and regulates cellular metabolism (80). IFN-γ can enhance the differentiation and activity of macrophages and has antitumor effects (80).

TABLE 27.2. *Factors produced by osteoclasts*

Factor	Effects on hematopoiesis
IL-1	Enhances growth of hematopoietic stem cells
IL-6	Enhances megakaryopoiesis
Annexin II	Induces GM-CSF production by stromal cells and T cells
MIP-1α	Inhibits hematopoiesis
TNF-α	Inhibits erythropoiesis
IFN-γ	Inhibits growth of CFU-GM

CFU-GM, Colony-forming unit. granulocyte macrophage; GM-CSF, granulocyte-macrophage colony-stimulating factor; γ-IFN, γ-interferon; IL, interleukin; MIP-1 α, macrophage inflammatory protein-1 α; TFN α, tumor necrosis factor-α.

SUMMARY

Skeletal cells produce growth factors and cytokines that can regulate their own activity and formation as well as that of other bone cells. Osteoblasts appear to play a critical role in modulating osteoclast formation, and osteoclasts release factors from the bone matrix that can regulate bone formation. In addition to these important effects on the skeleton, factors produced by osteoblasts and osteoclasts influence hematopoiesis and immune cell function through the production of cytokines such as IL-6, RANK ligand, IL-1β, IGF-I, and hematopoietic growth factors. Thus, cell-to-cell and paracrine interactions between skeletal cells and other cells in the bone microenvironment play a critical role in maintaining normal hematopoietic and immune cell function.

REFERENCES

1. Taichman RS, Reilly MJ, Emerson SG. Human osteoblasts support human hematopoietic progenitor cells *in vitro* bone marrow cultures. *Blood* 1996;87:518–524.
2. Taichman RS, Reilly MJ, Verma RS, et al. Augmented production of interleukin-6 by normal human osteoblasts in response to CD34$^+$ hematopoietic bone marrow cells *in vitro*. *Blood* 1997;89:1165–1172.
3. Williams DE, de Vries P, Namen AE, et al. The Steel factor. *Dev Biol* 1992;151:368.
4. Huang E, Nocka K, Beier DR, et al. The hematopoietic growth factor KL is encoded by the SI locus and is the ligand of the c-kit receptor, the gene product of the W locus. *Cell* 1990;63:225.
5. Metcalf D. The molecular biology and functions of the granulocyte-macrophage colony-stimulating factors. *Blood* 1986;67:257.
6. Weisbart RH, Golde DW, Clark SC, et al. Human granulocyte-macrophage colony-stimulating factor is a neutrophil activator. *Nature* 1985;314:361.
7. Lindemann A, Riedel D, Oster W, et al. Granulocyte-macrophage colony-stimulating factor induces cytokine secretion by human polymorphonuclear leukocytes. *J Clin Invest* 1989;83:1308.
8. Socinski MA, Cannistra SA, Sullivan R, et al. Granulocyte-macrophage colony-stimulating factor induces the expression of the CD11b surface adhesion molecule on human granulocytes *in vivo*. *Blood* 1988;72:691.
9. Furman WL, Crist WM. Potential uses of recombinant human granulocyte-macrophage colony-stimulating factor in children. *Am J Pediatr Hematol Oncol* 1991;13:388–399.
10. Platzer E, Welte K, Gabrilove JL, et al. Biological activities of a human pleuripotent hematopoietic colony-stimulating factor on normal and leukemic cells. *J Exp Med* 1985;162:1788–1801.
11. Yang Y-C, Kovacic S, Kriz R, et al. The human genes for GM-CSF and IL-3 are closely linked in tandem on chromosome 5. *Blood* 1988;71:958.
12. Gough NM, Gearing DP, Nicola NA, et al. Localization of the human GM-CSF receptor gene to the X-Y pseudoautosomal region. *Nature* 1990;345:734–736.
13. Gasson JC, Kaufman SE, Weisbart RH, et al. High affinity binding of granulocyte-macrophage colony-stimulating factor to normal and leukemic human myeloid cells. *Proc Natl Acad Sci USA* 1986;83:669.
14. Nicola NA. Hemopoietic cell growth factors and their receptors. *Annu Rev Biochem* 1989;58:45–77.
15. Whetton AD, Monk PN, Consalvey SD, et al. Interleukin 3 stimulates proliferation of protein kinase C activation without increasing inositol lipid turnover. *Proc Natl Acad Sci USA* 1988;85:3284–3288.
16. Socinski MA, Cannistra SA, Elias A, et al. Granulocyte-macrophage colony-stimulating factor expands the circulating haemopoietic progenitor cell compartment in man. *Lancet* 1988;1:1194.
17. Ohara A, Suca T, Saito M, et al. Effect of recombinant human granulocyte colony-stimulating factor on hemopoietic cells in serum-free culture. *Exp Hematol* 1987;15:695–699.
18. Suda T, Suda J, Kajigaya S, et al. Effects of recombinant murine granulocyte colony-stimulating factor on granulocyte macrophage and blast colony formation. *Exp Hematol* 1987;15:958–965.
19. Grosh WW, Quesenberry PJ. Recombinant human hematopoietic growth factors in the treatment of cytopenia. *Clin Immunol Immunopathol* 1992;62:S25–S38.
20. Groopman JE, Molina JM, Scadden DT. Hematopoietic growth factors. *N Engl J Med* 1989;321:1449–1459.
21. Ralph P, Warren MK, Nakoinz I, et al. Biological properties and molecular biology of the human macrophage growth factor, CSF-1. *Immunobiology* 1986;172:194.
22. Witmer-Pack MD, Hughes DA, Schuler G, et al. Identification of macrophages and dendritic cells in the osteopetrotic (op/op) mouse. *J Cell Sci* 1993;104:1021–1029.
23. Anderson DM, Lyman SD, Baird A, et al. Molecular cloning of mast cell growth factor, a hematopoietin that is active in both membrane bound and soluble forms. *Cell* 1990;63:235.
24. Bernstein ID, Andrews RG, Zsebo KM. Recombinant human stem cell factor enhances the formation of colonies of CD34$^+$ and CD34$^+$ lin$^-$ cells and the generation of colony forming cell progeny from CD34$^+$ lin$^-$ cell cultures with interleukin 3, granulocyte colony-stimulating factor or granulocyte-macrophage colony-stimulating factor. *Blood* 1991;77:2316.
25. Andrews RG, Knitter GH, Bartelmez SH, et al. Recombinant human stem cell factor, a c-kit ligand, stimulates hematopoiesis in primates. *Blood* 1991;78:1975.
26. McNiece IK, Langley KE, Zsebo KM. Recombinant human stem cell factor synergizes with GM-CSF, G-CSF, IL-3 and Epo to stimulate human progenitor cells of the myeloid erythroid lineages. *Exp Hematol* 1991;19:226–231.
27. Mei RL, Burstein SA. Megakaryocytic maturation in murine long-term bone marrow cultures: role of interleukin-6. *Blood* 1991;78:1438–1447.
28. Van de Ven C, Ishizawa L, Law P, et al. IL-11 in combination with SCF and G-CSF or GM-CSF significantly increases expansion of isolated CD34$^+$ cell population

from cord blood versus adult baboon marrow. *Exp Hematol* 1995;23:1289–1295.

29. Mii S, Khalil RA, Morgan KG, et al. Mitogen activated protein kinase and proliferation of human vascular smooth muscle cells. *Am J Physiol* 1996;270:H142–H150.

30. Heim MH. The Jak-STAT pathway: specific signal transduction from the cell membrane to the nucleus. *Eur J Clin Invest* 1996;26:1–12.

31. Claesson-Welsh L. Mechanism of action of platelet-derived growth factor. *Int J Biochem Cell Biol* 1996;28:373–385.

32. Delafontaine P. Growth factors and vascular smooth muscle cell growth responses. *Eur Heart J* 1998;19:G18–G22.

33. Stiles CD, Capone GT, Scher CD, et al. Dual control of cell growth by somatomedins and platelet-derived growth factor. *Proc Natl Acad Sci USA* 1979;76:1279–1283.

34. Takai K, Hara J, Matsumoto K, et al. Hepatocyte growth factor is constitutively produced by human bone marrow stromal cells and indirectly promotes hematopoiesis. *Blood* 1997;89:1560–1565.

35. Bezerra JA, Carrick TL, Degen JL, et al. Biological effects of targeted inactivation of hepatocyte growth factor-like protein in mice. *J Clin Invest* 1998;101:1175–1183.

36. Roodman GD, Bird A, Hutzler D, et al. Tumor necrosis factor-alpha and hematopoietic progenitors: effects of tumor necrosis factor on the growth of erythroid progenitors CFU-E and BFU-E and the hematopoietic cell lines K562, HL60, and HEL cells. *Exp Hematol* 1987;15:928.

37. Broxmeyer HE, Williams DE, Lu I, et al. The suppressive influences of human tumor necrosis factors on bone marrow hematopoietic progenitor cells from normal donors and patients with leukemia: synergism of tumor necrosis factor and interferon-gamma. *J Immunol* 1986;136:4487.

38. Sieff CA, Niemeyer CM, Mentzer SJ, et al. Interleukin-1, tumor necrosis factor, and the production of colony-stimulating factors by cultured mesenchymal cells. *Blood* 1988;72:1316.

39. Kaushansky K, Lin N, Adamson JW. Interleukin 1 stimulates fibroblasts to synthesize granulocyte-macrophage and granulocyte colony-stimulating factors. *J Clin Invest* 1988;81:92.

40. Walther Z, May LT, Sehgal PB. Transcriptional regulation of the interferon-β2/B cell differentiation factor BSF-2/hepatocyte-stimulating factor gene in human fibroblasts by other cytokines. *J Immunol* 1988;140:974.

41. Parker AN, Pragnell IB. Inhibitors of haemopoiesis and their potential clinical relevance. *Blood Rev* 1995;9:226–233.

42. Maltman J, Pragnell IB, Graham GJ. Specificity and reciprocity in the interactions between TGF-beta and macrophage inflammatory protein-1 alpha. *J Immunol* 1996;156:1566–1571.

43. Bruno E, Horrigan SK, Van Den Berg G, et al. The Smad5 gene is involved in the intracellular signaling pathways that mediate the inhibitory effects of transforming growth factor-beta on human hematopoiesis. *Blood* 1998;91:1917–1923.

44. Kishimoto T. The biology of interleukin-6. *Blood* 1989;74:1–10.

45. Ikebuchi K, Wong GC, Clark SC, et al. Interleukin-6 enhancement of interleukin 3-dependent proliferation of multipotential hemopoietic progenitors. *Proc Natl Acad Sci USA* 1987;84:9035.

46. Hodgkin PD, Bond MW, O'Garra A, et al. Identification of IL-6 as a T cell-derived factor that enhances the proliferative response of thymocytes to IL-4 and phorbol myristate acetate. *J Immunol* 1988;141:151.

47. Klein B, Zhang X-G, Jourdan M, et al. Paracrine rather than autocrine regulation of myeloma-cell growth and differentiation by interleukin-6. *Blood* 1989;73:517.

48. Miyaura C, He Jin C, Yamaguchi Y, et al. Production of interleukin 6 and its relation to the macrophage differentiation of mouse myeloid leukemia cells (MI) treated with differentiation-inducing factor and 1α,25-dihydroxyvitamin D$_3$. *Biochem Biophys Res Commun* 1989;158:660.

49. Satoh T, Nakamura S, Taga T, et al. Induction of neuronal differentiation in PC12 cells by B-cell stimulatory factor 2/interleukin 6. *Mol Cell Biol* 1988;8:3546.

50. Morrone G, Ciliberto G, Oliviero S, et al. Recombinant interleukin 6 regulates the transcriptional activation of a set of human acute phase genes. *J Biol Chem* 1988;263:12554.

51. Bauman H, Schendel P. Interleukin-11 regulates the hepatic expression of the same plasma protein genes as interleukin-6. *J Biol Chem* 1993;266:20424.

52. Du XX, Neben T, Goldman S, et al. Effects of recombinant human interleukin-11 on hematopoietic reconstitution in transplant mice: acceleration of recovery of peripheral blood neutrophils and platelets. *Blood* 1993;81:27.

53. Nakashima K, Taga T. gp130 and the IL-6 family of cytokines: signaling mechanisms and thrombopoietic activities. *Semin Hematol* 1998;35:210–221.

54. Gough NM, Gearing DP, King JA, et al. Molecular cloning and expression of the human homologue of the murine gene encoding myeloid leukemia-inhibitory factor. *Proc Natl Acad Sci USA* 1988;85:2623.

55. Metcalf D, Nicola NA, Gearing DP. Effects of injected leukemia inhibitory factor on hematopoietic and other tissues in mice. *Blood* 1990;76:50.

56. Smith AG, Heath JK, Donaldson DD, et al. Inhibition of pluripotential embryonic stem cell differentiation by purified polypeptides. *Nature* 1988;336:688.

57. Wallace PM, MacMaster JF, Rillema JR, et al. Thrombocytopoietic properties of oncostatin M. *Blood* 1995;86:1310–1315.

58. Baggiolini M, Walz M, Kunkel SL. Neutrophil-activating peptide-1/interleukin-8, a novel cytokine that activates neutrophils. *J Clin Invest* 1989;84:1045.

59. Peveri P, Walz A, Dewald B, et al. A novel neutrophil activating factor produced by human mononuclear phagocytes. *J Exp Med* 1988;167:1547.

60. Koch AE, Polverini PJ, Kunkel SL, et al. Interleukin-8 as a macrophage-derived mediator of angiogenesis. *Science* 1992;258:1798.

61. Broxmeyer HE, Cooper S, Cacalano G, et al. Involvement of interleukin 8 receptor in negative regulation of myeloid progenitor cells *in vivo*: evidence from mice lacking the murine IL-8 receptor homologue. *J Exp Med* 1996;184:1825–1832.

62. Dinarello CA, Novick D, Puren AJ, et al. Overview of interleukin-18: more than an interferon-gamma inducing factor. *J Leukoc Biol* 1998;63:658–664.

63. Martin TJ, Romas E, Gillespie MT. Interleukins in the

control of osteoclast differentiation. *Crit Rev Eukaryot Gene Expr* 1998;8:107–123.

64. Bagby GC, Dinarello CA, Wallace P, et al. Interleukin-1 stimulates granulocyte macrophage colony stimulating activity release by vascular endothelial cells. *J Clin Invest* 1986;78:1316.

65. Broudy VC, Kaushansky K, Harlan JM, et al. Interleukin-1 stimulates human endothelial cells to produce granulocyte macrophage colony-stimulating factor and granulocyte colony-stimulating factor. *J Immunol* 1987; 139:464.

66. Maury CP, Andersson LC, Teppo AM, et al. Mechanism of anaemia in rheumatoid arthritis: demonstration of raised interleukin 1 beta concentrations in anaemic patients and of interleukin 1 mediated suppression of normal erythropoiesis and proliferation of human erythroleukaemia (HEL) cells *in vitro*. *Ann Rheum Dis* 1988; 47:972–978.

67. Lee GR. The anemia of chronic disease. *Semin Hematol* 1983;20:61–80.

68. Zucali JR, Broxmeyer HE, Dinarello CA, et al. Regulation of early human hematopoietic (BFU-E and CFU-GEMM) progenitor cells *in vitro* by interleukin 1-induced fibroblast conditioned medium. *Blood* 1987;69: 33.

69. Kelley KW, Arkins S, Minshall C, et al. Growth hormone, growth factors and hematopoiesis. *Horm Res* 1996;45:38–45.

70. Arkins S, Rebeiz N, Brunke-Reese DL, et al. The colony-stimulating factors induce expression of insulin-like growth factor-I messenger ribonucleic acid during hematopoiesis. *Endocrinology* 1995;136:1153–1160.

71. Yasuda H, Shima N, Nakagawa N, et al. Osteoclast differentiation factor is a ligand for osteoprotegerin/osteoclastogenesis inhibitory factor and is identical to TRANCE/RANKL. *Proc Natl Acad Sci USA* 1998;95: 3597–3602.

72. Anderson DM, Maraskovsky E, Billingsley WL, et al.

A homologue of the TNF receptor and its ligand enhance T-cell growth and dendritic-cell function. *Nature* 1997; 390:175.

73. Mills BG, Frausto A. Cytokines expressed in multinucleated cells: Paget's disease and giant cell tumors versus normal bone. *Calcif Tissue Int* 1997;61:16–21.

74. Siever DA, Erickson HP. Extracellular annexin II. *Int J Biochem Cell Biol* 1997;29:1219–1223.

75. Menaa C, Devlin RD, Reddy SV, et al. Annexin II increases osteoclast formation by stimulating the proliferation of osteoclast precursors in human marrow cultures. *J Clin Invest* 1999;103:1603–1613.

76. Kukita T, Nomiyama H, Ohmoto Y, et al. Macrophage inflammatory protein-1 alpha (LD78) expressed in human bone marrow: its role in regulation of hematopoiesis and osteoclast recruitment. *Lab Invest* 1997;76: 399–406.

77. Fuller K, Owens JM, Chambers TJ. Macrophage inflammatory protein-1 alpha and IL-8 stimulate the motility but suppress the resorption of isolated rat osteoclasts. *J Immunol* 1995;154:6065–6072.

78. Cook DN. The role of MIP-1 alpha in inflammation and hematopoiesis. *J Leukoc Biol* 1996;59:61–66.

79. Alsina M, Choi SJ, Cruz JC, et al. Overexpression of the osteoclast stimulatory factor (OSF), macrophage inflammatory protein 1-alpha (MIP-1α) in multiple myeloma (MM). *Blood* 1998;92:681a (abst 2805).

80. Taylor JL, Grossberg SE. Recent advances in interferon research: molecular mechanisms of regulation, action, and virus circumvention. *Virus Res* 1990;15:1–26.

81. Young HA, Klinman DM, Reynolds DA, et al. Bone marrow and thymus expression of interferon-gamma results in severe B-cell lineage reduction, T-cell lineage alterations, and hematopoietic progenitor deficiencies. *Blood* 1997;89:583–595.

82. Murray PJ, Young RA, Daley GQ. Hematopoietic remodeling in interferon-gamma-deficient mice infected with mycobacteria. *Blood* 1998;91:2914–2924.

Skeletal Growth Factors,
edited by Ernesto Canalis.
Lippincott Williams & Wilkins, Philadelphia, © 2000.

28

Colony-Stimulating Factors and Bone

Eleanor C. Weir, Gang-Qing Yao, *Yan Chen, and *Karl L. Insogna

*Departments of Comparative Medicine and *Internal Medicine, Yale School of Medicine,
New Haven, Connecticut 06520-8020*

Since bone cells arise in the hematopoietic microenvironment, there is considerable interest in exploring the role of hematopoietic growth factors in skeletal metabolism. This chapter is an effort to summarize recent work relevant to the roles of five growth factors in bone, colony-stimulating factor-I (CSF-1), granulocyte-macrophage colony-stimulating factor (GM-CSF), granulocyte colony-stimulating factor (G-CSF), stem cell factor (SCF), interleukin-3 (IL-3), and megakaryocyte growth and development factor (MGDF).

While abundant data have established a role for several of these factors in influencing osteoclastogenesis and mature osteoclast function, with the exception GM-CSF, little data exist supporting a role for any of these in regulating osteoblast differentiation or function. An important unanswered question is whether these factors act in any hierarchical manner during osteoclastogenesis or, with the exception of CSF-1, whether their osteoclastogenic activity represents a redundant or "spillover" function.

A separate section is devoted to each growth factor, and an effort has been made to organize each section in a similar fashion to facilitate access to the information and comparisons among the growth factors.

In an effort to conserve space, only critical references that deal with molecular biology and protein chemistry are cited in the sections devoted to these topics for each growth factor.

COLONY STIMULATING FACTOR-1

CSF-1 is a multifunctional cytokine that supports the proliferation, differentiation, and survival of cells of the monocyte-macrophage lineage and enhances the function of mature hematopoietic cells. CSF-1 was initially purified from human urine and mouse L cells and is now known to be synthesized and secreted by activated monocytes, mesenchymal cells (fibroblasts, osteoblasts, stromal cells), and epithelial cells. The protein and/or its mRNA has been identified in a number of tissues in humans and mice, including the central nervous system (astrocytes), kidney (mesangial cells), liver, lung, heart, spleen, placenta, and uterus. While the precise function of CSF-1 in many of these sites is unclear, spatiotemporal coexpression of the ligand and receptor and characterization of the CSF-1, deficient osteopetrotic (*op/op*) mouse suggest a role for CSF-1 in reproduction, brain development, and bone metabolism. Thus, high levels of both CSF-1 receptor mRNA in mouse placental trophoblasts and CSF-1 protein in the pregnant mouse uterus indicate a role for CSF-1 in placental development (1). Additionally, the *op/op* mouse shows poor ovulatory rates, small litters, and failure to lactate, indicating a role for CSF-1 in follicular development and ovulation, placental development, and development of the mammary gland during pregnancy (2,3). Neurological abnormalities in *op/op* mice and coexpression of CSF-1 and its receptor in astrocytes and microglia, respectively, suggest a role for CSF-1 in the central nervous system. Reproductive abnormalities in male *op/op* mice are thought to be due to abnormalities in development and function of the hypothalamic–pituitary–gonadal axis (4).

The CSF-1 gene is located on human chromosome 1p13-p21 and on mouse chromosome 3 at the *op* locus. The human gene is approximately 21 kb in length, comprising ten exons. Multiple human CSF-1 mRNA species (4.0, 3.0, 2.3, 1.9, and 1.6 kb) are transcribed from the CSF-1 gene. Molecular cloning of cDNAs derived from these transcripts has demonstrated that the size differences are due to alternative splicing in exon 6 and the alternative use of the 3′-end of exon 9 (0.68 kb) or 10 (2 kb). A combination of nucleotide sequence analysis and transfection studies indicates that two distinct CSF-1 protein products are encoded by these transcripts: a 256–amino acid precursor, derived from the 1.6- and 3.0-kb cDNAs, and a 554–amino acid precursor, derived from the 1.9-, 2.3-, and 4.0-kb cDNAs. Both primary translation products are membrane-bound glycoproteins that are released by proteolysis. The 1.6- and 3.0-kb CSF-1 cDNAs, however, give rise by alternative splicing, to a short exon 6 in which the site for proteolytic cleavage of the CSF-1 precursor has been spliced out. Thus, the products are cell surface– or membrane-bound glycoproteins that are slowly and inefficiently released from the cell surface by extracellular proteolysis (5,6). By contrast, the products of the 1.9-, 2.3-, and 4.0-kb cDNAs have intermediate or long versions of exon 6, in which the proteolytic cleavage site is intact, thus giving rise to products that are cleaved within the cell and rapidly released into the extracellular compartment as soluble growth factors (6,7). For both soluble and cell surface forms of CSF-1 the precursor polypeptides are dimerized via disulfide bonds and translationally glycosylated. A proteoglycan form of soluble CSF-1 which carries chondroitin sulfate glycosaminoglycan has also been identified (8). The latter form of the protein has a molecular mass of over 200 kDa, binds to type V collagen and has been identified in osteoblast-conditioned media (9,10).

The recombinant human CSF-1 dimer contains two bundles of four α helices, in which the helices run up–up–down–down. This structure is unlike the more commonly observed up–down–up–down connectivity of most four-helical bundles (11). There are three intramolecular disulfide bonds in each monomer, all of which are at the ends distal to the dimer interface. Mutation analyses have shown that the six Cys residues involved in these bonds are essential for biological activity. CSF-1 that expresses as few as the first 150 amino acids retains biological activity, indicating that the C-terminal region is not required (12).

Receptor

The receptor for CSF-1, c-fms, is a single high-affinity transmembrane receptor with a cytoplasmic domain that includes a split tyrosine kinase cassette similar to that seen in the platelet-derived growth factor (PDGF) receptor (13). C-fms is a member of a family that includes the PDGF-β receptor and c-kit, the stem cell receptor. The c-fms gene maps to chromosome 5 at band q33.3 in close proximity to the PDGF-β receptor, as well as to the genes for CSF-1, GM-CSF, IL-3, IL-4, and IL-5. The receptor includes a 512–amino acid extracellular segment containing the ligand-binding region, a hydrophobic 25–amino acid transmembrane region, and a 435–amino acid intracellular tail that includes the tyrosine kinase domain.

Signal Transduction

Ligand binding leads to receptor oligomerization and activation of the receptor's tyrosine kinase domain. This results in rapid tyrosine phosphorylation of selected cellular proteins and the recruitment of signaling molecules to the receptor. A large number of these proteins appear to exist as preassembled cytosolic complexes in close proximity to the membrane. Receptor activation results in an increase in the size of these complexes (14). Among the proteins recruited to the receptor is c-src. In cells engineered to overexpress c-fms, CSF-1 treatment induces c-src binding to Tyr^{599} in the cytoplasmic domain of c-fms, resulting in both an increase in src kinase activity and tyrosine phosphorylation of the protein (15). Similar results have recently been reported in osteoclasts *(infra vida)*.

Four other tyrosine residues in the cytoplasmic tail of c-fms, Tyr^{697}, Tyr^{706}, Tyr^{721}, and Tyr^{807} (amino acid numbers refer to murine fms) have been identified as important for downstream signaling events. Tyr^{697} is essential for binding of the adaptor protein Grb-2 (16). Grb-2 exists in association with the nucleotide exchange factor mammalian son of sevenless (SOS). When this complex associates with c-fms, it recruits and activates ras. This, in turn, activates a signaling cascade that eventuates in activation of mitogen-activated protein (MAP) kinase and subsequent induction of nuclear transcription factors such as c-myc, c-jun, c-fos, and elk-1. For example, CSF-1 induces transcriptional activation of fos within minutes of addition to bone marrow macrophages (17). Tyr^{721} is important for recruitment of phosphoinositol-3-kinase (PI3-K) and subsequent induction of phosphoinositol turnover (18). PI3-K has been implicated in the regulation of cytoskeletal function in a number of cell types following CSF-1 stimulation, and evidence indicates that this is also the case for osteoclasts *(infra vida)*.

Colony-Stimulating Factor-1 and Bone Metabolism

Knockout Animals

The most definitive *in vivo* studies demonstrating a role for CSF-1 in bone metabolism are those in the spontaneously occurring osteopetrotic *(op/op)* mouse. Mice homozygous for this mutation have an osteopetrotic phenotype, characterized by increased bone density, an occluded bone marrow cavity, and reduced marrow hematopoiesis. They are devoid of serum and tissue CSF-1, have reduced macrophages and monocytes, and have no osteoclasts (19–21). The mutation involves a 1-bp (thymidine) insertion in the exon 4 coding region of the gene for CSF-

1, resulting in generation of a stop codon 21 bp downstream and production of a truncated, nonfunctional CSF-1 (22). Treatment of mutant mice with CSF-1 corrects the defect in bone remodeling and hematopoiesis (23). Osteoblasts derived from *op/op* mice do not support osteoclast development *in vitro* (24), while exogenously added CSF-1 induces osteoclast formation in *op/op* hematopoietic cells (25,26). This suggests that the defect in osteoclastogenesis in these animals is not in the osteoclast progenitor cells but is a result of defective osteoblast-derived CSF-1. Interestingly, osteopetrosis and macrophage deficiency appear to correct with age (27). While the mechanism for this correction is unclear, it suggests that the hematopoietic and skeletal systems have alternative mechanisms to compensate for CSF-1 deficiency.

Production by Bone Cells

Several groups have reported that mouse and rat primary osteoblasts and osteoblast-like cells release CSF-1 constitutively and in response to parathyroid hormone (PTH), tumor necrosis factor (TNF), and IL-1 (28–32). While osteoblasts have been shown to release several hematopoietic growth factors, including CSF-1, GM-CSF, and G-CSF, the colony-stimulating activity released from rat osteoblasts in response to PTH and PTH-related protein (PTHrP) is predominantly due to CSF-1 (33). Murine and human osteoblasts and osteoblast-like cells also express CSF-1 mRNA, and TNF and PTH enhance expression via a transcriptional mechanism which, at least for PTH, appears to involve a cyclic adenosine monophosphate (cAMP)–mediated pathway (32–35). Figure 28.1 illustrates PTHrP and TNF-induced upregulation of CSF-1 mRNA in osteoblast-like cells.

More recently, detailed analysis of the CSF-1 isoforms synthesized and released by osteoblasts has been conducted. Using a combination of quantitative reverse-transcriptase polymerase chain reaction, flow cytometry, and Western immunoblot analysis, human osteoblast-like cells and primary osteoblasts have been shown to express soluble and cell surface CSF-1 (mRNA and protein), both constitutively and in response to

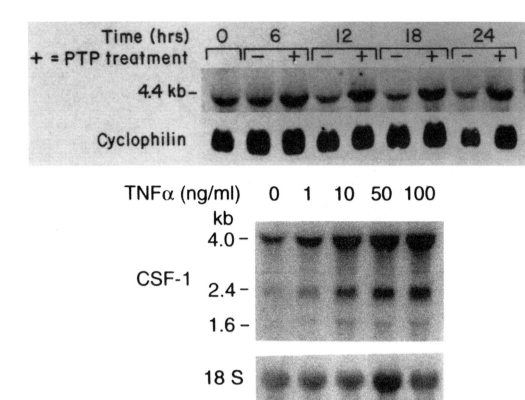

FIG. 28.1. **Upper Panel**: Time course of effect of parathyroid hormone–related protein (PTHrP) treatment on colony-stimulating factor-1 (CSF-1) transcript expression in ROS 17/2.8 cells. Cells were treated with 10^{-8} M PTHrP at the times indicated. An increase in transcript expression is seen at 6 hours and persists to 24 hours of treatment. (From ref. 33, with permission.) **Lower panel**: Dose-response of CSF-1 transcript expression to treatment with tumor necrosis factor-α *(TNF-α)* in MC3T3-E1 cells treated for 16 hours. (From ref. 32, with permission.)

TNF and PTH (34). Figure 28.2 illustrates flow-cytometric evidence for upregulation of cell surface CSF-1 by TNF and PTH in MG-63 and Saos-2 cells. Primary murine osteoblasts have also been reported to express cell surface CSF-1 constitutively and in response to dexamethasone (35,36). Limited studies on the protein structure of osteoblast-derived CSF-1 have revealed that a proteoglycan form is synthesized by murine and human osteoblasts and can be extracted from bone tissue and cultured osteoblast matrix (10).

Consistent with osteoblast expression of CSF-1 *in vitro, in situ* hybridization studies have revealed CSF-1 transcript expression in mouse metatarsal bones from day 18 of gestation. Expression increases throughout gestation, and postnatally, CSF-1 expression is detectable in

cells lining all bone surfaces. Expression of the CSF-1 receptor c-fms is also detectable in osteoclasts and mononuclear osteoclast precursors and appears to be spatiotemporally related to expression of the ligand (37,38). These findings suggest that locally produced CSF-1 plays a role in osteoclastogenesis and mature osteoclast function during bone development.

Recent intriguing observations have indicated that CSF-1 production is regulated by estrogen. These findings are covered in Chapter 29.

Role of CSF-1 in Osteoclastogenesis

In vitro data supporting a role for CSF-1 in bone remodeling were initially reported in the mid-1980s by MacDonald et al. (39), who ob-

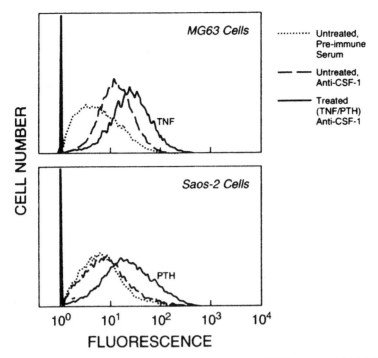

FIG. 28.2. Flow-cytometric analysis of tumor necrosis factor *(TNF)*–treated MG-63 cells **(upper panel)** and parathyroid hormone *(PTH)*–treated Saos-2 cells **(lower panel)** for cell surface colony-stimulating factor-1 *(CSF-1)*. Both osteotropic agents induce an increase in expression of cell surface CSF-1, as evidenced by an increase in fluorescence. (From ref. 34, with permission.)

served that CSF-1 stimulates formation of osteo-clast-like cells in long-term bone marrow culture. Following these initial studies, a variety of additional data have indicated that CSF-1 is critical for the proliferation and differentiation of osteoclast progenitors. Thus, in mouse osteoblast/bone marrow coculture systems, CSF-1 is the most effective CSF at stimulating osteoclast formation (39a) and, in a similar system, neutralization of endogenous CSF-1 during the proliferation or differentiation phase of osteoclastogenesis results in complete inhibition of osteoclast formation (25). CSF-1 has been shown to stimulate bone resorption in the fetal mouse metacarpal assay, which is designed to examine osteoclast formation (40); and a neutralizing antiserum to CSF-1 inhibits PTHrP-induced bone resorption in the fetal mouse metacarpal assay, suggesting a role for endogenous CSF-1 in PTHrP- (and presumably PTH-) induced bone resorption (41). While many earlier

studies indicated that CSF-1 plays a key role in osteoclastogenesis in mice, more recent *in vitro* studies also suggest a role in bone remodeling in humans. Primary human osteoblasts and osteoblast-like cells express the soluble and cell surface forms of CSF-1 constitutively and in response to TNF and PTH (34), and recombinant human CSF-1 has recently been shown to induce osteoclastogenesis and bone resorption in human marrow cultures (42).

In addition to a clear role for soluble CSF-1 in osteoclastogenesis, recent studies have suggested that the cell surface CSF-1 may mediate osteoclast formation via cell–cell contact with adjacent receptor-bearing cells in the bone microenvironment. Indirect evidence for such a role includes the observation of Takahashi et al. (24) that when osteoblasts from *op/op* (CSF-1-deficient) mice are cocultured with splenocytes, pharmacological amounts of CSF-1 are required to support osteoclast formation. Other studies have shown that much higher concentrations of soluble CSF-1 are required to induce osteo-clastogenesis in metatarsals from *op/op* mice than in metatarsals/metacarpals from normal mice (40,43). These findings suggest that cell surface CSF-1, either alone or in addition to sol-uble CSF-1, might be required for osteoclasto-genesis. Consistent with this hypothesis, it has recently been shown that glutaraldehyde-fixed NIH 3T3 cells transfected with the cDNA encod-ing the cell surface form of CSF-1 and glutaral-dehyde-fixed ST-2 stromal cells support forma-tion of osteoclast-like cells in an *in vitro* coculture system (34,44).

CSF-1 is also thought to play a role in mature osteoclast function. The CSF-1 receptor is ex-pressed by mature osteoclasts (33,37), and CSF-1 has been shown to induce c-fms autophosphor-ylation and to activate the cytoplasmic tyrosine kinase c-src in osteoclasts (45). Figure 28.3 shows the increases in plasma membrane phos-

photyrosine staining observed in authentic rat osteoclasts exposed to CSF-1. Figure 28.4 dem-onstrates CSF-1-dependent tyrosine phosphory-lation of c-src in murine osteoclast-like cells. This latter observation is of interest since c-src is known to be critically important for osteoclast function. Targeted disruption of the src gene leads to osteopetrosis in mice due to a defect in the resorptive function of mature osteoclasts (46). CSF-1 is one of the few growth factors re-ported to increase src-kinase activity (45). CSF-1 also increases osteoclast migration/chemotaxis and spreading and inhibits apoptosis (47). Re-cent work has suggested that PI-3K is required for the chemotactic and cytoskeletal changes in-duced by CSF-1 (48), and CSF-1 has been shown to activate PI-3K in osteoclast-like cells (49,50).

The precise effect of CSF-1 on mature osteo-clast resorptive function, however, is unclear. CSF-1 has been reported to directly inhibit re-sorption by isolated rat osteoclasts (51). Consis-

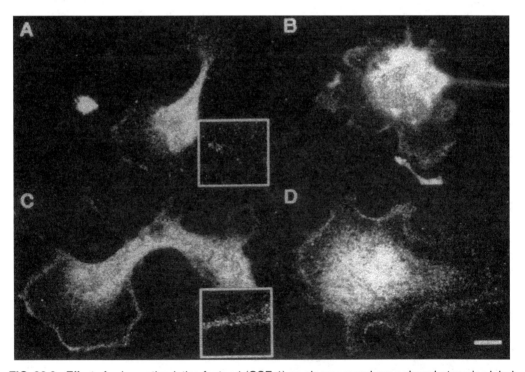

FIG. 28.3. Effect of colony-stimulating factor-1 (CSF-1) on plasma membrane phosphotyrosine label-ing in authentic rat osteoclasts. Control **(A)** and 30 seconds **(B),** 2 minutes **(C),** and 5 minutes **(D)** after treatment with 2.5 nM CSF-1. Note the increase in plasma membrane labeling highlighted in the **insert.** (From ref. 45, with permission.)

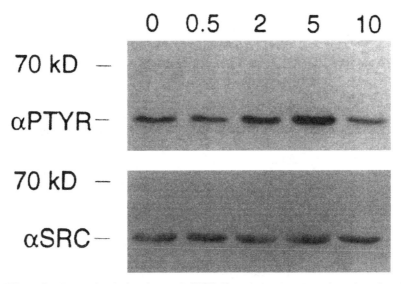

FIG. 28.4. Effect of colony-stimulating factor-1 (CSF-1) treatment on tyrosine phosphorylation of c-src in osteoclast-like cells. The **upper panel** shows phosphotyrosine staining of immunoprecipitated c-src at different times after CSF-1 treatment, and the **bottom panel** shows the same membrane stripped and reprobed for src. Increased phosphotyrosine staining noted at 5 minutes was associated with an increase in kinetic activity of the enzyme. (From ref. 45, with permission.)

tent with these findings, neutralizing antisera to CSF-1 increase PTH-induced bone resorption in the fetal rat long bone assay (40), suggesting that CSF-1 has a restraining effect on the resorptive function of mature osteoclasts. In contrast, Lees and Heersche (52) have reported an increase in size and resorptive activity in rabbit osteoclasts treated with CSF-1.

Osteoclast differentiation factor (ODF), also known as TNF-related activation-induced cytokine (TRANCE), receptor activator of NFκB (RANK) ligand, and osteoprotegerin (OPG) ligand, has been identified recently as a cytokine critically important for osteoclast differentiation and activation. Targeted disruption of the ODF gene results in severe osteopetrosis with a complete failure of osteoclast development. This is due to an osteoblast defect since osteoblasts isolated from ODF knockout mice cannot support osteoclast differentiation while the marrow of these animals can be shown to contain normal numbers of functional osteoclast precursors. ODF has been shown to be expressed on the surface of osteoblasts and to be regulated by osteotropic hormones. ODF and CSF-1 together appear to be both necessary and sufficient for osteoclastogenesis to occur (53,54). It has been suggested that CSF-1 is required only for osteoclast progenitor survival and proliferation and that ODF is capable of inducing the full differentiation program for osteoclasts. The finding that transgenic overexpression of Bcl-2 in monocyte-macrophage precursors corrects the osteopetrotic phenotype of *op/op* mice is consistent with the notion that CSF-1 simply promotes survival of osteoclast progenitors (55). However, *in vitro* data suggest that in cocultures of osteoblasts and murine marrow, CSF-1 is required for both early and late stages of differentiation (25).

In summary, of all of the growth factors discussed in this chapter, CSF-1 is the only one with a clear nonredundant role in bone. Its appropriate expression is absolutely required for normal osteoclastogenesis to occur. In addition, it appears to profoundly influence mature osteoclast function, although how it does so in the bone microenvironment remains unclear. There are several important unanswered questions about CSF-1. Is it simply a survival factor for osteoclast progenitors or does it play a role in the differentiation program of these cells? Does it stimulate or inhibit the resorptive activity of mature osteoclasts? Is it a chemoattractant for mature osteoclasts *in vivo* and, if so, how? Do its different isoforms have different biological actions in bone? What are the molecular targets downstream from activated c-fms in mature osteoclasts and osteoclast progenitors? The answers to these questions should help to clarify the role of this important growth factor in bone.

GRANULOCYTE-MACROPHAGE COLONY-STIMULATING FACTOR

GM-CSF is a monomeric glycoprotein which supports, *in vitro,* the proliferation of early progenitor cells for granulocytes, erythrocytes, megakaryocytes, macrophages, and eosinophils. GM-CSF also influences the function of mature cells of the granulocyte-macrophage series, including inhibition of neutrophil migration, induction of neutrophil phagocytosis, and enhancement of macrophage tumoricidal activity.

The molecular mass of the core protein is approximately 14 kDa, but due to variable glycosylation, purification of natural and recombinant GM-CSF yields proteins with a molecular mass of 14 to 35 kDa for humans and 18 to 25 kDa for the murine protein. The amino acid sequences for human and mouse GM-CSF are 60% homologous. Both contain four cysteine residues, suggesting that disulfide bridges may be a component of the molecule. GM-CSF is encoded by a single-copy gene, which is located on chromosome 5 in humans (region 5q21-32) and 11 in mice and consists of four exons and three introns. The nucleotide sequence in humans and mice is 70% homologous. The residues on the GM-CSF molecule involved in binding to its cellular receptor are located in four general regions: residues 18 to 22, 34 to 41, 52 to 61, and 94 to 115. Residues responsible for interaction with the β chain of the receptor are located within the first α helix (residues 18 to 22).

GM-CSF is produced by a wide range of cell types, including T lymphocytes, macrophages, endothelial cells, and fibroblasts in response to mediators of inflammation. Keratinocytes, tro- phoblasts, mesangial cells, and smooth muscle cells also produce GM-CSF.

Receptor

The biological effects of human GM-CSF are mediated through binding of the growth factor to high-affinity receptors expressed in relatively low numbers on responding cells. In addition to expression on hematopoietic cells, GM-CSF receptors have been identified on several nonhematopoietic cells, including small cell carcinoma and adenocarcinoma cell lines, COS cells, placenta, and melanoma. The human GM-CSF receptor consists of two subunits, a low-affinity α subunit and a β subunit which is shared among the receptor systems for GM-CSF, IL-3, and IL-5 but which does not by itself bind to any of these cytokines. Coexpression of the α and β chains, however, confers high-affinity GM-CSF binding to responsive cells (56).

Signal Transduction

The β subunit has a long intracytoplasmic tail that plays a major role in signal transduction (57). Signaling by the GM-CSF receptor depends on the activation of the tyrosine phosphorylation pathways mediated by the stimulation of tyrosine kinases, lyn, fes, and Jak2 (58–60). These subsequently interact with Src homology 2 (SH2) domains of signaling intermediates like Stat5, Grb2, and Shc as well as PI-3K (61–63). In contrast to the β chain, the α chain has a very small cytoplasmic domain that lacks tyrosine residues phosphorylated by Jak2 or other kinases and was originally believed to play little role in signaling. This, however, is being challenged by reports suggesting its involvement in regulating cell proliferation and differentiation (64).

Granulocyte-Macrophage Colony-Stimulating Factor and Bone Metabolism

Knockout Mice

While GM-CSF administration has been shown to stimulate hematopoiesis *in vivo,* characterization of a GM-CSF knockout mouse has suggested that the growth factor is not critical for basal hematopoiesis since homozygous mice have relatively normal populations of circulating and progenitor hematopoietic cells. However, knockout mice develop a progressive lung disorder, characterized by accumulation of surfactant lipids and proteins in the alveolar space, with an associated susceptibility to pulmonary infections, thus indicating a critical role for GM-CSF in pulmonary homeostasis (65).

Production by and Effects on Osteoblasts

As for CSF-1, a role for GM-CSF was originally proposed by MacDonald et al. (39), who showed that GM-CSF increases the formation of osteoclast-like cells in long-term marrow cultures. A number of studies subsequently demon-strated that osteoblasts release GM-CSF in response to osteotropic agents. Primary mouse osteoblasts and a clonal mouse osteoblast cell line were reported to release GM-CSF in response to lipopolysaccharide (LPS) and PTH, and clonal rat osteoblasts and osteoblast-like cells were shown to secrete GM-CSF constitu-tively and in response to PTH, LPS, and TNF (66–68). Figure 28.5 summarizes data demon-strating the release of GM-CSF from PTH-treated ROS 17/2.8 cells.

In addition to releasing GM-CSF, osteoblasts have been shown to respond to GM-CSF. Evans et al. (69) reported that GM-CSF induces prolif-eration of human osteoblast-like cells *in vitro*, while antagonizing the effect of 1,25(OH)$_2$D$_3$-induced osteocalcin synthesis and alkaline phos-phatase activity. GM-CSF also induces TNF re-

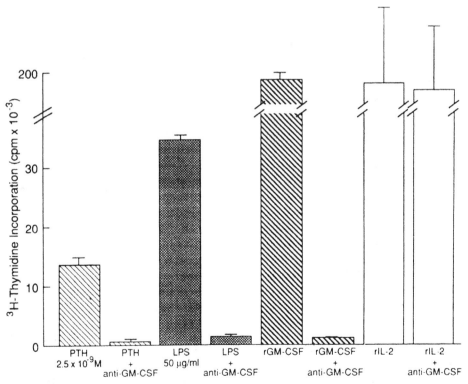

FIG. 28.5. Effect of anti-lipopolysaccharide granulocyte-macrophage colony-stimulating factor *(GM-CSF)* antibody on HT2 mitogenesis induced by parathyroid hormone *(PTH)* and lipopolysaccharide *(LPS)* in ROS cell–conditioned media or by recombinant murine GM-CSF or recombinant murine interleukin-2 *(IL-2)*. Neutralizing antisera to GM-CSF completely block the HT2 mitogenic activity in PTH- and LPS-treated media as well as the effect of GM-CSF but have no effect on the ability of IL-2 to induce mitogenesis. (From ref. 67, with permission.)

lease from primary human osteoblasts (70). Modrowski and coworkers (71) have reported that
GM-CSF is mitogenic for human osteoblasts.
This mitogenic activity was enhanced when
GM-CSF was exposed to matrix elaborated by
human osteoblasts, presumably due to binding to
glycosaminoglycans (71). Human osteosarcoma
cells have been reported to produce a cell-associated form of GM-CSF (72). Thus, in addition to
its potential osteoclastogenic activity, as described below, GM-CSF may play an autocrine
or paracrine role in regulating osteoblast activity.

Osteoclastogenesis

Since GM-CSF was first reported to induce
formation of osteoclast-like cells *in vitro*, a number of subsequent studies have led to conflicting
conclusions on the role of GM-CSF in osteoclastogenesis. Macrophage and osteoclast differentiation are regulated by several growth factors,
including GM-CSF. GM-CSF, like CSF-1, is
able to induce terminal macrophage differentiation, and GM-CSF has been reported to induce
the formation of osteoclast-like cells *in vitro* in
mouse osteoblast–bone marrow cocultures and
in long-term baboon marrow culture (39a,73).
GM-CSF also induces changes in expression of
the $\beta 3$ and $\beta 5$ integrin subunits in bone marrow
macrophages, which are consistent with early
differentiation toward an osteoclast phenotype
(74). Lee and coworkers (75) observed that
C57B16 mice treated with 450 ng per day of
GM-CSF evidenced an increase in osteoclast
numbers, with enlargement of the medullary
area and a decrease in bone thickness. Further,
Myint et al. (76) have recently reported that administration of 5 ng per day of GM-CSF to
young *op/op* mice led to an expansion of the
marrow cavity and an increase in the number of
tartrate-resistant acid phosphatase (TRAP)–positive cells present in bone.

By contrast, a number of other studies suggest
that GM-CSF does not induce, or even inhibits,
osteoclast formation. Thus, in an earlier report,
Wiktor-Jedrzejczak et al. (77) found that when
GM-CSF was administered to *op/op* mice at
higher doses (20 to 40 μg per day) than reported

above, it corrected the macrophage deficiency
but had no effect on bone abnormalities in these
animals. It is possible that a biphasic osteoclastogenic response to GM-CSF explains these
differences. The findings of Wiktor-Jedrzejczak
and coworkers (77) are consistent with those of
Hattersley et al. (26), who showed that while
GM-CSF induces macrophages in *op/op* hematopoietic cells, it is unable to induce osteoclast
formation. GM-CSF has also been shown to reduce bone resorption and inhibit formation of
calcitonin receptor–positive cells in mouse marrow cultures (78). Studies conducted by Shuto et
al. (79,80) indicate that, in mouse bone marrow
cultures, GM-CSF suppresses LPS-induced osteoclast formation and that dexamethasone stimulates osteoclast-like cell formation via inhibition of endogenous GM-CSF production. IL-18
is produced by osteoblasts and inhibits osteoclastogenesis. Two recent reports have indicated
that this inhibitory effect is mediated by IL-18-
induced GM-CSF production by T cells (81,82).

The reasons for these conflicting data are unclear, particularly since the experimental conditions in all studies are not identical. It has been
suggested that, assuming that osteoclasts and
macrophages are derived from a common precursor, GM-CSF diverts the progenitor population toward the macrophage or granulocyte lineage and away from osteoclast development. An
alternative explanation is that, since GM-CSF
has been shown to downregulate expression of
the CSF-1 receptor *c-fms*, GM-CSF may abro-
gate the response to CSF-1 (83). Since CSF-1
is known to be critical for osteoclast formation,
GM-CSF may thus inhibit osteoclastogenesis. A
third explanation suggested by Hattersley et al.
(26) is that the macrophage population induced
by GM-CSF cannot substitute for CSF-1-in-
duced macrophages and is unable to form osteoclasts.

In summary, GM-CSF appears to be the only
CSF that acts on osteoblasts, where it appears
to be mitogenic. However, its physiological role
in mediating osteoblast function remains unclear. Similarly, data on its osteoclastogenic
properties are conflicting, although most recent
data tend to suggest an inhibitory effect.

GRANULOCYTE COLONY-STIMULATING FACTOR

G-CSF is a lineage-specific growth factor that stimulates granulopoiesis. The cellular sources of G-CSF in the hematopoietic microenvironment are thought to be primarily macrophages and fibroblasts. Because of its widespread clinical use, G-CSF has been extensively studied and there have been several reports describing its effects in bone.

G-CSF is a glycoprotein with an estimated mass of 20 kDa. The gene for G-CSF is located on human chromosome 17q21-q22 and on mouse chromosome 11. The G-CSF transcript is approximately 1.5 kb in size, and the human, but not the mouse, G-CSF gene produces alternatively spliced mRNAs. The mature human G-CSF protein is 174 amino acids in length. An alternatively spliced transcript for human G-CSF encodes a 177–amino acid protein that has considerably reduced specific activity. Human G-CSF contains five cystine residues, four of which are connected by disulfide bonds. Mutational analysis of the cystine residues indicates that these disulfide bonds are essential for proper folding of the molecule and biological activity. Human and mouse G-CSF are 73.6% identical at the amino acid sequence level and can interact with each other's receptors. G-CSF has a four-α-helical bundle structure. Mutational analysis of human G-CSF and epitope mapping with neutralizing antibodies indicate that amino acid residues 20 to 46 as well as the C terminus are important for binding to the receptor.

Receptor

The human G-CSF receptor gene is located on chromosome 1p35-34.3 and is composed of 17 exons spanning about 17 kb. The mature protein has an estimated mass of 100 to 300 kDa. The extracellular region of the receptor comprises six structural domains: an N-terminal immunoglobulin (Ig)-like domain, a cytokine receptor homologous module (CRHM) containing two fibronectin type III-like (FNIII) domains, and three additional FNIII domains. The CRHM and Ig domain of the G-CSF receptor have been implicated in ligand binding, whereas the three membrane-proximal FNIII domains may play a role in receptor stability and/or signal transduction. The Ig domain is required for receptor dimerization. The cytoplasmic region of the G-CSF receptor carries no motif for enzymatic activities such as tyrosine kinase and phosphatase. A 76–amino acid stretch proximal to the transmembrane domain in the cytoplasmic region is essential for transducing the growth signal, while both N-terminal and C-terminal domains of the cytoplasmic region are indispensable for transducing the differentiation signal.

Signal Transduction

The G-CSF receptor forms homoligomeric complexes upon ligand binding. Important signaling molecules utilized by the G-CSF receptor include the Janus tyrosine kinases (JAKs), the src kinases p55lyn and p56/59hck; and STATs 1, 3, and 5 (84–87). The G-CSF receptor has no intrinsic tyrosine kinase activity but activates cytoplasmic tyrosine kinases such as lyn and hck. Ligation of the G-CSF receptor results in the rapid phosphorylation of tyrosine residues in the cytoplasmic tail of the β subunit, which serve as docking sites for complexes of signaling molecules such as Shc/Grb2/p140 (88). Analysis of signaling pathways downstream suggest a positive role for STAT 3 activation in both differentiation and survival signaling, whereas SHP-2, Grb2, and Shc appear to be important for proliferation signaling.

Granulocyte Colony-Stimulating Factor and Bone Metabolism

Knockout and Transgenic Mice

G-CSF knockout mice have been generated and are neutropenic with reduced hematopoietic progenitors in the bone marrow and spleen. They do not appear to have any bony abnormalities (89). However, overexpression of G-CSF has been reported to lead to osteoporosis in mice. Takahashi et al. (90) have found that animals with high-level transgenic G-CSF expression under the control of the SR-α promoter com-

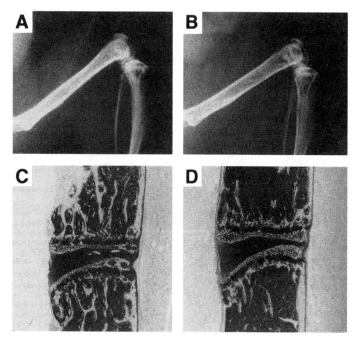

FIG. 28.6. Radiography and transverse sections of bones from transgenic mice overexpressing granulocyte colony-stimulating factor (G-CSF). Normal specimens are shown in **A** and **C** and specimens obtained from transgenic mice in **B** and **D**. Note the obvious cortical thinning in **B** versus **A** and the loss of trabecular bone in **D** versus **C**. (From ref. 90, with permission.)

prised of the SV40 early promoter and the HtLv-I-long terminal regeat have cortical thinning, enlarged bone marrow cavities in both vertebral bodies and long bones, and both biochemical and histomorphometric evidence for increased bone resorption and bone turnover (Fig. 28.6). Similar findings have been observed in rats administered high doses of recombinant human G-CSF (91). In these experiments, rats were treated with G-CSF for 28 days. Histological changes included accelerated osteoclastic bone resorption; focal areas of increased resorption and formation were observed throughout the skeleton. Earlier reports in rats and mice also documented increased resorptive activity in animals treated with recombinant human G-CSF. Using dexamethasone, Soshi et al. (92) have reported that rats treated with G-CSF have significantly reduced bone mineral density in the lumbar vertebrae and femora when compared with vehicle-treated animals.

Skeletal Effects in Humans

Evidence also exists for skeletal effects of G-CSF when given in therapeutic doses to humans. Osteopenia and osteoporosis have been reported in patients receiving chronic therapy with G-CSF for treatment of congenital neutropenia (93). Fifteen of 44 patients with severe congenital neutropenia treated for 4 to 6 years with G-CSF had reduced bone mass, while none of ten patients with cyclical neutropenia evidenced such changes. In the patients with severe congenital neutropenia, radiographic evidence existed in some individuals for reduced bone mass prior to the initiation of treatment. Thus, it is unclear whether the therapy per se or differences in severity of the underlying disease is responsible for these findings.

A number of malignant tumors have been described that overproduce G-CSF (94). Takeuchi et al. (95) reported the case of a patient with a lung carcinoma producing large amounts of G-

CSF, which was associated with scintigraphic evidence of increased bone turnover. These tumors have, in some patients, caused hypercalcemia; but when studied, the etiology of the hypercalcemia has been ascribed to other factors produced by the tumor, such as IL-1α or PTHrP (96).

In humans, a major side effect of G-CSF treatment is bone pain (97). Froberg et al. (98) reported that when seven healthy progenitor-cell donors were treated with recombinant G-CSF for 5 days, all developed bone pain with elevations in serum levels of bone-specific alkaline phosphatase. Interestingly, osteocalcin levels decreased and there were no significant changes in serum levels of TRAP. The authors concluded that effects on osteoblasts might be responsible for some of the bone pain observed with G-CSF treatment. Takamatsu et al. (99) showed that osteocalcin levels were reduced in individuals treated with G-CSF for 3 days, which was associated with biochemical evidence for increased bone resorption. In the same report, using a murine model, they observed increased excretion of urine deoxypyridinoline in association with evidence for increased osteoclast numbers on histomorphometric analysis of bone from treated mice. These changes were inhibited by treatment with the bisphosphonate pamidronate.

Production by Bone Cells

There are at least three reports indicating that osteoblasts and osteoblast-like cells produce G-CSF. Felix et al. (100) reported, using a bioassay, that conditioned media from LPS-treated mouse calvariae contained G-CSF-like bioactivity. This activity was also present in conditioned media from cultured calvarial cells prepared by serial collagenase digestion. The same group (66) reported the production of G-CSF by rat osteoblastic cells. These experiments did not employ specific neutralizing antibodies to G-CSF to confirm the nature of the bioactivity observed. More recently, Teichmann and Emerson (72) reported that two human osteosarcoma cell lines, MG-63 and Saos-2, expressed transcripts for G-CSF protein. These cell lines produced several species of G-CSF, including the 28- and 32-kDa cell-associated forms, suggesting that G-

CSF may be produced locally in bone by osteoblasts in a membrane-associated isoform.

Role in Osteoclastogenesis

The cellular targets in bone for G-CSF are unknown. Because of its effects on osteoclastogenesis, it is assumed that G-CSF may directly stimulate osteoclast progenitor proliferation or differentiation. Thus, G-CSF treatment facilitates clonogenic osteoclast progenitor formation from hematopoietic stem cells in lymphoid long-term cultures (100a), and normal peripheral blood mononuclear cells, mobilized with G-CSF, have increased osteoclastogenic potential (101). *In vitro,* G-CSF does not appear to stimulate bone resorption in traditional assays using fetal mouse long bones (102).

Whether G-CSF can exert effects on osteoclastogenesis indirectly by influencing osteoblast or stromal function is unclear. However, at least one report provides evidence that G-CSF may affect stromal cell function. Fukushima et al. (103) have found that splenic stromal cells isolated from mice treated with G-CSF specifically bound radiolabeled cytokine and had greater colony-stimulating activity than cells isolated from untreated mice. Further, at least one stromal line isolated from G-CSF-treated mice produced IL-6 and GM-CSF, two cytokines that are capable of influencing osteoclastogenesis.

In summary, G-CSF appears to significantly increase osteoclastogenesis *in vitro* and *in vivo*. This appears to be clinically relevant insofar as abnormalities are observed in patients receiving G-CSF in therapeutic doses. The mechanisms by which G-CSF induces osteoclastogenesis are obscure but may involve not only stimulation of osteoclast progenitor proliferation and/or survival but may also involve influencing the liberation of osteoclastogenic activities from stromal cells and osteoblasts.

STEM CELL FACTOR

SCF stimulates the growth of primitive hematopoietic progenitor cells. Murine and human SCF map to chromosomes 10 and 12, respectively. This gene yields predominantly a single mRNA species of 6.5 kb. SCF is expressed in different isoforms, determined by alternate splicing. Full-length SCF is 248 amino acids long; is comprised of extracellular, transmembrane, and cytoplasmic domains; and is initially expressed at the cell surface. Presumed proteolytic cleavage results in the production of a soluble form of the molecule, derived from the extracellular domain. Alternate splicing also leads to production of a shorter form, which lacks the proteolytic cleavage site and therefore tends to remain membrane-bound. Evidence exists for functional differences between soluble and membrane-bound SCFs *(infra vida)*. Soluble SCF is secreted as a glycoprotein monomer. The core protein is 18.4 kDa but contains both *N*-linked and *O*-linked carbohydrate residues, which increase the apparent molecular weight to 30 to 35 kDa and to approximately 45 kDa for the dimeric form. Glycosylation is not necessary for biological activity, as recombinant *Escherichia coli*–derived material is active *in vitro*. The protein sequence is highly conserved across species, and there is >80% amino acid homology between the murine and human forms.

Receptor

The cell surface receptor for SCF is the product of the protooncogene c-kit and is a transmembrane protein tyrosine kinase belonging to the subfamily which includes the PDGF receptor. In the hematopoietic system, c-kit mutations affect the stem cell compartment, erythroid precursors, tissue mast cells, and platelets (104). The human kit cDNA encodes a signal sequence (amino acids 1 to 23) followed by an extracellular domain (amino acids 24 to 520, five Ig-like domains), a hydrophobic transmembrane region (amino acids 521 to 543), and a cytoplasmic domain (residues 544 to 976) which includes a split kinase domain. Two forms of c-kit arise as a consequence of alternative mRNA splicing. The soluble form has been found in the conditioned media of cells that express c-kit and at high levels in human serum. The major expression product at the cell surface is a glycoprotein with a molecular weight of about 145 kDa.

Signal Transduction

The intracytoplasmic protein tyrosine kinase portion of c-kit transduces a diverse array of cellular responses, including proliferation, differentiation, and cell survival. After binding SCF, the receptor is autophosphorylated at a number of discrete sites within its C-terminal cytoplasmic domain. Following autophosphorylation at these sites, the src family members lyn, PI-3K, and phospholipase C1 are recruited to the activated receptor. Lyn has been found to associate with a juxtamembrane region of c-kit (amino acids 544 to 577), and SCF induces rapid increases in both tyrosine phosphorylation of lyn and its kinase activity *in vitro*.

Stem Cell Factor and Bone Metabolism

Knockout Animals

Naturally occuring mutations in the murine genes encoding SCF and c-kit have implicated these molecules in hematopoiesis, coat color, and gonadal development (105). Animals completely deficient in SCF, the Steel locus, die before birth, and detailed skeletal analyses have not been reported. Similarly, animals completely deficient in c-kit, the W locus, typically die in perinatal life. In *mi/mi* mice, which have molecular defects in the helix–loop–helix–leucine zipper transcription factor mi, c-kit expression is diminished (106). As described below, c-kit is expressed on osteoclasts and their progenitors, and it is therefore possible that reduced c-kit expression may play a role in the pathogenesis of the osteopetrotic phenotype observed in *mi/mi* mice.

Functionally different roles for the two forms of SCF have been identified by selective expression of these two isoforms in animals lacking SCF. The transgenic expression of the membrane form results in significant improvement in erythropoiesis and runting, while expression of the soluble form only improves myelopoiesis without effects on erythropoiesis or growth (107).

Transgenic overexpression of the membrane-associated isoform of human SCF leads to a "knockdown" phenotype because human SCF antagonizes endogenous murine SCF. These animals demonstrate abnormalities in coat color but have not been reported to have abnormalities in the skeleton or hematopoiesis.

Production by Bone Cells

Recent reports have identified SCF as a product of osteoblasts. Blair et al. (108) have reported that nontransformed osteoblasts as well as osteosarcoma cells express the membrane isoform of SCF. Expression of this isoform was stimulated by PTH but not by vitamin D (108). Consistent with this finding, this group has reported that in hyperparathyroid individuals *in situ* analysis of bone biopsy specimens demonstrated high-level expression of SCF by metabolically active osteoblasts (109,110). This expression was also observed in normal biopsies, but the extent of osteoblast activation, and therefore SCF expression, was proportionately less. Since SCF is critical for mast cell development, the authors postulated that enhanced mast cell expression in hyperparathyroid bone is a reflection of increased local SCF expression by activated osteoblasts.

Role in Osteoclastogenesis

Several studies have suggested a role for SCF in osteoclastogenesis (Fig. 28.7). In 1992, De-

mulder and colleagues (111) reported the effects of SCF on osteoclastogenesis in long-term human marrow cultures. They found that SCF could enhance osteoclast progenitor proliferation from unfractionated human marrow preparations. However, when a CD34$^+$-enriched population of cells was used, SCF was unable to increase osteoclast precursor colony formation. They concluded that SCF acted at an early step in osteoclastogenesis but other factors were required for the full differentiation program of osteoclasts to be effected. Consistent with this observation is the finding that preosteoclasts appear to express c-kit. Muguruma and Lee (112) found that cells in a marrow fraction enriched for osteoclast precursors express c-kit. However, the cells with the highest level of c-kit expression largely generated colony-forming unit–macrophage (CFU-M), CFU-GM, and CFU-SCF colonies, while hematopoietic progenitors of osteoclasts had lower levels of c-kit expression (112). The preosteoclast cell line FLG29.1 has also been reported to express c-kit, and SCF stimulated proliferation of these cells (113). Blair and colleagues (114), using an *in vitro* coculture that employed human macrophages and human osteosarcoma cells, found that antisera to SCF blocked osteoclast formation.

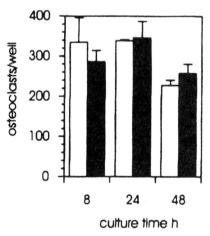
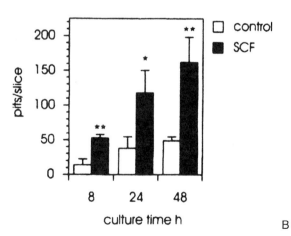

A   B

FIG. 28.7. Effect of stem cell factor *(SCF)* on osteoclast formation and activity. Osteoclasts were cultured on dentin slides for the indicated times and the cell number **(A)** as well as the pits per slice **(B)** quantitated. Note that over the 48-hour time course there is no increase in osteoclast number in SCF-treated wells as compared to control wells, while there is a marked increase in resorptive activity over the same time period. (From ref. 115, with permission.)

Mature osteoclasts also have been reported to express c-kit and to be activated by SCF. Thus, Gattei et al. (113) have reported, using immunohistochemical methods, that c-kit can be identified in human osteoclasts resident in bone. Avian SCF has been reported to enhance bone resorption by chicken osteoclasts, independent of an increase in cell number [Fig. 28.7] (115). Consistent with the findings of Blair et al. (114), these investigators also reported that chicken osteoblasts and periosteal fibroblasts express SCF and that PTH upregulates membrane-associated SCF expression in these cells.

In summary, SCF appears to be an important, but not indispensable, mediator of early osteoclastogenesis. It is expressed by osteoblasts and seems to be regulated by osteotropic hormones in these cells. Its receptor, c-kit, is expressed on osteoclast progenitors as well as on mature osteoclasts, although its precise role in mature osteoclasts remains to be clarified. Several downstream targets from activated c-kit are known to be important for mature osteoclast function, and exploring the effects of SCF on these molecules in mature osteoclasts may help to clarify this latter issue.

INTERLEUKIN-3

IL-3 is a multilineage hematopoietic growth factor that promotes the growth of most lineages of blood cell precursors. Its production is presumed to be largely from $CD4^+CD8^-$ T lymphocytes in the hematopoietic microenvironment (116,117). It was discovered independently by a number of laboratories studying different biological activities. The IL-3 gene is located on human chromosome 5 at position 5q23-q32 and on mouse chromosome 11. IL-3 is a relatively small molecule: the murine protein has a polypeptide chain length of 140 amino acids, while human IL-3 is 133 amino acids long. It is heavily glycosylated. IL-3 belongs to the helical cytokine superfamily, with structural similarities to GM-CSF and IL-5. The cytokine consists of four helical bundles in an up–up–down–down configuration. Studies have shown that the first 16 and the final 22 amino acids of IL-3 can be deleted with very little loss of biological activity, suggesting that residues 17 to 118 represent the

sequence necessary for interaction with, and activation of, the receptor (118).

Receptor

The human IL-3 receptor is a heterodimer made up of two members of the hemopoietin receptor superfamily. The 70-kDa ligand-specific α chain binds IL-3 with low affinity and is homologous with two other ligand-specific chains that bind GM-CSF and IL-5, respectively. The 120-kDa common β chain (β_c) is shared by the human IL-3, IL-5, and GM-CSF receptors. The α chain does not by itself transduce any biological activities. The β_c subunit converts the ligand-bound α chain to a high-affinity state and is important for most, if not all, signaling events (114).

Signal Transduction

Binding of IL-3 to its receptor rapidly induces activation of multiple intracellular signaling pathways. IL-3 has been shown to induce activation of both Jak2 and Src family tyrosine kinases, which correlate with the rapid tyrosine phosphorylation of a number of cellular proteins and activation of intracellular signaling cascades, including the Ras/extracellular signal-regulated kinase kinase pathway, p38 and stress-activated protein kinase, STAT5, SHP2, and PI-3K (121–124). Both GM-CSF and IL-3 stimulate PI-3K activation (122,123). Over a period of 10 minutes, the β chain of the IL-3 receptor increases in apparent molecular weight, shifting from 125 kDa in unstimulated cells to 135 to 150 kDa. Much of this increase in apparent molecular weight appears to result from concomitant serine/threonine phosphorylation (125).

Interleukin-3 and Bone Metabolism

Knockout Animals

The IL-3 knockout animal appears to have no specific defect in bone metabolism, although detailed studies have not been reported (126). Further, these animals have apparently normal hematopoiesis, presumably due to redundancy of function between IL-3 and other CSFs, such as GM-CSF. Using overexpression of antisense RNA to IL-3, selective suppression of T-cell IL-3 production has been achieved (127). These animals develop progressive neurological dysfunction with apparently no bony abnormalities.

Production by Bone Cells

These is little evidence that cells committed to either the osteoblast or osteoclast lineage produce IL-3. One report has indicated that small amounts of IL-3 are produced by cultured murine calvariae (100). However, in cells prepared by sequential collagenase digestion from these calvariae, there was no evidence of IL-3 production. This suggests that the source of IL-3 in these organ cultures is cells other than osteoblasts or osteoblast precursors. Little work has focused on the effects of IL-3 on osteoblasts.

Role in Osteoclastogenesis

There has been ongoing interest in the role of IL-3 in the process of osteoclastogenesis. In 1989, Barton and Mayer (128) reported that IL-3 induced production of multinucleated, TRAP-positive cells in IL-3-treated murine marrow cultures. These cells were reported to be somewhat smaller than those induced by 1,25-$(OH)_2$ D, and no data on the bone-resorbing capacity of these cells were provided. A subsequent study by Hattersley and Chambers (78) reported that, while IL-3 was able to induce the appearance of cells expressing the calcitonin receptor, these cells were unable to induce bone resorption. Further, the cells were uniformly mononuclear. In the presence of 1,25-$(OH)_2$ D, however, the appearance of bone-resorbing, calcitonin receptor–positive, multinucleated cells was enhanced, suggesting an additive or synergistic effect between the two compounds. Since the doses of IL-3 used in the two studies are difficult to compare, it is unclear whether the failure to observe multinucleation and bone resorption is related to the dose used or to other differences in experimental design. Hattersley and Chambers (78) concluded that IL-3 promoted differentia-

tion of osteoclasts to a step short of a fully mature osteoclast. However, treatment of young *op/op* mice, which lack osteoclasts and are osteopetrotic, with IL-3 and GM-CSF improves the osteopetrosis and leads to the appearance of mononuclear, TRAP-positive cells (76).

Recent work has suggested that, together with other cytokines, IL-3 can induce the formation of human osteoclasts from peripheral blood cells (129,130). CSF-1, GM-CSF, and IL-3 can induce cultured human monocytes to form fully functioning osteoclasts when cocultured with osteoblasts in the presence of 1,25$(OH)_2$ vitamin D and dexamethasone (130). By itself, the potency of IL-3 was severely diminished, and the addition of neutralizing antibodies to CSF-1 completely abolished IL-3 osteoclastogenic activity, suggesting that CSF-1 was necessary for IL-3-induced osteoclastogenesis. Consistent with a role for IL-3 in inducing osteoclast differentiation from circulating mononuclear precursors in humans is a report by Weitzmann et al. (131) that CD34$^+$-enriched peripheral blood stem cells, when cultured with IL-1, IL-3, and GM-CSF, differentiated to mononuclear, TRAP-positive preosteoclasts. With continued culture, multinucleated, TRAP-positive cells appeared, which expressed the calcitonin receptor and high levels of c-src and were able to resorb bone. These same workers found that all three cytokines, when combined, can induce the expression of $\alpha_v\beta_3$ integrin in these cells, a key marker for mature osteoclast differentiation. Individually, none of the cytokines was as effective as the combination (131).

IL-3-induced proliferation of hematopoietic cells involves activation of activator protein-1 (AP-1)/ets family members among other signaling cascades. Preliminary data suggest that this transcriptional machinery is, at least in part, modulated by estrogen, which may have relevance to estrogen-deficiency bone loss. Specifically, a preliminary report has indicated that estrogen suppressed AP-1/ets-mediated, but not NFκB- or STAT2-mediated, transactivation of reporter constructs containing these response elements (132). What downstream targets, in the IL-3 signaling pathway, are responsible for its effects on osteoclastogenesis remain unclear, although expression of the transcription factor mi, which is required for normal osteoclastogenesis (133,134), is upregulated by IL-3 (135).

In summary, these data suggest that IL-3 has a lesser role to play in inducing osteoclastogenesis. Studies in human cells suggest that, at least in conjunction with other cytokines, IL-3 may participate in a program of differentiation that leads to completely mature osteoclasts. The murine data suggest, however, that as a single agent it is not capable of fully inducing this pathway. The exact details of the mechanisms by which this osteoclastogenic potential is effected remain unclear.

MEGAKARYOCYTE GROWTH AND DEVELOPMENT FACTOR

MGDF, also known as thrombopoietin, is a cytokine that regulates megakaryocyte development and exerts its action by binding to a specific cell surface receptor encoded by the protooncogene c-mpl (136). The human MGDF gene has been mapped to chromosome 3q26.3 and consists of seven exons and six introns spanning 8 kb. The human and murine MGDF genes produce two alternatively spliced mRNAs which encode membrane-associated species (137). The human MGDF protein can be divided into an amino-terminal domain of 153 amino acids and a carboxyl-terminal domain of 179 amino acids containing six potential N-linked glycosylation sites. The amino-terminal domain is highly conserved among mice, rats, dogs, and humans, whereas the carboxyl-terminal domain is not required for receptor binding and displays wide species divergence. Sequence analysis shows that the amino-terminal domain of MGDF has homology with erythropoietin and is a member of the four-helix bundle cytokine family. Four alanine substitutions, at Arg[10], Pro[42], Glu[50], and Lys[138], nearly or completely abolish the activity, whereas a mutation at Arg[14] slightly decreases the activity, suggesting that these residues are functionally important in interacting with its receptor (138).

Receptor

The receptor of MGDF, c-mpl, is classified as a member of the cytokine receptor superfamily.

This rapidly growing group of type I transmembrane proteins is characterized by a 200–amino acid motif containing four conserved cysteines and a Trp-Ser-X-Trp-Ser sequence near its carboxyl end. C-mpl contains a duplication of the entire cytokine receptor domain (139). The intracytoplasmic domain of the murine mpl receptor is 121 amino acids long and does not encode any recognized kinase domain or enzymatic motif. Like gp130 and other cytokine receptors, the membrane-proximal region of the c-mpl cytoplasmic domain has a potential box 1/box 2 sequence, thought to be important for mitogenic signaling (140). Experiments with truncated cytokine receptors have shown that this membrane-proximal region (50 to 60 amino acids) is necessary and sufficient to support proliferation of cytokine-dependent cell lines (140,141). The carboxyl terminus of the intracytoplasmic domain seems to direct cytokine-specific differentiation. Mpl homodimerization is sufficient for signaling (141).

Signal Transduction

In general, homodimeric receptors utilize a single JAK, whereas heterodimeric receptors require two distinct JAKs. Thus, it is surprising that several reports have demonstrated that MGDF induces phosphorylation of two distinct Janus family members, JAK2 and TYK2 (142–144). Recent studies have confirmed that JAK2-deficient cells are unable to initiate MGDF-mediated signaling. In contrast, cells that are TYK2-deficient are able to induce tyrosine phosphorylation of Mpl, JAK2, STAT3, and Shc as efficiently as parental cells can. These data indicate that JAK2 is an essential component of Mpl signaling and that, in the absence of JAK2, TYK2 is incapable of initiating MGDF-induced tyrosine phosphorylation (145).

Megakaryocyte Growth and Development Factor and Bone Metabolism

Both MGDF and its receptor, c-mpl, have been knocked out using homologous recombination techniques (146). In both cases, animals demonstrate marked reduction in megakaryocytes and platelet levels. Further, in mpl(−/−) mice, there are reduced numbers of pleuripotent stem cells. Thus, Kimura and coworkers (147) have demonstrated that marrow from mice with targeted disruption of the mpl gene has reduced repopulating capacity when used as donor tissue to reconstitute the marrow of irradiated mice. Mpl(−/−) bone marrow generated eight- to tenfold fewer spleen colonies than wild-type marrow. These data suggest that normal signaling through c-mpl is important for normal hematopoietic stem cell survival and proliferation.

Overexpression of MGDF in the liver leads to thrombocytosis but no bone phenotype (148).

However, Yan and coworkers (149,150) reported that transgenic overexpression of MGDF in marrow leads to findings reminiscent of those in some patients with myelodysplastic syndromes. In these experiments, murine bone marrow was infected with a retroviral vector encompassing the coding region for MGDF under the control of a viral long terminal repeat promoter. Mice repopulated with these cells developed increased numbers of megakaryocytes and platelets (149). Interestingly, these animals also demonstrated a marked increase in marrow myelofibrosis with increased reticulin, as well as pronounced osteosclerosis. Circulating levels of

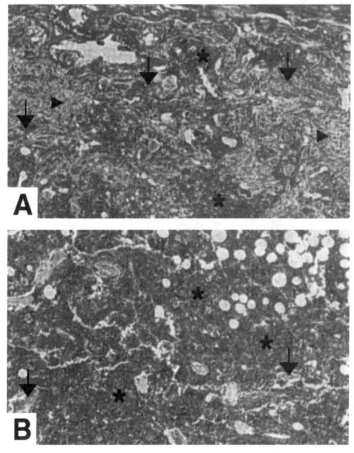

FIG. 28.8. Changes in bone induced by transgenic overexpression of megakaryocyte growth and development factor (MGDF) **(A)** and the reversal of those changes by reimplantation of transgenic mice with normal marrow **(B).** Note in **A** marked osteosclerosis and marrow fibrosis, with a return to normal in **B. Arrows** indicate bone; *arrowheads,* regions of marrow fibrosis; and *asterisks,* marrow. (From ref. 150, with permission.)

transforming growth factor-β1 (TGF-β1) and PDGF, cytokines previously speculated to play a role in the pathogenesis of myelofibrosis were elevated in these animals. Retransplantation in MGDF-overexpressing mice of normal bone marrow resulted in a return to normal of mega-karyocyte and platelet levels and a complete correction of the myelofibrosis and osteosclerosis (150). Figure 28.8 shows representative bone histology before and after correction of the my-elofibrosis and osteosclerosis in these animals. Whether the high PDGF and TGF-β1 levels seen in these animals are solely responsible for this syndrome or whether other factors contribute is unclear. Nonetheless, this model provides intriguing insight into the pathogenesis of a heretofore obscure syndrome, the osteosclerotic syndrome associated with some myelodysplastic disorders.

Apart from this report, little other data are available about potential roles for MGDF in bone. However, these observations suggest that MGDF may have important physiological and/ or pathophysiological roles in bone that warrant further study.

ACKNOWLEDGMENTS

This work was supported by grants from the National Institutes of Health, including AG-15345 (KLI); DE12459 (KLI), and DK45228 (KLI), and in part by the Yale Core Center for Musculo-skeletal Disorders, P30 AR46032 (GQY, KLI). The authors gratefully acknowledge the administrative and secretarial assistance of Ms. Marilyn Feldman and Ms. Nancy Canetti.

REFERENCES

1. Areci RJ, Shanahan F, Stanley ER, et al. Temporal expression and location of colony-stimulating factor-1 (CSF-1) and its receptor in the female reproductive tract are consistent with CSF-1-regulated placental development. *Proc Natl Acad Sci USA* 1989;86: 8818–8822.
2. Cohen PE, Zhu L, Pollard JW. The absence of CSF-1 in osteopetrotic (csfmop/csfmop) mice disrupts estrous cycles and ovulation. *Biol Reprod* 1997;56:110–118.
3. Pollard JW, Hennighausen L. Colony stimulating factor-1 is required for mammary gland development during pregnancy. *Proc Natl Acad Sci USA* 1994;91: 9312–9316.
4. Cohen PE, Hardy MP, Pollard JW. Colony stimulating factor-1 plays a major role in the development of reproductive function in male mice. *Mol Endocrinol* 1997; 11:1636–1650.
5. Pampfer S, Tabibzadeh S, Chuan FC, et al. Expression of colony-stimulating factor-1 (CSF-1) messenger RNA in human endometrial glands during the menstrual cycle: molecular cloning of a novel transcript that predicts a cell surface form of CSF-1. *Mol Endocrinol* 1991;5:1931–1938.
6. Rettenmier CW, Roussel MF, Ashmun RA, et al. Synthesis of membrane-bound colony stimulating factor 1 (CSF-1) and down-modulation of CSF-1 receptors in NIH-3T3 cells transformed by co-transfection of the human CSF-1 and c-fms (CSF-1 receptor) genes. *Mol Cell Biol* 1987;7:2378–2387.
7. Rettenmier CW. Biosynthesis of macrophage colony-stimulating factor (CSF-1): differential processing of CSF-1 precursors suggests alternative mechanisms for stimulating CSF-1 receptors. *Cur Top Microbiol Immunol* 1989;149:129–141.
8. Price LKH, Choi HU, Rosenberg L, et al. The predominant form of secreted colony stimulating factor-1 is a proteoglycan *J Biol Chem* 1992;267:2190–2199.
9. Suzu S, Ohtsuki T, Yanai N, et al. Identification of a high molecular weight macrophage colony-stimulating factor as a glycosaminoglycan-containing species. *J Biol Chem* 1992;267:4345–4348.
10. Ohtsuki T, Suzu S, Hatake K, et al. A proteoglycan form of macrophage colony-stimulating factor that binds to bone-derived collagens and can be extracted from bone matrix. *Biochem Biophys Res Commun* 1993;190:15–22.
11. Presnell SR, Cohen FE. Topological distribution of four-α-helix bundles. *Proc Natl Acad Sci USA* 1989; 86:6592–6596.
12. Kawasaki ES, Ladner MB. Molecular biology of macrophage colony-stimulating factor. *Immunol Ser* 1990;49:155–176.
13. Sherr C. Colony-stimulating factor-1 receptor. *Blood* 1990;75:1–12.
14. Yeung YG, Wang Y, Einstein D, et al. Colony-stimulating factor-1 stimulates the formation of multimeric cytosolic complexes of signaling proteins and cytoskeletal components in macrophages. *J Biol Chem* 1998;273:17128–17137.
15. Courtneidge SA, Dhand R, Pilat D, et al. Activation of src family kinases by colony stimulating factor-1, and their association with its receptor. *EMBO J* 1993; 12:943–950.
16. van der Geer P, Hunter T. Mutation of Tyr697, a GRB2-binding site, and Tyr721, a PI 3-kinase binding site, abrogates signal transduction by the murine CSF-1 receptor expressed in Rat-2 fibroblasts. *EMBO J* 1993;12:5161–5172.
17. Bravo R, Neuberg M, Burckhardt J, et al. Involvement of common and cell type-specific pathways in *c-fos* gene control: stable induction by cAMP in macrophages. *Cell* 1987;48:251–260.
18. Roussel MF. Signal transduction by the macrophage-colony-stimulating factor receptor (CSF-1R). *J Cell Sci* 1994;[Suppl 18]:105–108.
19. Wiktor-Jedrzejczak W, Ahmed A, Szcylik C, et al. Hematological characterization of congenital osteopetrosis in op/op mouse. Possible mechanism for

abnormal macrophage differentiation. *J Exp Med* 1982; 156:1516–1527.

20. Wiktor-Jedrzejczak W, Bartocci A, Ferrante F Jr, et al. Total absence of colony-stimulating factor 1 in the macrophage-deficient osteopetrotic (op/op) mouse. *Proc Natl Acad Sci USA* 1990;87:4828–4832.

21. Felix R, Cecchini MG, Hofstetter W, et al. Impairment of macrophage colony-stimulating factor production and lack of resident bone marrow macrophages in the osteopetrotic op/op mouse. *J Bone Miner Res* 1990;5: 781–789.

22. Yoshida H, Hayashi SI, Kunisada T. The murine mutation osteopetrosis is in the coding region of the macrophage colony stimulating gene. *Nature* 1990;345: 442–444.

23. Felix R, Cecchini MG, Fleisch H. Macrophage colony stimulating factor restores *in vivo* bone resorption in the op/op osteopetrotic mouse. *Endocrinology* 1990; 127:2592–2594.

24. Takahashi N, Udagawa N, Akatsu T, et al. Deficiency of osteoclasts in osteopetrotic mice is due to a defect in the local microenvironment provided by osteoblastic cells. *Endocrinology* 1991;128:1792–1796.

25. Tanaka S, Takahashi N, Udagawa N, et al. Macrophage colony-stimulating factor is indispensable for both proliferation and differentiation of osteoclast progenitors. *J Clin Invest* 1993;91:257–263.

26. Hattersley G, Owens J, Flanagan AM, et al. Macrophage colony stimulating factor (M-CSF) is essential for osteoclast formation *in vitro*. *Biochem Biophys Res Commun* 1991;177:526–531.

27. Begg SK, Bertoncello I. The haematopoietic deficiencies in osteopetrotic (op/op) mice are not permanent, but progressively correct with age. *Exp Hematol* 1993; 21:493–495.

28. Felix R, Fleisch H, Elford PR. Bone-resorbing cytokines enhance release of macrophage colony-stimulating activity by the osteoblastic cell MC3T3-E1. *Calcif Tissue Int* 1989;44:356–360.

29. Elford PR, Felix R, Cecchini M, et al. Murine osteoblast-like cells and the osteogenic cell MC3T3-E1 release macrophage colony-stimulating activity in culture. *Calcif Tissue Int* 1987;41:151–156.

30. Shiina-Ishimi Y, Abe E, Tanaka H, et al. Synthesis of colony-stimulating factor (CSF) and differentiation-inducing factor (D-factor) by osteoblastic cells, clone MC3T-E1. *Biochem Biophys Res Commun* 1986;134: 400–406.

31. Sato K, Kasono K, Fujii Y, et al. Tumor necrosis factor type α (cachectin) stimulates mouse osteoblast-like cells (MC3T3) to produce macrophage-colony stimulating activity and prostaglandin E2. *Biochem Biophys Res Commun* 1987;145:323–329.

32. Kaplan DL, Eielson CM, Horowitz MC, et al. Tumor necrosis factor-α induces transcription of the colony-stimulating factor-1 gene in murine osteoblasts. *J Cell Physiol* 1996;168:199–208.

33. Weir E, Horowitz M, Baron R, et al. Macrophage colony-stimulating factor release and receptor expression in bone cells. *J Bone Miner Res* 1993;8:1507–1517.

34. Yao G-Q, Sun B-H, Hammond E, et al. The cell surface form of colony stimulating factor-1 is regulated by osteotropic agents and supports formation of multinucleated osteoclast-like cells. *J Biol Chem* 1998;273: 4119–4128.

35. Felix R, Halasy-Nagy J, Wetterwald A, et al. Synthesis of membrane and matrix-bound colony-stimulating factor-1 (CSF-1) by cultured osteoblasts. *J Cell Physiol* 1996;166:311–322.

36. Rubin J, Bishkobing DM, Jadhav L, et al. Dexamethasone promotes expression of membrane-bound colony-stimulating factor in murine osteoblast-like cells. *Endocrinology* 1998;139:1006–1012.

37. Hofstetter W, Wetterwald A, Cecchini M, et al. Detection of transcripts for the receptor for macrophage colony-stimulating factor, c-fms, in murine osteoclasts. *Proc Natl Acad Sci USA* 1992;89:9637–9641.

38. Felix R, Hofstetter W, Wetterwald A, et al. Role of colony-stimulating factor-1 in bone metabolism. *J Cell Biochem* 1994;55:340–349.

39. MacDonald BR, Mundy GR, Clark S, et al. Effects of human recombinant CSF-GM and highly purified CSF-1 on the formation of multinucleated cells with osteoclast characteristics in long-term bone marrow cultures. *J Bone Miner Res* 1986;1:227–233.

39a. Takahashi N, Udagawa N, Akatsu T, et al. Role of colony-stimulating factors in osteoclast development. *J Bone Miner Res* 1991;6:977–985.

40. Antonioli-Corboz VA, Cecchini MG, Felix R, et al. Effect of macrophage colony stimulating factor (M-CSF) on *in vitro* osteoclast generation and bone resorption (BR). *Endocrinology* 1992;130:437–442.

41. Weir EC, Lowik CWGM, Paliwal I, et al. Colony stimulating factor-1 plays a role in osteoclast formation and function in bone resorption induced by parathyroid hormone and parathyroid hormone–related protein. *J Bone Miner Res* 1996;11:1474–1481.

42. Sarma U, Flanagan AM. Macrophage colony-stimulating factor induces substantial osteoclast generation and bone resorption in human bone marrow cultures. *Blood* 1996;88:2531–2540.

43. Morohashi T, Antonioli-Corboz V, Fleisch H, et al. Macrophage colony-stimulating factor (M-CSF) restores bone resorption in op/op bone *in vitro* in conjunction with PTH or 1,25(OH)$_2$D$_3$. *J Bone Miner Res* 1994;9:401–407.

44. Fan X, Fan D, Horwitz M, et al. Membrane-bound MCSF is more potent than secreted MCSF in supporting osteoclast formation. *Bone* 1998;23[Suppl]:S432.

45. Insogna KL, Sahni M, Grey AB, et al. Colony-stimulating factor-1 induces cytoskeletal reorganization and c-src-dependent tyrosine phosphorylation of selected cellular proteins in rodent osteoclasts. *J Clin Invest* 1997;100:2476–2485.

46. Soriano P, Montgomery P, Gese R, et al. Targeted disruption of the c-src proto-oncogene leads to osteopetrosis in mice. *Cell* 1991;64:693–702.

47. Fuller K, Owens MJ, Jager CJ, et al. M-CSF suppresses osteoclastic apoptosis and switches function from bone resorption to migration/chemotaxis. *J Bone Miner Res* 1993;8[Suppl 1]:1068.

48. Pilkington MF, Sims SM, Dixon SJ. Wortmannin inhibits spreading and chemotaxis of rat osteoclasts *in vitro*. *J Bone Miner Res* 1998;13:688–694.

49. Felix R, Hofstetter W, Cecchini M, et al. Colony stimulating factor-1 induces cell spreading and pinocytosis by stimulating phosphoinositol 3-kinase. *J Bone Miner Res* 1996;11[Suppl 1]:S287.

50. Grey A, Carlberg K, Rohrschneider L, et al. C-src associates directly with the 85 kD subunit of phosphoinosi-

tol 3-kinase in osteoclast-like cells via its SH3 domain. *J Bone Miner Res* 1997;12[Suppl 1]:S155.

51. Hattersley G, Dorey E, Horton MA, et al. Human macrophage colony stimulating factor inhibits bone resorption by osteoclasts disaggregated from rat bone. *J Cell Physiol* 1988;137:199–203.

52. Lees R, Heersche J. Macrophage colony stimulating factor increases bone resorption in dispersed osteoclast cultures by increasing osteoclast size. *J Bone Miner Res* 1999;14:937–945.

53. Kong Y-Y, Yoshida H, Sarosi I, et al. OPGL is a key regulator of osteoclastogenesis, lymphocyte development and lymph-node organogenesis. *Nature* 1999; 397:315–323.

54. Lacey DL, Timms E, Tan H-L, et al. Osteoprotegerin ligand is a cytokine that regulates osteoclast differentiation and activation. *Cell* 1998;93:165–176.

55. Lagasse E, Weissman I. Enforced expression of Bcl-2 in monocytes rescues macrophages and partially reverses osteopetrosis in op/op mice. *Cell* 1997;89: 1021–1031.

56. Sasaki K, Chiba S, Hanazono Y, et al. Coordinate expression of the alpha and beta chains of human granulocyte-macrophage colony-stimulating factor receptor confers ligand-induced morphological transformation in mouse fibroblasts. *J Biol Chem* 1993;268: 13697–13702.

57. Sakamaki K, Miyajima I, Kitamura T, et al. Critical cytoplasmic domains of the common beta subunit of the human GM-CSF, IL-3 and IL-5 receptors for growth signal transduction and tyrosine phosphorylation. *EMBO J* 1992;11:3541–3549.

58. Li Y, Shen BF, Karanes C, et al. Association between Lyn protein tyrosine kinase (p53/56lyn) and the beta subunit of the granulocyte-macrophage colony-stimulating factor (GM-CSF) receptors in a GM-CSF-dependent human megakaryocytic leukemia cell line (M-07e). *J Immunol* 1995;155:2165–2174.

59. Brizzi MF, Aronica MG, Rosso A, et al. Granulocyte-macrophage colony-stimulating factor stimulates JAK2 signaling pathway and rapidly activates p93fes, STAT1 p91, and STAT3 p92 in polymorphonuclear leukocytes. *J Biol Chem* 1996;271:3562–3567.

60. Hanazono Y, Chiba S, Sasaki K, et al. c-fps/fes protein-tyrosine kinase is implicated in a signaling pathway triggered by granulocyte-macrophage colony-stimulating factor and interleukin-3. *EMBO J* 1993;12: 1641–1646.

61. al-Shami A, Bourgoin SG, Naccache PH. Granulocyte-macrophage colony-stimulating factor-activated signaling pathways in human neutrophils. I. Tyrosine phosphorylation-dependent stimulation of phosphatidylinositol 3-kinase and inhibition by phorbol esters. *Blood* 1997;89:10–44.

62. Lanfrancone L, Pelicci G, Brizzi MF, et al. Overexpression of Shc proteins potentiates the proliferative response to the granulocyte-macrophage colony-stimulating factor and recruitment of Grb2/SoS and Grb2/p140 complexes to the beta receptor subunit. *Oncogene* 1995;10:907–917.

63. Pratt JC, Weiss M, Sieff CA, et al. Evidence for a physical association between the Shc-PTB domain and the beta c chain of the granulocyte-macrophage colony-stimulating factor receptor. *J Biol Chem* 1996;271: 12137–12140.

64. Matsuguchi T, Zhao Y, Lilly MB, et al. The cytoplasmic domain of granulocyte-macrophage colony-stimulating factor (GM-CSF) receptor alpha subunit is essential for both GM-CSF-mediated growth and differentiation. *J Biol Chem* 1997;272:17450–17459.

65. Stanley E, Lieschke GJ, Grail D, et al. Granulocyte-macrophage colony-stimulating factor–deficient mice show no major perturbation of hematopoiesis but develop a characteristic pulmonary pathology. *Proc Natl Acad Sci USA* 1994;91:5592–5596.

66. Horowitz MC, Coleman DL, Flood PM, et al. Parathyroid hormone and lipopolysaccharide induce murine osteoblast-like cells to secrete a cytokine indistinguishable from granulocyte-macrophage colony-stimulating factor. *J Clin Invest* 1989;83:149–157.

67. Weir EC, Insogna KL, Horowitz MC. Osteoblast-like cells secrete granulocyte-macrophage colony-stimulating factor in response to parathyroid hormone and lipopolysaccharide. *Endocrinology* 1989;124:899–904.

68. Felix R, Cecchini G, Hofstetter W, et al. Production of granulocyte-macrophage (GM-CSF) and granulocyte colony-stimulating factor (G-CSF) by rat clonal osteoblastic cell population CRP 10/30 and the immortalized cell line IRC 10/30-mycl stimulated by tumor necrosis factor. *Endocrinology* 1991;128:661–667.

69. Evans DB, Bunning RAD, Russell RGG. The effects of recombinant human granulocyte-macrophage colony-stimulating factor (rhGM-CSF) on human osteoblast-like cells. *Biochem Biophys Res Commun* 1989;160: 588–595.

70. Gowen M, Chapman K, Littlewood A, et al. Production of tumor necrosis factor by human osteoblasts is modulated by other cytokines, but not by osteotropic hormones. *Endocrinology* 1990;126:1250–1255.

71. Modrowski D, Lomri A, Marie P. Glycosaminoglycans bind granulocyte-macrophage colony-stimulating factor and modulate its mitogenic activity and signaling in human osteoblastic cells. *J Cell Physiol* 1998;177: 187–195.

72. Taichman R, Emerson S. Human osteosarcoma cell lines MG-63 and SaOS-2 produce G-CSF and GM-CSF: identification and partial characterization of cell-associated isoforms. *Exp Hematol* 1996;24:509–517.

73. Kurihara N, Suda T, Miura Y, et al. Generation of osteoclasts from isolated hematopoietic progenitor cells. *Blood* 1989;74:1295–1302.

74. Inoue M, Namba N, Chappel J, et al. Granulocyte macrophage-colony stimulating factor reciprocally regulates alpha v associated integrins on murine osteoclast precursors. *Mol Endocrinol* 1998;12:1955–1962.

75. Lee MY, Fukunaga R, Lee TJ, et al. Bone modulation in sustained hematopoietic stimulation in mice. *Blood* 1991;77:2135–2141.

76. Myint Y, Miyaka K, Naito M, et al. Granulocyte/macrophage colony-stimulating factor and interleukin-3 correct osteopetrosis in mice with osteopetrosis mutation. *Am J Pathol* 1999;1564:553–566.

77. Wiktor-Jedrzejczak W, Urbanowska E, Szperl M. Granulocyte-macrophage colony-stimulating factor corrects macrophage deficiencies, but not osteopetrosis, in the colony-stimulating factor-1-deficient op/op mouse. *Endocrinology* 1994;134: 1932–1935.

78. Hattersley G, Chambers TJ. Effects of interleukin 3

and of granulocyte-macrophage and macrophage colony stimulating factors on osteoclast deafferentation from mouse hemopoietic tissue. *J Cell Physiol* 1990; 142:201–209.

79. Shuto T, Kukita T, Hirata M, et al. Dexamethasone stimulates osteoclast-like cell formation by inhibiting granulocyte-macrophage colony-stimulating factor production in mouse bone marrow culture. *Endocrinology* 1994;134:1121–1126.

80. Shuto T, Jimi E, Kukita T, et al. Granulocyte-macrophage colony-stimulating factor suppresses lipopolysaccharide-induced osteoclast-like cell formation in mouse bone marrow cultures. *Endocrinology* 1994; 134:831–837.

81. Udagawa N, Horwood N, Elliott J, et al. Interleukin-18 (interferon-gamma-inducing factor) is produced by osteoblasts and acts via granulocyte/macrophage colony-stimulating factor and not via interferon-gamma to inhibit osteoclast formation. *J Exp Med* 1997;185: 1005–1012.

82. Horwood J, Udagawa N, Elliott J, et al. Interleukin 18 inhibits osteoclast formation via T cell production of granulocyte macrophage colony-stimulating factor. *J Clin Invest* 1998;101:595–603.

83. Gliniak BC, Rohrschneider LR. Expression of the M-CSF receptor is controlled posttranscriptionally by the dominant actions of GM-CSF or multi-CSF. *Cell* 1990; 63:1073–1083.

84. Novak U, Ward AC, Hertzog PJ, et al. Aberrant activation of JAK/STAT pathway components in response to G-CSF, interferon-alpha/beta and interferon-gamma in NFS-60 cells. *Growth Factors* 1996;13:251–260.

85. Corey SJ, Burkhardt AL, Bolen JB, et al. Granulocyte colony-stimulating factor receptor signaling involves the formation of a three-component complex with Lyn and Syk protein-tyrosine kinases. *Proc Natl Acad Sci USA* 1994;91:4683–4687.

86. Ward AC, Monkhouse JL, Csar XF, et al. The Src-like tyrosine kinase Hck is activated by granulocyte colony-stimulating factor (G-CSF) and docks to the activated G-CSF receptor. *Biochem Biophys Res Commun* 1998; 251:117–123.

87. Tian SS, Tapley P, Sincich C, et al. Multiple signaling pathways induced by granulocyte colony-stimulating factor involving activation of JAKs, STAT5, and/or STAT3 are required for regulation of three distinct classes of immediate early genes. *Blood* 1996;88: 4435–4444.

88. de Koning JP, Schelen AM, Dong F, et al. Specific involvement of tyrosine 764 of human granulocyte colony-stimulating factor receptor in signal transduction mediated by p145/Shc/GRB2 or p90/GRB2 complexes. *Blood* 1996;87:132–140.

89. Lieschke G, Grail D, Hodgson G, et al. Mice lacking granulocyte colony stimulating factor have neutropenia granulocyte and macrophage progenitor cell deficiency, and impaired neutrophil mobilization. *Blood* 1994;84:1737.

90. Takahashi T, Wada T, Mori M, et al. Overexpression of the granulocyte colony-stimulating factor gene leads to osteoporosis in mice. *Lab Invest* 1996;74:827–834.

91. Suzuki M, Sakamaki Y, Miyoshi A, et al. Histopathological study on bone changes induced by recombinant granulocyte colony-stimulating factor in rats. *Exp Toxicol Pathol* 1997;49:253–259.

92. Soshi S, Takahashi HE, Tanizawa T, et al. Effect of recombinant human granulocyte colony-stimulating factor (rh G-CSF) on rat bone: inhibition of bone formation at the endosteal surface of vertebra and tibia. *Calcif Tissue Int* 1996;58:337–340.

93. Bonilla M, Dale D, Zeidler C, et al. Long-term safety of treatment with recombinant human granulocyte colony-stimulating factor (r-metHuG-CSF) in patients with severe congenital neutropenias. *Br J Haematol* 1994;88:723–730.

94. Iwasa K, Noguchi M. Anaplastic thyroid carcinoma producing the granulocyte colony-stimulating factor (G-CSF): report of a case. *Surg Today* 1995;25: 158–160.

95. Takeuchi R, Kasagi K, Ohta H, et al. Diffuse bony uptake of thallium-201-chloride in the granulocyte colony-stimulating factor-producing lung carcinoma. *J Nucl Med* 1998;39:241–242.

96. Sato K, Fujii Y, Kakiuchi T, et al. Paraneoplastic syndrome of hypercalcemia and leukocytosis caused by squamous carcinoma cells (T3M-1) producing parathyroid hormone–related protein, interleukin 1α, and granulocyte colony-stimulating factor. *Cancer Res* 1989;49:4740–4746.

97. Gudi R, Krishnamurthy M, Pachter BR. Astemizole in the treatment of granulocyte colony-stimulating factor-induced bone pain [Letter]. *Ann Intern Med* 1995;123: 236–237.

98. Froberg MK, Garg UC, Stroncek DF, et al. Changes in serum osteocalcin and bone-specific alkaline phosphatase are associated with bone pain in donors receiving granulocyte colony-stimulating factor for peripheral blood stem and progenitor cell collection. *Transfusion* 1999;39:410–414.

99. Takamatsu Y, Simmons PJ, Moore RJ, et al. Osteoclast-mediated bone resorption is stimulated during short-term administration of granulocyte colony-stimulating factor but is not responsible for hematopoietic progenitor cell mobilization. *Blood* 1998;92:3465–3473.

100. Felix R, Elford PR, Stoerckle C, et al. Production of hematopoietic growth factors by bone tissue and bone cells in culture. *J Bone Miner Res* 1988;3:27–36.

100a. Lee MY, Fevold KL, Muguruma Y, et al. Conditions that support long-term production of osteoclast progenitors *in vitro*. *Stem Cells* 1997;15:340–346.

101. Purton LE, Lee MY, Torok-Storb B. Normal human peripheral blood mononuclear cells mobilized with granulocyte colony-stimulating factor have increased osteoclastogenic potential compared to nonmobilized blood. *Blood* 1996;87:1802–1808.

102. Lorenzo J, Sousa S, Fonseca J, et al. Colony-stimulating factors regulate the development of multinucleated osteoclasts from recently replicated cells *in vitro*. *J Clin Invest* 1987;80:160–164.

103. Fukushima N, Nishina H, Koishihara Y, et al. Enhanced hematopoiesis *in vivo* and *in vitro* by splenic stromal cells derived from the mouse with recombinant granulocyte colony-stimulating factor. *Blood* 1992;80: 1914–1922.

104. Yarden Y, Kuang WJ, Yang-Feng T, et al. Human proto-oncogene c-kit: a new cell surface receptor tyrosine kinase for an unidentified ligand. *EMBO J* 1987; 6:3341–3351.

105. Loveland KL, Schlatt S. Stem cell factor and c-kit in

the mammalian testis: lessons originating from Mother Nature's gene knockouts. *J Endocrinol* 1997;153: 337–344.

106. Isozaki K, Tsujimura T, Nomura S, et al. Cell type-specific deficiency of c-kit gene expression in mutant mice of mi/mi genotype. *Am J Pathol* 1994;145:827.

107. Kapur R, Majumdar M, Xiao X, et al. Signaling through the interaction of membrane-restricted stem cell factor and c-kit receptor tyrosine kinase: genetic evidence for a differential role in erythropoiesis. *Blood* 1998;91:879–889.

108. Blair HC, Julian BA, Cao X, et al. Parathyroid hormone–regulated production of stem cell factor in human osteoblasts and osteoblast-like cells. *Biochem Biophys Res Commun* 1999;255:778–784.

109. Dong S-S, Julian BA, Blair HC. Membrane-associated stem cell factor in PTH-stimulated human osteoblasts: correlation with activity state. *J Bone Miner Res* 1996; 11[Suppl 1]:S175.

110. Dong S-S, Julian BA, Blair HC. Stem cell factor (c-kit ligand) expression by osteoblasts guides terminal osteoclast differentiation to nearby sites. *Bone* 1998; 23[Suppl 1]:S334.

111. DeMulder A, Suggs SV, Zsebo KM, et al. Effects of stem cell factor on osteoclast-like cell formation in long-term human marrow cultures. *J Bone Miner Res* 1992;7:1337–1344.

112. Muguruma Y, Lee M. Isolation and characterization of murine clonogenic osteoclast progenitors by cell surface phenotype analysis. *Blood* 1998;91:1272–1279.

113. Gattei V, Aldinucci D, Quinn J, et al. Human osteoclasts and preosteoclast cells (FLG 29.1) express functional c-kit receptors and interact with osteoblast and stromal cells via membrane-bound stem cell factor. *Cell Growth Differ* 1996;7:753–763.

114. Blair HC, Julian BA, Dong S-S. Formation of human osteoclasts *(in vitro)* is blocked by antibody to stem cell factor (c-kit ligand) expressed by osteoblasts supporting differentiation. *J Bone Miner Res* 1997; 12[Suppl 1]:S196.

115. Van'T Hof R, Von Linden M, Nijweide P, et al. Stem cell factor stimulates chicken osteoclast activity *in vitro*. *FASEB J* 1997;11:287–293.

116. Ihle J, Pepersack L, Rebar L. Regulation of T cell differentiation: *in vitro* induction of 20-hydrosteroid dehydrogenase in splenic lymphocytes from athymic mice by a unique lymphokine. *J Immunol* 1981;126: 2184–2189.

117. Ihle J. Interleukin-3 and hematopoiesis. *Chem Immunol* 1992;51:65–106.

118. Clark-Lewis I, Aebersold R, Ziltener H, et al. Automated chemical synthesis of a protein growth factor for hemopoietic cells, interleukin-3. *Science* 1986;231: 134–139.

119. Robb L, Drinkwater CC, Metcalf D, et al. Hematopoietic and lung abnormalities in mice with a null mutation of the common beta subunit of the receptors for granulocyte-macrophage colony-stimulating factor and interleukins 3 and 5. *Proc Natl Acad Sci USA* 1995;92: 9565–9569.

120. Bagley CJ, Woodcock JM, Stomski FC, et al. The structural and functional basis of cytokine receptor activation: lessons from the common beta subunit of the granulocyte-macrophage colony-stimulating factor, in-

terleukin-3 (IL-3), and IL-5 receptors. [Review]. *Blood* 1997;89:1471–1482.

121. de Groot RP, Coffer PJ, Koenderman L. Regulation of proliferation, differentiation and survival by the IL-3/IL-5/GM-CSF receptor family. *Cell Signal* 1998;10: 619–628.

122. Sato N, Sakamaki K, Terada N, et al. Signal transduction by the high-affinity GM-CSF receptor: two distinct cytoplasmic regions of the common beta subunit responsible for different signaling. *EMBO J* 1993;12: 4181–4189.

123. Jucker M, Feldman RA. Identification of a new adapter protein that may link the common beta subunit of the receptor for granulocyte/macrophage colony-stimulating factor, interleukin (IL)-3, and IL-5 to phosphatidylinositol 3-kinase. *J Biol Chem* 1995;270:27817–27822.

124. Welham MJ, Duronio V, Leslie KB, et al. Multiple hemopoietins, with the exception of interleukin-4, induce modification of Shc and mSos1, but not their translocation. *J Biol Chem* 1994;269:21165–21176.

125. Duronio V, Clark-Lewis I, Federspiel B, et al. Tyrosine phosphorylation of receptor beta subunits and common substrates in response to interleukin-3 and granulocyte-macrophage colony-stimulating factor. *J Biol Chem* 1992;267:21856–21863.

126. Mach N, Lantz CS, Galli SJ, et al. Involvement of interleukin-3 in delayed-type hypersensitivity. *Blood* 1998;91:778–783.

127. Sugita Y, Zhao B, Shankar P, et al. CNS interleukin-3 (IL-3) expression and neurological syndrome in antisense-IL-3 transgenic mice. *J Neuropathol Exp Neurol* 1999;58:480–488.

128. Barton BE, Mayer R. IL-3 induces differentiation of bone marrow precursor cells to osteoclast-like cells. *J Immunol* 1989;143:3211–3216.

129. Pierelli L, Scambia G, d'Onofrio G, et al. Generation of multinuclear tartrate-resistant acid phosphatase positive osteoclasts in liquid culture of purified human peripheral blood CD34+ progenitors. *Br J Haematol* 1997;96:64–69.

130. Sabokbar A, Fujikawa Y, Athanasou NA. IL-3 and GM-CSF support human monocyte-osteoclast differentiation. *Bone* 1998;23[Suppl]:S215.

131. Weitzmann MN, Srivastava SK, Ross FP, et al. The integrin $\alpha v \beta 3$, initially absent, is induced by cytokine treatment. *Bone* 1998;23[Suppl]:S217.

132. Bendixen A, Maruyama M, Pike JW, et al. Estrogen receptor–mediated interference in cytokine signaling: a novel perspective in negative regulation of hematopoiesis. *Bone* 1998;23[Suppl]:S267.

133. Marks CR, Seifert MF, Marks SC III. Osteoclast populations in congenital osteopetrosis: additional evidence of heterogeneity. *Metab Bone Dis Rel Res* 1984;5: 259–264.

134. Steingrimsson E, Moore KJ, Lamoreux ML, et al. Molecular basis of mouse *microphthalmia (mi)* mutations helps explain their developmental and phenotypic consequences. *Nat Genet* 1994;8:256–263.

135. Nechushtan H, Zhang Z, Razin E. Microphthalmia (mi) in murine mast cells: regulation of its stimuli-mediated expression on the translational level. *Blood* 1997;89: 2999–3008.

136. Bartley TD, Bogenberger J, Hunt P, et al. Identification and cloning of a megakaryocyte growth and develop-

ment factor that is a ligand for the cytokine receptor Mpl. *Cell* 1994;77:1117–1124.

137. Chang M, McNinch J, Basu R, et al. Cloning and characterization of the human megakaryocyte growth and development factor (MGDF) gene. *J Biol Chem* 1995; 270:511–514.

138. Park H, Park SS, Jin EH, et al. Identification of functionally important residues of human thrombopoietin. *J Biol Chem* 1998;273:256–261.

139. Vigon I, Florindo C, Fichelson S, et al. Characterization of the murine Mpl proto-oncogene, a member of the hematopoietic cytokine receptor family: molecular cloning, chromosomal location and evidence for a function in cell growth. *Oncogene* 1993;8:2607–2615.

140. Murakami M, Narazaki M, Hibi M, et al. Critical cytoplasmic region of the interleukin 6 signal transducer gp 130 is conserved in the cytokine receptor family. *Proc Natl Acad Sci USA* 1991;88:11349–11353.

141. Skoda RC, Seldin DC, Chiang MK, et al. Murine c-mpl: a member of the hematopoietic growth factor receptor superfamily that transduces a proliferative signal. *EMBO J* 1993;12:2645–2653.

142. Sattler M, Durstin MA, Frank DA, et al. The thrombopoietin receptor c-MPL activates JAK2 and TYK2 tyrosine kinases. *Exp Hematol* 1995;23:1040–1048.

143. Morita H, Tahara T, Matsumoto A, et al. Functional analysis of the cytoplasmic domain of the human Mpl receptor for tyrosine-phosphorylation of the signaling molecules, proliferation and differentiation. *FEBS Lett* 1996;395:228–234.

144. Ezumi Y, Takayama H, Okuma M. Thrombopoietin, c-Mpl ligand, induces tyrosine phosphorylation of Tyk2, JAK2, and STAT3, and enhances agonist-induced aggregation in platelets *in vitro*. *FEBS Lett* 1995;374: 48–52.

145. Drachman JG, Millett KM, Kaushansky K. Thrombopoietin signal transduction requires functional JAK2, not TYK2. *J Biol Chem* 1999;274:13480–13484.

146. Murone M, Carpenter DA, de Sauvage FJ. Hematopoietic deficiencies in c-mpl and TPO knockout mice. *Stem Cells* 1998;16:1–6.

147. Kimura S, Roberts AW, Metcalf D, et al. Hematopoietic stem cell deficiencies in mice lacking c-mpl, the receptor for thrombopoietin. *Proc Natl Acad Sci USA* 1998;95:1195–1200.

148. Zhou W, Toombs CF, Zou T, et al. Transgenic mice overexpressing human c-mpl ligand exhibit chronic thrombocytosis and display enhanced recovery from 5-fluorouracil or antiplatelet serum treatment. *Blood* 1997;89:1551–1559.

149. Yan X-G, Lacey D, Fletcher F, et al. Chronic exposure to retroviral vector encoded MGDF (mpl-ligand) induces lineage-specific growth and differentiation of megakaryocytes in mice. *Blood* 1995;86:4025–4033.

150. Yan X-Q, Lacey D, Hill D, et al. A model of myelofibrosis and osteosclerosis in mice induced by overexpressing thrombopoietin (mpl ligand): reversal of disease by bone marrow transplantation. *Blood* 1996;88: 402–409.

Skeletal Growth Factors,
edited by Ernesto Canalis.
Lippincott Williams & Wilkins, Philadelphia, © 2000.

29

Role of Cytokines in Postmenopausal Osteoporosis

Roberto Pacifici

Washington University School of Medicine and Barnes-Jewish Hospital, St. Louis, Missouri 63110

CYTOKINES AND CONTROL OF BONE REMODELING

Postmenopausal osteoporosis is a heterogeneous disorder characterized by a progressive loss of bone tissue which begins after natural or surgical menopause and leads to fracture within 15 to 20 years from the cessation of ovarian function. Although suboptimal skeletal development ("low peak bone mass") and age-related bone loss may be contributing factors, a hormone-dependent increase in bone resorption and accelerated loss of bone mass in the first 5 or 10 years after menopause appear to be the main pathogenetic factors.

A large number of immune and hematopoietic factors have been shown to have complex and overlapping effects on both bone formation and resorption. Among these are interleukin-1 α (IL-1α), IL-1β (1–5), IL-6 (6–8), tumor necrosis factor (TNF) α and β (9,10), macrophage colony-stimulating factor (M-CSF) (11,12), and granulocyte-macrophage CSF (GM-CSF) (13, 14). Osteoclast differentiation is also specifically regulated by a group of recently described factors related to the TNF and TNF receptor families. Among these factors are osteoprotegerin (OPG) and OPG ligand (OPGL), also known as osteoclast differentiation factor (ODF) or receptor activator of NFκB ligand (RANKL).

IL-1 and TNF are among the most powerful stimulators of bone resorption known and are well-recognized inhibitors of bone formation (5,9,15). These cytokines promote bone resorption *in vitro* (1,2) and cause bone loss and hypercalcemia when infused *in vivo* (16–18). IL-1 and TNF activate mature osteoclasts indirectly via a primary effect on osteoblasts (10,19) and inhibit osteoclast apoptosis. In addition, they markedly enhance osteoclast formation by stimulating osteoclast precursor proliferation both directly (20) and by stimulating the proosteoclastogenic activity of stromal cells. IL-1 and TNF are also powerful inducers of other cytokines which regulate the differentiation of osteoclast precursor cells into mature osteoclasts, such as IL-6 (6,21), M-CSF (22), and GM-CSF (23). Therefore, with respect to osteoclastogenesis, IL-1 and TNF should be regarded as "upstream" cytokines necessary for inducing the secretion of "downstream" factors which stimulate hematopoietic osteoclast precursors. This cascade mechanism assures that small changes in IL-1 and TNF levels result in large changes in osteoclast production.

DNA cloning has revealed two independent species of IL-1, IL-1α and IL-1β, which, despite a distant homology, exert the same biological effects (24). In human cells, there is a preponderant expression of the IL-1β gene, which after antigenic stimulation can increase 200 to 300 times within 2 to 3 hours (24).

A specific competitive inhibitor of IL-1, known as IL-1 receptor antagonist (IL-1ra), has been purified from the supernatant of immunoglobulin G (IgG)–stimulated monocytes (25) and from the myelomonocytic cell line U937 (26). This substance exists in two forms, a 22-kDa glycosylated form and a 17-kDa nonglycosylated form. The 17-kDa form has been cloned and expressed in *Escherichia coli* (26). This recombinant molecule, which has 26% amino acid sequence homology with IL-1β, binds to cells expressing primarily the 87-kDa type I IL-1 receptor with nearly the same affinity as IL-1 and competes with either IL-1α or IL-1β on these cells without detectable IL-1 agonist effects (27,28). The type I IL-1 receptor is expressed in T cells, tissue macrophages, endothelial cells, and bone cells (29,30). IL-1ra also binds, although with a lower affinity, to the type II IL-1 receptor, which is expressed mainly in blood neutrophils and B cells (29). Since the binding of five molecules of IL-1 per cell is sufficient to induce a full biological response, a 50% IL-1 inhibition in bone cells requires amounts of IL-1ra up to 100 times in excess of the amounts of IL-1α or IL-1β present.

IL-6 stimulates the early stages of osteoclastogenesis in human and murine cultures (31,32). IL-6 increases bone resorption in systems rich in osteoclast precursor, such as the mouse fetal metacarpal assay (33), whereas it has no effect in organ cultures where more mature cells predominate, such as murine fetal radii (32). This suggests that IL-6 increases the formation of osteoclasts from hemopoietic precursors but does not activate mature osteoclasts.

The essential role of CSFs in the proliferation and differentiation of osteoclast precursors is best demonstrated by the presence of osteopetrosis in a natural M-CSF knockout, the *op/op* mouse (34). These mice, which are cured by administration of M-CSF (35), have an extra thymidine inserted within the coding region of the M-CSF gene, a mutation that generates a stop codon within the coding sequence (36), thereby resulting in the production of a defective M-CSF (34). The formation of osteoclasts in bone marrow cultures is also increased by GM-CSF (23,37). This factor stimulates the early stages of osteoclastogenesis in cooperation with IL-3 (14,38). Although in the mouse, osteoclast formation is completely blocked by anti-M-CSF, but not anti-GM-CSF, antibodies (12), GM-CSF

is critical for the proliferation and differentiation of human osteoclast precursors (39).

OPGL is a membrane-bound factor produced by stromal cells and osteoblasts that bind to a receptor known as RANK or osteoclast differentiation–activating receptor (ODAR), which is expressed on the surface of osteoclasts and osteoclast precursors of the monocytic lineage (40). In the presence of M-CSF, OPGL induces the differentiation of monocytic cells into osteoclasts (40). Since M-CSF and OPGL are capable of inducing osteoclast formation in the absence of stromal cells, these factors are regarded as the true essential osteoclastogenic cytokines. OPGL also binds to OPG, a soluble and membrane-bound factor produced by numerous hematopoietic cells. Thus, OPG, by functioning as a decoy for OPGL, is currently recognized as a potent antiosteoclastogenic cytokine (41) (Fig. 29.1).

Although most bone cell–targeting cytokines are produced by either bone or bone marrow cells, mononuclear cells of the monocyte/macrophage lineage are recognized as the major source of IL-1 and TNF (29). In contrast, preosteoclastogenic downstream cytokines are produced mainly by stromal cells and osteoblasts (42,43). Thus, osteoclastogenesis requires the hierarchical interaction of mononuclear cells, stromal cells, and/or osteoblasts and hematopoietic osteoclast precursors.

The main consequence of increased cytokine production in the bone microenvironment is an expansion of the osteoclastic pool due to increased osteoclast formation and elongation of their life span (44). In addition, enhanced cytokine production results in increased activity of mature osteoclasts and increased osteoblastic activity. The latter compensates in part for the consequences of increased bone formation on bone mass.

Cytokines exert their regulatory effects on bone turnover by stimulating both the secretory and proliferative activities of mature cells. However, they also condition the differentiation of immature cells, leading to the emergence of new phenotypes which favor osteoclastogenesis. Examples of this phenomenon are the differentiation of stromal cell precursors in "high osteoclastogenic" stromal cells as a result of the

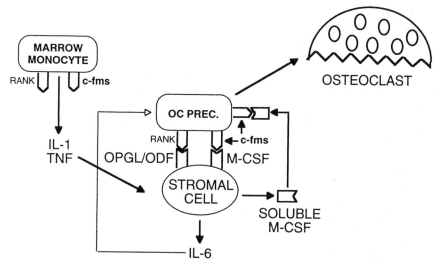

FIG. 29.1. Cells and cytokines critical for osteoclast formation. Estrogen decreases osteoclast formation by downregulating the monocytic production of interleukin-1 *(IL-1)* and tumor necrosis factor *(TNF)* and the stromal cell production of macrophage colony-stimulating factor *(M-CSF)* and IL-6.

increased bone marrow levels of IL-1 and TNF induced by estrogen deficiency (45) and the differentiation of cells of the monocytic lineage into osteoclasts in response to factors produced by stromal cells such as IL-6, IL-11 (46), and M-CSF (12).

Among the cytokines known to be regulated by estrogen are IL-1, IL-6, and TNF (46,47).

EFFECTS OF MENOPAUSE ON CYTOKINE PRODUCTION

The cytokines first recognized to be regulated by estrogen were IL-1 and TNF. This observation was promoted by the finding that monocytes of patients with "high-turnover" osteoporosis, the histological hallmark of postmenopausal osteoporosis, secrete increased amounts of IL-1 (48). Cross-sectional and prospective comparisons of pre- and postmenopausal women revealed that monocytic production of IL-1 and TNF increases after natural and surgical menopause and is decreased by treatment with estrogen and progesterone (49,50). Subsequent observations showed that the postmenopausal increase in IL-1 activity results from an effect of estrogen on the production of both IL-1 and

IL-1ra (51). Studies in women undergoing ovariectomy (OVX) (52,53) revealed that estrogen withdrawal is associated with increased production not only of IL-1 and TNF but also of GM-CSF. The changes in these cytokine levels occur in a temporal sequence consistent with a causal role of IL-1, TNF, and GM-CSF in the pathogenesis of OVX-induced bone loss (52). Moreover, since the increase in GM-CSF production precedes the increase in IL-1 and TNF (52), the data suggest that the inreased production of GM-CSF is not a result of enhanced secretion of IL-1 and TNF but rather a direct effect of estrogen withdrawal (52).

The *in vitro* production of cytokines from cultured monocytes reflects phenotypic characteristics acquired from local stimuli during their maturation in the bone marrow (54). This phenomenon is thought to play an important role in providing the basis for tissue and functional specificity. Consequently, monocyte cytokine secretion is relevant to postmenopausal bone loss, as it mirrors cytokine secretion from marrow-resident cells of the monocyte-macrophage lineage or monocytes that have homed to bone (54). This hypothesis was proved correct by studies showing that the secretion of IL-1 from blood monocytes correlates with that from bone marrow mononuclear cells in subjects with Paget's disease and osteoporosis (55,56) and by observations in rats and mice, where OVX and estrogen replacement were found to regulate the bone marrow mononuclear cell production of IL-1 and TNF (57,58).

It is also important to recognize that monocytes are the major source of IL-1 and TNF in the bone marrow (59). Moreover, the anatomical proximity of mononuclear cells to remodeling loci, the capacity to secrete numerous products recognized for their effects in bone remodeling, and the expression of integrin receptors (60), which make these cells capable of adhering to the bone matrix, make them likely candidates as participants in skeletal remodeling.

More direct evidence in favor of a cause–effect relationship between increased production of IL-1, TNF, and IL-6 and postmenopausal osteoporosis is provided by the findings of Ralston (61) demonstrating that IL-1, TNF, and IL-6 mRNAs are expressed more frequently in bone cells from untreated postmenopausal women than in those from women on estrogen replacement. That the increased monocytic production of cytokines plays a direct role in inducing bone resorption was later demonstrated by Cohen-Solal et al. (62) by examining the bone-resorption activity of culture supernatants from monocytes obtained from pre- and postmenopausal women. Using this approach, it was found that the culture media of monocytes obtained from postmenopausal women have increased *in vitro* bone-resorption activity, which is blocked by addition of IL-1ra and anti-TNF antibody.

Recent studies have provided new insight about the molecular mechanism by which estrogen regulates the production of inflammatory cytokines.

The genomic effects of estradiol (E_2) are mediated by a ligand-inducible transcription factor known as estrogen receptor (ER). Following the discovery of a second ER phenotype (ERβ) (63–65), the first identified ER became known as ERα (63). ERα is expressed primarily in the uterus, testis, ovary, and pituitary, while ERβ is expressed mostly in the prostate, ovary, lung, bladder, brain, uterus, and testis (66). Although

ERα and ERβ have similar DNA-binding domains, their A/B domains and activation-function region 1 (AF-1) is quite different, suggesting they that may differentially regulate ER-responsive genes (66). Recent studies have indeed demonstrated that ERα and ERβ respond differently to ligands, leading to opposite effects on activator protein-1 (AP-1)-induced gene expression (67). Specifically, while the ERα-mediated effects of E_2 lead to stimulation of AP-1-induced gene expression, E_2 acts as a repressor of AP-1-induced transcription when bound to ERβ (67).

Cells of the monocytic lineage are known to express both ERα and ERβ. Estrogen binding to ERβ leads to decreased production of c-Jun and JunD, two members of the AP-1 family of transcription factors. Decreased AP-1 production results in decreased AP-1-induced TNF gene expression and lower TNF production (68). Interestingly, binding of E_2 to ERα results in stimulation of TNF gene expression. Recently, Ruh et al. (69,70) have reported that E_2 stimulates IL-1β gene expression in cells overexpressing ERα. While the ERβ-mediated effects of E_2 on IL-1 remain to be determined, one can speculate that ERβ mediates the inhibitory effects of E_2 on the IL-1 gene.

Interestingly, the association between estrogen deficiency and increased IL-1 and TNF activity was confirmed by others when IL-1 activity was measured by bioassay (53,71–74). Conversely, this association was not observed when IL-1 was measured by enzyme-linked immunosorbent assay (ELISA) or immunoradiometric assay (IRMA) (75,76). It should be noted that IL-1 bioactivity reflects the relative amounts of biologically active IL-1 and IL-1 antagonists present in the test sample. Consequently, IL-1 bioassays provide a reliable estimate of target cell response to IL-1. In contrast, ELISAs and IRMAs, although more specific, do not provide information on the amount of biologically active IL-1 which binds to the signal-transducing type I IL-1 receptor. The binding of IL-1 to the type I receptor is, in fact, antagonized by IL-1ra (29,77), soluble type I (sIL-1 RI) and type II (sIL-1 RII) IL-1 receptors (78,79), anti-IL-1β autoantibodies (80), and IL-1β binding proteins

(81). Moreover, while sIL-1 RI antagonizes the effects of IL-1ra (79), sIL-1 RII binds IL-1β but does not bind IL-1ra (78,79). Thus, sIL-1 RII can compete with cell-associated receptors for IL-1β and potentiate the inhibitory action of IL-1ra. Since estrogen could regulate IL-1 bioactivity by modulating factors which antagonize the binding of IL-1 to its active receptor, investigations on the effects of estrogen on production of IL-1ra, sIL-1 receptors, and IL-1 binding proteins are likely to provide important information on the effect of estrogen on IL-1 bioactivity.

Recent studies have also shown that estrogen increases expression of the decoy type II IL-1 receptor in bone marrow cells and osteoclasts (82). Thus, upregulation of cell responsiveness to IL-1 via downregulation of IL-1 RII is also likely to be a key mechanism by which estrogen deficiency induces bone loss.

Subsequent studies conducted to determine if estrogen regulates the production of IL-6 revealed that in murine stromal and osteoblastic cells IL-6 production is inhibited by the addition of estrogen (6) and stimulated by estrogen withdrawal (8). *In vivo* studies also revealed that the production of IL-6 is increased in cultures of bone marrow cells from OVX mice (7). This effect is mediated, at least in the mouse, by an indirect effect of estrogen on the transcription activity of the proximal 225-bp sequence of the IL-6 promoter (83,84).

Interestingly, although studies with human cell lines have demonstrated inhibitory effects of estrogen on the human IL-6 promoter (85), three independent groups have failed to demonstrate an inhibitory effect of estrogen on IL-6 production from human bone cells and stromal cells expressing functional estrogen receptors (43,86,87). These data raise the possibility that the production of human IL-6 protein does not increase in conditions of estrogen deficiency. This is further supported by a report that in humans surgical menopause is not followed by an increase in IL-6, although it causes an increase in sIL-6 receptor (88).

Another possible intermediate in estrogen action is transforming growth factor-β (TGF-β). This growth factor is a multifunctional protein produced by many mammalian cells, including osteoblasts, and has a wide range of biological activities. TGF-β is a potent osteoblast mitogen (89). In specific experimental conditions, TGF-β decreases both osteoclastic resorptive activity and osteoclast recruitment.

Oursler et al. (90) have reported that estrogen increases the steady-state level of TGF-β mRNA and release of TGF-β protein. This mechanism provides the first example of positive effects of estrogen in bone which may result in decreased bone turnover.

Recent studies have shown that one of the key mechanisms by which estrogen regulates osteoclastogenesis is by modulating the stromal cell production of M-CSF.

In conditions of E_2 deficiency, the high bone marrow levels of IL-1 and TNF lead to the expansion of a stromal cell population which produces larger amounts of soluble M-CSF (45). These high M-CSF-producing stromal cells have an increased capacity to support osteoclastogenesis (Fig. 29.2). Interestingly, estrogen has no direct regulatory effects on the production of soluble M-CSF, as it regulates M-CSF secretion exclusively by conditioning the differentiation of stromal cells toward a phenotype characterized by lower production of M-CSF. The high M-CSF-producing stromal cells found in estrogen-deficient mice are characterized by increased phosphorylation of the transcription factor Egr-1. While Egr-1 binds and sequesters the nuclear protein Sp-1, phosphorylated Egr-1 does not bind to Sp-1. As a result, cells from estrogen-deficient mice are characterized by increased levels of free Sp-1. This protein binds to the M-CSF promoter and stimulates M-CSF gene expression (91) (Fig. 29.3).

In addition to an indirect effect on soluble M-CSF, E_2 has been shown to decrease the production of membrane-bound M-CSF via a direct effect on bone marrow cells (92,93). Thus, estrogen regulates the key osteoclastogenic cytokine with at least two distinct mechanisms.

Little information on the effects of menopause on the production of OPG and OPGL is available. However, Lacey et al. (unpublished observations) have shown that circulating levels of OPGL increase with aging. Moreover, estrogen

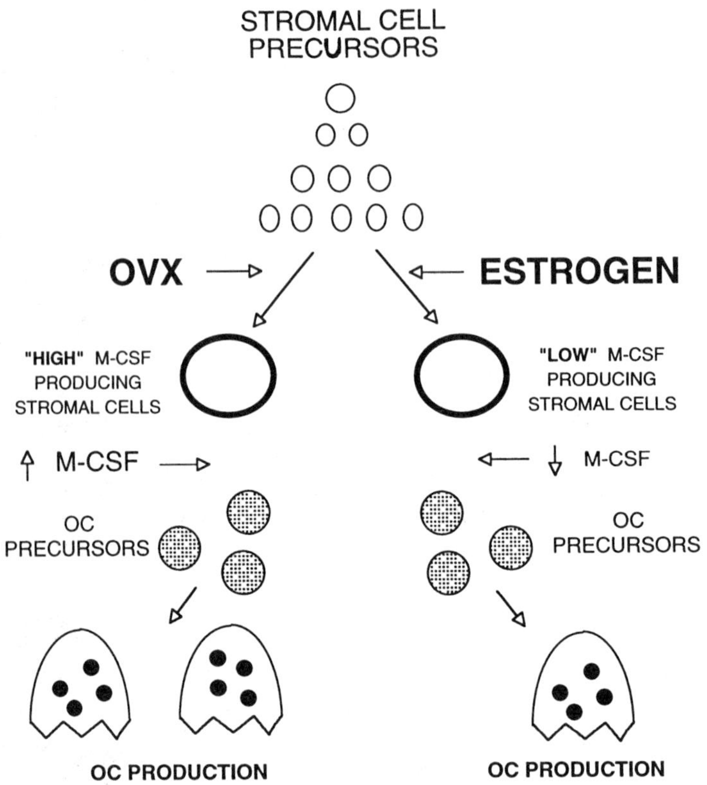

FIG. 29.2. Estrogen regulates the differentiation of stromal cell precursors and leads to the formation of "low" macrophage colony-stimulating factor *(M-CSF)*–producing stromal cells.

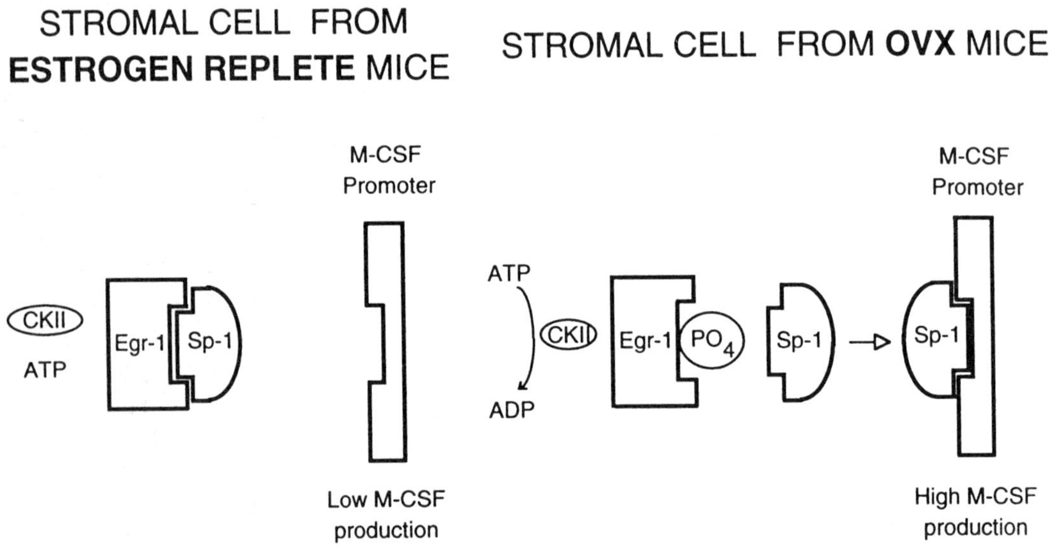

FIG. 29.3. Mechanism by which stromal cells from estrogen-deficient mice produce low levels of macrophage colony-stimulating factor *(M-CSF)*. Stromal cells from estrogen-deficient mice exhibit increased creatine kinase II *(CKII)*–dependent phosphorylation of the nuclear protein Egr-1. Phosphorylated Egr-1 binds less avidly to the transcriptional activator Sp-1, and the resulting higher levels of free Sp-1 stimulate M-CSF gene expression.

has been shown to increase the production of OPG. Thus, it appears that OPG and OPGL are subjected to regulatory mechanisms similar to those described for other bone-regulating cytokines.

Attempts to demonstrate that menopause increases circulating levels of IL-1, TNF, and IL-6 have been, for the most part, unsuccessful, presumably because only a small fraction of the cytokine produced in the bone marrow "leaks" into the peripheral circulation. The lack of increased serum cytokine levels in estrogen-deficient women is also consistent with the notion that since cytokine release requires the adherence of cells to a solid substrate (94,95), estrogen deficiency is unlikely to stimulate cytokine production from circulating cells.

INTERLEUKINS 1 AND 6 AND TUMOR NECROSIS FACTOR ARE POTENT INDUCERS OF BONE LOSS IN CONDITIONS OF ESTROGEN DEFICIENCY

The development of specific cytokine inhibitors and transgenic mice lacking a cytokine or a cytokine receptor has made it possible to link genes to specific phenotypes and to determine the function of numerous proteins.

Lorenzo et al. (96) have shown that mice insensitive to IL-1 due to the lack of IL-1 receptor type I are protected against OVX-induced bone loss.

These findings confirm earlier studies demonstrating that treatment with IL-1ra prevents bone loss in OVX rats (57). Together, these observations establish IL-1 as an essential mediator of the effects of estrogen deficiency in bone.

Substantial evidence supports the notion that TNF (either alone or in cooperation with IL-1) is also a key mediator of the effects of estrogen deficiency in bone. Treatment of OVX mice with TNF binding protein, a potent inhibitor of TNF, completely prevents the bone loss and the increase in osteoclast formation and bone resorption induced by OVX, while it has no effect in sham-operated mice (97). Moreover, Ammann et al. (98) have demonstrated that transgenic mice insensitive to TNF due to over-

expression of soluble TNF receptor are also protected against OVX-induced bone loss. Finally, an orally active inhibitor of IL-1 and TNF production has been shown to completely prevent bone loss in OVX rats (99). Although the finding that functional block of either IL-1 or TNF is sufficient to prevent OVX-induced bone loss may appear to be difficult to reconcile, it should be emphasized that in most biological systems IL-1 and TNF have potent synergistic effects. Thus, the functional block of one of these two cytokines elicits biological effects identical to those induced by blockade of both IL-1 and TNF. The long-term stimulation of bone resorption which follows OVX is sustained primarily by an expansion of the osteoclastic pool. Since osteoclast formation is synergistically stimulated by IL-1 and TNF (58), it is not surprising that long-term inhibition of either IL-1 or TNF results in complete prevention of OVX-induced bone loss.

While studies with transgenic mice and inhibitors of IL-1 and TNF have consistently demonstrated that IL-1 and TNF are key inducers of bone loss in OVX animals, investigations aimed at assessing the contribution of IL-6 to OVX-induced bone loss have yielded conflicting results. In favor of a causal role for IL-6 in OVX-induced bone loss is the report of Poli et al. (100), indicating that IL-6 knockout mice are protected against the loss of trabecular bone induced by OVX. Against a significant pathogenetic role of IL-6 are studies demonstrating that osteoporosis is not a feature of transgenic mice overexpressing IL-6 (101). Studies have also been conducted by injecting an antibody to neutralize IL-6 in OVX mice. Neutralizing IL-6 prevents the increase in osteoclast formation induced by estrogen deficiency (7,97) but does prevent OVX-induced bone loss and does not decrease *in vivo* bone resorption (97). These findings confirm that IL-6 contributes to the expansion of the osteoclastic pool induced by OVX; however, this cytokine does not appear to be the dominant factor in inducing bone loss in estrogen-deficient mice.

SUMMARY AND CONCLUSIONS

The mechanisms of the bone-sparing effects of estrogen appear to be particularly complex as they involve the regulated production of up-stream cytokines from mononuclear cells and bone cells and the responsiveness of stromal cells to these cytokines. Although many details of this process remain to be defined, it is now clearly established that estrogen downregulates the production of IL-1 and TNF from bone marrow mononuclear cells. Since the production of these cytokines is triggered by bone matrix fragments via integrin receptors (94,95,102), estrogen appears to regulate the functional communication between mononuclear cells and the bone matrix. IL-1 and TNF target stromal cells and induce the production of two essential osteoclastogenic factors, OPGL and M-CSF, whose production is also regulated by estrogen. Thus, both lower IL-1 and TNF levels and a decreased stromal cell response to IL-1 and TNF likely account for the ability of estrogen to block osteoclastogenesis.

Numerous other local and systemic factors are likely to participate in the hormonal regulation of bone turnover. Probable candidates are IL-6 and TGF-β. The exact contribution of IL-6 remains unclear because of insufficient data demonstrating that blockade of IL-6 decreases bone resorption *in vivo* and bone loss in a bona fide experimental model of postmenopausal osteoporosis. However, the exact role of IL-6, as well as that of TGF-β, is likely to be defined in the near future.

Remarkable progress has been made in clarifying the mechanism of the bone-sparing effect of estrogen in animal models. A more challenging task will be to demonstrate the relevance of the mechanisms described above in human subjects.

REFERENCES

1. Gowen M, Wood DD, Ihrie EJ, et al. An interleukin-1-like factor stimulates bone resorption *in vitro*. *Nature* 1983;306:378–380.
2. Lorenzo JA, Sousa SL, Alander C, et al. Comparison of the bone-resorbing activity in the supernatants from phytohemaglutinin-stimulated human peripheral blood mononuclear cells with that of cytokines through the use of an antiserum to interleukin 1. *Endocrinology* 1987;121:1164–1170.
3. Gowen M, Wood DD, Russell RGG. Stimulation of the proliferation of human bone cells *in vitro* by human monocyte products with interleukin-1 activity. *J Clin Invest* 1985;75:1223–1229.
4. Canalis E. Interleukin-1 has independent effects on deoxyribonucleic acid and collagen synthesis in cultures of rat calvariae. *Endocrinology* 1986;118:74–81.
5. Stashenko P, Dewhirst FE, Rooney ML, et al. Interleukin-1β is a potent inhibitor of bone formation *in vitro*. *J Bone Miner Res* 1987;2:559–565.
6. Girasole G, Jilka RL, Passeri G, et al. 17β-Estradiol inhibits interleukin-6 production by bone marrow–derived stromal cells and osteoblasts *in vitro:* a potential mechanism for the antiosteoporotic effect of estrogens. *J Clin Invest* 1992;89:883–891.
7. Jilka RL, Hangoc G, Girasole G, et al. Increased osteoclast development after estrogen loss: mediation by interleukin-6. *Science* 1992;257:88–91.
8. Passeri G, Girasole G, Jilka RL, et al. Increased interleukin-6 production by murine bone marrow and bone cells after estrogen withdrawal. *Endocrinology* 1993;133:822–828.
9. Bertolini DR, Nedwin GE, Bringman TS, et al. Stimulation of bone resorption and inhibition of bone formation *in vitro* by human tumor necrosis factor. *Nature* 1986;319:516–518.
10. Thomson BM, Mundy GR, Chambers TJ. Tumor necrosis factor α and β induce osteoblastic cells to stimulate osteoclastic bone resorption. *J Immunol* 1987;138:775–779.
11. Takahashi N, Udagawa N, Akatsu T, et al. Role of colony-stimulating factors in osteoclast development. *J Bone Miner Res* 1991;6:977–985.
12. Tanaka S, Takahashi N, Udagawa N, et al. Macrophage colony-stimulating factor is indispensable for both proliferation and differentiation of osteoclast progenitors. *J Clin Invest* 1993;91:257–263.
13. Schneider GB, Relfson M. Pluripotent hemopoietic stem cells give rise to osteoclasts in vitro: effect of rGM-CSF. *Bone Miner* 1989;5:129–138.
14. Kurihara N, Suda T, Miura Y, et al. Generation of osteoclasts from isolated hematopoietic progenitor cells. *Blood* 1989;74:1295–1302.
15. Nguyen L, Dewhirst FE, Hauschka PV, et al. Interleukin-1β stimulates bone resorption and inhibits bone formation *in vivo*. *Lymphokine Cytokine Res* 1991;10:15–21.
16. Boyce BF, Aufdemorte TB, Garrett IR, et al. Effects of interleukin-1 on bone turnover in normal mice. *Endocrinology* 1989;125:1142–1150.
17. Sabatini M, Boyce B, Aufdemorte TB, et al. Infusions of recombinant human interleukin 1 alpha and beta cause hypercalcemia in normal mice. *Proc Natl Acad Sci USA* 1988;85:5235–5239.
18. Johnson RA, Boyce BF, Mundy GR, et al. Tumors producing human tumor necrosis factor induce hypercalcemia and osteoclastic bone resorption in nude mice. *Endocrinology* 1989;124:1424–1427.
19. Thomson BM, Saklatvala J, Chambers TJ. Osteoblasts mediate interleukin 1 stimulation of bone resorption by rat osteoclasts. *J Exp Med* 1986;164:104–112.
20. Pfeilschifter J, Chenu C, Bird A, et al. Interleukin-1 and tumor necrosis fator stimulate the formation of human osteoclast-like cells *in vitro*. *J Bone Miner Res* 1989;4:113–118.
21. Elias JA, Lentz V. IL-1 and tumor necrosis factor synergistically stimulate fibroblast IL-6 production and

stabilize IL-6 messenger RNA. *J Immunol* 1990;145: 161–166.

22. Felix R, Fleish H, Elford PR. Bone-resorbing cytokines enhance release of macrophage colony-stimulating activity by osteoblastic cell MC3T3-E1. *Calcif Tissue Int* 1989;44:356–360.

23. Lorenzo JA, Sousa SL, Fonseca JM, et al. Colony-stimulating factors regulate the development of multinucleated osteoclasts from recently replicated cells *in vitro. J Clin Invest* 1987;160:164–160.

24. Dinarello CA. Biology of interleukin 1. *FASEB J* 1988; 2:108–115.

25. Hannum CH, Wilcox CJ, Arend WP, et al. Interleukin-1 receptor antagonist activity of a human interleukin-1 inhibitor. *Nature* 1990;343:336–340.

26. Carter DB, Deibel MR Jr, Dunn CJ, et al. Purification, cloning, expression and biological characterization of an interleukin-1 receptor antagonist protein. *Nature* 1990;344:633–638.

27. Arend WP, Joslin FG, Thompson RC, et al. An IL-1 inhibitor from human monocytes. *J Immunol* 1989; 143:1851–1858.

28. Arend WP. Interleukin 1 receptor antagonist: a new member of the interleukin 1 family. *J Clin Invest* 1991; 88:1445–1451.

29. Dinarello CA. Interleukin-1 and interleukin-1 antagonism. *Blood* 1991;77:1627–1652.

30. Seckinger P, Klein-Nulend J, Alander C, et al. Natural and recombinant human IL-1 receptor antagonists block the effects of IL-1 on bone resorption and prostaglandin production. *J Immunol* 1990;145:4181–4184.

31. Kurihara N, Civin C, Roodman GD. Osteotropic factor responsiveness of highly purified populations of early and late precursors for human multinucleated cells expressing the osteoclast phenotype. *J Bone Miner Res* 1991;6:257–261.

32. Roodman GD. Interleukin-6: an osteotropic factor? *J Bone Miner Res* 1992;7:475–478.

33. Lowik CWGM, van der Pluijm G, Bloys H, et al. Parathyroid hormone (PTH) and PTH-like protein (PLP) stimulate IL-6 production by osteogenic cells: a possible role of interleukin-6 in osteoclastogenesis. *Biochem Biophys Res Commun* 1989;162:1546–1552.

34. Suda T, Takahashi N, Martin TJ. Modulation of osteoclast differentiation. *Endocr Rev* 1992;13:66–80.

35. Felix R, Cecchini MG, Fleish H. Macrophage colony-stimulating factor restores *in vivo* bone resorption in the op/op osteopetrotic mouse. *Endocrinology* 1990; 127:2592–2597.

36. Yoshida HS, Hayashi S, Kunisada T, et al. The murine mutation osteopetrosis is in the coding region of macrophage colony stimulating factor gene. *Nature* 1990;345:442–444.

37. Macdonald BR, Mundy GR, Clark S, et al. Effects of human recombinant CSF-GM and highly purified CSF-1 on the formation of multi-nucleated cells with osteoclast characteristics in long-term bone marrow cultures. *J Bone Miner Res* 1986;1:227–232.

38. Kurihara N, Chenu C, Miller M, et al. Identification of committed mononuclear precursors for osteoclast-like cells formed in long term human marrow cultures. *Endocrinology* 1990;126:2733–2741.

39. Matayoshi A, Brown C, DiPersio J, et al. Human blood-mobilized hematopoietic precursors differentiate into osteoclasts in the absence of stromal cells. *Proc Natl Acad Sci USA* 1996;93:10785–10790.

40. Lacey DL, Timms E, Tan HL, et al. Osteoprotegerin ligand is a cytokine that regulates osteoclast differentiation and activation. *Cell* 1998;93:165–176.

41. Simonet WS, Lacey DL, Dunstan CR, et al. Osteoprotegerin: a novel secreted protein involved in the regulation of bone density [see comments]. *Cell* 1997;89: 309–319.

42. Fibbe WE, Van Damme J, Billiau A, et al. Interleukin-1 induces human marrow stromal cells in long term cultures to produce G-CSF and M-CSF. *Blood* 1988; 71:431–435.

43. Rifas L, Kenney JS, Marcelli M, et al. Production of interleukin-6 in human osteoblasts and human bone marrow stromal cells: evidence that induction by interleukin-1 and tumor necrosis factor-α is not regulated by ovarian steroids. *Endocrinology* 1995;136:4056–4067.

44. Roodman GD. Advances in bone biology: the osteoclast. *Endocr Rev* 1996;17:308–332.

45. Kimble RB, Srivastava S, Ross FP, et al. Estrogen deficiency increases the ability of stromal cells to support osteoclastogenesis via an IL-1 and TNF mediated stimulation of M-CSF production. *J Biol Chem* 1996;271: 28890–28897.

46. Manolagas SC, Jilka RL. Bone marrow, cytokines, and bone remodeling. *N Engl J Med* 1995;332:305–311.

47. Pacifici R. Estrogen, cytokines and pathogenesis of postmenopausal osteoporosis. *J Bone Miner Res* 1996; 11:1043–1051.

48. Pacifici R, Rifas L, Teitelbaum S, et al. Spontaneous release of interleukin 1 from human blood monocytes reflects bone formation in idiopathic osteoporosis. *Proc Natl Acad Sci USA* 1987;84:4616–4620.

49. Pacifici R, Rifas L, McCracken R, et al. Ovarian steroid treatment blocks a postmenopausal increase in blood monocyte interleukin 1 release. *Proc Natl Acad Sci USA* 1989;86:2398–2402.

50. Pacifici R, Brown C, Rifas L, et al. TNFα and GM-CSF secretion from human blood monocytes: effect of menopause and estrogen replacement. *J Bone Miner Res* 1990;5:(abst 145).

51. Pacifici R, Vannice JL, Rifas L, et al. Monocytic secretion of interleukin-1 receptor antagonist in normal and osteoporotic women: effect of menopause and estrogen/progesterone therapy. *J Clin Endocrinol Metab* 1993;77:1135–1141.

52. Pacifici R, Brown C, Puscheck E, et al. Effect of surgical menopause and estrogen replacement on cytokine release from human blood mononuclear cells. *Proc Natl Acad Sci USA* 1991;88:5134–5138.

53. Fiore CE, Falcidia E, Foti R, et al. Differences in the time course of the effects of oophorectomy in women on parameters of bone metabolism and interleukin-1 levels in the circulation. *Bone Miner* 1993;20:79–85.

54. Horowitz M. Cytokines and estrogen in bone: anti-osteoporotic effects. *Science* 1993;260:626–627.

55. Pioli G, Girasole G, Pedrazzoni M, et al. Spontaneous release of interleukin 1 (IL-1) from medullary mononuclear cells of Pagetic subjects. *Calcif Tissue Int* 1989; 45:257–259.

56. Choen-Solal ME, Graulet AM, Guerris J, et al. Bone resorption at the femoral neck is dependent on local factors in nonosteoporotic late postmenopausal

women: an *in vitro–in vivo* study. *J Bone Miner Res* 1995;10:307–314.

57. Kimble RB, Vannice JL, Bloedow DC, et al. Interleukin-1 receptor antagonist decreases bone loss and bone resorption in ovariectomized rats. *J Clin Invest* 1994; 93:1959–1967.

58. Kitazawa R, Kimble RB, Vannice JL, et al. Interleukin-1 receptor antagonist and tumor necrosis factor binding protein decrease osteoclast formation and bone resorption in ovariectomized mice. *J Clin Invest* 1994;94: 2397–2406.

59. Dinarello CA. Interleukin-1 and its biologically related cytokines. *Adv Immunol* 1989;44:153–205.

60. Hynes RO. Integrins: versatility, modulation, and signaling in cell adhesion. *Cell* 1992;69:11–25.

61. Ralston SH. Analysis of gene expression in human bone biopsies by polymerase chain reaction: evidence for enhanced cytokine expression in postmenopausal osteoporosis. *J Bone Miner Res* 1994;9:883–890.

62. Cohen-Solal ME, Graulet AM, Denne MA, et al. Peripheral monocyte culture supernatants of menopausal women can induce bone resorption: involvement of cytokines. *J Clin Endocrinol Metab* 1993;77: 1648–1653.

63. Kuiper GG, Enmark E, Pelto-Huikko M, et al. Cloning of a novel receptor expressed in rat prostate and ovary. *Proc Natl Acad Sci USA* 1996;93:5925–5930.

64. Mosselman S, Polman J, Dijkema R. ER beta: identification and characterization of a novel human estrogen receptor. *FEBS Lett* 1996;392:49–53.

65. Tremblay GB, Tremblay A, Copeland NG, et al. Cloning, chromosomal localization, and functional analysis of the murine estrogen receptor beta. *Mol Endocrinol* 1997;11:353–365.

66. Couse JF, Lindzey J, Grandien K, et al. Tissue distribution and quantitative analysis of estrogen receptor-alpha (ERalpha) and estrogen receptor-beta (ERbeta) messenger ribonucleic acid in the wild-type and ERalpha-knockout mouse. *Endocrinology* 1997;138: 4613–4621.

67. Paech K, Webb P, Kuiper GG, et al. Differential ligand activation of estrogen receptors ERalpha and ERbeta at AP1 sites [see comments]. *Science* 1997;277:1508–1510.

68. Srivastava S, Weitzmann MN, Cenci S, et al. Estrogen decreases TNF gene expression by blocking JNK activity and the resulting production of c-jun and junD. *J Clin Invest* 1999;104:503–513.

69. Ruh MF, Bi Y, Cox L, et al. Effect of environmental estrogens on IL-1beta promoter activity in a macrophage cell line. *Endocrine* 1998;9:207–211.

70. Ruh MF, Bi Y, D'Alonzo R, et al. Effect of estrogens on IL-1beta promoter activity. *J Steroid Biochem Mol Biol* 1998;66:203–210.

71. Pioli G, Basini G, Pedrazzoni M, et al. Spontaneous release of interleukin-1 and interleukin-6 by peripheral blood monocytes after ovariectomy. *Clin Sci* 1992;83: 503–507.

72. Ralston SH, Russell RGG, Gowen M. Estrogen inhibits release of tumor necrosis factor from peripheral blood mononuclear cells in postmenopausal women. *J Bone Miner Res* 1990;5:983–988.

73. Matsuda T, Matsui K, Shimakoshi Y, et al. 1-Hydroxyethilidene-1,1-bisphosphonate decreases the postovariectomy-enhanced interleukin 1 production by peritoneal macrophages in adult rats. *Calcif Tissue Int* 1991; 49:403–406.

74. Kaneki M, Nakamura T, Masuyama A, et al. The effect of menopause on IL-1 and IL-6 release from peripheral blood monocytes. *J Bone Miner Res* 1991;6:76.

75. Zarrabeitia MT, Riancho JA, Amado JA, et al. Cytokine production by blood cells in postmenopausal osteoporosis. *Bone Miner* 1991;14:161–167.

76. Hustmyer FG, Walker E, Yu XP, et al. Cytokine production and surface antigen expression by peripheral blood mononuclear cells in postmenopausal osteoporosis. *J Bone Miner Res* 1993;8:51–59.

77. Thompson RC, Dripps DJ, Eisenberg SP. IL-1ra: properties and uses of an interleukin-1 receptor antagonist. *Agents Actions Suppl* 1991;35:41–49.

78. Symons JA, Young PR, Duff GW. Soluble type II interleukin 1 (IL-1) receptor binds and blocks processing of IL-1-beta precursor and loses affinity for IL-1 receptor antagonist. *Proc Natl Acad Sci USA* 1995;92: 1714–1718.

79. Burger D, Chicheportiche R, Giri JG, et al. The inhibitory activity of human interleukin-1 receptor antagonist is enhanced by type II interleukin-I soluble receptor and hindered by type I interleukin-1 soluble receptor. *J Clin Invest* 1995;96:38–41.

80. Hansen MB, Svenson M, Bendtzen K. Human anti-interleukin 1α antibodies. *Immunol Lett* 1990;30:133–140.

81. Simon JA, Eastgate JA, Duff GW. A soluble binding protein specific for interleukin 1β is produced by activated mononuclear cells. *Cytokine* 1990;2:190–198.

82. Sunyer T, Lewis J, Osdoby P. Estrogen decreases the steady state levels of the IL-1 signaling receptor (type I) while increasing those of the IL-1 decoy receptor (type II) in human osteoclast-like cells. *J Bone Miner Res* 1997;12[Suppl 1]:(abst 131).

83. Pottratz ST, Bellido T, Mocharia H, et al. 17β-Estradiol inhibits expression of human interleukin-6 promoter-reporter constructs by a receptor-dependent mechanism. *J Clin Invest* 1994;93:944–950.

84. Ray A, Prefontaine KE, Ray P. Down-modulation of interleukin-6 gene expression by 17 beta-estradiol in the absence of high affinity DNA binding by the estrogen receptor. *J Biol Chem* 1994;269:12940–12946.

85. Stein B, Yang MX. Repression of the interleukin-6 promoter by estrogen receptor is mediated by NF-kappa-B and C/EBP-BETA. *Mol Cell Biol* 1995;15: 4971–4979.

86. Rickard D, Russell G, Gowen M. Oestradiol inhibits the release of tumour necrosis factor but not interleukin 6 from adult human osteoblasts *in vitro*. *Osteoporos Int* 1992;2:94–102.

87. Chaudhary LR, Spelsberg TC, Riggs BL. Production of various cytokines by normal human osteoblast-like cells in response to interleukin-1β and tumor necrosis factor-α: lack of regulation by 17β-estradiol. *Endocrinology* 1992;130:2528–2534.

88. Girasole G, Pedrazzoni M, Giuliani N, et al. Increased serum soluble interleukin-6 receptor levels are induced by ovariectomy, prevented by estrogen replacement and reversed by alendronate administration. *J Bone Miner Res* 1995;10:A86.

89. Oursler MJ. Osteoclast synthesis and secretion and activation of latent transforming growth factor beta. *J Bone Miner Res* 1994;9:443–452.

90. Oursler MJ, Cortese C, Keeting P, et al. Modulation of transforming growth factor-beta production in normal human osteoblast-like cells by 17 beta-estradiol and parathyroid hormone. *Endocrinology* 1991;129:3313–3320.

91. Srivastava S, Weitzmann MN, Kimble RB, et al. Estrogen blocks M-CSF gene expression and osteoclast formation by regulating CKII-induced phosphorylation of Egr-1 and its interaction with Sp-1. *J Clin Invest* 1998; 102:1850–1859.

92. Sarma U, Edwards M, Motoyoshi K, et al. Inhibition of bone resorption by 17beta-estradiol in human bone marrow cultures. *J Cell Physiol* 1998;175:99–108.

93. Lea CK, Sarma U, Flanagan AM. Macrophage colony stimulating-factor transcripts are differentially regulated in rat bone-marrow by gender hormones. *Endocrinology* 1999;140:273–279.

94. Pacifici R, Carano A, Santoro SA, et al. Bone matrix constituents stimulate interleukin-1 release from human blood mononuclear cells. *J Clin Invest* 1991; 87:221–228.

95. Pacifici R, Basilico C, Roman J, et al. Collagen-induced release of interleukin 1 from human blood mononuclear cells. Potentiation by fibronectin binding to the alpha 5 beta 1 integrin. *J Clin Invest* 1992;89: 61–67.

96. Lorenzo JA, Naprta A, Rao Y, et al. Mice lacking the type I interleukin-1 receptor do not lose bone mass after ovariectomy. *Endocrinology* 1998;139:3022–3025.

97. Kimble R, Bain S, Pacifici R. The functional block of TNF but not of IL-6 prevents bone loss in ovariectomized mice. *J Biomed Mater Res* 1997;12:935–941.

98. Ammann P, Rizzoli R, Bonjour JP, et al. Transgenic mice expressing soluble tumor necrosis factor-receptor are protected against bone loss caused by estrogen deficiency. *J Clin Invest* 1997;99:1699–1703.

99. Bradbeer JN, Stroup SJ, Hoffman JC, et al. An orally active inhibitor of cytokine synthesis prevents bone loss in the ovariectomized rat. *J Bone Miner Res* 1996; 11[Suppl 1]: (abst 123).

100. Poli V, Balena R, Fattori E, et al. Interleukin-6 deficient mice are protected from bone loss caused by estrogen depletion. *EMBO J* 1994;13:1189–1196.

101. Kitamura H, Kawata H, Takahashi F, et al. Bone marrow neutrophilia and suppressed bone turnover in human interleukin-6 transgenic mice. *Am J Pathol* 1995;147:1682–1692.

102. Pacifici R, Roman J, Kimble R, et al. Ligand binding to monocyte $\alpha_5\beta_1$ integrin activates the $\alpha_2\beta_1$ receptor via the α_5 subunit cytoplasmic domain and protein kinase C. *J Immunol* 1994;153:2222–2233.

Skeletal Growth Factors,
edited by Ernesto Canalis.
Lippincott Williams & Wilkins, Philadelphia, © 2000.

30

Role of Cytokines in Osteopetrosis

L. Lyndon Key, Jr., *William Ries, and Prema Madyastha

*Departments of Pediatrics and of *Dentistry, Medical University of South Carolina,
Charleston, South Carolina 29425*

Osteopetrosis results from a reduction in bone resorption relative to bone formation, leading to an accumulation of excessive amounts of bone. The relative decrease in resorption is a consequence of inadequate osteoclastic bone resorption. This imbalance leads to a thickening of the cortical region and a decrease in the size of the medullary space in the long bones, with sclerosis of the base of the skull (1,2) and vertebral bodies. There are a number of serious consequences resulting from the excessive accumulation of bone. A reduced marrow space results in a decrease in hematopoiesis, even to the point of complete bone marrow failure. Extramedullary hematopoiesis occurs but is unable to compensate for the reduction in medullary blood cell production. A decrease in the caliber of the cranial nerve and vascular canals leads to nerve compression and vascular compromise. Dense bones are subject to fracture and are poorly vascularized, predisposing the bones to necrosis and infection.

The ability to correct the osteopetrotic defect by bone marrow transplantation established the role of hematopoietic cells in controlling bone resorption and demonstrated that hematopoietic stem cells were the precursors of osteoclasts (3). In one of the first descriptions of a successful transplantation, the excessive bone in osteopetrotic *mi (microphthalmic)* mice was found to disappear within weeks after irradiation and transplantation of spleen or bone marrow cells from normal littermates. Because the excessive bone in the *mi* mutation is the result of reduced

bone resorption (3,4), this pioneering study suggested that a subpopulation of the transplanted cells was necessary for the formation of osteoclasts (5). Bone marrow transplantation does not universally correct skeletal defects in animal models (4). Subsequently, bone marrow transplantation has become the only curative therapy for osteopetrosis (6–9). Recently, two cases of human malignant osteopetrosis suggested a role for cytokines in human disease (10). In both of these cases, isolated osteoblast-like cells expressed defective phenotypic features. Cells from both patients responded abnormally to vitamin D and inflammatory cytokines *in vitro*. Following bone marrow transplantation, the osteoclasts, although still of recipient origin, functioned normally. While these results demonstrated that the interaction between osteoclasts and the microenvironment was crucial for controlling function, they also suggested that replacing microenvironmental factors controlling osteoclasts may allow for the function of osteoclasts.

A variety of animal models for osteopetrosis have been explored. The macrophage colony-stimulating factor (M-CSF) deficiency in the *op/op* mouse seems to be the most clearly related defect (11–16); however, replacing the M-CSF with exogenous cytokine does not result in complete remission (17). Several possible explanations have been suggested. The timing of the administration may not be the most advantageous (17–19). Alternatively, there may be other related factors which must interact. One of the most plausible ideas is that, in addition to circulating levels of M-CSF, there is the need for membrane-bound M-CSF (20) on the osteoblast or embedded in the bone surface (21) to be presented to the osteoclast or its precursors. A less clear-cut defect, but a demonstrated role for M-CSF therapy in improving the phenotypic abnormalities in the *tl/tl (toothless)* rat (22), has suggested some involvement with M-CSF production or the M-CSF receptor in the genesis of this mutant phenotype. To date, the precise defect has not been reported. Thus, humans and other species with few macrophages and osteoclasts may be found to have a defect in M-CSF production or response.

A number of cytokine transgenic and knockout animals have been useful in identifying possible roles for cytokines. The discovery of the osteoclast differentiation factor (ODF, also known as the osteoprotegerin ligand) and its inhibitor, osteoprotegerin, led to the demonstration that both the knockout of the ligand and the overexpression of the inhibitor protein resulted in an osteopetrotic phenotype (23–25). A knockout of tumor necrosis factor (TNF) receptor–associated factor, a postreceptor factor necessary for downstream activation of TNF-mediated [also interleukin-1 (IL-1)-, CD40-mediated] activation, is osteopetrotic (25). The dependence on a functional TNF receptor (the class of receptors mediating the effects of ODF) corroborates the importance of this pathway in osteoclastic bone resorption. The specificity for ODF is suggested by the fact that the knockout mutations of other members of the TNF family and IL-1 do not result in an osteopetrotic phenotype (R. Jilka, personal communication).

No specific defect in cytokine production has been established in patients with severe congenital osteopetrosis. While several patients have been found to have a reduced number of osteoclasts, suggesting a deficiency in M-CSF, the M-CSF production in 13 osteopetrotic patients screened was normal (26). We have screened 48 patients with osteopetrosis for abnormalities in interferon-γ1b production. Indeed in most patients, the interferon levels are at least two times higher than the upper limit of normal for age (Key et al. unpublished data, 1994). Despite the

fact that no specific defects have been found, therapy with cytokines has been tried with some success.

Three therapeutic modalities, involving cytokines, M-CSF, interferon-γ1b, and calcitriol, have been studied. In each case, preclinical trials suggested that the therapy could be beneficial. These studies have been done in animals where there was no deficiency of the cytokine being tested. Thus, these therapies have taken advantage of the pharmacological effects of the cytokines. Calcitriol is known to increase the generation of osteoclasts, apparently through increasing the ODF–ODF receptor interaction (27).

In work done by Grise et al. (28), osteopetrotic rabbits improved bone resorption on calcitriol. In this model, the mutation is not lethal and mimics the milder forms of osteopetrosis (intermediate forms). The *mi/mi* mouse model normally survives only a few months, although prolonged survival may be possible with adequate nutrition (29). These animals are blind, become profoundly anemic, and have no teeth. In this model, both interferon-γ1b and M-CSF were administered, with an improvement in bone resorption and a restoration of the marrow space (30). The combination of M-CSF and interferon-γ1b resulted in an even greater improvement. The *mi/mi* mutant contains both M-CSF (31) and interferon-γ1b receptors (unpublished data from our laboratory). While both receptors appear to activate the production of oxygen radicals in osteoclasts (32,33), M-CSF was found to increase the number of osteoclasts present in the cells even in the face of concomitant treatment with interferon-γ1b (30). Schneider et al. (34) have shown that the vitamin D binding protein–macrophage activating factor (DBP-MAF) stimulates bone resorption in the *op/op* and *ia/ia* rat models of osteopetrosis. This therapy has not been tried in humans, but this along with ODF therapy may provide additional treatment regimens in the future.

Calcitriol was introduced as a therapeutic modality for osteopetrosis in the early 1980s (35), following the seminal observation that calcitriol increased the number and activity of osteoclasts (36). The strategy was to stimulate bone resorption and thus increase osteoclast numbers; however, the osteoclast numbers are generally already increased in most patients prior to the start of therapy (37). This may be due to the fact that the 1,25-dihydroxyvitamin D_3 levels are elevated at baseline (38). While there is an increase in osteoclast numbers with calcitriol therapy and with therapeutic administration of M-CSF, these therapies alone rarely cause improvement patients with the severe malignant forms of osteopetrosis (39). However, high-dose calcitriol has reversed the clinical syndrome in three patients with the intermediate form of the disease. Success in adults with the condition has also been noted, with a decrease in bone pain and an increase in the cranial nerve foraminal diameter. Since calcitriol also stimulates osteoclastic activity, the precise reason for improvement is unknown (35). We have had no side effects from high-dose calcitriol (1 mcg/kg per day in severe malignant and intermediate forms and 8 mcg per day in adult forms).

One of the major problems with osteopetrosis is infection. Septicemia, osteomyelitis, and pneumonia are common occurrences for patients with severe congenital osteopetrosis. Indeed, the rate of infection in six children followed for 1 year on calcitriol therapy was seven infections per year that required hospitalization and/or intravenous antibiotics. The explanation for this propensity in infection does not appear to be marrow failure but rather an intrinsic white cell defect (40). In osteopetrotic patients, superoxide generation is reduced (41). Based on this observation, it was reasoned that increasing superoxide generation should improve white cell function and reduce the rate of infection. Since the osteoclast is derived from the white cell lineage, it was also speculated that bone resorption may be improved. With the introduction of inter-

feron-γ1b to treat patients with chronic granulomatous disease, based on the ability of this cytokine to stimulate neutrophilic superoxide generation, a treatment strategy for osteopetrosis became available (42).

To date, we have data on up to 48 months of therapy with interferon-γ in a cohort of 23 patients (39). The data (Table 30.1) show that there has been an increase in the nitroblue tetrazolium (NBT) reduction by white cells, a marker of superoxide production. This change is sustained and represents the reason that the incidence of new infections drops from 6.9 infections per year to 0.7, $p < 0.01$. The result is a 4-year survival rate of 72% compared to 30% for untreated patients with a similar degree of severity (43). Recently, we have performed an interim analysis of the first 20 patients enrolled in a prospective, randomized trial of interferon-γ. The data shown in Figure 30.1 show that there have been five infections in the four children who were not treated with interferon-γ1b (average duration of therapy 9 months). Conversely, no infections have occurred in the children on interferon-γ (average duration of therapy 1 year). These data suggest that interferon-γ1b increases white cell function, reducing infections. In addition, the decrease in bone mass suggests that there is an increase in osteoclastic activity, resulting in an increased bone marrow space and an increased size of cranial foramina. Despite the improved clinical condition leading to increased survival, interferon therapy does not reverse all of the deformities of osteopetrosis. Thus, this therapy is best used when bone marrow transplantation is not available, when there is a delay prior to transplantation, or when the bone marrow space needs to be expanded to improve the odds of engraftment.

TABLE 30.1. *Clinical effects of interferon-γ at 24 months of therapy*

Parameter (n = 23)	Before therapy	After therapy	p value
Neutrophil NBT reduction	0.30 ± 0.05	0.85 ± 0.08	<0.0005
Trabecular bone volume	56.4 ± 2.9%	39.6% ± 2.7	<0.05
Hemoglobin	8.8 ± 1.5%	10.2 ± 2.3%	0.07
Platelet count	143K ± 15K	228K ± 26K	0.06
Optic nerve canal area (mm²)	6.9 ± 2.2	11.9 ± 1.8	<0.05
Auditory canal area (mm²)	8.9 ± 1.9	10.4 ± 2.4	0.1

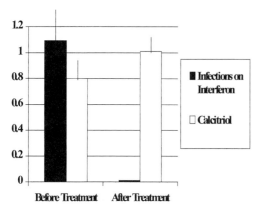

FIG. 30.1. Infections in osteopetrosis during phase III trial of interferon. Sixteen patients with osteopetrosis were randomly assigned to two treatment groups: calcitriol therapy alone (1 μg/kg per day) and calcitriol + interferon-γ-1b (1.5 μg/kg 3 times per week). No infections were seen in the group treated with interferon-γ1b. The statistical difference between groups was negligible prior to therapy (*p* = 0.77, slightly higher for the interferon-γ1b group) and markedly different after therapy (*p* < 0.0000001). These numbers are small but corroborate the data collected in the phase II trial previously reported (39).

An absence of M-CSF has been found to produce osteopetrosis in the *op/op* mouse mutant (18). In this mutation, there are reduced numbers of osteoclasts. While this state of affairs is not commonly seen in patients with severe malignant osteopetrosis, patients whose biopsy shows a reduction in the number of osteoclasts should be studied for a deficiency in M-CSF. Limited trials of M-CSF have been carried out (44). While some improvement in bone marrow space has been observed, no other clinical improvement was noted. Three patients were treated with interferon-γ1b plus M-CSF. All three developed a severe respiratory ailment after minor surgical procedures, leading to their death from a syndrome similar to adult respiratory distress syndrome or transfusion-related lung injury (despite the absence of transfusions). Patients with osteopetrosis have subsequently been studied on and off interferon-γ1b and found to have an increased amount of cytophilic immunoglobulin G bound to their neutrophils (45).

As noted, we have found that interferon-γ1b increases osteoclastic bone resorption in osteopetrotic animals and patients with malignant osteopetrosis. The treatment effect has been studied recently *in vitro* in osteoclasts generated by culturing peripheral white blood cells from osteopetrotic patients and normal controls (46). These osteoclasts exhibited multinuclearity and tartrate-resistant acid phosphatase (TRAP) staining. Unstimulated osteoclasts generated from peripheral white blood cells of normal donors expressed calcitonin receptors and generated resorption pits on bovine bone slabs. Interferon-γ1b enhanced superoxide production (*p* < 0.0001) in osteoclasts from normal subjects, measured by NBT staining. NBT staining was reduced by 80% in the presence of superoxide dismutase but not by catalase, demonstrating that this assay measured predominantly superoxide. Unstimulated osteoclasts from six osteopetrotic patients revealed a reduced baseline level of NBT staining (*p* < 0.0001) compared to unstimulated osteoclasts generated from normal subjects (Fig. 30.2). Stimulation with interferon-γ markedly increased (*p* < 0.001) superoxide production. The formation of multinucleated cells with an increased intensity of TRAP staining was observed in interferon-γ-stimulated cultures of white blood cells obtained from patients compared with those unstimulated (*p* < 0.0001). The increase in TRAP staining suggests a global effect on osteoclast activation. Osteoclasts expressed receptors for interferon-γ, suggesting that the stimulation of superoxide production may be mediated directly through interferon-γ receptor activation. Thus, the stimulation of osteoclasts may not be dependent on the presence of accessory cells. Increased superoxide production may explain how interferon-γ increases bone resorption in osteopetrotic patients.

Thus, a variety of cytokines may play a role in osteopetrosis (Table 30.2). The only cytokine shown to cause a natural mutation is M-CSF. A variety of cytokines have been implicated as possible causes of osteopetrosis using transgenic and/or knockout mice. Three cytokines (M-CSF, interferon-γ1b, and DBP-MAF) and calcitriol

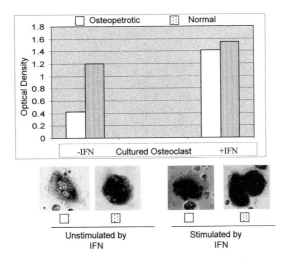

FIG. 30.2. Superoxide production stimulated in osteoclasts harvested from peripheral blood mononuclear cells of osteopetrotic patients and normal controls. This figure shows the nitroblue tetrazolium (NBT) staining in four osteoclasts: two normal and two control with and without interferon-γ1b stimulation. The bar graph assesses 15 cells from each group. There is a marked increase in NBT staining between patients and controls. The interferon-γ1b stimulation normalizes the NBT staining. This suggests, based on our other studies demonstrating that over 90% of NBT staining results from superoxide generation, that interferon-γ1b stimulates superoxide generation in osteoclasts derived from osteopetrotic patients.

TABLE 30.2. *Cytokines having a relationship with osteopetrosis*

Cytokine[a]	Action	Osteopetrotic condition	References
M-CSF	Stimulates osteoclast formation and function	*op/op* mouse mutation causes M-CSF? relationship to *tl/tl* rat	18 3
M-CSF	Stimulates bone formation and osteoclast formation in humans	Little effect on clinical course, may cause respiratory distress	39 45
OPG	Inhibits bone resorption	Overexpression in transgenic model is osteopetrotic	24 23
Osteoclast Differention factor (OPG ligand)	Stimulates osteoclast formation and action	Knockout is osteopetrotic, OPG ligand recovers	23 24
Interferon-γ1b	Stimulates osteoclastic superoxide production; inhibits osteoclast formation	Reduces infection and improves survival	39
DBP-MAF	Stimulates osteoclast activity and macrophage activity	Used as treatment for osteopetrotic rats	34
IL-1, IL-11, IL-18, IL-6	Stimulate osteoclast formation and/or activity	Knockouts do not cause osteopetrosis	

DBP-MAF, vitamin D binding protein–macrophage activating factor; IL, interleukin; [a] M-CSF, macrophage colony-stimulating factor; OPG, osteoprotegerin.

have been used in animals with osteopetrosis, with some reversal of the illness. To date, only interferon-γ1b used in conjunction with calcitriol has been shown to improve survival. Although promising, these treatments have not cured the osteopetrotic condition. The use of DBP-MAF and ODF may ultimately result in improved therapies. In addition, understanding the cytokines involved may ultimately lead us to an understanding of the defects present in this disorder.

ACKNOWLEDGMENTS

Support for the original studies supported in this chapter came from the Food and Drug Administration Orphan Drug Grant Program, grant FD-R-000768. The study was also supported by General Clinical Research Center (GCRC) grant 5MO1RR-01070-21.

REFERENCES

1. Elster AD, Theros EG, Key LL, et al. Cranial imaging in autosomal recessive osteopetrosis. Part I. Facial bones and calvarium. *Radiology* 1992;183:129–135.
2. Elster AD, Theros EG, Key LL, et al. Cranial imaging in autosomal recessive osteopetrosis. Part II. Skull base and brain. *Radiology* 1992;183:137–144.
3. Marks SC. Pathogenesis of osteopetrosis in the microphthalmic mouse: reduced bone resorption. *Am J Anat* 1977;149:269–276.
4. Popoff SN, Schneider GB. Animal models of osteopetrosis: the impact of recent molecular developments on novel strategies for therapeutic intervention. *Mol Med Today* 1986;2:349–358.
5. Schneider GB, Relfson M, Nicolas J. Pluripotent hemopoietic stem cells give rise to osteoclasts. *Am J Anat* 1986;177:505–511.
6. Ballet JJ, Griscelli C, Courtris C, et al. Bone-marrow transplantation in osteopetrosis. *Lancet* 1977;2: 1137–1140.
7. Coccia PF, Krivit W, Cervenka J, et al. Successful bone-marrow transplantation for infantile malignant osteopetrosis. *N Engl J Med* 1985;302:701–708.
8. Gerritsen EJ, Vossen JM, Fasth A, et al. Bone marrow transplantation for autosomal recessive osteopetrosis. A report from the Working Party on Inborn Errors of the European Bone Marrow Transplantation Group. *J Pediatr* 1994;125:896–902.
9. Solh H, DaCunha AM, Giri N, et al. Bone marrow transplantation for infantile malignant osteopetrosis. *J Pediatr Hematol Oncol* 1995;17:350–355.
10. Lajeunesse D, Busque L, Menard P, et al. Demonstration of an osteoblast defect in two cases of human malignant osteopetrosis. Correction of the phenotype after bone marrow transplant. *J Clin Invest* 1996;98:1835–1842.
11. Begg SK, Radley JM, Pollard JW, et al. Delayed hema-

topoietic development in osteopetrotic (op/op) mice. *J Exp Med* 1993;177:237–242.
12. Lowe C, Yoneda T, Boyce BF, et al. Osteopetrosis in Src-deficient mice is due to an autonomous defect of osteoclasts. *Proc Natl Acad Sci USA* 1993;90: 4485–4489.
13. Marks SC, Wojtowicz A, Szperl M, et al. Administration of colony stimulating factor-1 corrects some macrophage, dental, and skeletal defects in an osteopetrotic mutation (toothless, tl) in the rat. *Bone* 1992;13:89–93.
14. Nilsson SK, Bertoncello I. The development and establishment on hemopoiesis in fetal and newborn osteopetrotic (op/op) mice. *Dev Biol* 1994;164:456–462.
15. Philippart C, Tzehoval E, Moricard Y, et al. Immune cell defects affect bone remodelling in osteopetrotic op/op mice. *Bone Miner* 1993;23:317–332.
16. Wiktor-Jedrezejczak W, Urbanowska E, Szperl M. Granulocyte-macrophage colony-stimulating factor corrects macrophage deficiences, but not osteopetrosis, in the colony-stimulating factor-1-deficient op/op mouse. *Endocrinology* 1994;134:1932–1935.
17. Sundquist KT, Cecchini MG, Marks SC. Colony-stimulating factor-1 injections improve but do not cure skeletal sclerosis in osteopetrotic (op) mice. *Bone* 1995;16: 39–46.
18. Hofstetter W, Wetterwald A, Cecchini MG, et al. Detection of transcripts and binding sites for colony-stimulating factor 1 during bone development. *Bone* 1995;17: 145–151.
19. Lee TH, Fevold KL, Muguruma Y, et al. Relative roles of osteoclast colony-stimulating factor and macrophage colony-stimulating factor in the course of osteoclast development. *Exp Hematol* 1994;22:66–73.
20. Stanley ER, Berg KL, Einstein DB, et al. The biology and action of colony stimulating factor-1. *Stem Cells* 1994;12[suppl 1]:15–25.
21. Ohtsuki T, Hatake K, Suzu S, et al. Immunohistochemical identification of proteoglycan form of macrophage colony-stimulating factor on bone surface. *Calcif Tissue Int* 1995;57:213–217.
22. Marks SC, MacKay CA, Jackson ME, et al. The skeletal effects of colony-stimulating factor-1 in toothless (osteopetrotic) rats: persistent metaphyseal sclerosis and the failure to restore subepiphyseal osteoclasts. *Bone* 1993;14:675–680.
23. Boyle W, Kung Y, Lace D, et al. Osteoprotegerin ligand (OPGL) is required for murine osteoclastogenesis. *J Bone Miner Res* 1998;[Suppl 1]:1169.
24. Simonet WS, Lacey DL, Dunstan CR, et al. Osteoprotegerin: a novel secreted protein involved in the regulation of bone density. *Cell* 1998;89:159–161.
25. Lomaga MA, Yeh WC, Sarosi I, et al. TRAF6 deficiency results in osteopetrosis and defective interleukin-1, CD40, and LPS signaling. *Genes Dev* 1999;13: 1015–1024.
26. Orchard PJ, Dahl N, Aukerman L, et al. Circulating macrophage colony-stimulating factor is not reduced in malignant osteopetrosis. *Exp Hematol* 1992;20: 103–105.
27. Hofbauer LC, Dunstan CR, Spelsberg TC, et al. Osteoprotegerin production by human osteoblast lineage cells is stimulated by vitamin D, bone morphogenetic protein-2, and cytokines. *Biochem Biophys Res Commun* 1998; 250:776–781.
28. Grise MA, Marks SC Jr, MacKay CA, et al. Effects of 1,25 dihydroxyvitamin D on osteoclast number and

cytochemistry in normal and osteopetrotic (os) rabbits. *Am J Anat* 1990;189:261–266.

29. Darden AG, Oexman JM, Key LL. Increased longevity of osteopetrotic mice resulting from nutritional intervention in the microphthalmic model of osteopetrosis. *J Bone Miner Res* 1993;8:S291.

30. Rodriquiz RM, Key LL, Ries WL. Combination macrophage-colony stimulating factor and interferon gamma administration ameliorates the osteopetrotic condition in microphthalmic mice. *Pediatr Res* 1993;33:284–389.

31. Yang S, Zhang Y, Ries WL, et al. Characterization of the M-CSF and its receptor in microphthalmic mice. *Exp Hematol* 1995;23:126–132.

32. Yang S, Zhang Y, Ries WL, et al. Functions of the M-CSF receptor on osteoblasts. *Bone* 1996;18:355–360.

33. Darden AG, Ries WL, Wolf WC, et al. Osteoclastic superoxide production and bone resorption: stimulation and inhibition by modulators of NADPH oxidase. *J Bone Miner Res* 1996;11:671–675.

34. Schneider GB, Benis KA, Flay NW, et al. Effects of vitamin D binding protein-macrophage activating factor (DBP-MAF) infusion on bone resorption in two osteopetrotic mutations. *Bone* 1995;16:657–662.

35. Key LL, Carnes D, Cole S, et al. Treatment of osteopetrosis with high-dose calcitriol. *N Engl J Med* 1984;310:410–415.

36. Holtrop ME, Raisz LG. Comparisons of the effects of 1,25 dihydroxycholecalciferol, prostaglandin E_2, and osteoclast-activating factor with parathyroid hormone on the ultrastructure of osteoclasts in cultured long bone fetal rats. *Calcif Tissue Int* 1979;29:201–205.

37. Shapiro F, Key LL Jr, Anast C. Variable osteoclast appearance in human infantile osteopetrosis. *Calcif Tissue Int* 1988;43:67–76.

38. Key LL Jr. Osteopetrosis: a genetic window into osteoclast function. ACPC Series. *Cases Metab Bone Dis* 1987;2.

39. Key LL Jr, Rodriguiz RM, Willi SM, et al. Long-term treatment of osteopetrosis with recombinant human interferon gamma. *N Engl J Med* 1995;332:1594–1599.

40. Reeves JD, August CS, Humbert JR, et al. Host defense in infantile osteopetrosis. *J Pediatr* 1978;64:202–206.

41. Key LL Jr, Ries WL. Osteopetrosis: the pharmaco-physiologic basis of therapy. *Clin Orthop Rel Res* 1993;294:85–89.

42. Ezekowitz RA, Dinauer MC, Jaffe HS, et al. Partial correction of the phagocyte defect in patients with X-linked chronic granulomatous disease by subcutaneous interferon gamma. *N Engl J Med* 1988;318:146–151.

43. Gerritsen EJA, Vossen JM, van Loo IHG, et al. Autosomal recessive osteopetrosis: variability of findings at diagnosis and during the natural course. *Pediatrics* 1994;93:247–253.

44. Key LL, Rodriguiz RM, Wang WC. Cytokines and bone resorption in osteopetrosis. *Int J Pediatr Hematol Oncol* 1995;2:143–149.

45. Madyastha PR, Jeter EK, Key LL. Cytophilic immunoglobulin G binding on neutrophils from a child with malignant osteopetrosis who developed fatal acute respiratory distress mimicking transfusion-related lung injury. *Am J Hematol* 1996;53:196–200.

46. Madyastha PR, Yang S, Ries, et al. Normalization of superoxide generation in human osteopetrotic osteoclasts is mediated by the direct binding of interferon-α to the osteoclastic cell surface receptors. *J Bone Miner Res* 1999;14:SA203.

Skeletal Growth Factors,
edited by Ernesto Canalis.
Lippincott Williams & Wilkins, Philadelphia, © 2000.

31

Cytokines, Growth Factors, and Malignancy

Gregory R. Mundy

Department of Medicine/Endocrinology, University of Texas Health Science Center,
San Antonio, Texas 78284-7877

Cancers frequently involve the skeleton to cause osteolytic or osteoblastic metastases. Although the precise mechanisms are still not well understood, the effects of tumors on the skeleton are due to tumor factors which influence osteoblast and osteoclast activity and whose effects are superimposed on the normal remodeling process. Table 31.1 shows the spectrum of changes which occur in bone in patients with varying types of malignancy. At one end of the spectrum is the discrete osteolytic metastasis frequently associated with myeloma, in which there is bone resorption with little or no bone formation. At the other end of the spectrum is the osteoblastic metastasis frequently associated with prostate cancer, in which osteoblast activity occurs on resting bone surfaces without prior bone resorption. The majority of malignancies have an osteolytic response with a partial but impaired osteoblastic response. In all cases, the disturbances are due to excess production of factors which influence the activity of osteoclasts and osteoblasts and disrupt normal bone remodeling. In this chapter, the factors implicated in this process are reviewed.

TYPES OF BONE METASTASES

When cancers involve the skeleton, they cause a spectrum of effects ranging from discrete bone loss (osteolysis) to osteosclerosis. The pattern of changes seen with common malignancies is depicted in Table 31.1.

Osteolytic Metastases

Osteolytic metastases are due to increased osteoclastic bone resorption. They are apparent radiologically as lytic lesions which are undermineralized. They are usually discrete and local but may also be more diffuse and general. There are serious clinical consequences associated with osteolytic bone disease due to malignancy, including intractable bone pain, pathological fracture following trivial injury or possibly even no injury at all, and hypercalcemia and deformity, which may result in nerve-compression syndromes or spinal cord compression. Involvement of the bone marrow cavity by tumor cells adjacent to cancers frequently leads to bone marrow suppression and occasionally a leukoerythroblastic response. Recent data indicate that osteolysis can even enhance the growth of aggressive behavior of tumor cells in the bone microenvironment (1). The osteoblastic response to the osteolytic lesion is variable. In malignancies such as myeloma, there may be marked impairment of the osteoblastic response, whereas in the majority of malignancies such as breast and lung cancer, the osteoblastic response may be present but impaired. Nevertheless, the osteoblastic response is how the bone metastasis is recognized clinically. Radionuclide uptake at the site of the metastasis or an increase in serum alkaline phosphatase is a reflection of the osteoblastic response to the osteolytic lesions.

The factors which have been implicated in the osteolytic response include parathyroid hormone (PTH)-related peptide (PTHrP) and a

TABLE 31.1. *Spectrum of bone lesions seen in malignancy*

	Myeloma	Breast cancer	Prostate cancer
X-rays	Osteolytic	Mixed	Osteosclerotic
Histology	Osteoclasts increased	Mixed osteoclastic and osteoblastic	Osteoblastic bone formation
Serum alkaline phosphatase	Normal	Increased	Markedly increased
Bone scans	Normal	Increased activity	Markedly increased activity

number of other cytokines generated in the bone microenvironment, including transforming growth factor-α (TGF-α), interleukin-6 (IL-6), IL-2, and tumor necrosis factor (TNF). The precise role of these cytokines is not clear in the majority of malignancies at the present time. However, there are increasing numbers of malignancies in which PTHrP has been implicated not just as a systemic factor but also as a local factor (see below).

Osteoblastic Metastases

Osteoblastic (also called osteosclerotic) metastases are less common than osteolytic metastases. However, they occur frequently in patients with prostate cancer and malignancies involving the urinary tract. In some patients, the osteoblastic response occurs on a previously resting bone surface and without any evidence of prior resorption. In others, there appears to be an exaggeration of the formation phase of the normal bone-remodeling process, and the osteoblastic metastasis occurs at the site of previous resorption but is markedly exaggerated. One interesting piece of information which has become apparent in the last few years as a consequence of widespread use of markers of bone resorption is that in essentially all patients with prostate cancer and osteoblastic metastases there is a marked increase in bone-resorption markers such as urinary deoxypyridinoline.

These are even more enhanced than in patients with osteolytic metastases. The reason for this increase in bone-resorption markers is not clear. Although in some cases it may be due to bone resorption occuring prior to the osteoblastic lesion and at the same site, in some patients it is obvious that this increase in bone resorption is

distinct and possibly related to a systemic increase in bone resorption mediated by circulating factors.

The consequences of osteoblastic metastasis are probably not as dramatic as those of osteolytic metastasis. In some patients, they include pain that may also be intractable and, in some patients, deformities caused by bone overgrowth, which may lead to nerve-compression syndromes such as spinal cord compression. Pathological fracture also occurs but not as commonly as with osteolytic metastases. Hypercalcemia is rare in patients with osteoblastic metastases, but occasionally patients develop hypocalcemia, presumably due to shifts of calcium from the extracellular fluid into bone.

Mixed Osteolytic and Osteoblastic Metastases

This is the most frequent type of bone metastasis, occurring often in common tumors such as carcinoma of the lung and carcinoma of the breast. These patients have predominantly osteolytic metastases but with an osteoblastic response, as exemplified by increases in serum alkaline phosphatase and radionuclide scan uptake. Patients with these tumors have the same clinical consequences as patients with discrete osteolytic metastases.

CYTOKINES AND GROWTH FACTORS AND THE ROLE IN OSTEOLYTIC BONE DISEASE

Parathyroid Hormone-related Protein and Parathyroid Hormone

PTHrP was first discovered using *in vitro* bioassays for PTH in tumors derived from lung, breast, and kidney (2–4). This factor is now known to be expressed by many squamous cell carcinomas and has also been described in some T-cell lymphomas which present with humoral hypercalcemia (5). It is a 141–amino acid peptide which bears considerable homology to PTH in the first 13 amino acids. It binds to and activates the PTH receptor and, thus, may mimic the biological effects of PTH on bone, kidney, and gut. These effects include stimulation of osteoclastic bone resorption and promotion of renal tubular calcium reabsorption in concentrations similar to that of native PTH (6). In some models of hypercalcemia associated with increased plasma PTHrP, hypercalcemia can be reversed by passive inoculation with neutralizing antibodies to PTHrP (7). PTHrP is produced by about 50% of primary breast cancers, and its production may be enhanced locally in bone by bone-derived factors such as TGF-β (8,9). More recently, excess production of PTHrP has been implicated in myeloma (10).

Radioimmunoassays have been developed for PTHrP, although these assays have not shown a perfect relationship between the presence and severity of hypercalcemia and the expression of the protein (3,11,12).

It is not surprising that there is a less than perfect correlation between circulating PTHrP concentrations and hypercalcemia. The work of Guise et al. (9) shows that PTHrP may be an important local mediator of bone resorption, particularly in breast cancer. Here, it may cause local osteolysis with or without hypercalcemia. Thus, PTHrP may cause two distinct tumor-related syndromes, humoral hypercalcemia of malignancy (HHM) or localized osteolysis. The latter may or may not be associated with hypercalcemia, depending on the extent of the bone lesions.

We have created a model of PTHrP-induced hypercalcemia in nude mice by transfecting Chinese hamster ovarian (CHO) cells with the human PTHrP gene (13). These cells are stably transfected with PTHrP and express it in a constant manner. When these tumors are inoculated into nude mice, the tumor-bearing nude mice develop hypercalcemia and increased plasma PTHrP. In addition, they have other features

which are identical to those seen with PTH excess, namely, increased osteoclastic bone resorption associated with increased bone formation and increased plasma 1,25-dihydroxyvitamin (13). Since these features are not seen in the majority of patients dying with the syndrome of HHM, tumor-increased production of PTHrP alone cannot explain the syndrome. Our hypothesis is that other factors produced in conjunction with PTHrP may modify the effects of PTHrP on target tissues. Other data suggest that TGF-α, IL-1α, IL-6, and TNF-α may be synergistic with PTHrP *in vivo* (13–16).

PTHrP may have roles other than as a mediator of cancer hypercalcemia which have not yet been clearly determined. It has been found in lactating rat breast tissue as well as in human milk (11,17). It has been suggested that it may be involved in placental calcium transport (18). PTHrP has also been demonstrated in increased amounts in the amniotic fluid and is produced by amniotic cells (19). Its expression in amniotic cells decreases when the membranes rupture. It may have a role as a smooth muscle relaxant in this situation and be involved in labor and delivery. On the basis of these studies, it is possible that it may be important during embryonic life for calcium transport in the fetus.

Null mutant mice with absent production of PTHrP have been studied in an attempt to identify the normal physiological functions of PTHrP (20). Homozygous mice deficient in PTHrP expression do not survive embryonic life. These mice show marked abnormalities at the growth plate, with enhanced differentiation of chondrocytes probably mediated, at least in part, by the Indian hedgehog gene product produced by perichondral cells (21). Thus, PTHrP expression may be important for normal endochondral bone formation.

This has been further emphasized in more recent studies. Point mutations in the PTH/PTHrP receptor which are activating cause the condition Jansen's metaphyseal chondrodysplasia, a rare genetic disorder characterized by short-limbed dwarfism and severe, agonist-independent hypercalcemia (22). Moreover, the recent finding that PTH/PTHrP receptor deficiency due to targeted gene disruption causes premature differentiation of chondrocytes, leading to abnormalities in endochondral bone formation, which can be reversed by adding PTHrP further emphasizes this point (23).

Recently, PTH itself has been implicated as a tumor mediator in several nonparathyroid tumors (24–26). However, this is a rare occurrence (27). These tumors were a small cell lung cancer, a neuroectodermal tumor, and an ovarian carcinoma. In one of these tumors, a DNA rearrangement in the region of the promoter was presumably responsible for overexpression of the PTH gene by the tumor. Most patients with nonparathyroid cancer who develop hypercalcemia and increased immunoreactive serum PTH have coexistent primary hyperparathyroidism.

Interleukins 1α and 1β

ILs 1α and 1β are powerful bone-resorbing cytokines produced by not only activated monocytes but also many other cells. ILs 1α and 1β seem to have identical effects on bone-resorbing and bone-forming cells (28–30). IL-1α is expressed by many solid tumors as well as lymphomas (14,31,32). It has been shown to work in concert with PTHrP to provoke hypercalcemia (14). It has powerful effects on osteoclastic bone resorption in vivo (28–30). It inhibits differentiation of osteoblasts in vitro but may promote their proliferation (33). Unlike IL-1α, IL-1β has not been implicated in solid tumors associated with hypercalcemia, but several groups have recently shown that freshly isolated cells from the marrow of patients with myeloma produce IL-1β (34,35). Bone-resorbing activity present in these cultured cell supernatants has been blocked by neutralizing antibodies to IL-1β. Whether this mechanism may explain the unique form of bone destruction associated with myeloma remains uncertain.

Both IL-1α and IL-1β are powerful hypercalcemic agents. This has been shown by infusions in normal intact mice as well as by repeated subcutaneous injections (28–30). The effects of IL-1 to cause hypercalcemia are clearly mediated by the effects of IL-1 on osteoclastic bone resorption. In osteopetrotic mice in which osteoclasts are nonfunctional, hypercalcemia does not occur, in contrast to when PTH or PTHrP is injected into osteopetrotic mice and hypercalcemia occurs, presumably due to renal effects of the hormones (36).

Transforming Growth Factor-α

TGF-α is produced by many solid tumors as well as breast carcinomas. TGF-α is a powerful stimulator of osteoclast precursor proliferation and causes osteoclastic bone resorption and hypercalcemia in vivo (37–39). It has synergistic effects with PTH and, more importantly, with PTHrP both on bone resorption and on hypercalcemia (13,40). TGF-α is a cell membrane–associated protein and may exert biological effects while still incorporated into the cell membrane (41). However, it is also clear that it can produce systemic effects on osteoclastic bone resorption and hypercalcemia since CHO cells expressing and secreting TGF-α cause hypercalcemia when inoculated into nude mice (40).

The effects of TGF-α on osteoclastic bone resorption may be exerted primarily on osteoclast progenitors (42,43). It stimulates progenitors to replicate but not to differentiate. It exerts identical effects on osteoclasts as epidermal growth factor (EGF). In nude mice carrying CHO tumors overexpressing TGF-α, hypercalcemia is associated with osteoclasts, which are small and have fewer nuclei than the osteoclasts formed in response to PTH or PTHrP (40). This suggests that these osteoclasts have been generated in response to a growth-regulatory factor and are consistent with the in vitro studies that indicate a primary proliferative effect of TGF-α on osteoclast progenitor cells.

Synergism has been demonstrated between PTH or PTHrP and IL-1α in vivo, causing hypercalcemia (14), and in vitro, causing bone resorption (44). Similarly, there may also be complicated interactions between PTH and TGF-α, IL-1, and TGFβ. TGF-α, EGF, IL-1, and TNF inhibit the capacity of PTH (and presumably PTHrP) to cause increases in adenylate cyclase activity in bone and renal tubular cells (45), whereas TGF-β enhances PTH-mediated adenylate cyclase activity (46). Whether these responses have biological significance is not entirely clear, although Pizurki et al. (47) have shown that the effects of PTHrP and PTH on renal phosphate transport may be enhanced by TGF-α.

Tumor Necrosis Factor

TNF has biological effects on osteoclasts similar to those of IL-1. It stimulates proliferation of precursors, enhances differentiation of committed precursors, and activates the mature cell indirectly to stimulate the resorption of bone (48–50). It is not known to be produced by solid tumors, although some soluble members of the TNF receptor family may be (see later). It may play a role in the bone destruction associated with solid tumors by being produced by normal host cells in excess amounts in response to the tumor (51). In this way, it may be associated with the paraneoplastic syndromes of cachexia, hypercalcemia, and leukocytosis. There are several experimental examples in which this mechanism seems to be important. In the MH-85 tumor, a squamous cell carcinoma of the maxilla, both the original patient and nude mice carrying this tumor develop hypercalcemia, leukocytosis, and cachexia (51). The tumor-bearing nude mice have increased circulating concentrations of TNF, although the tumor itself does not produce TNF; and when nude mice are treated with neutralizing antibodies to TNF, the hypercalcemia is markedly reduced. In these animals, it appears that tumor cells themselves produce a circulating factor, which in turn is responsible for provoking TNF production. This mechanism has also been examined in two other models of hypercalcemia, the rat Leydig cell tumor and the A375 tumor. The rat Leydig cell tumor produces both PTHrP and TGF-α in large amounts. This is a tumor which causes profound hypercalcemia. However, the tumor-bearing rats also develop profound cachexia and hypertriglyceridemia, which is associated with increased circulating concentrations of TNF (52,53). Similarly, in the A375 human melanoma, nude mice bearing this tumor develop severe cachexia and hypercalcemia. These mice also have increased circulating concentrations of TNF. In this tumor, the factor responsible for provoking TNF production by the tumor cells has been purified and shown to

be colony-stimulating factor (CSF) for the granulocyte macrophage series (GM-CSF) (52,53). The activity responsible for provoking TNF production in the MH-85 tumor cannot be ascribed to GM-CSF and has still not been identified.

Lymphotoxin

Lymphotoxin has biological effects similar to those of TNF. It is also a powerful stimulator of osteoclastic bone resorption and causes hypercalcemia when infused or injected *in vivo*. It has been implicated in the hypercalcemia and bone destruction associated with myeloma (54). Long-term cultures of human myeloma cells express lymphotoxin mRNA. Moreover, there is lymphotoxin biological activity in conditioned media of cultured cells, and bone-resorbing activity in the culture media of these cells can be blocked by neutralizing antibodies to lymphotoxin (54). Thus, lymphotoxin may be important in the bone destruction associated with myeloma, possibly in association with other cytokines such as IL-1β and IL-6.

Interleukin-6

IL-6 is a ubiquitous cytokine which is a powerful B-cell mitogen. It is an important growth-regulatory factor in myeloma, although its major cellular source is still debated. Some investigators believe it has an important paracrine or autocrine role in the pathophysiology of the disease (55). Its effects on bone resorption are more controversial. It stimulates bone resorption in some systems but seems to be ineffective in other organ culture systems (56–58). Its effects may depend on the presence of precursors for osteoclasts in the organ cultures. IL-6 causes mild hypercalcemia *in vivo*, although not as marked as that caused by IL-1 or PTrP. CHO cells which have been transfected with the IL-6 gene and stably overexpress it cause hypercalcemia when inoculated into nude mice (59). In addition, the nude mice develop leukocytosis, thrombocytosis, and cachexia which can be ascribed to IL-6 (59). It may be a stimulator of bone resorption by acting early in the bone-resorption process (60) but is probably effective only in combination with the soluble IL-6 receptor. IL-6 is produced by many solid tumors and must be a potential mediator of hypercalcemia and other paraneoplastic syndromes associated with malignancy. Neutralizing antibodies to IL-6 have been shown to reduce hypercalcemia in one human tumor model (61).

However, the major role for IL-6 may not be as an independent factor but rather as a subsidiary factor enhancing the effects of other mediators. De La Mata et al. (15) showed that IL-6 markedly enhanced the effects of PTHrP both on osteoclast formation and on generation of hypercalcemia in tumor-bearing mice. Since IL-6 is produced by bone cells in the presence of PTH and PTHrP (62), this may be an important mechanism for hypercalcemia in some patients.

We have found that in a solid human tumor (a squamous cell carcinoma) which causes hypercalcemia in tumor-bearing nude mice, hypercalcemia may be reversed by treatment with neutralizing antibodies to IL-6 (51). The source of the IL-6 is the tumor cells. Thus, IL-6 may be a contributory factor in hypercalcemia and other paraneoplastic syndromes associated not only with myeloma but also with some solid tumors.

Prostaglandins of the E Series

Prostaglandins of the E series have long been known to be relatively powerful bone-resorbing factors (63). Their role in the bone destruction associated with malignancy remains unclear (64). However, it is known that at least some of the effects of the cytokines on osteoclastic bone resorption *in vivo* as well as *in vitro* are mediated through prostaglandin synthesis. Boyce et al. (29,30) showed this by intermittent subcutaneous injections of IL-1 over the calvariae of mice, some of which were treated with indomethacin, which inhibits prostaglandin synthesis. They found that some of the effects of IL-1 on bone *in vivo*, as assessed by histomorphometry, could be blocked by indomethacin. However, it is also possible that prostaglandins of the E series exert more direct effects on osteoclastic bone resorption. They are produced by cultured tumor cells *in vitro*. Whether a similar phenomenon happens *in vivo* or not is unknown. One possibility is

that prostaglandins, like cytokines such as TNF, could be produced by host immune cells in response to tumor.

1,25-Dihydroxyvitamin D

Serum 1,25-dihydroxyvitamin D is suppressed in most patients with bone destruction associated with hypercalcemia. However, in a small subset of patients with T-cell lymphomas, 1,25-dihydroxyvitamin D_3 production by the tumor tissue is increased, and this is associated with increased calcium absorption from the gut (65). This mechanism is important in the pathophysiology of the hypercalcemia in these cases. This mechanism probably represents a minority of all patients with T-cell lymphomas. An atypical metabolite of 1,25-dihydroxyvitamin D_3 has also been invoked in one solid tumor associated with hypercalcemia (66). This also appears to be an uncommon mechanism responsible for hypercalcemia of malignancy.

Osteoprotegerin and Related Molecule

Recently, a member of the TNF receptor superfamily which inhibits bone resorption independently of the stimulus has been identified by two groups independently (67,68). This protein has been named osteoclastogenesis inhibitory factor (OCIF) or osteoprotegerin (OPG) and represents a peptide which is a soluble secreted form of the TNF receptor that acts as an antagonist to osteoclastic bone resorption both *in vitro* and *in vivo*. Even more recently, the ligand for this endogenous antagonist has been identified as the putative osteoclastogenesis differentiation-inducing factor (ODIF), which acts directly on osteoclasts. It appears to be identical, or at the very least related, to receptor activator of NFκB ligand [RANKL, also called TNF-related, activation-induced cytokine (TRANCE)] (69). This peptide, which has a membrane-bound form, is also a ligand for OPG/OCIF (70) and has been shown to stimulate osteoclastic bone resorption in marrow cultures by acting directly on cells in the osteoclast lineage. This has led to the concept that OPG or OCIF inhibits bone resorption by binding directly to TRANCE/

ODIF, the final common mediator of osteoclastic bone resorption. Although a role for this ligand and receptor has not yet been described in malignancy, it seems very likely that one may eventually be identified.

POTENTIAL FACTORS INVOLVED IN BONE DESTRUCTION IN MYELOMA

The pathogenesis of the bone lesions is related to increased production of a local bone-resorbing factor in the bone marrow of patients with myeloma. This bone-resorbing factor has characteristics similar to the bone-resorbing activity produced by activated peripheral blood leukocytes that was formerly called osteoclast-activating factor (OAF) (71). OAF represents a family of bone-resorbing factors that are produced by lymphocytes and monocytes following exposure to an antigen to which they have previously been exposed or a nonspecific mitogen such as phytohemagglutinin (72). The OAFs, which have been implicated in myeloma, are lymphotoxin, IL-1β, and IL-6.

Lymphotoxin

Lymphotoxin is a normal activated lymphocyte product which is also produced by lymphoid cell lines in culture. Lymphotoxin increases bone resorption (48) and stimulates the formation of osteoclasts from precursors in marrow cell cultures (73). In addition, lymphotoxin can activate mature osteoclasts to form resorption pits (74). Lymphotoxin has effects identical to those of TNF on bone resorption and overlapping those of ILs 1α and 1β. Repeated injections of recombinant human lymphotoxin cause hypercalcemia in normal mice (54).

B-lymphoblastoid cell lines often express and secrete lymphotoxin. It has now been shown that in a number of cell culture lines isolated from patients with myeloma the tumor cells express lymphotoxin mRNA and contain cytotoxic activity in the conditioned medium (54). This cytotoxic activity can be ascribed to lymphotoxin. The conditioned medium also contains bone-resorbing activity, which can be partially neutralized by lymphotoxin-neutralizing antibodies.

Interleukin-1β

ILs 1α and 1β are powerful stimulators of osteoclastic bone resorption (75–77). In addition, IL-1 can cause hypercalcemia (28) and markedly increased osteoclastic bone resorption *in vivo* (28–30). Freshly isolated marrow cells from patients with myeloma, which contain myeloma cells plus stromal cells, have been shown to produce IL-1β in the conditioned medium (34,35). Bone-resorbing activity produced by these cultures can be neutralized by antibodies to IL-1β. In contrast, established cell lines from patients with myeloma do not express IL-1β (54). The reason for these discrepancies probably relates to the nature of the cells studied. Artifacts could occur in both models. Established cell lines could have changed in culture to produce factors that the parent cells *in situ* did not. Alternatively, the freshly isolated cells (which contain dead and dying elements) likely release factors that they did not release *in situ* (as has been shown previously for prostaglandins).

IL-1 stimulates the formation of osteoclasts from progenitor cells (73). IL-1 also activates mature osteoclasts to resorb bone (78). This is probably the most powerful peptide bone-resorbing factor known.

Interleukin-6

IL-6 is a recently described multifunctional cytokine which may play an important role in the pathophysiology of myeloma. Considerable evidence suggests that it may be an important growth factor in myeloma, and recently it has been suggested that neutralizing antibodies to IL-6 may have important effects on the course of the disease (55). We have tested IL-6 for its effects on bone resorption and calcium homeostasis *in vitro* and *in vivo* (59). IL-6 has effects which are different from those of IL-1 and TNF. IL-6 does not stimulate osteoclastic bone resorption in organ cultures of fetal rat long bones. Its effects in neonatal mouse calvariae are also minor or possibly nonexistent. However, in other types of organ culture, it has been shown to stimulate osteoclastic bone resorption (56,57). IL-6 causes hypercalcemia *in vivo*. When IL-6 is stably transfected into CHO cells from tumors in nude mice, the cells express IL-6. Mice carrying tumors with CHO cells expressing IL-6 develop increasing levels of IL-6 in the serum as the tumor grows. These mice become progressively hypercalcemic and develop leukocytosis, thrombocytosis, and cachexia (59). This increase in serum calcium is due to an increase in osteoclastic bone resorption *in vivo*.

IL-6 may also have effects in the bone microenvironment which are different from those of the other cytokines. Although bone cells isolated from trabecular bone surfaces (bone-lining cells) express cytokines such as IL-1, TNF, CSF, and IL-6, it is only in the case of IL-6 that these bone cells produce more of a cytokine when exposed to osteotropic factors such as PTH, IL-1, and TNF (62). In the case of the other cytokines, production by bone cells may be enhanced by nonphysiological stimuli such as lipopolysaccharide. In addition, it has recently been shown that bone cell expression of IL-6 can be decreased by exposure of the bone cells to estrogen (79,80).

Recently, PTHrP has also been implicated in the bone destruction associated with myeloma (10,11,81). It is demonstrated in about one-third of patients in increased amounts in the circulation and in marrow myeloma cells by immunohistochemistry.

Which of these cytokines is the most important in bone lesions associated with myeloma is at present unknown. It is possible in myeloma that some combination of these cytokines enhances bone resorption. Other mechanisms may also be important, particularly interactions between marrow stromal cells and myeloma cells in the production of both IL-6 and the cytokines responsible for bone resorption (82).

FACTORS INVOLVED WITH OSTEOBLASTIC METASTASES

A number of factors have been suggested to be potential mediators of osteoblastic metastasis associated with prostate cancer.

1. TGF-β2 is abundant in PC3 human prostatic cancer cells and was purified from the human prostate cancer cell line PC3 (83). TGF-β2 stimulates proliferation of osteoblasts *in vitro* as well as bone formation *in vivo*.

2. Prostatic cancer cells express large amounts of both acidic and basic fibroblast growth factors (FGFs) (84,85), and these are potential mediators of osteoblast proliferation in patients with this disease (86,87). Both acidic and basic FGFs (also called FGFs 1 and 2) cause profound stimulation of bone formation *in vivo* (88,89). Izbicka et al. (90) have shown that a human tumor cell line causes bone formation *in vivo* and produces a mitogenic factor for osteoblastic cells which was identified as an extended form of FGF-2.

3. There have been several reports of purification of mitogenic activity for rat calvarial osteoblastic cells present in the conditioned medium of the human prostatic cancer cell line PC3 (91,92). The first ten amino acids were sequenced and shown to be identical to the serine protease urokinase plasminogen activator (u-PA). Overexpression of u-PA in rat prostate cancer cells leads to bone metastases *in vivo* (93). An amino-terminal fragment of u-PA which contains EGF-like repeats has been shown to have mitogenic activity for osteoblasts (94). The carboxy-terminal proteolytic domain may be responsible for tumor invasiveness or growth factor activation. The expression of proteases in the microenvironment of growth factors such as TGF-β may be very important for their activation in bone (95,96). Plasmin-sensitive cleavage sites which mask TGF-β activity are present in the latent TGF-β binding protein.

4. We have found that both normal and neoplastic prostate tissues express a variety of bone morphogenetic proteins (BMPs). We have examined human and rat neoplastic prostate tissues and found evidence of BMPs 2, 3, 4, and 6 mRNA (97).

5. Cultured prostatic cancer cells frequently express PTHrP, which in appropriate doses has an anabolic effect on bone (98). This tumor peptide may be related to the anabolic effect of prostate cancers (L. McCauley, personal communication). There are no direct data as yet to support this notion.

6. The serine protease prostate-specific antigen (PSA), which is expressed by prostate cancer cells, can cleave PTHrP at the amino terminus (99) and could also potentially activate other growth factors produced by prostate carcinomas. PSA is produced in excessive amounts by prostate carcinoma cells and is used as a marker of tumor burden. Whether it has harmful effects is unknown, but one possibility is that its enzymatic action could be responsible for activating anabolic agents such as IGF-I and TGF-β, by cleaving them from their binding proteins or by cleaving PTHrP to an anabolic fragment. It has been shown to cleave PTHrP (99).

7. Endothelin-1 has recently been implicated as an osteoblast stimulant in metastatic prostate cancer (100). It is a powerful mitogenic factor for osteoblasts (101,102) and is produced in large amounts by the prostatic epithelium (103). Circulating concentrations are increased in patients with metastatic prostate cancer (100). However, whether it has more pathophysiological significance than the numerous other growth-regulatory factors for bone cells produced by prostate carcinomas remains unknown.

ACKNOWLEDGMENTS

Some of the work described here was supported in part by grants CA-40035, RR-01346, AR-28149, and AR-07464.

REFERENCES

1. Yin JJ, Spinks TJ, Cui Y, et al. Clonal variation in parathyroid hormone–related protein (PTH-rP) secretion by a human breast cancer cell line alters severity of osteolytic metastases. *J Bone Miner Res* 1997; 12[Suppl 1]:19.
2. Moseley JM, Kubota M, Diefenbach-Jagger H, et al. Parathyroid hormone–related protein purified from a human lung cancer cell line. *Proc Natl Acad Sci USA* 1987;84:5048–5052.
3. Stewart AF, Wu T, Goumas D, et al. N-terminal amino acid sequence of two novel tumor-derived adenylate cyclase–stimulating proteins: identification of parathyroid hormone-like and parathyroid hormone-unlike domains. *Biochem Biophys Res Commun* 1987;146: 672–678.
4. Strewler GJ, Stern PH, Jacobs JW, et al. Parathyroid hormone-like protein from human renal carcinoma cells: structural and functional homology with parathyroid hormone. *J Clin Invest* 1987;80:1803–1807.
5. Motokura T, Fukumoto S, Matsumoto T, et al. Parathyroid hormone related protein in adult T-cell leukemia-lymphoma. *Ann Intern Med* 1989;111:484–488.
6. Yates AJP, Gutierrez GE, Smolens P, et al. Effects of a synthetic peptide of a parathyroid hormone–related protein on calcium homeostasis, renal tubular calcium reabsorption and bone metabolism. *J Clin Invest* 1988; 81:932–938.
7. Kukreja SC, Shevrin DH, Wimbiscus SA, et al. Antibodies to parathyroid hormone–related protein lower serum calcium in athymic mouse models of malignancy-associated hypercalcemia due to human tumors. *J Clin Invest* 1988;82:1798–1802.
8. Powell GJ, Southby J, Danks JA, et al. Localization of parathyroid hormone–related protein in breast cancer metastases: increased incidence in bone compared with other sites. *Cancer Res* 1991;51:3059–3061.
9. Guise TA, Yin JJ, Taylor SD, et al. Evidence for a causal role of parathyroid hormone–related protein in the pathogenesis of human breast cancer–mediated osteolysis. *J Clin Invest* 1996;98:1544–1549.
10. Firkin F, Seymour JF, Watson AM, et al. Parathyroid hormone–related protein in hypercalcemia associated with haematological malignancy. *Br J Haematol* 1996; 94:486–492.
11. Budayr AA, Halloran BP, King JC, et al. High levels of a parathyroid hormone-like protein in milk. *Proc Natl Acad Sci USA* 1989;86:7183–7185.
12. Henderson B, Pettipher ER. Arthritogenic actions of recombinant IL-1 and tumour necrosis factor alpha in the rabbit: evidence for synergistic interactions between cytokines *in vivo. Clin Exp Immunol* 1989;75: 306–310.
13. Guise TA, Yoneda T, Yates AJ, et al. The combined effect of tumor-produced parathyroid hormone–related protein and transforming growth factor alpha enhance hypercalcemia *in vivo* and bone resorption *in vitro. J Clin Endocrinol Metab* 1993;77:40–45.
14. Sato K, Fujii Y, Kasono K. Parathyroid hormone–related protein and interleukin-1α synergistically stimulate bone resorption *in vitro* and increase the serum calcium concentration in mice *in vivo. Endocrinology* 1989;124:2172–2178.
15. De La Mata J, Uy H, Guise TA, et al. IL-6 enhances hypercalcemia and bone resorption mediated by PTH-rP *in vivo. J Clin Invest* 1995;95:2846–2852.
16. Uy HL, Mundy GR, Boyce BF, et al. Tumor necrosis factor enhances parathyroid hormone related protein (PTH-rP)–induced hypercalcemia *in vivo. J Bone Miner Res* 1996;11[Suppl 1]:S447.
17. Thiede MA, Rodan GA. Expression of a calcium-mobilizing parathyroid hormone-like peptide in lactating mammary tissue. *Science* 1988;242:278–280.
18. Rodda CP, Kubota M, Heath JA, et al. Evidence for a novel parathyroid hormone–related protein in fetal lamb parathyroid glands and sheep placenta: comparisons with a similar protein implicated in humoral hypercalcemia of malignancy. *J Endocrinol* 1988;117: 261–271.
19. Bruns DE, Ferguson JE, Weir EC, et al. Parathyroid hormone–related protein (PTH-rP): a novel hormone in human pregnancy. *J Bone Miner Res* 1992;7[Suppl 1]:6.

20. Karaplis AC, Luz A, Glowacki J, et al. Lethal skeletal dysplasia from targeted disruption of the parathyroid-related peptide gene. *Genes Dev* 1994;8:277–289.

21. Vortkamp A, Lee K, Lanske B, et al. Regulation of rate of cartilage differentiation by Indian hedgehog and PTH-related protein. *Science* 1996;273:613–622.

22. Schipani E, Kruse K, Juppner H. A competitively active mutant PTH-PTHrP receptor in Jansen-type metaphyseal chondrodysplasia. *Science* 1995;268:98–100.

23. Lanske B, Karaplis AC, Lee K, et al. PTH/PTHrP receptor in early development and Indian hedgehog–related bone growth. *Science* 1996;273:663–666.

24. Yoshimoto K, Yamasaki R, Sakai H, et al. Ectopic production of parathyroid hormone by small cell lung cancer in a patient with hypercalcemia. *J Clin Endocrinol Metab* 1989;68:976–981.

25. Strewler GJ, Budayr AA, Bruce RJ. Secretion of authentic parathyroid hormone by a malignant tumor. *Clin Res* 1990;38:462A.

26. Nussbaum SR, Gaz RD, Arnold A. Hypercalcemia and ectopic secretion of parathyroid hormone by an ovarian carcinoma with rearrangement of the gene for parathyroid hormone. *N Engl J Med* 1990;323:1324–1328.

27. Simpson EL, Mundy GR, D'Souza SM, et al. Absence of parathyroid hormone messenger RNA in non-parathyroid tumors associated with hypercalcemia. *N Engl J Med* 1983;309:325–330.

28. Sabatini M, Boyce B, Aufdemorte TB, et al. Infusions of recombinant human interleukin-1α and β cause hypercalcemia in normal mice. *Proc Natl Acad Sci USA* 1988;85:5235–5239.

29. Boyce BF, Aufdemorte TB, Garrett IR, et al. Effects of interleukin-1 on bone turnover in normal mice. *Endocrinology* 1989;125:1142–1150.

30. Boyce BF, Yates AJP, Mundy GR. Bolus injections of recombinant human interleukin-1 cause transient hypocalcemia in normal mice. *Endocrinology* 1989;125:2780–2783.

31. Fried RM, Voelkel EF, Rice RH, et al. Two squamous cell carcinomas not associated with humoral hypercalcemia produce a potent bone resorption–stimulating factor which is interleukin-1 alpha. *Endocrinology* 1989;125:742–751.

32. Nowak RA, Morrison NE, Goad DL, et al. Squamous cell carcinomas often produce more than a single bone resorption–stimulating factor—role of interleukin-1 alpha. *Endocrinology* 1990;127:3061–3069.

33. Gowen M, Wood DD, Russell RGG. Stimulation of the proliferation of human bone cells *in vitro* by human monocyte products with interleukin-1 activity. *J Clin Invest* 1985;75:1223–1229.

34. Cozzolino F, Torcia M, Aldinucci D, et al. Production of interleukin-1 by bone marrow myeloma cells. *Blood* 1989;74:380–387.

35. Kawano M, Tanaka H, Ishikawa H, et al. Interleukin-1 accelerates autocrine growth of myeloma cells through interleukin-6 in human myeloma. *Blood* 1989;73:2145–2148.

36. Boyce BF, Yoneda T, Lowe C, et al. Requirement of pp60[c-src] expression of osteoclasts to form ruffled borders and resorb bone. *J Clin Invest* 1992;90:1622–1627.

37. Ibbotson KJ, Twardzik DR, D'Souza SM, et al. Stimulation of bone resorption *in vitro* by synthetic transforming growth factor-alpha. *Science* 1985;228:1007–1009.

38. Tashjian AH, Voelkel EF, Lazzaro M, et al. Alpha and beta transforming growth factors stimulate prostaglandin production and bone resorption in cultured mouse calvaria. *Proc Natl Acad Sci USA* 1985;82:4535–4538.

39. Takahashi N, Mundy GR, Kuehl TJ, et al. Osteoclast like formation in fetal and newborn long term baboon marrow cultures is more sensitive to 1,25-dihydroxyvitamin D3 than adult long term marrow cultures. *J Bone Miner Res* 1987;2:311–317.

40. Yates AJP, Favarato G, Aufdemorte TB, et al. Expression of human transforming growth factor α by Chinese hamster ovarian tumors in nude mice causes hypercalcemia and increased osteoclastic bone resorption. *J Bone Miner Res* 1992;7:847–853.

41. Massagué J. Transforming growth factor alpha. A model for membrane-anchored growth factors. *J Biol Chem* 1990;265:21393–21396.

42. Takahashi N, MacDonald BR, Hon J, et al. Recombinant human transforming growth factor alpha stimulates the formation of osteoclast-like cells in long term human marrow cultures. *J Clin Invest* 1986;78:894–898.

43. Takahashi N, Mundy GR, Roodman GD. Recombinant human interferon-γ inhibits formation of human osteoclast-like cells. *J Immunol* 1986;137:3544–3549.

44. Dewhirst FE, Ago JM, Peros WJ, et al. Synergism between parathyroid hormone and interleukin-1 in stimulating bone resorption in organ culture. *J Bone Miner Res* 1987;2:127–134.

45. Gutierrez GE, Mundy GR, Derynck R, et al. Inhibition of parathyroid hormone-responsive adenylate cyclase in clonal osteoblast-like cells by transforming growth factor alpha and epidermal growth factor. *J Biol Chem* 1987;262:15845–15850.

46. Gutierrez GE, Mundy GR, Manning DR, et al. Transforming growth factor β enhances parathyroid hormone stimulation of adenylate cyclase in clonal osteoblast-like cells. *J Cell Physiol* 1990;144:438–447.

47. Pizurki L, Rizzoli R, Bonjour JP. Inhibition by (D-Trp[12], Tyr[34])bPTH(7–34)amide of PTH and PTHrP effects on P_i transport in renal cells. *Am J Physiol* 1990;259:F389–F392.

48. Bertolini DR, Nedwin GE, Bringman TS, et al. Stimulation of bone resorption and inhibition of bone formation *in vitro* by human tumour necrosis factors. *Nature* 1986;319:516–518.

49. Johnson RA, Boyce BF, Mundy GR, et al. Tumors producing human TNF induce hypercalcemia and osteoclastic bone resorption in nude mice. *Endocrinology* 1989;124:1424–1427.

50. Uy HL, Dallas M, Calland JW, et al. Use of an *in vivo* model to determine the effects of interleukin-1 on cells at different stages in the osteoclast lineage. *J Bone Miner Res* 1995;10:295–301.

51. Yoneda T, Alsina MM, Chavez JB, et al. Evidence that splenic cytokines play a pathogenetic role in the paraneoplastic syndromes of cachexia, hypercalcemia and leukocytosis in a human tumor in nude mice. *J Clin Invest* 1991;87:977–985.

52. Sabatini M, Yates AJ, Garrett IR, et al. Increased production of tumor necrosis factor by normal immune cells in a model of the humoral hypercalcemia of malignancy. *Lab Invest* 1990;63:676–682.

53. Sabatini M, Chavez J, Mundy GR, et al. Stimulation of tumor necrosis factor release from monocytic cells by the A375 human melanoma via granulocyte-macrophage colony stimulating factor. *Cancer Res* 1990;50: 2673–2678.

54. Garrett IR, Durie BGM, Nedwin GE, et al. Production of the bone resorbing cytokine lymphotoxin by cultured human myeloma cells. *N Engl J Med* 1987;317: 526–532.

55. Bataille R, Jourdan M, Zhang XG, et al. Serum levels of interleukin-6, a potent myeloma cell growth factor, as a reflection of disease severity in plasma cell dyscrasias. *J Clin Invest* 1989;84:2008–2011.

56. Lowik CW, Van der Pluijm G, Bloys H, et al. Parathyroid hormone (PTH) and PTH-like protein (Plp) stimulate interleukin-6 production by osteogenic cells—a possible role of interleukin-6 in osteoclastogenesis. *Biochem Biophys Res Commun* 1989;162:1546–1552.

57. Ishimi Y, Miyaura C, Jin CH, et al. IL-6 is produced by osteoblasts and induces bone resorption. *J Immunol* 1990;145:3297–3303.

58. Gowen M, Chapman K, Littlewood A, et al. Production of tumor necrosis factor by human osteoblasts is modulated by other cytokines but not by osteotropic hormones. *Endocrinology* 1990;126:1250–1255.

59. Black K, Garrett IR, Mundy GR. Chinese hamster ovarian cells transfected with the murine interleukin-6 gene cause hypercalcemia as well as cachexia, leukocytosis and thrombocytosis in tumour-bearing nude mice. *Endocrinology* 1991;128:2657–2659.

60. Kukita A, Bonewald L, Rosen D, et al. Osteoinductive factor inhibits formation of human osteoclast-like cells. *Proc Natl Acad Sci USA* 1990;87:3023–3026.

61. Yoneda T, Nakai M, Moriyama K, et al. Neutralizing antibodies to human interleukin-6 reverse hypercalcemia associated with a human squamous carcinoma. *Cancer Res* 1993;53:737–740.

62. Feyen JHM, Elford P, Di Padova FE, et al. Interleukin-6 is produced by bone and modulated by parathyroid hormone. *J Bone Miner Res* 1989;4:633–638.

63. Klein DC, Raisz LG. Prostaglandins: stimulation of bone resorption in tissue culture. *Endocrinology* 1970; 86:1436–1440.

64. Mundy GR. *Calcium homeostasis: hypercalcemia and hypocalcemia.* London: Martin Dunitz, 1990.

65. Breslau NA, McGuire JL, Zerwekh JE, et al. Hypercalcemia associated with increased serum calcitriol levels in three patients with lymphoma. *Ann Intern Med* 1984; 100:1–6.

66. Shigeno C, Yamamoto I, Dokoh S, et al. Identification of 1,24(R)-dihydroxyvitamin D3-like bone-resorbing lipid in a patient with cancer-associated hypercalcemia. *J Clin Endocrinol Metab* 1985;61:761–768.

67. Simonet WS, Lacey DL, Dunstan CR, et al. Osteoprotegerin: a novel secreted protein involved in the regulation of bone density. *Cell* 1997;89:309–319.

68. Tsuda E, Goto M, Mochizuki S, et al. Isolation of a novel cytokine from human fibroblasts that specifically inhibits osteoclastogenesis. *Biochem Biophys Res Commun* 1997;234:137–142.

69. Wong BR, Josien R, Lee SY, et al. TRANCE (tumor necrosis factor (TNF)–related activation-induced cytokine), a new TNF family member predominantly expressed in T cells, is a dendritic cell-specific survival factor. *J Exp Med* 1997;186:2075–2080.

70. Yasuda H, Shima N, Nakagawa N, et al. Osteoclast differentiation factor is a ligand for osteoprotegerin/osteoclastogenesis-inhibitory factor and is identical to TRANCE/RANKL. *Proc Natl Acad Sci USA* 1998;95:3597–3602.

71. Mundy GR, Raisz LG, Cooper RA, et al. Evidence for the secretion of an osteoclast stimulating factor in myeloma. *N Engl J Med* 1974;291:1041–1046.

72. Horton JE, Raisz LG, Simmons HA, et al. Bone resorbing activity in supernatant fluid from cultured human peripheral blood leukocytes. *Science* 1972;177: 793–795.

73. Pfeilschifter J, Chenu C, Bird A, et al. Interleukin-1 and tumor necrosis factor stimulate the formation of human osteoclast-like cells *in vitro. J Bone Miner Res* 1989;4:113–118.

74. Thomson BM, Mundy GR, Chambers TJ. Tumor necrosis factors alpha and beta induce osteoblastic cells to stimulate osteoclastic bone resorption. *J Immunol* 1987;138:775–779.

75. Gowen M, Wood DD, Ihrie EJ, et al. An interleukin-1 like factor stimulates bone resorption *in vitro. Nature* 1983;306:378–380.

76. Gowen M, Meikle MC, Reynolds JJ. Stimulation of bone resorption *in vitro* by a non-prostanoid factor released by human monocytes in culture. *Biochem Biophys Acta* 1983;762:471–474.

77. Gowen M, Nedwin G, Mundy GR. Preferential inhibition of cytokine stimulated bone resorption by recombinant interferon gamma. *J Bone Miner Res* 1986;1: 469–474.

78. McSheehy PMJ, Chambers TJ. Osteoblastic cells mediate osteoclastic responsiveness to parathyroid hormone. *Endocrinology* 1986;118:824–828.

79. Girasole G, Jilka RL, Passeri G, et al. 17β-Estradiol inhibits interleukin-6 production by bone marrow–derived stromal cells and osteoblasts *in vitro*. A potential mechanism for the antiosteoporotic effect of estrogens. *J Clin Invest* 1992;89:883–891.

80. Jilka RL, Hangoc G, Girasole G, et al. Increased osteoclast development after estrogen loss—mediation by interleukin-6. *Science* 1992;257:88–91.

81. Suzuki A, Takahashi T, Okuno Y, et al. Production of parathyroid hormone–related protein by cultured human myeloma cells. *Am J Hematol* 1994;45:88–90.

82. Michigami T, Dallas SL, Mundy GR, et al. Interaction of myeloma cells with bone marrow stromal cells via α4β1 integrin-VCAM-1 is required for the development of osteolysis. *J Bone Miner Res* 1997;12[Suppl 1]:104.

83. Marquardt H, Lioubin MN, Ikeda T. Complete amino acid sequence of human transforming growth factor type beta 2. *J Biol Chem* 1987;262:12127–12130.

84. Matuo Y, Nishi N, Matsui S, et al. Heparin binding affinity of rat prostate growth factor in normal and cancerous prostate: partial purification and characterization of rat prostate growth factor in the Dunning tumor. *Cancer Res* 1987;47:188–192.

85. Mansson PE, Adams P, Kan M, et al. HBGF1 gene expression in normal rat prostate and two transplantable rat prostate tumors. *Cancer Res* 1989;49: 2485–2494.

86. Canalis E, Lorenzo J, Burgess WH, et al. Effects of endothelial cell growth factor on bone remodeling *in vitro. J Clin Invest* 1987;79:52–58.

87. Canalis E, Centrella M, McCarthy T. Effects of basic fibroblast growth factor on bone formation *in vitro*. *J Clin Invest* 1988;81:1572–1577.

88. Mayahara H, Ito T, Nagai H, et al. *In vivo* stimulation of endosteal bone formation by basic fibroblast growth factor in rats. *Growth Factors* 1993;9:73–80.

89. Dunstan CR, Garrett IR, Adams R, et al. Systemic fibroblast growth factor (FGF-1) prevents bone loss, increases new bone formation, and restores trabecular microarchitecture in ovariectomized rats. *J Bone Miner Res* 1995;10[Suppl 1]:P279.

90. Izbicka E, Dunstan CR, Esparza J, et al. Human amniotic tumor which induces new bone formation *in vivo* produces a growth regulatory activity *in vitro* for osteoblasts identified as an extended form of basic fibroblast growth factor (bFGF). *Cancer Res* 1996;56:633–636.

91. Rabbani SA, Desjardins J, Bell AW, et al. An aminoterminal fragment of urokinase isolated from a prostate cancer cell line (PC-3) is mitogenic for osteoblast-like cells. *Biochem Biophys Res Commun* 1990;173:1058–1064.

92. Rabbani SA, Desjardins J, Bell AW, et al. Identification of a new osteoblast mitogen from a human prostate cancer cell line, PC-3. *J Bone Miner Res* 1990;5:549.

93. Achbarou A, Kaiser S, Tremblay G, et al. Urokinase overproduction results in increased skeletal metastasis by prostate cancer cells *in vivo*. *Cancer Res* 1994;54:2372–2377.

94. Rabbani SA, Mazar AP, Bernier SM, et al. Structural requirements for the growth factor activity of the amino-terminal domain of urokinase. *J Biol Chem* 1992;267:14151–14156.

95. Dallas SL, Park-Snyder S, Miyazono K, et al. Characterization and autoregulation of latent TGFβ complexes in osteoblast-like cell lines: production of a latent complex lacking the latent TGFβ-binding protein (LTBP). *J Biol Chem* 1994;269:6815–6822.

96. Dallas SL, Miyazono K, Skerry TM, et al. Dual role for the latent transforming growth factor-beta binding protein in storage of latent TGF-beta in the extracellular matrix and as a structural matrix protein. *J Cell Biol* 1995;131:539–549.

97. Harris SE, Bonewald LF, Harris MA, et al. Effects of transforming growth factor beta on bone nodule formation and expression of bone morphogenetic protein 2, osteocalcin, osteopontin, alkaline phosphatase, and type 1 collagen mRNA in long-term cultures of fetal rat calvarial osteoblasts. *J Bone Miner Res* 1994;9:855–863.

98. Stewart AF. PTHrP(1–36) as a skeletal anabolic agent for the treatment of osteoporosis. *Bone* 1996;19:303–306.

99. Cramer SD, Chen Z, Peehl DM. Prostate specific antigen cleaves parathyroid hormone–related protein in the PTH-like domain: inactivation of PTH-rP stimulated cAMP accumulation in mouse osteoblasts. *J Urol* 1996;156:526–531.

100. Nelson JB, Hedican SP, George DJ, et al. Identification of endothelin-1 in the pathophysiology of metastatic adenocarcinoma of the prostate. *Nat Med* 1995;1:944.

101. Takuwa Y, Ohue Y, Takuwa N, et al. Endothelin-1 activates phospholipase C and mobilizes Ca^{2+} from extra- and intracellular pools in osteoblastic cells. *Am J Physiol* 1989;257:E797–E803.

102. Takuwa Y, Masaki T, Yamashita K. The effects of the endothelin family peptides on cultured osteoblastic cells from rat calvariae. *Biochem Biophys Res Commun* 1990;170:998–1005.

103. Langenstroer P, Tang R, Shapiro E, et al. Endothelin-1 in the human prostate: tissue levels, source of production and isometric tension studies. *J Urol* 1993;150:495–499.

Skeletal Growth Factors,
edited by Ernesto Canalis.
Lippincott Williams & Wilkins, Philadelphia, © 2000.

32

Clinical Use of Growth Factors

Gemma Sesmilo and Anne Klibanski

Neuroendocrine Unit, Massachusetts General Hospital, Boston, Massachusetts 02114

During recent years, there have been important advances in our understanding of the role of growth factors in the processes of bone formation and bone resorption. Growth regulatory factors are produced locally in bone and act in a paracrine and autocrine fashion to control cellular events involved in bone remodeling. These factors act in concert with systemic hormones in the maintenance of bone homeostasis and may play a role in the pathogenesis of osteoporosis. Recent studies have begun to elucidate the possible use of growth factors in the treatment of conditions associated with bone loss. One of the most interesting aspects of these new anabolic agents in the treatment of osteoporosis is their potential role in increasing bone formation. This chapter reviews the use of growth factors in experimental clinical models and disease states. Potential future strategies using growth factors in the treatment of osteoporosis are discussed.

USE OF GROWTH FACTORS IN GROWTH HORMONE DEFICIENCY SYNDROMES

Insulin-like Growth Factor-I Administration in Growth Hormone Insensitivity Syndrome

One of the earliest uses of recombinant insulin-like growth factor-I (IGF-I) was in the treatment of patients with Laron dwarfism, a rare autosomal-recessive disorder caused by a deficiency of functional growth hormone (GH) receptors. This disorder is characterized by the clinical features of GH deficiency but normal or elevated serum GH concentrations and low IGF-I levels. Classically, there is clinical unresponsiveness to GH therapy as defined by an inability to generate endogenous IGF-I. Laron dwarfism is termed primary GH insensitivity syndrome (GHIS), in contrast to secondary GHIS, in which attenuated growth responses to exogenous GH occur in children with GH deficiency due to a deletion in the GH gene. Several groups have reported the long-term effects of recombinant human IGF-I (rhIGF-I) administration in these conditions.

The principal endpoint in evaluating the long-term administration of rhIGF-I in GHIS is the promotion of longitudinal growth (1–4). Such patients represent an interesting model in which to investigate the potential independent effects of GH and IGF-I in bone physiology. Ranke et al. (1) reported the results of 26 GHIS patients (ages 3 to 11 years) who received long-term IGF-I therapy at a dose of 40 to 120 μg/kg subcutaneously twice daily. During the first year of therapy, the mean growth velocity increased from 3.9 $\pm$ 1.8 to 8.5 $\pm$ 2.1 cm and was 6.4 $\pm$ 2.2 cm during the second year in the 18 patients who continued therapy (Fig. 32.1). The overall improvement in height score at the end of the second year was 1.2 standard deviation (SD). As expected, IGF-I levels, low at baseline, rose above pretreatment concentrations, but a dose-response effect of IGF-I on linear growth was not noted. There was considerable heterogeneity in the response seen, and in the majority of patients, IGF-I remained below the normal

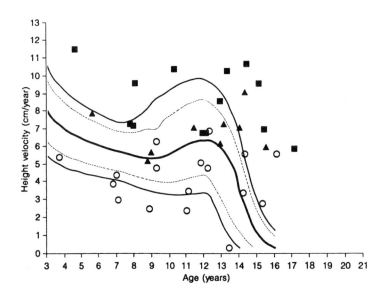

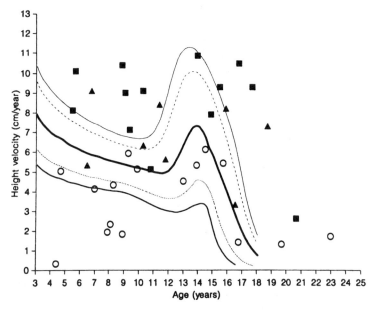

FIG. 32.1. Height velocity of girls **(top)** and boys **(bottom)** with growth hormone insensitivity syndrome (GHIS) treated with insulin-like growth factor-I (IGF-I) before and during the first and second years of treatment in comparison with normal standards. *Graphs* show the third, tenth, fiftieth, ninetieth, and ninety-seventh percentiles; *open circles* give pretreatment height velocities; *squares* give first-year and *triangles* second-year height velocities. (From ref. 1, with permission.)

age-adjusted range. In addition, IGF binding protein-3 (IGFBP-3) remained low and unchanged from pretreatment levels. A number of adverse events at these doses were reported, including headache, hypoglycemia, reversible papilledema, and Bell's palsy. These adverse events as well as a decrease in serum potassium concentrations have been reported by other groups (2,3). In another study of 22 patients with GHIS, Guevara-Aguirre et al. (4) evaluated growth velocity during administration of two doses of IGF-I. Fifteen patients received 120 μg/kg IGF-I subcutaneously twice daily and seven patients received 80 μg/kg twice daily (group ages 3.1 to 17.1 years, height SD scores -5.8 to -11.5). There was no difference in either the IGF-I levels or the clinical effects between the two groups, suggesting a plateau effect beyond 80 μg/kg twice daily. The investigators reported that IGF-I levels rose from a subnormal to a therapeutic range despite unchanged levels of IGFBP-3, postulating an alternative mechanism for sustaining and avoiding rapid clearance of rhIGF-I levels. The results for the first-year growth velocity were 8.9 $\pm$ 1.5 cm (more than doubled from baseline) and 6.1 $\pm$ 1.5 cm for the second year, and a significant correlation between the increases over baseline in serum IGF-I levels and annual increments in height age was noted. As in the previous study by Ranke et al. (1), there was a decrease in growth velocity during the second year of therapy compared to the first. However, a small subgroup receiving the highest dose followed during a third year demonstrated that growth velocity was sustained compared to the previous year. When Guevara-Aguirre et al. compared the results with a group of 11 children with GH deficiency treated with GH, growth velocity was higher in GH-treated patients, consistent with a direct effect of GH on bone (4). Similar effects on longitudinal growth have been reported by other groups (2,5). Therefore, one can conclude that the growth-promoting effect is more pronounced in the first year of treatment, reduced by 33% in the second year, and maintained in the third. Finally, these data indicate that systemically administered IGF-I acts by endocrine mechanisms and its effect is not solely dependent on autocrine or paracrine actions.

The effects of IGF-I on bone mineral density (BMD) are more difficult to elucidate based on the data obtained from the models studied to date. Backeljauw et al. (2) measured BMD in six children with GHIS before and after receiving treatment with IGF-I 80 to 120 μg/kg twice daily for up to 3 years. Although they found an increase in spinal BMD compared with age-related standards, the results could not be statistically analyzed due to the small patient number. Bach-

rach et al. (6) studied a group of 11 adults with GHIS Laron subtype and controls using dual-energy x-ray absorptiometry (DEXA), bone biopsies, and surrogate bone turnover markers. They found a lower BMD in patients than controls but not when adjusted for the differences in bone thickness in the two groups. Histomorphometric data confirmed the maintenance of volumetric bone density and cortical widths in adults with GHIS, and the only difference found was a reduction in bone connectivity. Because the calculated volumetric bone density was an estimate, the authors postulated that it would be inaccurate due to the extremely small bone size of subjects with GHIS. More data in this regard will elucidate the contribution of IGF-I to the acquisition and maintenance of bone mineral density. Other reported effects of IGF-I that could influence bone mass include increases in lean body mass and in urinary calcium excretion, probably due to a parathyroid hormone (PTH)–independent effect on renal 1α-hydroxylation of vitamin D (2,3).

Insulin-like Growth Factor-I in Acquired Growth Hormone Deficiency

Acquired GH deficiency (GHD) is associated with low BMD and osteoporosis. Bone turnover has been shown to be decreased in GHD states. Johansson et al. (7), in a cross-sectional study of 29 patients with GHD, showed a correlation between serum IGF-I levels and both spinal and total BMD, suggesting the importance of the endocrine effects of IGF-I in the maintenance of bone mass. Although BMD also correlated with mean pulsatile GH secretion, a multivariate analysis showed IGF-I to be the major factor explaining variations in spinal bone mass. Long-term administration of GH has been shown to increase BMD in these patients in association with increases in serum IGF-I levels. Baum et al. (8) reported the results of an 18-month placebo-controlled trial in a group of 32 men with adult-onset GHD who received physiological doses of GH [mean 4 μg/kg subcutaneously (sc) daily]. BMD increased in the lumbar spine and femoral neck (5.1 $\pm$ 43.1% and 2.4 $\pm$ 3.5%, respectively). Data from a number of other groups have supported these findings (9–12).

The short-term effects of IGF-I have been tested in GHD adults by Bianda et al. (13), who compared the effects of short-term administration of rhIGF-I (5 μg/kg daily in a continuous sc infusion) with those of sc GH (0.03 IU/kg daily). Both hormones stimulated bone formation and resorption, as shown by biochemical serum markers. However, the increase in formation markers was not preceded by an increase in those of resorption with IGF-I treatment. Therefore, they hypothesized that there may be a direct anabolic effect of IGF-I in bone cells *in vivo*. In addition, as has been previously described in healthy humans (14) and GH-resistant states (2,15), they found a direct stimulatory effect of IGF-I on renal 1α-hydroxylation of vitamin D.

GROWTH FACTORS AND OSTEOPOROSIS

Insulin-like Growth Factor-I in Age-related Osteoporosis

The aging process is associated with a decline in trabecular and cortical bone that leads to osteoporotic fractures in both men and women. Cross-sectional studies have shown a parallel decrease in the serum concentrations of IGF-I with aging in different populations (16–21). Although systemic circulating IGF-I levels do not necessarily reflect local concentrations of IGF-I, bone biopsies have shown an age-dependent decline in bone IGF-I content which parallels that seen in circulating IGF-I levels. The magnitude of the decline in bone IGF-I levels differs in individual studies and is likely attributable to differences in technique and population studied. In a cross-sectional study in women and men, Nicolas et al. (22) found a 60% reduction in IGF-I and a 25% reduction in transforming growth factor-β (TGF-β) in cortical bone between the second and sixth decades. Similarly, a decline in both cortical and trabecular bone IGF-I content, more marked for trabecular bone (net loss of 41% of IGF-I for trabecular, 35% for cortical) was described in a postmortem study (23). Seck et al. (24) reported the results of IGF-I and IGF-II concentrations in the bone matrix of 533 human bone biopsies obtained from the iliac crest during surgery for early breast cancer. In addition to the inverse relationship between IGF-I and age, they found a positive correlation between IGF-I matrix content and histomorphometric and biochemical parameters of bone formation and bone resorption, as well as cancellous bone volume. These data suggest that age-associated osteoporosis may be related to the decline in IGF-I with age.

A number of epidemiological studies have shown a correlation between serum IGF-I concentrations and BMD (17–20,25,26) (Fig. 32.2). The results of cross-sectional studies have been consistent with the hypothesis that IGF-I may be a factor determining bone density. However, gender effects remain less certain. Kelly et al. (17) found that IGF-I levels correlated with BMD at the lumbar spine, femoral neck, and distal radius in both pre- and postmenopausal women and that the results were dependent on physical fitness. Langlois et al. (18) studied the association between IGF-I levels and BMD in 682 women and men aged 72 to 94 years. IGF-I levels were positively associated with BMD at three femoral sites (Ward's area, femoral neck, trochanter) at the radius and the lumbar spine only in women after adjusting for other factors such as age, weight loss, physical activity, and protein intake. Barret-Connor et al. (19) studied a group of 483 men and 455 postmenopausal women not receiving estrogen therapy 55 years and older. They found an association between BMD and IGF-I levels in women but not in men after considering a number of confounding factors, including physical activity, smoking, alcohol use, body mass index, age, and diuretic use. The gender-specific relationship of IGF-I levels and BMD differs from that reported in other reports. For example, in the study by Janssen et al. (25) in healthy men and women aged 55 to 80 years, a correlation of IGF-I levels and BMD of the lumbar spine was found in men but not in women. Two other studies with fewer patients (26,27) showed a positive correlation of BMD with IGF-I in men. Therefore, although the gender specificity of the relationship between serum IGF-I levels and bone density remains somewhat controversial, the results of numerous studies provide strong evidence for a role of IGF-I directly or as a marker of other factors important in the maintenance of bone mass.

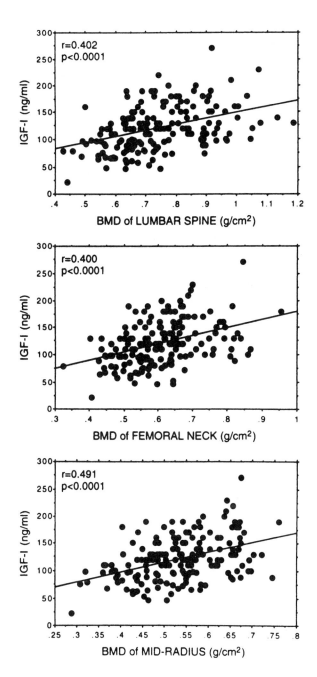

FIG. 32.2. Relationship between serum insulin-like growth factor-I *(IGF-I)* level and bone mineral density *(BMD)* at various sites. (From ref. 20, with permission.)

A more direct experimental approach in the investigation of IGF-I effects on bone has been the administration of IGF-I to humans. A small number of studies have assessed the effect of IGF-I administration on bone metabolism in men and women of different ages receiving different doses of IGF-I. Based on previous animal studies which showed a selective increase in markers of bone formation without an increase in bone resorption after IGF-I administration in rats (28), Ebeling et al. (29) conducted one of the first short-term studies of IGF-I administration in normal human volunteers. Eighteen postmenopausal women received either 30,60,120, or 180 μg/kg daily of IGF-I sc for 6 days. They found significant dose-dependent increases in procollagen I carboxyl-terminal propeptide (PICP), a surrogate marker of bone formation in all four dosage groups. Urinary excretion of pyridinoline (PYR) and deoxypyridinoline (DPYR), both markers of bone resorption, increased significantly only in the two and the three highest dosage groups, respectively. Although side effects were noted in the two highest treatment groups, minimal or no side effects were reported in the lower-dosage groups. Therefore, these data were important in showing that a selective effect on bone formation could be achieved at a low dose without significant side effects. Short-term effects of rhIGF-I in healthy men have been reported by Bianda et al. (14), who administered 8 μg/kg hourly by a continuous sc infusion for 5 days to seven young male subjects and compared its effects to 5 days

of GH (6 U twice daily). Increases in markers of bone turnover were rapidly noted in both groups. In contrast to IGF-I, GH increased renal phosphate absorption as well as serum phosphate. IGF-I increased the free calcitriol index, which is consistent with a direct stimulatory effect on 25-OHD-1α-hydroxylase. Supporting the concept of a dose-dependent effect of rhIGF-I on bone turnover, Ghiron et al. (30) conducted a study comparing IGF-I to GH in 16 healthy elderly women who were divided into three treatment groups. Five women received rhIGF-I 60 μg/kg, five received rhIGF-I 15 μg/kg twice daily, and six women received GH 25 μg/kg daily for 28 days. GH and high-dose IGF-I caused a progressive increase in both markers of bone formation and resorption, whereas low-dose IGF-I showed an increase in markers of bone formation without increases in those of bone resorption (Fig. 32.3). The uncoupled bone

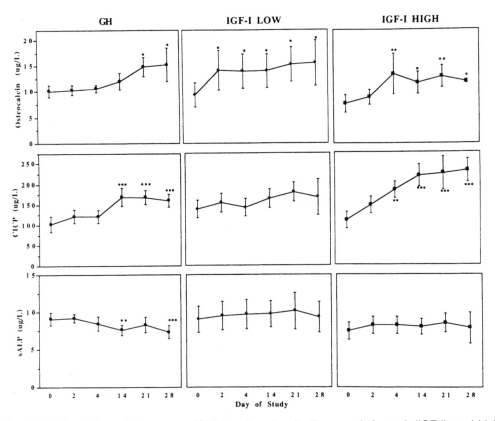

FIG. 32.3. Effect of growth hormone *(GH)* low-dose insulin-like growth factor-I *(IGF-I),* and high-dose *IGF-I* on markers of bone formation. *$p < 0.05$, **$p < 0.01$, ***$p < 0.001$ versus baseline. (From ref. 30, with permission.)

formation was an important observation suggesting a rationale for the use of IGF-I in states of reduced bone mass, especially those with reduced bone formation. The unique dose-dependent effect of rhIGF-I to stimulate bone turnover is of potential relevance. Of note as well is that, based on these data, the dose required for this effect is unassociated with clinically important side effects.

In conclusion, short-term administration of IGF-I has been shown to stimulate bone formation and, depending on dose and mode of administration, both formation and resorption. Long-term studies are necessary to assess the long-term effects of IGF-I administration in increasing bone formation and bone density in osteopenic patients.

Insulin-like Growth Factor-I in Idiopathic Osteoporosis

Idiopathic osteoporosis encompasses all forms of decreased bone mass without an identifiable underlying cause of bone loss and affects both men and women. It typically presents with spontaneous fractures, and several studies have shown a reduction in plasma levels of IGF-I in this condition. Ljunghall et al. (31) studied 12 men with symptomatic idiopathic osteoporosis and found lower plasma IGF-I concentrations in patients than in controls. IGF-I levels also correlated with BMD of the spine and the forearm in the whole group independently of age and weight. Studies of GH secretion with 24-hour sampling and stimulation tests ruled out subclinical GHD in these patients, supporting the concept that both systemic and locally produced IGF-I may have a role in the pathogenesis of this disease. Similarly, in a study by Reed et al. (32), IGF-I serum concentrations were reported to be lower in men and women with idiopathic osteoporosis than in controls. Studies of bone biopsies in these patients showed a significant correlation between serum IGF-I levels and osteoblastic surface, mineralization, and bone formation rate. Kurland et al. (33) also confirmed the reduced IGF-I levels (Fig. 32.4) and reduced histomorphometric parameters of bone formation in a group of 24 men with idiopathic

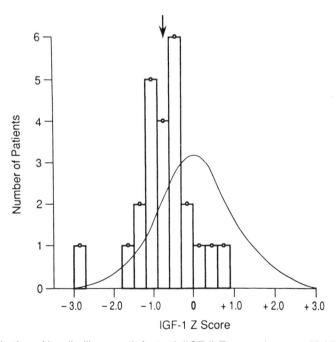

FIG. 32.4. Distribution of insulin-like growth factor-I *(IGF-I) Z* scores in men with idiopathic osteoporosis. The graph shows that the mean *Z* score, -0.75, is significantly lower ($p + 0.0002$) than the theoretical Gaussian distribution of the normal population (mean $Z = 0$). (From ref. 33, with permission.)

osteoporosis. Therefore, using published norma- tive control data, these studies suggest, but do not prove, an etiological role for IGF-I in this disease.

Based on these data, Johansson et al. (34) per- formed a randomized double-blind crossover trial in 12 patients with idiopathic osteoporosis (32 to 57 years of age), who received daily sc injections of rhIGF-I (80 μg/kg) or GH (2 IU/m^2) for 7 days. Serum levels of IGF-I in- creased during both treatments but more mark- edly with GH (171% vs. 119%). In both groups, the relatively high IGF-I levels and the high inci- dence of side effects suggested that the adminis- tered doses were too high. There was an increase in surrogate markers of bone formation (osteo- calcin and PICP) and resorption (DPYR) during administration of both GH and IGF-I compara- ble to previous studies using higher IGF-I doses. Comparison of the treatments suggested that IGF-I enhanced formation of collagen type I more than GH did, but again, there were proba- bly dose-dependent differences.

In summary, the data available are insufficient to define the precise role of IGF-I in the treat- ment of idiopathic osteoporosis, but the studies point to a promising effect of IGF-I in increasing bone turnover in this condition.

Growth Factors in Estrogen-related Bone Loss

Loss of gonadal function, in both men and women, is associated with an increase in bone turnover, with bone resorption exceeding bone formation and ultimately leading to bone loss. Local factors including cytokines such as in- terleukin-6 (IL-6), IL-1, and tumor necrosis fac- tor-α (TNF-α) have been implicated in this pro- cess (35–37). However, growth factors such as IGF-I and TGF-β may also play roles in the pathogenesis of estrogen-related bone loss (38–41).

Experiments in rats have shown a beneficial effect of systemic rhIGF-I and combined rhIGF- I and IGFBP-3 in increasing bone formation after ovariectomy-induced bone loss (42–44). Short-term trials of rhIGF-I in late postmeno- pause have shown a dose-dependent stimulation in bone formation as assessed by biochemical

markers with dose-differential effects in bone re- sorption [(29,30), discussed above]. Further stud- ies in humans are warranted to assess the potential benefits of IGF-I or the combination of IGF-I and IGFBP-3 in estrogen-related bone loss.

Intermittently administered PTH has been one of the few treatments capable of increasing bone formation and BMD in estrogen-related bone loss. The effects of intermittent PTH are thought to be mediated by local production of IGF-I and TGF-β (45,46). Finkelstein et al. (47) adminis- tered PTH (sc 40 μg daily) to women receiving gonadotropin-releasing hormone (GnRH) ana- logue therapy for endometriosis. The use of in- termittent PTH prevented the decrease in BMD at the lumbar spine seen with the analogue treat- ment alone. Lindsay et al. (48) studied the ef- fects of the 1–34 amino-terminal fragment of human PTH (25 μg daily sc) in 17 postmenopau- sal women with osteoporosis taking hormone- replacement therapy and controls. They found a 13% increase in vertebral BMD, a 2.7% increase at the hip, and an 8% increase in total body bone mineral at the end of 3 years in the group of women taking PTH. Moreover, this was associ- ated with a reduction in vertebral fractures. PTH-related protein (PTHrP) acts through the PTH receptor and in rats increases bone mineral content when administered sc. Plotkin et al. (49) tested the effects of PTHrP-(1–36) (1.64, 3.28, or 6.56 μg/kg as a single sc daily dose for 14 days) in 13 postmenopausal women (mean age 58 years). Formation markers increased, whereas resorption markers (N-telopeptide and DPYR) significantly decreased in the highest- dose group. This unique action of PTHrP makes it an interesting tool in the investigation of the accelerated bone resorption seen in postmeno- pausal women.

In conclusion, intermittent PTH seems to in- crease BMD and to reduce fracture rates in post- menopausal women. More data are needed to define the role of rhIGF-I and PTHrP-(1–36) in the treatment of this condition.

Insulin-like Growth Factor-I in Osteopenic Women with Anorexia Nervosa

Anorexia nervosa is associated with severe osteopenia and increased bone resorption (50,

51). It represents an increasing problem in adolescents, affecting the achievement of peak bone mass and leading to profound and often irreversible osteopenia in adulthood. Estrogen therapy alone in this group of patients cannot prevent the accelerated bone loss (52), suggesting that additional factors are involved in the pathogenesis of the osteoporosis seen in these patients. Nutritional factors likely play a critical role, and IGF-I may be implicated given the decline in IGF-I levels seen in undernutrition. Grinspoon et al. (53) studied the role of IGF-I treatment in an experimental model of IGF-I deficiency. Decreased bone turnover markers as well as IGF-I levels were found in a group of 14 normal women after 4 days of fasting. Pa-

tients were randomly assigned to receive either IGF-I (100 μg/kg daily) or placebo during 6 days while they continued fasting; IGF-I administration increased bone formation markers (Fig. 32.5). These data suggested a role for IGF-I treatment in pathological states of undernutrition. Based on these previous results, they conducted a study in 23 women (aged 18 to 29 years) with anorexia nervosa who received placebo or IGF-I in two different doses (30 or 100 μg/kg sc twice daily for 6 days) (51). The group receiving the higher dose of IGF-I showed an increase in both markers of bone formation (osteocalcin and PICP) and resorption (PYR and DPYR), but the lower-dosage group showed increases only in markers of bone formation

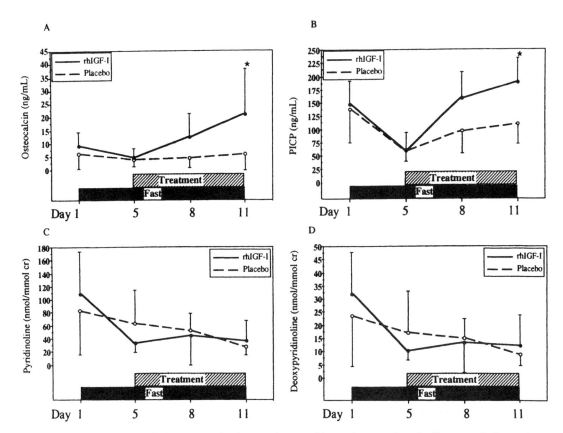

FIG. 32.5. The effects of short-term fasting and recombinant human insulin-like growth factor-I *(rhIGF-I)* administration on biochemical indices of bone turnover. **A:** Serum levels of osteocalcin at baseline and days 5,8, and 11 of the study. **B:** Serum levels of procollagen I carboxyl-terminal propeptide *(PICP)* at baseline and days 5, 8, and 11 of the study. **C:** Urinary excretion of pyridinoline at baseline and days 5, 8, and 11 of the study. Error bars represent mean $\pm$ 1 SD. *$p < 0.05$ versus placebo by the Mann-Whitney test. (From ref. 53, with permission.)

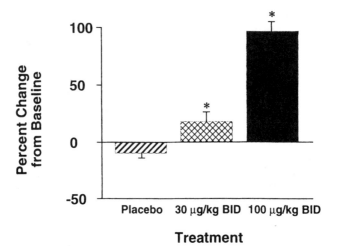

Treatment

FIG. 32.6. Percent change in procollagen I carboxyl-terminal propeptide *(PICP)* from baseline by treatment group. Error bars represent the mean $\pm$ SEM. *$p < 0.05$ versus placebo by analysis of variance. (From ref. 51, with permission.)

(Fig. 32.6). In summary, short-term administration of IGF-I has been demonstrated to increase bone formation in patients with anorexia nervosa but more data are needed to assess the long-term effects and the effects of IGF-I on bone density in this group of patients.

GROWTH FACTORS IN BONE HEALING AND REPAIR

Pseudoathrosis secondary to impaired bone healing, the need of extensive bone grafts in bone tumor surgery, and loosening of endoprotheses are problems in orthopedics. Bone reconstruction or the radiation-induced impairment of bone repair are important aspects in plastic reconstructive surgery. The mitogenic and angiogenic properties of different growth factors as well as their effects in the differentiation of mesenchymal stem cells into chondroblastic and osteoblastic cell lineages have raised interest in the potential use of these factors in the stimulation of bone formation and bone healing.

Although no human studies are available, the effects of different growth factors have been assessed in a number of different animal models of fracture healing. Bone morphogenetic proteins (BMPs), with their differentiating properties,

have been shown to be potent stimulators of bone formation in different models of bone healing in rats, rabbits, sheep, monkeys, and pigs (54–59), although they need a carrier in order to be effective at low doses. BMPs have also been useful in cartilage repair in rabbits (60) and in a model of radiation impairment of bone healing (61). TGF-β and fibroblast growth factor (FGF) are mitogens for bone cells, and FGF also has angiogenic properties. They stimulate bone formation in different animal models of bone healing (62–64). Less successful has been the use of IGF-I in studies of bone repair (65,66), although positive results have been reported by some investigators (67).

In summary, more needs to be done to determine the exact role of the use of growth factors in human bone healing and repair, but this represents a novel therapeutic future strategy in this field with promising results in animal studies.

SUMMARY AND FUTURE PERSPECTIVES

Bone growth factors, because of their effects on proliferation and differentiation of bone cells and on bone matrix formation, are promising tools in the treatment of osteoporosis and bone repair. The effects of growth factors have been assessed in different *in vitro* and *in vivo* models, but limited studies in humans have been performed to determine their exact role in the treatment of disease states. To date, IGF-I has been shown to be useful in the treatment of GHIS. Its effects in increasing bone formation uncoupled to bone resorption have been assessed in short-term studies in humans, suggesting the rationale for long-term clinical trials of IGF-I in the treatment of different conditions associated with osteoporosis (68). IGF-I has been implicated in the pathogenesis of glucocorticoid-induced osteoporosis, representing an interesting theoretical strategy in the treatment of this condition, especially in children in whom glucocorticoid effects on linear growth and bone mass are observed. Although no human studies are available, TGF-β is a potent mitogen *in vitro* and has been shown to stimulate bone formation in animal models (69). Bone content of TGF-β has also been found to decrease with age in biopsy studies and has been associated with histomorphometric and serum parameters of bone formation and resorption (22,70), suggesting a possible role in the future treatment of bone loss states. BMPs, FGF, and TGF-β could have roles in bone healing and repair, but human studies need to be done to define the precise role of these factors in clinical disease states.

In conclusion, local growth factors are critical for bone remodeling and repair and represent a possibly useful tool in the treatment of different bone disease states. Clinical research studies are needed to assess the exact role of both endocrine and autocrine/paracrine effects of growth factors on bone physiology.

ACKNOWLEDGMENTS

This work was supported by National Institutes of Health grants ROI-DK 52625 and MOI-RR-01066. Gemma Sesmilo is a recipient of the "Fundacio La Caixa" Fellowship.

REFERENCES

1. Ranke MB, Savage MO, Chatelain PG, et al. Insulin-like growth factor I improves height in growth hormone insensitivity: two years' results. *Horm Res* 1995;44:253–264.
2. Backeljauw PF, Underwood LE, GHIS Collaborative Group. Prolonged treatment with recombinant insulin-like growth factor-I in children with growth hormone insensitivity syndrome—a Clinical Research Center study. *J Clin Endocrinol Metab* 1996;81:3312–3317.
3. Laron Z, Anin S, Klipper-Aurbach Y, et al. Effects of insulin-like growth factor on linear growth, head circumference, and body fat in patients with Laron-type dwarfism. *Lancet* 1992;339:1258–1261.
4. Guevara-Aguirre J, Rosenbloom AL, Vasconez O, et al. Two-year treatment of growth hormone (GH) receptor deficiency with recombinant insulin-like growth factor I in 22 children: comparison of two dosage levels and to GH-treated GH deficiency. *J Clin Endocrinol Metab* 1997;82:629–633.
5. Klinger B, Laron Z. Three year IGF-I treatment of children with Laron syndrome. *J Pediatr Endocrinol Metab* 1995;8:149–158.
6. Bachrach LK, Marcus R, Ott SM, et al. Bone mineral, histomorphometry, and body composition in adults with growth hormone receptor deficiency. *J Bone Miner Res* 1998;13:415–421.
7. Johansson AG, Burman P, Westermark K, et al. The bone mineral density in acquired growth hormone deficiency correlates with circulating levels of insulin-like growth factor I. *J Intern Med* 1992;232:447–452.
8. Baum HBA, Biller BMK, Finkelstein JS, et al. Effects of physiologic growth hormone therapy on bone density and body composition in patients with adult-onset growth hormone deficiency. *Ann Intern Med* 1996;125:883–890.
9. Johannsson G, Rosen T, Bosaeus I, et al. Two years of growth hormone (GH) treatment increases bone mineral content and density in hypopituitary patients with adult-onset GH deficiency. *J Clin Endocrinol Metab* 1996;81:2865–2873.
10. Janssen YJH, Hamdy NAT, Frolich M, et al. Skeletal effects of two years of treatment with low physiological doses of recombinant human growth hormone (GH) in patients with adult-onset GH deficiency. *J Clin Endocrinol Metab* 1998;83:2143–2148.
11. Finkenstedt GF, Gasser RW, Hofle G, et al. Effects of growth hormone (GH) replacement on bone metabolism and mineral density in adult onset of GH deficiency: results of a double-blind placebo-controlled study with open follow-up. *Eur J Endocrinol* 1997;136:282–289.
12. Rahim A, Holmes SJ, Adams JE, et al. Long-term change in the bone mineral density of adults with adult onset growth hormone (GH) deficiency in response to short or long-term GH replacement therapy. *Clin Endocrinol (Oxf)* 1998;48:463–469.
13. Bianda T, Glatz Y, Bouillon R, et al. Effects of short-term insulin-like growth factor-I (IGF-I) or growth hormone (GH) treatment on bone metabolism and on production of 1,25-dihydroxycholecalciferol in GH-deficient adults. *J Clin Endocrinol Metab* 1998;83:81–87.
14. Bianda T, Hussain MA, Glatz Y, et al. Effects of short-term insulin-like growth factor-I on growth hormone treatment on bone turnover, renal phosphate reabsorption and 1,25 dihydroxyvitamin D$_3$ production in healthy man. *J Intern Med* 1997;241:143–150.
15. Vaccarello MA, Diamond FB Jr, Guevara-Aguirre J, et al. Hormonal and metabolic effects and pharmacokinetics of recombinant insulin-like growth factor-I in

growth hormone receptor deficiency/Laron syndrome. *J Clin Endocrinol Metab* 1993;77:273–280.

16. Clemmons DR, Van Wyk JJ. Factors controlling blood concentration of somatomedin C. *Clin Endocrinol Metab* 1984;13:113–143.

17. Kelly PJ, Eisman JA, Stuart MC, et al. Somatomedin-C, physical fitness, and bone density. *J Clin Endocrinol Metab* 1990;70:718–723.

18. Langlois JA, Rosen CJ, Visser M, et al. Association between insulin-like growth factor I and bone mineral density in older women and men: the Framingham Heart Study. *J Clin Endocrinol Metab* 1998;83:4257–4262.

19. Barret-Connor E, Goodman-Gruen D. Gender differences in insulin-like growth factor and bone mineral density association in old age: the Rancho Bernardo Study. *J Bone Miner Res* 1998;13:1343–1349.

20. Sugimoto T, Nishiyama K, Kuribayashi F, et al. Serum levels of insulin-like growth factor (IGF) I, IGF-binding protein (IGFBP)-2 and IGFBP-3 in osteoporotic patients with and without spinal fractures. *J Bone Miner Res* 1997;12:1272–1279.

21. Bennet AE, Wahner HW, Riggs BL, et al. Insulin-like growth factors I and II: aging and bone density in women. *J Clin Endocrinol Metab* 1984;59:701–704.

22. Nicolas V, Prewett A, Bettica P, et al. Age-related decreases in insulin-like growth factor-I and transforming growth factor-beta in femoral cortical bone from both men and women: implications for bone loss with aging. *J Clin Endocrinol Metab* 1994;78:1011–1016.

23. Boonen S, Aerssens J, Dequeker J, et al. Age-associated decline in human femoral neck cortical and trabecular content of insulin-like growth factor-I: potential implications for age-related (type II) osteoporotic fracture occurrence. *Calcif Tissue Int* 1997;61:173–178.

24. Seck T, Scheppach B, Scharla S, et al. Concentration of insulin-like growth factor (IGF)-I and II in iliac crest bone matrix from pre- and postmenopausal women: relationship to age, menopause, bone turnover, bone volume, and circulating IGFs. *J Clin Endocrinol Metab* 1998;83:2331–2337.

25. Janssen JAMJL, Burger H, Stolk RP, et al. Gender-specific relationship between serum free and total IGF-I and bone mineral density in elderly men and women. *Eur J Endocrinol* 1998;138:627–632.

26. Fall C, Hindmarsh P, Dennison E, et al. Programming of growth hormone secretion and bone mineral density in elderly men: a hypothesis. *J Clin Endocrinol Metab* 1998;83:135–139.

27. Johansson AG, Forslund A, Hambraeus L, et al. Growth hormone–dependent insulin-like growth factor binding protein is a major determinant of bone mineral density in healthy men. *J Bone Miner Res* 1994;9:915–921.

28. Spencer EM, Liu CC, Si ECC, et al. *In vivo* actions of insulin-like growth factor-I (IGF-I) on bone formation and resorption in rats. *Bone* 1991;12:21–26.

29. Ebeling PR, Jone JD, O'Fallon WM, et al. Short-term effects of recombinant human insulin-like growth factor I on bone turnover in normal women. *J Clin Endocrinol Metab* 1993;77:1384–1387.

30. Ghiron LJ, Thompson JL, Holloway L, et al. Effects of recombinant human insulin-like growth factor-I and growth hormone on bone turnover in elderly women. *J Bone Miner Res* 1995;10:1844–1852.

31. Ljunghall S, Johansson AG, Burman P, et al. Low plasma insulin-like growth factor 1(IGF-1) in male pa-

tients with idiopathic osteoporosis. *J Intern Med* 1992; 232:59–64.

32. Reed BY, Zerwekh JE, Sakhaee K, et al. Serum IGF 1 is low and correlated with osteoblastic surface in idiopathic osteoporosis. *J Bone Miner Res* 1995;10: 1218–1224.

33. Kurland ES, Rosen CJ, Cosman F, et al. Insulin-like growth factor-I in men with idiopathic osteoporosis. *J Clin Endocrinol Metab* 1997;82:2799–2805.

34. Johansson AG, Lindh E, Blum WF, et al. Effects of growth hormone and insulin-like growth factor I in men with idiopathic osteoporosis. *J Clin Endocrinol Metab* 1996;81:44–48.

35. Manolagas SC, Jilka RL. Bone marrow, cytokines, and bone remodeling. *N Engl J Med* 1995;332:305–311.

36. Kimble RB, Vannice JL, Bloedow DC, et al. Interleukin-1 receptor antagonist decreases bone loss and bone resorption in ovariectomized rats. *J Clin Invest* 1994;93: 1959–1967.

37. Kimble RB, Matayoshi AB, Vannice JL, et al. Simultaneous block of interleukin-1 and tumor necrosis factor is required to completely prevent bone loss in the early postovariectomy period. *Endocrinology* 1995;136: 3054–3061.

38. Yokose S, Ishizuya T, Ikeda T, et al. An estrogen deficiency caused by ovariectomy increases plasma levels of systemic factors that stimulate proliferation and differentiation of osteoblasts in rats. *Endocrinology* 1996; 137:469–478.

39. Raisz LG. Estrogen and bone: new pieces to the puzzle. *Nat Med* 1996;2:1077–1078.

40. Hughes DE, Dai A, Tiffee JC, et al. Estrogen promotes apoptosis of murine osteoclasts mediated by TGF-β. *Nat Med* 1996;2:1132–1136.

41. Finkelman RD, Bell NH, Strong DD, et al. Ovariectomy selectively reduces the concentration of transforming growth factor β in rat bone: implications for estrogen deficiency–associated bone loss. *Proc Natl Acad Sci USA* 1992;89:12190–12193.

42. Bagi CM, Brommage R, Deleon L, et al. Benefit of systemically administered rhIGF-I and rhIGF-I/IGFBP-3 on cancellous bone in overiectomized rats. *J Bone Miner Res* 1994;9:1301–1312.

43. Verhaeghe J, Van Bree R, Van Herck E, et al. Effects of recombinant human growth hormone and insulin-like growth factor-1, with or without 17 β-estradiol, on bone and mineral homeostasis of aged ovariectomized rats. *J Bone Miner Res* 1996;11:1723–1735.

44. Narusawa K, Nakamura T, Suzuki K, et al. The effects of recombinant human insulin-like growth factor (rhIGF)-1 and rhIGF-1/IGF binding protein-3 administration on rat osteopenia induced by ovariectomy with concomitant bilateral sciatic neurectomy. *J Bone Miner Res* 1995;10:1853–1864.

45. Canalis E, Centrella M, Burch W, et al. Insulin-like growth factor I mediates selective anabolic effects of parathyroid hormone in bone cultures. *J Clin Invest* 1989;83:60–65.

46. Pfeilschifter J, Laukhuf F, Muller-Beckman B, et al. Parathyroid hormone increases the concentration of insulin-like growth factor I and transforming growth factor beta in rat bone. *J Clin Invest* 1995;96:767–774.

47. Finkelstein JS, Klibanski A, Schaefer EH, et al. Parathyroid hormone for the prevention of bone loss induced

by estrogen deficiency. *N Engl J Med* 1994;331: 1618–1623.

48. Lindsay R, Nieves J, Formica C, et al. Randomized controlled study of effect of parathyroid hormone on vertebral-bone mass and fracture incidence among postmenopausal women on oestrogen with osteoporosis. *Lancet* 1997;350:550–555.

49. Plotkin H, Gundberg C, Mitnick M, et al. Dissociation of bone formation from resorption during 2-week treatment with human parathyroid hormone–related peptide-(1–36) in humans: potential as an anabolic therapy for osteoporosis. *J Clin Endocrinol Metab* 1998;83: 2786–2791.

50. Biller BMK, Saxe V, Herzog DB, et al. Mechanisms of osteoporosis in adult and adolescent women with anorexia nervosa. *J Clin Endocrinol Metab* 1989;68: 548–554.

51. Grinspoon SK, Baum HBA, Lee K, et al. Effects of short-term recombinant human insulin-like growth factor I administration on bone turnover in osteopenic women with anorexia nervosa. *J Clin Endocrinol Metab* 1996;81:3864–3870.

52. Klibanski A, Biller BMK, Schoenfeld DA, et al. The effects of estrogen administration on trabecular bone loss in young women with anorexia nervosa. *J Clin Endocrinol Metab* 1995;80:898–903.

53. Grinspoon SK, Baum HBA, Peterson S, et al. Effects of rhIGF-I administration on bone turnover during short-term fasting. *J Clin Invest* 1995;96:900–906.

54. Bostrom M, Lane JM, Tomin E, et al. Use of bone morphogenetic protein-2 in the rabbit ulnar nonunion model. *Clin Orthop* 1996;327:272–282.

55. Gerhart TN, Kirker-Head CA, Kriz MJ, et al. Healing segmental femoral defects in sheep using recombinant human bone morphogenetic protein. *Clin Orthop* 1993; 293:317–326.

56. Lindholm TC, Lindholm TS, Marttinen A, et al. Bovine bone morphogenetic protein (bBMP/NCP)-induced repair of skull trephine defects in pigs. *Clin Orthop* 1994; 301:263–270.

57. Lind M. Growth factors: possible new clinical tools. *Acta Orthop Scand* 1996;67:407–417.

58. Cook SD, Baffes GC, Wolfe MW, et al. Recombinant human bone morphogenetic protein-7 induces healing in a canine long-bone segmental defect model. *Clin Orthop* 1994;301:302–312.

59. Wozney JM, Rosen V. Bone morphogenetic protein and bone morphogenetic protein gene family in bone formation and repair. *Clin Orthop* 1998;346:26–37.

60. Sellers RS, Peluso D, Morris EA. The effects of recombinant human bone morphogenetic protein-2 (rhBMP-2) on the healing of full-thickness defects of articular cartilage. *J Bone Joint Surg Am* 1997;79:1452–1463.

61. Wurzler KK, Deweese TL, Sebald W, et al. Radiation-induced impairment of bone healing can be overcome by recombinant human bone morphogenetic protein-2. *J Craniofac Surg* 1998;9:131–137.

62. Noda M, Camilliere JJ. *In vivo* stimulation of bone formation by transforming growth factor β. *Endocrinology* 1989;124:2991–2994.

63. Varghese S, Ramsby ML, Jeffrey JJ, et al. Basic fibroblast growth factor stimulates expression of interstitial collagenase and inhibitors of metalloproteinases in rat bone cells. *Endocrinology* 1995;136:2156–2162.

64. Sumner DR, Turner TM, Purchio AF, et al. Enhancement of bone ingrowth by transforming growth factor-β. *J Bone Joint Surg Am* 1995;77-A:1135–1147.

65. Kirkeby OJ, Ekeland A. No effect of systemic administration of somatomedin C on bone repair in rats. *Acta Orthop Scand* 1990;61:335–338.

66. Kirkeby OJ, Ekeland A. No effect of local somatomedin C on bone repair. *Acta Orthop Scand* 1992;63:447–450.

67. Kobayashi K, Agrawal K, Jackson IT, et al. The effect of insulin-like growth factor 1 on craniofacial bone healing. *Plast Reconstr Surg* 1996;97:1129–1135.

68. Olbricht T, Benker G. Glucocorticoid-induced osteoporosis: pathogenesis, prevention and treatment, with special regard to the rheumatic disease. *J Intern Med* 1993; 234:237–244.

69. Rosen D, Miller S, Deleon E, et al. Systemic administration of recombinant transforming growth factor-β₂ stimulates parameters of cancellous bone formation in juvenile and adult rats. *Bone* 1994;15:355–358.

70. Pfeilschifter J, Diel I, Scheppach B, et al. Concentration of transforming growth factor beta in human bone tissue: relationship to age, menopause, bone turnover and bone volume. *J Bone Miner Res* 1998;13:716–730.

Skeletal Growth Factors,
edited by Ernesto Canalis.
Lippincott Williams & Wilkins, Philadelphia, © 2000.

33

Use of Growth Factors for Osteoporotic Therapy

Gideon A. Rodan

*Department of Bone Biology and Osteoporosis, Merck Research Laboratories,
West Point, Pennsylvania 19486*

This chapter discusses the potential use of growth factors as bone-forming agents for the treatment of osteoporosis. It starts by discussing the current concepts on the remodeling imbalance which leads to bone loss, the possible role of apoptosis in bone formation, the limitations of current osteoporotic therapies, the potential risk associated with mitogenic agents and increased bone turnover, and the logistical challenges faced in the development of bone-forming agents and concludes with a brief discussion of known growth factors as potential therapeutic agents.

IMBALANCE BETWEEN BONE RESORPTION AND BONE FORMATION

Osteoporosis is defined as a reduction in bone mass and microstructural deterioration that increases the risk of bone fractures. The bone loss that leads to osteoporosis results from an imbalance between osteoclastic bone resorption and osteoblastic bone formation. This bone loss is rapidly accelerated after menopause, when estrogen deficiency causes an increase in osteoclast number. Early postmenopausal women can lose up to 3% to 4% of spine bone mineral density (BMD) per year. This bone loss substantially increases the risk of fractures, which doubles for each 10% loss in BMD. The increased rate of bone resorption (destruction) is associated with an increase in bone formation, relative to premenopausal women, resulting in an overall increase in bone turnover. However, although bone formation may increase by as much as threefold, when estimated by biochemical markers, such as bone-specific alkaline phosphatase or osteocalcin (1), it does not fully compensate for the increase in bone resorption. The reason for this imbalance is not clear and is briefly discussed following.

The reason for persistent bone remodeling throughout life is inherent in the functions of bone. To release calcium from the skeleton and optimize skeletal structure for mechanical function, about 2 million packets of bone are being removed by osteoclastic bone resorption and replaced by osteoblastic bone formation in the skeleton at any given time (2). Resorption of a packet lasts about 3 weeks, while its rebuilding takes 3 to 4 months. Under physiological conditions, the bone removed is on average fully replaced and bone balance or bone homeostasis is maintained. The reason for disturbance of this balance in osteoporosis and the potential role of growth factors in the imbalance is not known.

It has been suggested that the amount of bone at a specific skeletal site is determined by the mechanical loads exerted on that bone, decreased load or mechanical usage promoting bone resorption and reducing bone formation, while increased loads have the opposite effect, i.e., more formation and less resorption. It was further suggested that estrogen may influence the ''set point'' level at which this homeostasis is maintained (3). The molecular basis for the change in set point, if it indeed exists, is not known. If it is mediated by the abundance of a growth factor, administration of such factors as replacement therapy could provide effective treatment. In the uterus and in isolated bone cells, estrogen stimulates insulin-like growth factor-I (IGF-I) expression, and high doses of estrogen were shown to stimulate bone formation *in vivo* in rodents. However, at this time, there is not sufficient evidence of anabolic effects of estrogen on bone in humans (4).

Another hypothesis for maintaining bone balance is based on the "coupling" phenomenon, whereby bone destruction releases growth factors which recruit and stimulate the bone-forming osteoblasts. Transforming growth factor-β (TGF-β) and IGF-II have been suggested to play such a role (5,6). If these growth factors indeed participate in maintaining bone balance, there is no compelling evidence so far that their release is locally reduced in estrogen deficiency.

A third simple possibility is that in the face of increased bone resorption, bone formation, a much slower process, cannot effectively replace the lost bone, even when proceeding at maximal efficiency (7). If this were the case, attempts to further stimulate bone formation with exogenous growth factors, especially during the early postmenopausal period, may not be successful unless bone resorption is inhibited at the same time. It is therefore likely and probably advisable that if and when bone-forming treatments become available, they will be given in conjunction with bone-resorption inhibitors.

To summarize this section, the mechanism for maintaining bone balance under healthy conditions is not understood at the molecular level. We know that mechanical forces play a role since immobilization causes bone loss; however, we do not know if the deficiency of a particular local growth factor is involved in this process. In effect, we assume that certain growth factors participate in the normal bone formation which is part of bone remodeling. However, there is no direct *in vivo* evidence supporting this assumption, and the role of specific growth factors in this process remains unknown.

ROLE OF APOPTOSIS IN THE CONTROL OF BONE FORMATION

Recent studies which examined the mechanism for prostaglandin (PGE) and parathyroid hormone (PTH) stimulation of bone formation *in vivo* and their inhibition by glucocorticoids pointed to the control of osteoblast apoptosis as a possible regulatory mechanism. Accordingly, the rate of bone formation, which is related to the number of osteoblasts on the bone surface, is not determined by the birth rate of bone-forming cells but by their survival.

For PGE, a potent stimulator of bone formation in all species examined including humans, the hypothesis is based on the fact that the bone-forming PGE_1 and PGE_2, while increasing cyclic adenosine monophosphate (cAMP) accumulation in osteoblastic cells *in vitro*, are not strongly mitogenic, whereas $PGF_{2\alpha}$, which is mitogenic *in vitro*, does not stimulate bone formation *in vivo*. Experiments on periosteum-derived cells showed that PGE, acting via cAMP, suppresses apoptosis by stimulating sphingosine-1-kinase and increasing the level of sphingosine-1-phosphate (8).

In the case of PTH, a potent bone anabolic agent, which incidentally also stimulates cAMP in osteoblast lineage cells, stimulation of bone formation was not accompanied by evidence for increased osteoblast mitogenesis *in vivo* (9). Recent data show that PTH also suppresses apoptosis in osteoblastic cells (10).

Glucocorticoids, known for a long time to suppress the rate of bone formation in humans, were shown to increase the rate of apoptosis in osteoblastic cells (11).

Taken together, these observations support the hypothesis that increased bone formation is the result of a decrease in osteoblast apoptosis. Since the rate of bone formation was shown by histomorphometric studies to be directly related to the number of osteoblasts on the bone surface, rather than the output of individual osteoblasts, it was assumed that bone formation–promoting agents stimulate the proliferation, differentiation, and recruitment to the bone surface of osteoprogenitor cells. The alternative possibility is that the increase in osteoblast number is the result of suppression of apoptosis in osteoblasts or osteoblast precursors, which would translate into an increase in the number of differentiating osteoblasts and/or extension of the osteoblast life span. More extensive data, primarily from *in vivo* experiments, are needed to test this hypothesis. Of interest, in the context of this volume, is the fact that a major action of growth factors is suppression of apoptosis, usually mediated by stimulation of mitogen-activated protein kinases (MAPKs).

ADVANTAGES AND LIMITATIONS OF CURRENT THERAPIES FOR OSTEOPOROSIS

As mentioned preceding, in the majority of cases, osteoporosis is associated with increased bone resorption and high turnover, which is most pronounced in the early postmenopausal years. Moreover, bone resorption markers were shown to be elevated in most osteoporotic women, regardless of age (1). Inhibition of bone resorption is therefore first-line therapy for osteoporotic patients.

The therapies approved in the United States are inhibitors of bone resorption and include estrogen, available in several forms, the most widely used being Premarin, conjugated equine estrogen; the bisphosphonate alendronate, approved for the prevention and treatment of osteoporosis and the treatment of glucocorticoid-induced osteoporosis; and calcitonin, available as an intranasal preparation of 200 IU.

In many countries, etidronate is approved for cyclical treatment, 2 weeks of 400 mg/day at 13-week intervals. Other bisphosphonates, such as clodronate, are approved in specific countries, e.g., Italy and Finland. Fluoride has been used in the past but is not approved in North America and, due to its safety and efficacy profile (see below), has very limited use today in the United States. However, it is still used in Europe, Germany for example, although such use is in decline. Additional medicines approved and used outside the United States include anabolic androgenic agents, such as durabolin; tibolone, a synthetic compound which has mixed estrogenic, progestogenic, and androgenic activity; and norethisterone, a progestogen with some androgenic activity, used in Europe in hormone-replacement therapy instead of the medroxyprogesterone used in the United States. This compound is currently in clinical development in the United States. Ipriflavone, a flavonoid, is approved in many countries. Several forms of vitamin D are approved for osteoporosis in a limited number of countries, e.g., calcitriol in Australia and 1α-calcidiol in Japan. In addition, a plethora of calcium medications are prescribed or purchased over the counter. This list is not exhaustive and is presented here only to illustrate the diversity of treatments used for osteoporosis.

Based on their effect on remodeling, therapies either inhibit bone resorption or stimulate bone formation. Most osteoporotic therapies are inhibitors of bone resorption and reduce bone turnover. This includes estrogens, bisphosphonates, calcitonin, and probably flavonoids, which have some estrogenic activity, as well as calcium and vitamin D.

The efficacy of these therapies varies widely. Estrogen is generally considered first-line therapy for osteoporosis, especially during the early postmenopausal period, since epidemiological studies suggest that current or long-term estrogen therapy (over 8 years) reduces the incidence of fractures, including hip fractures (12,13). So far, no large randomized, double-blind, placebo-controlled study has shown that estrogen reduces fracture risk. Such a study is currently in progress. Interestingly, a large placebo-controlled study, conducted to evaluate the efficacy of estrogen in secondary prevention of cardiovascular disease, evaluated effects on fractures as a secondary endpoint and found no differences between estrogen- and placebo-treated women (14). These negative results were attributed to the fact that this patient population was not at high risk for fractures or that the duration of treatment (4 years) and the average age of the patients were not optimal for showing estrogen efficacy against fractures.

Raloxifene, a selective estrogen receptor modulator, inhibits bone resorption in women at the administered dose of 60 mg per day by only half as much as 0.625 mg of Premarin, produces smaller increases in bone mass, and was shown to reduce morphometric fractures (diagnosed by lateral x-rays regardless of patient symptoms) by 37% to 44% but did not significantly reduce symptomatic fractures (15,16). No fracture data have been reported so far for flavonoids. Percutaneous estrogen (17) was shown in a relatively small study to reduce the number of morphometric vertebral fractures but not significantly the number of patients with fractures.

Bisphosphonates have the best documented efficacy for fracture reduction so far. Alendronate has been shown to reduce the risk of vertebral fractures by approximately 50%, multiple vertebral fractures by approximately 90%, all other fractures by about 30%, and hip fractures by about 50% (18).

Risedronate, another potent bisphosphonate, administered at 5 mg, was also reported to reduce vertebral fractures by 40% to 50% and other fractures by about 30%, although a reduction in hip fractures was not reported (19).

Calcitonin at 200 U intranasal showed very modest antiresorptive activity, based on biochemical markers and BMD increases, and was reported to reduce morphometric vertebral fractures at 200 IU but not at either 100 IU or 400 IU (20).

The increase in BMD by bone resorption inhibitors was at most 1 standard deviation (SD) (8% to 9% spine BMD for alendronate) after 3 to 5 years of treatment (18). Extensive studies conducted with multiple bone resorption inhibitory agents have not exceeded that effect. The risk of osteoporotic fractures in 50-year-old white women in the United States in their remaining lifetime was estimated at 54% (21). It is not known at this time if complete prevention of bone loss, e.g., by starting therapy with resorption inhibitors at menopause, would prevent almost all fractures in the future.

Some elderly osteoporotic patients may have lost over 4 SD (40%) of their BMD. Such patients could benefit from agents that stimulate bone formation, which could be used in addition to inhibitors of bone resorption and further increase BMD. It remains, however, to be shown that increasing bone density, as a result of stimulation of bone formation, indeed reduces fracture risk and that additional fracture risk reduction can be obtained on top of that produced by inhibitors of bone resorption.

The positive effects of fluorides or PTH on BMD were much more pronounced in the spine than in the hip, which raises the question of site specificity for the action of anabolic agents. It is highly possible that some agents could have a selective effect on cortical bone where accretion is related to periosteal bone growth. Such agents could be very beneficial in combined therapy with inhibitors of resorption, which have a much larger effect on the spine.

To summarize this section, although effective inhibitors of bone resorption, such as potent bisphosphonates, represent a landmark advance in the management of osteoporosis, alendronate having shown for the first time a substantial reduction in fracture incidence in prospective randomized double-blind trials (18), these agents cannot "cure" the disease in patients with advanced osteoporosis. Increased bone mass by stimulation of bone formation could be of significant additional benefit in these patients.

POTENTIAL RISKS ASSOCIATED WITH GROWTH FACTOR THERAPY

Based on data from clinical trials showing prevention of vertebral fractures associated with relatively small increases in bone density (20), it was suggested that reduced bone turnover produces an independent beneficial effect on fracture risk. *In vivo* stimulation of bone formation by PGE, PTH, TGF-β, IGF, growth hormone (GH), etc. was shown to be accompanied by increased bone turnover (see Chapter 32). It remains to be determined if increased bone turnover in itself constitutes a risk factor for fractures; if so, within what limits; and if it would outweigh the benefits of increased bone mass.

Fluoride treatment, which markedly increases spine BMD, did not reduce the risk of vertebral fractures (22–24). This was established in randomized, double-blind, placebo-controlled trials, both in the United States and in Europe, where the dose was lower and presumably devoid of toxic effects, attributed to osteomalacia or to changes in the structural properties of the bone resulting from replacement of calcium hydroxyapatite by fluoroapatite (25).

The other potent anabolic agent which was administered to humans is PTH; however, reported studies using this agent were not large enough to generate evidence on fractures.

The other major risk relates to general safety. Growth factors can stimulate the growth of tumors, even if they were not shown to be protooncogenes, and could increase the incidence of detectable tumors in test animals. It is not clear if this risk is equally applicable to humans since very high drug concentrations and highly susceptible animals are used in these studies.

To summarize this section, the two potential risks associated with growth factor therapy for stimulation of bone formation are the possibility that increased bone turnover may be a risk factor for bone fractures and the risk of tumorigenesis.

CHALLENGES IN THE DEVELOPMENT OF BONE-FORMING AGENTS

Preclinically, the challenge is to identify an animal model that predicts the response of the human skeleton to growth factor treatment. There are several well-known differences between humans and rodents. Rodents grow almost throughout life, albeit very slowly after the age of 9 months. The cortical bone in rodents has no haversian canals and is not subject to the type of remodeling occurring in human cortical bone. IGF-I seems to be the most abundant IGF in rat bone and IGF-II in human bone. The reproductive endocrinology between the species is different; e.g., women cycle approximately every 28 days and rodents every 4 days. The natural cessation of the estrous cycle in rodents is not accompanied by the endocrine changes seen in humans. These aspects are relevant since the sex steroids modulate secretion of pituitary growth factors and potentially growth factors produced in peripheral tissues, including bone. The limited examples where certain growth factors have been used both in rats and humans have highlighted potential differences. For example,

GH and IGF produce increases in bone mass in rats, whereas in humans they were shown to increase bone turnover without producing a positive bone balance (26–29). On the other hand, PTH was shown to increase bone mass in both rats and humans (30–32), although in humans this effect was localized primarily to the vertebrae (cancellous bone). PGE, not a classical growth factor, was also shown to be anabolic to bone in several species, including rats, dogs, and humans (33,34).

Some growth factors have a different sequence in different species, e.g., GH, which should be kept in mind.

The challenges in clinical development have several aspects. An important consideration is the mode of administration. All of the growth factors are peptides or proteins, best delivered parenterally, which puts some limitations on long-term usage. The smallest growth factors considered in this context are probably the IGFs, of about 6 kDa, and so far no methods have been proven effective in therapeutically delivering molecules of this size, except by injection.

An additional consideration is pharmacokinetics. Natural molecules have their characteristic physiological half-life, which would determine the frequency of required administration for producing optimal effects. Some growth factors, such as GH, are released in a pulsatile fashion and work best when such a regimen is followed.

A most critical question is the size of clinical studies. The accepted criteria for evaluating antiosteoporotic therapy is reduction of fractures, ideally hip fractures. A new therapy has to be compared to existing therapy. As discussed above, it is very likely and desirable to use bone-formation agents in combination with inhibitors of bone resorption. Combined therapy has to be compared with single therapy. Power calculations suggest that such studies would have to enroll many thousands of patients. Retention of patients in a multiyear trial with parenteral medication for a condition which is not immediately life-threatening is certainly a significant challenge, in addition to the resources needed to conduct such a study. There is generally some resistance to developing combined therapy for this reason; however, combined therapy has become routine for cancer, acquired immunodeficiency syndrome, hypertension, etc. and will probably be more widely used in the future for other diseases as well.

For any drug, safety is a major consideration. A regulatory challenge is to prove the safety of growth factors in preclinical studies. Specific risks for individual growth factors are discussed below; however, each growth factor, even those not known to be protooncogenes, could potentially increase tumor growth and the incidence of tumors in experimental animals during carcinogenicity testing. Current regulations stipulate that carcinogenicity studies (the incidence of tumors in susceptible mice and rats) have to be conducted at the maximum tolerated dose. It is very possible, even likely, that any of the growth factors known today would increase the growth of tumors, hence their appearance in the test animals, which were selected for these studies based on their high susceptibility to tumors.

To summarize this section, one faces several challenges in the development of growth factors for stimulation of bone formation: (a) identifying a growth factor involved in bone formation which is relatively selective and proving its efficacy in an animal model; (b) establishing its safety, especially with respect to tumorigenicity, and (c) designing and carrying out large clinical studies which demonstrate the superiority of combined treatment versus antiresorptive therapy alone in the prevention of (hip) fractures.

SPECIFIC GROWTH FACTORS AS CANDIDATES FOR OSTEOPOROTIC THERAPY

Each of the growth factors which acts on the skeleton or on skeletal cells has been reviewed separately in this volume, and the respective chapters should be consulted. The following comments briefly address aspects of potential therapeutic utility for some of the growth factors. In considering their uses for stimulation of bone formation, one should differentiate between fracture repair and bone remodeling in osteoporotic patients.

Bone Morphogenetic Protein Family

This family of TGF-β-related growth and differentiation factors (GDFs) was discovered, as the name indicates, based on the factors' bone-forming ability. They are therefore natural candidates to be considered for therapeutic application in the stimulation of bone formation. BMPs play a critical role in development in general, and specific BMPs have been shown to affect skeletal development (e.g., BMP-7, BMP-5, GDF-5). However, animals surviving until birth the deletion of specific BMPs by homologous recombination (knockout) usually had a complete skeleton, albeit sometimes with malformations (35).

Experimentally, local administration of BMP stimulates osteogenesis, and in many preclinical studies, local administration of BMPs was shown to promote the healing of a so-called critical-sized bone defect (a defect that would not spontaneously heal and ossify) (36). Several BMPs are now in phase III clinical trials for stimulation of bone formation during the repair of nonunion fractures.

Proof of concept is still lacking for the systemic use of BMPs in osteoporosis. So far, there is no convincing evidence that systemic administration of BMPs to animals increases bone mass.

Regarding TGF-β, similar to BMPs, there is not extensive evidence for systemic stimulation of bone formation by one of the known TGF-βs under conditions relevant to human osteoporosis, such as estrogen deficiency. However, TGF-β administration has been reported to maintain bone mass in non-weight-bearing limbs of tail-suspended rats (37). A significant safety limitation in the use of TGF-β is its immunosuppressive action. To my knowledge, there are no current attempts to develop TGF-β for therapeutic application in the bone area.

Growth Hormone and Insulin-like Growth Factors

Given the effects of GH on the skeleton during growth, development, and disease (acromegaly); the reported correlations between IGF-I levels and BMD and the possible role of IGF-II as a coupling factor, it was logical to consider GH and IGFs for osteoporotic therapy (see Chapter 32). Furthermore, PTH and PGE, potent stimulators of bone formation, were shown to stimulate IGF-I production in osteoblastic cells *in vitro* (38,39).

However, the limited clinical studies conducted so far showed that although GH and IGF increased bone turnover, as documented by biochemical markers, they produced no significant increase in bone mass (29). The actions of GH and IGF are complicated by the IGF binding proteins (IGFBPs), which can either increase or decrease IGF activity. It was shown, for example, that combined administration of IGF-I with IGFB-3 increased bone formation in ovariectomized rats (40). Comparable human studies have not been conducted and would be complicated by the need to administer two separate proteins, which may have different half-lives, etc. If GH and IGF affect primarily cortical bone, a highly desirable outcome, demonstration of a positive effect in humans may require longer trials, given the slow turnover of the cortical envelope.

An attractive mode of engaging the GH/IGF axis is via administration of GH-releasing factors (secretagogues). Such compounds could potentially be taken orally to stimulate a GH release that mimics the physiological pattern (41). Such a study was actually conducted with a GH secretagogue administered in conjunction with alendronate for 18 months. Combined treatment produced a significant increase in femoral neck BMD, relative to alendronate alone (42); however, no differences were observed at other sites. As mentioned above, longer and larger studies may be required to document such differences, if present.

Fibroblast Growth Factors

Another group of growth factors for which there is substantial evidence for effects on skeletal cells and on bone formation *in vivo* is comprised of the fibroblast growth factors (FGFs). FGFs may play a physiological role in bone formation since FGF-2 was shown to be produced by osteoblasts (43,44) and by endothelial cells.

A relationship between angiogenesis and osteogenesis has been established. It was reported that osteoblastic cells also produce vascular endothelial growth factor (VEGF), which is stimulated by PGE (45). One can envisage a positive-feedback loop whereby osteoblastic cells stimulate angiogenesis, and FGFs, produced by endothelial cells, increase the population of osteoprogenitors by stimulating proliferation or by inhibiting apoptosis. Interestingly, it was also reported that FGFs stimulate the production of TGF-β in osteoblastic cells (46), which may promote the differentiation or maturation of osteoblastic cells and increase bone formation.

To summarize this section, the growth factors known to stimulate the proliferation of osteoblastic cells *in vitro,* some of which were shown to stimulate bone formation or fracture repair *in vivo,* probably lack the specificity required for systemic use in osteoporotic therapy. Combined with the need for parenteral administration, the challenges for developing some of these growth factors for treatment are significant, as mentioned above. The stimulation of endogenous secretion of growth factors, either systemically or even better locally, is a very attractive alternative, especially if small bioavailable molecules can be developed for that purpose.

SUMMARY AND CONCLUSIONS

Osteoporosis is a widespread disease, which causes substantial morbidity and increases mortality in the elderly population. It is caused by a reduction in bone mass that starts in the fourth decade of life and can reach 50% in octogenarian women. Inhibitors of bone resorption can increase bone mass by at most 9% (alendronate over 5 years), suggesting that stimulation of bone formation could be of significant added benefit. No effective bone formation therapy, shown to reduce the incidence of bone fractures, is available. There are several difficulties associated with the development of growth factors for stimulation of bone formation:

1. The specific growth factors involved in bone remodeling have not been firmly identified and there is need for proof that such

factors increase bone mass in models of human osteoporosis.

2. There is uncertainty about the effect of high bone turnover on fracture risk.

3. Growth factors can stimulate the growth of tumors.

4. Growth factors are proteins which require parenteral administration, and effects may depend on the pharmacokinetic profile.

5. Last but not least, there is a need for skeletal selectivity.

These challenges seem daunting, but so were those which preceded other medical developments, and if a bone growth factor is identified, especially one which has bone specificity and is documented to play a physiological role in remodeling, it will probably be developed for osteoporotic therapy.

REFERENCES

1. Garnero P, Somay-Rendu E, Chapuy MC, et al. Increased bone turnover in late postmenopausal women is a major determinant of osteoporosis. *J Bone Miner Res* 1996;11:337–349.
2. Parfitt M. Stereologic basis of bone histomorphometry: theory of quantitative microscopy and reconstruction of the third dimension. In: Recker RR (ed) *Bone histomorphometry: techniques and interpretation.* Boca Raton, FL: CRC Press, 1983:53–87.
3. Frost H. The role of changes in mechanical usage set points in the pathogenesis of osteoporosis. *J Bone Miner Res* 1992;7:253–261.
4. Patel S, Pazianas M, Tobias J, et al. Early effects of hormone replacement therapy on bone. *Bone* 1999;24:245–248.
5. Mundy GR. The effects of TGFβ on bone. *Ciba Found Symp* 1991;157:137–143.
6. Mohan S, Baylink DJ. Insulin-like growth factor system components and the coupling of bone formation to resorption. *Horm Res* 1996;45[Suppl 1]:59–62.
7. Rodan GA. Bone mass homeostasis and bisphosphonate action. *Bone* 1997;20:1–4.
8. Machwate M, Rodan SB, Rodan GA, et al. Sphingosine kinase mediates cyclic AMP suppression of apoptosis in rat periosteal cells. *Mol Pharmacol* 1998;54:70–77.
9. Dobnig H, Turner RT. Evidence that intermittent treatment with parathyroid hormone increases bone formation in adult rats by activation of bone lining cells. *Endocrinology* 1995;136:3632–3638.
10. Bellido T, Plotkin L, Han L, et al. PTH prevents glucocorticoid-induced apoptosis of osteoblasts and osteocytes *in vitro:* direct interference with a private death pathway upstream from caspase-3. *Bone* 1998;23:S518.
11. Weinstein RS, Jilka RL, Parfitt AM, et al. Inhibition of osteoblastogenesis and promotion of apoptosis of osteoblasts and osteocytes by glucocorticoids. Potential mechanisms of their deleterious effects on bone. *J Clin Invest* 1998;102:274–282.
12. Michaelsson K, Baron JA, Farahmand BY, et al. Oral contraceptive use and risk of hip fracture: a case-control study. *Lancet* 1999;353:1481–1484.
13. Cauley JA, Seeley DG, Ensrud K, et al. Estrogen replacement therapy and fractures in older women. Study of osteoporotic fractures research group. *Ann Intern Med* 1995;122:9–16.
14. Hulley S, Grady D, Bush T, et al. Randomized trial of estrogen plus progestin for secondary prevention of coronary heart disease in postmenopausal women. Heart and estrogen/progestin replacement study (HERS) research group. *JAMA* 1998;280:605–613.
15. Lufkin EG, Whitaker MD, Nickelsen T, et al. Treatment of established postmenopausal osteoporosis with raloxifene: a randomized trial. *J Bone Miner Res* 1998;13:1747–1754.
16. Freedman LP, Razhez C, Suldan Z, et al. A novel protein complex that interacts with the vitamin D receptor in the presence of ligand and coactivates transcription. *J Bone Miner Res* 1998;23:S176.
17. Lufkin EG, Wahner HW, O'Fallon WM, et al. Treatment of postmenopausal osteoporosis with transdermal estrogen. *Ann Intern Med* 1992;117:1–9.
18. Black DM, Cummings SR, Karpf DB, et al. Randomised trial of effect of alendronate on risk of fracture in women with existing vertebral fractures. Fracture intervention trial research group. *Lancet* 1996;348:1535–1541.
19. Watts N, Hangartner T, Chestnut C, et al. Risedronate treatment prevents vertebral and non-vertebral fractures in women with postmenopausal osteoporosis. *Calcif Tissue Int* 1999;64[Suppl 1]:S42.
20. Silverman SL, Moniz C, Andriano K, et al. Salmon-calcitonin nasal spray prevents vertebral fractures in established osteoporosis. Final world wide results of the "PROOF" study. *Calcif Tissue Int* 1999;64:S43.
21. Chrischilles EA, Butler CD, Davis CS, et al. A model of lifetime osteoporosis impact. *Arch Intern Med* 1991;151:2026–2032.
22. Meunier PJ, Sebert JL, Reginster JY, et al. Fluoride salts are no better at preventing new vertebral fractures than calcium-vitamin D in postmenopausal osteoporosis: the FAVOStudy. *Osteoporos Int* 1998;8:4–12.
23. Riggs BL, Hodgson SF, O'Fallon WM, et al. Effect of fluoride treatment on the fracture rate in postmenopausal women with osteoporosis. *N Engl J Med* 1990;322:802–809.
24. Kleerekoper M, Peterson EL, Nelson DA, et al. A randomized trial of sodium fluoride as a treatment for postmenopausal osteoporosis. *Osteoporos Int* 1991;1:155–161.
25. Fratzl P, Roschger P, Eschberger J, et al. Abnormal bone mineralization after fluoride treatment in osteoporosis: a small-angle x-ray-scattering study. *J Bone Miner Res* 1994;9:1541–1549.
26. Mosekilde L, Tomsen JS, Orhii PB, et al. Growth hormone increases vertebral and femoral bone strength in osteopenic, ovariectomized, aged rats in a dose-dependent and site-specific manner. *Bone* 1998;23:343–352.
27. Ohlsson C, Bengtsson BA, Isaksson OG, et al. Growth hormone and bone. *Endocr Rev* 1998;19:55–79.
28. Marcus R, Hoffman AR. Growth hormone as therapy

for older men and women. *Annu Rev Pharmacol Toxicol* 1998;38:45–61.

29. Marcus R. Skeletal effects of growth hormone and IGF-I in adults. *Horm Res* 1997;48[Suppl 5]:60–64.

30. Lane NE, Sanchez S, Modin GW, et al. Parathyroid hormone treatment can reverse corticosteroid-induced osteoporosis. Results of a randomized controlled clinical trial. *J Clin Invest* 1998;102:1627–1633.

31. Finkelstein JS, Klibanski A, Arnold AL, et al. Prevention of estrogen deficiency–related bone loss with human parathyroid hormone-(1–34): a randomized controlled trial. *JAMA* 1998;280:1067–1073.

32. Ma Y, Jee WS, Yuan Z, et al. Parathyroid hormone and mechanical usage have a synergistic effect in rat tibial diaphyseal cortical bone. *J Bone Miner Res* 1999;14: 439–448.

33. Ma Y, Chen YY, Jee WS, et al. Co-treatment of PGE2 and risedronate is better than PGE2 alone in the long-term treatment of ovariectomized-induced osteopenic rats. *Bone* 1995;17[Suppl 4]:267S–272S.

34. Jorgensen HR, Svanholm H, Host A. Bone formation induced in an infant by systemic prostaglandin E2 administration. *Acta Orthop Scand* 1988;59:464–466.

35. Wozney JM, Rosen V. Bone morphogenetic protein and bone morphogenetic protein gene family in bone formation and repair. *Clin Orthop* 1998;346:26–37.

36. Ripamonti U, Van Den Heever B, Sampath TK, et al. Complete regeneration of bone in the baboon by recombinant human osteogenic protein-1 (hOP-1, bone morphogenetic protein-7). *Growth Factors* 1996;13: 273–289.

37. Machwate M, Zerath E, Holy X, et al. Systemic administration of transforming growth factor-beta 2 prevents the impaired bone formation and osteopenia induced by unloading in rats. *J Clin Invest* 1995;96:1245–1253.

38. Pereira RC, Canalis E. Parathyroid hormone increases mac25/insulin-like growth factor-binding protein–related protein-1 expression in cultured osteoblasts. *Endocrinology* 1999;140:1998–2003.

39. Pash JM, Delany AM, Adamo ML, et al. Regulation of insulin-like growth factor I transcription by prostaglandin E2 in osteoblast cells. *Endocrinology* 1995;136: 33–38.

40. Bagi C, van der Meulen M, Brommage R, et al. The effect of systemically administered rhIGF-I/IGFBP-3 complex on cortical bone strength and structure in ovariectomized rats. *Bone* 1995;16:559–565.

41. Hickey G, Jacks T, Judity F, et al. Efficacy and specificity of L-692,429, a novel nonpeptidyl growth hormone secretagogue, in beagles. *Endocrinology* 1994;134: 695–701.

42. Murphy G, Weiss S, Balske A, et al. Treatment of postmenopausal osteoporosis with alendronate and MK-677 (a growth hormone secretagogue) individually and in combination. *J Bone Miner Res* 1998;23:S468.

43. Globus RK, Plouet J, Gospodarowicz D. Cultured bovine bone cells synthesize basic fibroblast growth factor and store it in their extracellular matrix. *Endocrinology* 1989;124:1539–1547.

44. Lafage-Proust M-H, Wesolowski G, Ernst M, et al. Retinoic acid effects on an SV-40 large T antigen immortalized adult rat bone cell line. *J Cell Physiol* 1999;179: 267–275.

45. Harada S, Nagy JA, Sullivan KA, et al. Induction of vascular endothelial growth factor expression by prostaglandin E2 and E1 in osteoblasts. *J Clin Invest* 1994; 93:2490–2496.

46. Noda M, Vogel R. Fibroblast growth factor enhances type beta 1 transforming growth factor gene expression in osteoblast-like cells. *J Cell Biol* 1989;109: 2529–2535.

Subject Index

Page numbers in *italics* indicate figures; page numbers followed by t indicate tables.